Evidence-Based Nursing Guide to

Sign & Symptom Management

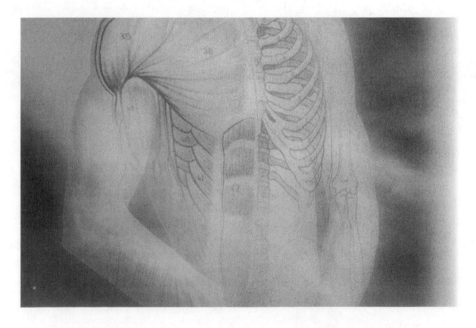

 Wolters Kluwer | Lippincott Williams & Wilkins
Health

Philadelphia · Baltimore · New York · London
Buenos Aires · Hong Kong · Sydney · Tokyo

STAFF

EXECUTIVE PUBLISHER
Judith A. Schilling McCann, RN, MSN

EDITORIAL DIRECTOR
H. Nancy Holmes

CLINICAL DIRECTOR
Joan M. Robinson, RN, MSN

EDITORIAL PROJECT MANAGER
Sean Webb

CLINICAL PROJECT MANAGER
Kathryn Henry, RN, BSN, CCRC

EDITOR
Catherine Harold

CLINICAL EDITOR
Jana L. Sciarra, RN, CRNP, MSN

COPY EDITORS
Leslie Dworkin, Jeannine Fielding,
Marna Poole, Jenifer Walker,
Pamela Wingrod

DIGITAL COMPOSITION SERVICES
Diane Paluba (Manager),
Joyce Rossi Biletz, Donna S. Morris

DESIGNER
Debra Moloshok

MANUFACTURING
Beth J. Welsh

EDITORIAL ASSISTANTS
Karen J. Kirk, Jeri O'Shea,
Linda K. Ruhf

DESIGN ASSISTANT
Kate Zulak

INDEXER
Deborah Tourtlotte

The clinical procedures described and recommended in this publication are based on research and consultation with nursing, medical, pharmaceutical, and legal authorities. To the best of our knowledge, these procedures reflect currently accepted practice; nevertheless, they can't be considered absolute and universal recommendations. For individual application, all recommendations must be considered in light of the patient's clinical condition and, before the administration of new or infrequently used drugs, in light of the latest package-insert information. The authors and publisher disclaim any responsibility for any adverse effects resulting directly or indirectly from the suggested procedures, from any undetected errors, or from the reader's misunderstanding of the text.

EBSS010908

Library of Congress
Cataloging-in-Publication Data

The evidence-based nursing guide to sign & symptom management.
    p. ; cm.
Includes bibliographical references and index.
    1. Nursing assessment—Handbooks, manuals, etc.
2. Nursing diagnosis—Handbooks, manuals, etc.
3. Symptoms—Handbooks, manuals, etc. 4. Evidence-based nursing—Handbooks, manuals, etc.   I.
Lippincott Williams & Wilkins. II. Title: Evidence-based nursing guide to sign and symptom management.
    [DNLM: 1. Nursing Assessment—methods—
Handbooks. 2. Signs and Symptoms—Handbooks.
3. Diagnostic Techniques and Procedures—Handbooks.
4. Evidence-Based Medicine—methods—Handbooks.
5. Physical Examination—Handbooks.
WY 49 E93 2008]
    RT48.E95 2008
    616.07'5—dc22
    ISBN-13: 978-0-7817-8827-4 (alk. paper)
    ISBN-10: 0-7817-8827-7 (alk. paper)
                                          2008021816

CONTENTS

CONTRIBUTORS AND CONSULTANTS

CHERYL BRADY, RN, MSN
Assistant Professor
Kent State University
Salem, Ohio

NATALIE BURKHALTER, RN, MSN, FNP, ACNP, CS, CCRN
Interim Director/Associate Professor,
Canseco School of Nursing
Texas A&M International University
Laredo

LAURA M. CRIDDLE, RN, MS, CEN, CNRN, CCRN
Clinical Nurse Specialist
Premier Jets/Lifeguard Air Ambulance
Portland, Ore.

SUSAN DENMAN, RN, PhD, FNP-C, APRNB-BC
Assistant Professor
Duke School of Nursing
Durham, N.C.

SHELBA DURSTON, RN, MSN, CCRN
Nursing Instructor
San Joaquin Delta College
Stockton, Calif.

M. SUSAN EMERSON, RN, PhD, BC, ANP, ACNP, CNS
Nurse Practitioner
Truman Medical Center—Hospital Hill
Kansas City, Mo.

VIVIAN GAMBLIAN, RN, MSN
Nursing Faculty
Baylor University
Louise Harrington School of Nursing
Dallas

v

KATHRYN H. HAUGH, RN, MSN, PhD
Assistant Professor
University of Virginia School of Nursing
Charlottesville

JANICE J. HOFFMAN, RN, PhD
Faculty
Johns Hopkins University School of Nursing
Baltimore

BRIDGET HOWARD, APRN-BC, MSN
Nurse Practitioner
Midwest Gastroenterology
Lee's Summit, Mo.

TIMOTHY L. HUDSON, RN, PhD(ABD), FACHE, CCRN, CHE
Chief, Evening/Night Nursing Supervision
Martin Army Community Hospital
Fort Benning, Ga.

SHARON KUMM, RN, MN, CCRN
Clinical Associate Professor
University of Kansas School of Nursing
Kansas City

GINA MAIOCCO, RN, PhD, CCRN, CCNS
Assistant Professor/CNS
West Virginia University School of Nursing
Morgantown

CYNTHIA MICULAN, RN, MSN, ONC, CNA, BC
Clinical Manager
The University Hospital
Cincinnati

MARCELLA A. MIKALAITIS, RN, MSN, CCRN
Staff Nurse
Doylestown (Pa.) Hospital

DARRELL OWENS, ARNP, PhD
Clinical Assistant Professor & Director of Palliative Care
Harborview Medical Center
Seattle

CONCHA SITTER, APN, MS, CGRN, FNP-BC
Gastroenterology Nurse Practitioner
Sterling Rock Falls Clinic
Sterling, Ill.

NORA D. YAN, RN, BSN
Staff Nurse
Stanford (Calif.) Hospital & Clinics

FOREWORD

The *Evidence-Based Nursing Guide to Sign & Symptom Management* is a new book written especially for practicing nurses that provides authoritative information on more than 130 clinical signs and symptoms that nurses encounter and need to interpret and respond to in their everyday work.

Terms are organized alphabetically for easy location. The scope is impressive including common conditions such as conjuctival injection and constipation, uncommon ones like decerebrate posture and Kernig's sign, and acute (such as stridor) and chronic (such as pruritus) signs and symptoms. Each term is carefully defined, appropriate history taking and examination is described, potential differential diagnoses are listed, special issues relevant to pediatric and older patients are reviewed, and references are provided.

For each sign or symptom discussed, there's also information on immediate nursing treatment measures that should be undertaken and patient counseling topics that should be reviewed. Illustrations, charts, and tables highlight important information. The editors have worked to ensure that the writing is succinct and straightforward using easy-to-understand language. The standardized format allows the reader to readily identify specific terms included and easily locate relevant information. The result is a text that provides users with accessible clinical information they can use directly in patient care.

The book contains other features that will be of interest to practicing nurses. The *Drug watch* logo highlights important drug information. Recent medical news reports on nursing topics are identified by the *In the news* logo, and information on health and safety issues such as infection control, injury, and risk reduction are identified by the *Health and safety* logo. An *Evidence-based practice* logo identifies pieces that provide evidence-based reviews, organized in a standard format, which summarizes recent patient-oriented research findings such as methods to improve dyspnea management in COPD patients. The appendices provide additional useful evidence-based nursing practice information and a helpful listing of evidence-based practice resources.

For nursing professionals and students looking for a wide ranging, well-written, and well-organized book that provides quick access to diagnostic and treatment information that will help them with patient care, the *Evidence-Based Nursing Guide to Sign & Symptom Management* is a valuable new resource.

Eric Henley, MD, MPH
Professor and Head
Department of Family and Community Medicine
University of Illinois College of Medicine
Rockford

ABDOMINAL DISTENTION

Abdominal distention refers to increased abdominal girth—the result of increased intra-abdominal pressure forcing the abdominal wall outward. Depending on the amount of pressure, distention may be mild or severe. It may be localized or diffuse and may occur gradually or suddenly.

Abdominal distention may result from fat, flatus, a fetus (including in ectopic pregnancy), or fluid. Fluid and gas are normal in the GI tract but not in the peritoneal cavity. However, if fluid and gas cannot pass freely through the GI tract, abdominal distention occurs. In the peritoneal cavity, distention may reflect acute bleeding, accumulation of ascitic fluid, or air from perforation of an abdominal organ. Acute abdominal distention may signal life-threatening peritonitis or acute bowel obstruction.

Abdominal distention doesn't always signal pathology. For example, in anxious patients or those with digestive distress, localized distention in the left upper quadrant can result from aerophagia—the unconscious swallowing of air. Generalized distention can result from ingestion of fruits or vegetables that contain large quantities of unabsorbable carbohydrates, such as legumes, or from abnormal food fermentation by microbes. Make sure to rule out pregnancy in all women with abdominal distention.

In acute abdominal distention, quickly check for signs of hypovolemia, such as pallor, diaphoresis, hypotension, rapid and thready pulse, rapid and shallow breathing, decreased urine output, poor capillary refill, and altered mentation. Ask the patient if he has severe abdominal pain or is having trouble breathing. Ask about any recent accidents, and check for signs of trauma and peritoneal bleeding, such as Cullen's sign or Turner's sign.[1] Then auscultate all abdominal quadrants, noting rapid and high-pitched, diminished, or absent bowel sounds. (If you don't hear bowel sounds immediately, listen for at least 5 minutes per quadrant.) Gently palpate the abdomen for rigidity. Avoid deep or extensive palpation, which may increase pain.

If you detect abdominal distention and rigidity along with abnormal bowel sounds, and the patient complains of pain, begin emergency interventions. Place the patient in the supine position, administer oxygen, and insert an I.V. line for fluid replacement.

Prepare to insert a nasogastric tube to relieve acute intraluminal distention and prevent aspiration.[1] Reassure the patient, and prepare him for surgery.

History and physical examination

If the patient's abdominal distention isn't acute, ask about its onset, duration, and related signs and symptoms. A patient with localized distention may report a sensation of pressure, fullness, or tenderness in the affected area. A patient with generalized distention may report a bloated feeling, a pounding heartbeat, and difficulty breathing deeply, especially when lying flat. The patient may also feel unable to bend at the waist. Be sure to ask about abdominal pain, fever, nausea, vomiting, anorexia, altered bowel habits, and weight gain or loss.

Obtain a medical history, noting GI or biliary disorders that may cause peritonitis or ascites, such as cirrhosis, hepatitis, or inflammatory bowel disease. (See *Detecting ascites*.) Ask about the patient's bowel elimination pattern, and note chronic constipation. Has the patient recently had abdominal surgery, which can lead to abdominal distention? Ask about recent accidents, even minor ones, such as falling off a stepladder.

Perform a complete physical examination. Don't restrict your examination to the abdomen because you could miss important clues to the cause of abdominal distention. Next, stand at the foot of the bed and observe the recumbent patient for abdominal asymmetry to determine if distention is localized or generalized. Then assess abdominal contour by stooping at the patient's side. Inspect for tense, glistening skin and bulging flanks, which may indicate ascites. Observe the umbilicus. Eversion may indicate ascites or an umbilical hernia. An inverted umbilicus may indicate distention from gas; it's also common in obese people.

Inspect the abdomen for signs of inguinal or femoral hernia and for incisions that may point to adhesions; both may lead to intestinal obstruction. Then auscultate for bowel sounds, abdominal friction rubs (indicating peritoneal inflammation), and bruits (indicating an aneurysm). Listen for a succussion splash—a splashing sound normally heard in the stomach when the patient moves or when palpation disturbs the viscera. An abnormally loud splash indicates fluid accumulation, suggesting gastric dilation or obstruction.

Next, percuss and palpate the abdomen to determine if distention results from air, fluid, or both. A tympanic note in the left lower quadrant suggests an air-filled descending or sigmoid colon. A tympanic note throughout a generally distended abdomen suggests an air-filled peritoneal cavity. A dull percussion note throughout a generally distended abdomen suggests a fluid-filled peritoneal cavity. Shifting of dullness laterally when the patient is in the decubitus position also indicates a fluid-filled abdominal cavity. A pelvic or intra-abdominal mass causes local dullness with percussion and should be palpable. Obesity causes a large abdomen with generalized rather then localized dullness and without shifting dullness, prominent tympany, or palpable bowel or other masses.

Palpate the abdomen for tenderness, noting whether it's localized or generalized. Watch for peritoneal signs and symptoms, such as rebound tenderness, guarding, rigidity, McBurney's point, obturator sign, and psoas sign. Female patients should undergo a pelvic examination; males, a genital examination. All patients who report abdominal pain should undergo a digital rectal examination with fecal occult blood testing.

Finally, measure abdominal girth for a baseline value. Mark the flanks with a felt-tipped pen as a reference point for subsequent measurements.

Medical causes

▶ *Abdominal cancer.* An indication of advanced disease, generalized abdominal distention may occur when cancer—most commonly ovarian, hepatic, or pancreatic cancer—produces ascites (usually in a patient with a known tumor). Shifting dullness and a fluid wave accompany the distention. Related signs and symptoms may include severe abdominal pain, an abdominal mass, anorexia, jaundice, GI hemorrhage (hematemesis or melena), dyspepsia, and weight loss that progresses to muscle weakness and atrophy.

▶ *Abdominal trauma.* When brisk internal bleeding accompanies trauma, abdominal distention may be acute and dramatic. Related signs and symptoms of this life-threatening disorder include abdominal rigidity with guarding, decreased or absent bowel sounds, vomiting, tenderness, and abdominal bruising. The patient may feel pain over the trauma site or, if abdominal bleeding irritates the phrenic nerve, over the scapula. Signs of hypovolemic shock (such as hypotension and a rapid, thready pulse) appear with significant blood loss.

▶ *Bladder distention.* Various disorders cause bladder distention, which in turn causes lower abdominal distention. Slight dullness on percussion above the symphysis indicates mild bladder distention. A palpable, smooth,

Detecting ascites

Ascites is an accumulation of fluid in the abdominal cavity. To differentiate ascites from other causes of distention, check for shifting dullness, a fluid wave, and the puddle sign, as described below.

SHIFTING DULLNESS

Step 1. With the patient in a supine position, percuss from the umbilicus outward to the flank, as shown. Draw a line on the patient's skin to mark the change from tympany to dullness.

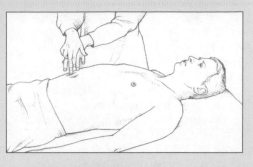

Step 2. Turn the patient onto his side, which would cause ascitic fluid to shift. Percuss again, and mark the change from tympany to dullness. Any difference between these lines can indicate ascites.

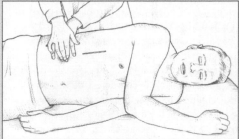

FLUID WAVE

Have another person press deep into the patient's midline to prevent vibration from traveling along the abdominal wall. Place one of your palms on one of the patient's flanks. Strike the opposite flank with your other hand. If you feel the blow in the opposite palm, ascitic fluid is present.

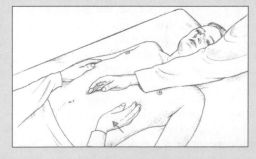

PUDDLE SIGN

Position the patient on his elbows and knees; ascitic fluid will pool in the most dependent part of the abdomen. Percuss the abdomen from the flank to the midline. The percussion note becomes louder at the edge of the puddle of ascetic fluid.

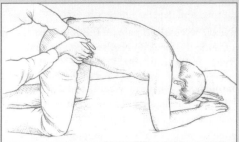

rounded, fluctuant suprapubic mass suggests severe distention. A fluctuant mass extending to the umbilicus indicates extremely severe distention. Urinary dribbling, frequency, or urgency may occur with urinary obstruction. Suprapubic discomfort is also common.

▶ *Cirrhosis.* In cirrhosis, ascites causes generalized distention and is confirmed by a fluid wave, shifting dullness, and a puddle sign. Umbilical eversion and caput medusae (dilated veins around the umbilicus) are common. The patient may report a feeling of fullness or weight gain. Related findings include vague abdominal pain, fever, anorexia, nausea, vomiting, constipation or diarrhea, bleeding tendencies, severe pruritus, palmar erythema, spider angiomas, leg edema, and possibly splenomegaly. Hematemesis, encephalopathy, gynecomastia, or testicular atrophy also may occur. Jaundice is usually a late sign. Hepatomegaly occurs initially, but the liver may not be palpable in advanced disease.

▶ *Gastric dilation (acute).* Left-upper-quadrant distention is characteristic in acute gastric dilation, but the presentation varies. The patient usually complains of epigastric fullness or pain and nausea with or without vomiting. Physical examination reveals tympany, gastric tenderness, and a succussion splash. Initially, peristalsis may be visible. Later, hypoactive or absent bowel sounds confirm ileus. The patient may be pale and diaphoretic and may have tachycardia or bradycardia.

▶ *Heart failure.* Generalized abdominal distention caused by ascites typically accompanies severe cardiovascular impairment and is confirmed by shifting dullness and a fluid wave. Signs and symptoms of heart failure are numerous and depend on the disease stage and degree of cardiovascular impairment. Hallmarks include peripheral edema, jugular vein distention, dyspnea, and tachycardia. Common related signs and symptoms include hepatomegaly (which may cause right-upper-quadrant pain), nausea, vomiting, productive cough, crackles, cool extremities, cyanotic nail beds, nocturia, exercise intolerance, nocturnal wheezing, diastolic hypertension, and cardiomegaly.

▶ *Irritable bowel syndrome (IBS).* IBS may produce intermittent, localized distention—the result of periodic intestinal spasms. Lower abdominal pain or cramping typically accompanies these spasms. The pain is usually relieved by defecation or by passage of intestinal gas and is aggravated by stress. Other possible signs and symptoms include diarrhea that may alternate with constipation or normal bowel function; nausea; dyspepsia; straining and urgency at defecation; feeling of incomplete evacuation; and small, mucus-streaked stools.

▶ *Large-bowel obstruction.* Dramatic abdominal distention is characteristic in large-bowel obstruction, a life-threatening disorder; in fact, loops of the large bowel may become visible on the abdomen. Constipation precedes distention and may be the only symptom for days. Related findings include tympany, high-pitched bowel sounds, and sudden onset of colicky lower abdominal pain that becomes persistent. Fecal vomiting and diminished peristaltic waves and bowel sounds are late signs.

▶ *Mesenteric artery occlusion (acute).* In mesenteric artery occlusion—a life-threatening disorder—abdominal distention usually occurs several hours after the sudden onset of severe, colicky periumbilical pain accompanied by rapid (even forceful) bowel evacuation. The pain later becomes constant and diffuse. Related signs and symptoms include severe abdominal tenderness with guarding and rigidity, absent bowel sounds and, occasionally, a bruit in the right iliac fossa. The patient also may have vomiting, anorexia, diarrhea, or constipation. Late signs include fever, tachycardia, tachypnea, hypotension, and cool, clammy skin. Abdominal distention or GI bleeding may be the only clue if pain is absent.

▶ *Nephrotic syndrome.* This syndrome may produce massive edema, causing generalized abdominal distention with a fluid wave and shifting dullness. It also may cause increased blood pressure, hematuria or oliguria, fatigue, anorexia, depression, pallor, periorbital edema, scrotal swelling, and skin striae.

▶ *Ovarian cysts.* Typically, large ovarian cysts produce lower abdominal distention accompanied by umbilical eversion. Because they're thin walled and fluid filled, these cysts produce a fluid wave and shifting dullness—

signs that mimic ascites. Lower abdominal pain and a palpable mass may be present.

▶ *Paralytic ileus.* Paralytic ileus, which produces generalized distention with a tympanic percussion note, is accompanied by absent or hypoactive bowel sounds and, occasionally, mild abdominal pain and vomiting. The patient may be severely constipated or may pass flatus and small, liquid stools.

▶ *Peritonitis.* In peritonitis—a life-threatening disorder—abdominal distention may be localized or generalized, depending on the extent of peritonitis. Fluid accumulates first within the peritoneal cavity and then within the bowel lumen, causing a fluid wave and shifting dullness. Typically, distention is accompanied by rebound tenderness, abdominal rigidity, and sudden and severe abdominal pain that worsens with movement.

The skin over the patient's abdomen may appear taut and shiny. Related signs and symptoms usually include hypoactive or absent bowel sounds, fever, chills, hyperalgesia, nausea, and vomiting. Signs of shock, such as tachycardia and hypotension, appear with significant fluid loss into the abdomen.

▶ *Small-bowel obstruction.* Abdominal distention is characteristic in small-bowel obstruction—a life-threatening disorder—and is most pronounced during late obstruction, especially in the distal small bowel. Auscultation reveals hypoactive or hyperactive bowel sounds, whereas percussion produces a tympanic note.[2] Related signs and symptoms include colicky periumbilical pain, constipation, nausea, and vomiting; the higher the obstruction, the earlier and more severe the vomiting.[2] Rebound tenderness reflects intestinal strangulation with ischemia. Related signs and symptoms include drowsiness, malaise, and signs of dehydration. Signs of hypovolemic shock appear with progressive dehydration and plasma loss.

▶ *Toxic megacolon (acute).* Toxic megacolon is a life-threatening complication of infectious or ulcerative colitis that produces dramatic abdominal distention. The distention usually develops gradually and is accompanied by a tympanic percussion note, diminished or absent bowel sounds, and mild rebound tenderness. The patient also has abdominal pain and

tenderness, fever, tachycardia, and dehydration.

Other causes

DRUG WATCH *Opioids such as morphine delay gastric emptying and slow peristalsis, promoting abdominal distention.[3]*

Special considerations

If abdominal distention impairs the patient's ability to breathe, monitor his respiratory status closely, including respiratory rate, pulse oximetry, and breath sounds. Administer oxygen as needed.[2]

Position the patient comfortably, using pillows for support. Place him on his left side to help flatus escape or, if he has ascites, elevate the head of the bed to ease his breathing. Administer drugs to relieve pain or gas, and offer emotional support.

Prepare the patient for diagnostic tests, such as abdominal X-rays, endoscopy, laparoscopy, ultrasonography, computed tomography scan, or possibly paracentesis.

Pediatric pointers

Because a young child's abdomen is normally rounded, distention may be difficult to observe. However, a child's abdominal wall is less well developed than an adult's, so palpation is easier. When percussing the abdomen, remember that children normally swallow air when eating and crying, resulting in louder-than-normal tympany. Minimal tympany with abdominal distention may result from fluid accumulation or solid masses. To check for abdominal fluid, test for shifting dullness instead of for a fluid wave. (In a child, air swallowing and incomplete abdominal muscle development make the fluid wave difficult to interpret.)

Some children won't cooperate with a physical examination. Try to gain the child's confidence, and consider letting him sit in the parent's or caregiver's lap. You can gather clues by observing the child while he's coughing, walking, or even climbing on office furniture. Remove all the child's clothing to avoid missing any diagnostic clues. Also, perform a gentle rectal examination.

In neonates, ascites usually results from GI or urinary perforation; in older children, from heart failure, cirrhosis, or nephrosis. Besides ascites, congenital malformations of the GI tract (such as intussusception and volvulus) may cause abdominal distention. A hernia may cause distention if it produces an intestinal obstruction. In addition, overeating and constipation can cause distention.

Geriatric pointers

As people age, fat tends to accumulate in the lower abdomen and near the hips, even when body weight is stable. This accumulation, together with weakening abdominal muscles, commonly produces a potbelly, which some elderly patients interpret as fluid collection or evidence of disease. Aging also increases the patient's risk of gallstones, which may produce abdominal distention, as well as right-upper-quadrant pain, flatus, nausea, and vomiting.[4]

Patient counseling

If anxiety triggers air swallowing or deep breathing that causes discomfort, advise the patient to take slow breaths. If he has an obstruction or ascites, explain food and fluid restrictions. Stress good oral hygiene to prevent dry mouth.

REFERENCES

1. Blank-Reid, C. "Abdominal Trauma: Dealing with the Damage," *Nursing* 37(ED Insider):4-11, Spring 2007.
2. Freeman, L. "Responding to Small-Bowel Obstruction," *Nursing* 37(5):56hn1-56hn4, 56hn6, May 2007.
3. Steele, A. and Carlson, K. "Nausea and Vomiting: Applying Research to Bedside Practice," *AACN Advanced Critical Care* 18(1):61-73, January-March 2007.
4. Neal-Boylan, L. "Health Assessment of the Very Old Person at Home." *Home Healthcare Nurse* 25(6):388-398, June 2007.

ABDOMINAL MASS

Commonly detected on routine physical examination, an abdominal mass is a localized swelling in one abdominal quadrant. Typically, this sign develops insidi-ously and may represent an enlarged organ, a neoplasm, an abscess, a vascular defect, or a fecal mass.

Distinguishing an abdominal mass from a normal structure requires skillful palpation. At times, palpation must be repeated with the patient in a different position or performed by a second examiner to verify initial findings. A palpable abdominal mass is an important clinical sign and usually represents a serious—perhaps life-threatening—disorder.

If the patient has a pulsating midabdominal mass and severe abdominal, back, or flank pain, suspect an aortic aneurysm.[1] Quickly take his vital signs. Because the patient may need emergency surgery, withhold food or fluids until he's examined. Prepare to give oxygen and to start two large-bore I.V. lines for fluid and blood replacement. Obtain routine preoperative tests, and prepare the patient for angiography. Provide drugs for pain control. Monitor blood pressure, pulse rate, respirations, and urine output often.[2]

Be alert for signs of shock, such as tachycardia, hypotension, and cool, clammy skin, which may indicate significant blood loss.

History and physical examination

If the patient's abdominal mass doesn't suggest an aortic aneurysm, take a detailed history. Ask the patient if the mass is painful. If so, ask if the pain is constant or if it occurs only on palpation. Is it localized or generalized? Determine if the patient was already aware of the mass. If so, find out if he noticed any change in its size or location.

Next, review the patient's medical history, paying special attention to GI disorders. Ask about GI symptoms, such as constipation, diarrhea, rectal bleeding, abnormally colored stools, and vomiting. Has the patient noticed a change in appetite or bowel habits? If the patient is female, ask whether her menstrual cycles are regular and when the first day of her last menstrual period was.

Perform a complete physical examination. Next, auscultate for bowel sounds in each quadrant. Listen for bruits or friction rubs, and check for enlarged veins. Lightly palpate and then deeply palpate the abdomen, assessing any painful or suspicious areas last. Note the patient's position when you locate the mass. Some masses can be detected only with the patient in a supine position; others require a side-lying position.

Estimate the size of the mass in centimeters, and describe its shape, contour (smooth, rough, sharply defined, nodular, irregular), and consistency (doughy, soft, solid, hard). Also, percuss the mass. A dull sound indicates a fluid-filled mass; a tympanic sound, an air-filled mass.

Next, determine if the mass moves with your hand or in response to respiration. Is it free-floating or attached to intra-abdominal structures? To determine whether the mass is located in the abdominal wall or the abdominal cavity, ask the patient to lift his head and shoulders off the examination table, thereby contracting his abdominal muscles. While these muscles are contracted, try to palpate the mass. If you can, the mass is in the abdominal wall; if you can't, it's in the abdominal cavity.

After the abdominal examination is complete, perform pelvic, genital, and rectal examinations.

Medical causes

▶ *Abdominal aortic aneurysm.* An abdominal aortic aneurysm may persist for years, producing only a pulsating periumbilical mass with a systolic bruit over the aorta. However, it may become life-threatening if the aneurysm expands and its walls weaken. In such cases, the patient initially reports constant upper abdominal pain or, less often, low back or dull abdominal pain. If the aneurysm ruptures, he'll report severe abdominal and back pain. And after rupture, the aneurysm no longer pulsates.

Related signs and symptoms of rupture include mottled skin below the waist, absent femoral and pedal pulses, lower blood pressure in the legs than in the arms, mild to moderate tenderness with guarding, and abdominal rigidity. Signs of shock—such as tachycardia and cool, clammy skin—appear with significant blood loss.

▶ *Bladder distention.* A smooth, rounded, fluctuant suprapubic mass is characteristic. In extreme distention, the mass may extend to the umbilicus. Severe suprapubic pain and urinary frequency and urgency also may occur.

▶ *Cholecystitis.* Deep palpation below the liver border may reveal a smooth, firm, sausage-shaped mass. However, in acute inflammation, the gallbladder is usually too tender to be palpated. Cholecystitis can cause severe right-upper-quadrant pain that may radiate to the right shoulder, chest, or back; abdominal rigidity and tenderness; fever; pallor; diaphoresis; anorexia; nausea; and vomiting. Recurrent attacks usually occur 1 to 6 hours after meals. Murphy's sign (inspiratory arrest when you palpate the right upper quadrant as the patient takes a deep breath) is common.[3]

▶ *Cholelithiasis.* A stone-filled gallbladder usually produces a painless right-upper-quadrant mass that's smooth and sausage-shaped. However, passage of a stone through the bile or cystic duct may cause severe right-upper-quadrant pain that radiates to the epigastrium, back, or shoulder blades. Related signs and symptoms include anorexia, nausea, vomiting, chills, diaphoresis, restlessness, and low-grade fever. Jaundice may occur with obstruction of the common bile duct. The patient also may have intolerance of fatty foods and frequent indigestion.

▶ *Colon cancer.* A right-lower-quadrant mass may occur in cancer of the right colon, which may also cause occult bleeding with anemia and abdominal aching, pressure, or dull cramps. Related findings include weakness, fatigue, exertional dyspnea, vertigo, and signs and symptoms of intestinal obstruction, such as obstipation and vomiting.

Occasionally, cancer of the left colon also causes a palpable mass. Usually though, it produces rectal bleeding, intermittent abdominal fullness or cramping, and rectal pressure. The patient may also report fremitus and pelvic discomfort. Later, he develops obstipation, diarrhea, or pencil-shaped, grossly bloody, or mucus-streaked stools. Typically, defecation relieves pain.

▶ *Crohn's disease.* In Crohn's disease, tender, sausage-shaped masses are usually palpable in the right lower quadrant and, at times, in the left lower quadrant. Attacks of colicky right-lower-quadrant pain and diarrhea are common. Related signs and symptoms include fever, anorexia, weight loss, hyperactive bowel sounds, nausea, abdominal tenderness with guarding, and perirectal, skin, or vaginal fistulas.

▶ *Diverticulitis.* Most common in the sigmoid colon, diverticulitis may produce a left-lower-quadrant mass that's usually tender, firm, and fixed. It also produces intermittent abdominal pain that's relieved by defecation or passage of flatus. Other findings may include alternating constipation and diarrhea, nausea, low-grade fever, and a distended and tympanic abdomen.

▶ *Gallbladder cancer.* Gallbladder cancer may produce a moderately tender, irregular mass in the right upper quadrant. Accompanying it is chronic, progressively severe epigastric or right-upper-quadrant pain that may radiate to the right shoulder. Related signs and symptoms include nausea, vomiting, anorexia, weight loss, jaundice, and possibly hepatosplenomegaly.

▶ *Gastric cancer.* Advanced gastric cancer may produce an epigastric mass. Early findings include chronic dyspepsia and epigastric discomfort, whereas late findings include weight loss, a feeling of fullness after eating, fatigue, and occasionally coffee-ground vomitus or melena.

▶ *Hepatic cancer.* Hepatic cancer produces a tender, nodular mass in the right upper quadrant or right epigastric area, possibly accompanied by severe pain. Other effects include weight loss, weakness, anorexia, nausea, fever, dependent edema, and occasionally jaundice and ascites. A large tumor also may cause a bruit or hum.

▶ *Hepatomegaly.* Hepatomegaly produces a firm, blunt, irregular mass in the epigastric region or below the right costal margin. Related signs and symptoms vary with the causative disorder but commonly include ascites, right-upper-quadrant pain and tenderness, anorexia, nausea, vomiting, leg edema, jaundice, palmar erythema, spider angiomas, gynecomastia, testicular atrophy, and possibly splenomegaly.

▶ *Hydronephrosis.* By enlarging one or both kidneys, hydronephrosis produces a smooth, boggy mass in one or both flanks. Other findings vary with the degree of hydronephrosis. The patient may have severe colicky renal pain or dull flank pain that radiates to the groin, vulva, or testes. Hematuria, pyuria, dysuria, alternating oliguria and polyuria, nocturia, accelerated hypertension, nausea, and vomiting may also occur.

▶ *Ovarian cyst.* A large ovarian cyst may produce a smooth, rounded, fluctuant mass resembling a distended bladder in the suprapubic region. Large or multiple cysts also may cause mild pelvic discomfort, low back pain, menstrual irregularities, and hirsutism. A twisted or ruptured cyst may cause abdominal tenderness, distention, and rigidity.

▶ *Pancreatic abscess.* Occasionally, a pancreatic abscess may produce a palpable epigastric mass with epigastric pain and tenderness. The patient's temperature usually rises abruptly but may climb steadily. Nausea, vomiting, diarrhea, tachycardia, and hypotension may also occur.

▶ *Pancreatic pseudocysts.* After pancreatitis, pseudocysts may form on the pancreas, causing a palpable nodular mass in the epigastric area. Other findings include nausea, vomiting, diarrhea, abdominal pain and tenderness, low-grade fever, and tachycardia.

▶ *Renal cell carcinoma.* Usually occurring in only one kidney, renal cell carcinoma produces a smooth, firm, nontender mass near the affected kidney. Accompanying it are dull, constant abdominal or flank pain and hematuria. Other signs include elevated blood pressure, fever, and urine retention. Weight loss, nausea, vomiting, and leg edema occur in late stages.

▶ *Splenomegaly.* Lymphomas, leukemias, hemolytic anemias, and inflammatory diseases are among the many disorders that may cause splenomegaly. Typically, the smooth edge of the enlarged spleen is palpable in the left upper quadrant. Related signs and symptoms vary with the causative disorder but often include a feeling of abdominal fullness, left-upper-quadrant abdominal pain and tenderness, splenic friction rub, splenic bruits, and low-grade fever.

▶ *Uterine leiomyomas (fibroids).* If large enough, these common, benign uterine tumors produce a round, multinodular mass in the suprapubic region. The patient's chief complaint is usually menorrhagia; she also may have a feeling of heaviness in the abdomen, and pressure on surrounding organs may cause back pain, constipation, and urinary frequency or urgency. Leg edema and varicosities may develop. Rapid fibroid growth in perimenopausal or postmenopausal women needs further evaluation.

Special considerations

Discovery of an abdominal mass commonly causes anxiety. Offer emotional support to the patient and his family as they await the diagnosis. Position the patient comfortably, and give drugs for pain or anxiety as needed.

If an abdominal mass causes bowel obstruction, watch for indications of peritonitis—abdominal pain and rebound tenderness—and for signs of shock, such as tachycardia and hypotension.

Pediatric pointers

Detecting an abdominal mass in an infant can be quite a challenge. However, these tips will make palpation easier for you: Allow an infant to suck on his bottle or pacifier to prevent crying, which causes abdominal rigidity and interferes with palpation. Avoid tickling him because laughter also causes abdominal rigidity. Also, reduce his apprehension by distracting him with cheerful conversation. Warm your hands, and rest one hand on the infant's abdomen for a few moments before palpation. If he's still sensitive, place his hand under yours as you palpate. Consider letting the child sit on the parent's or caregiver's lap. Also perform a gentle rectal examination.

In neonates, most abdominal masses result from renal disorders, such as polycystic kidney disease or congenital hydronephrosis. In older infants and children, abdominal masses usually are caused by enlarged organs, such as the liver and spleen.

Other common causes include Wilms' tumor, neuroblastoma, intussusception, volvulus, Hirschsprung's disease (congenital megacolon), pyloric stenosis, and abdominal abscess. (See *Wilms' tumor*.)

Geriatric pointers

Ultrasonography should be used to evaluate a prominent midepigastric mass in thin elderly patients.

HEALTH & SAFETY

Wilms' tumor

Wilms' tumor is the most common kidney tumor in children and usually is diagnosed in children younger than age five.[4] Typically, the child has a nontender mass on one side of the abdomen. Other signs may include an enlarged abdomen, hypertension, hematuria, and anemia.

When assessing a child with Wilms' tumor, don't palpate the abdomen because doing so may rupture the tumor's capsule, allowing cancer cells to metastasize.[5]

Consider placing a notice at the child's bedside warning other health care providers not to palpate his abdomen. Also instruct the child's parents to handle and bathe the child carefully to avoid injuring or rupturing the capsule.[5]

Patient counseling

Carefully explain diagnostic tests, which may include blood and urine studies, abdominal X-rays, barium enema, computed tomography scan, ultrasonography, radioisotope scan, and gastroscopy or sigmoidoscopy. A pelvic or rectal examination is usually indicated.

REFERENCES

1. Gendreau-Webb, R. "Is It a Kidney Stone or Abdominal Aortic Aneurysm?" *Nursing* 36(5) ED Insider:22-24, Spring 2006.
2. Irwin, G.H. "How to Protect A Patient with Aortic Aneurysm." *Nursing* 37(2):36-42, February 2007.
3. Baltimore, J.J. and Davidson, J. "Caring For a Patient with Acute Cholecystitis." *Nursing* 37(3):64hn1-64hn4, March 2007.
4. Castellino, S.M. and McLean, T.W. "Pediatric Genitourinary Tumors." *Current Opinion in Oncology* 19(3):248-253, May 2007.
5. Hockenberry, M.J. and Wilson, D. (Eds.) *Wong's Nursing Care of Infants and Children*, 8th ed. St. Louis: Mosby, 2007.

ABDOMINAL PAIN

Abdominal pain usually results from a GI disorder, but it also may be caused by a reproductive, genitourinary (GU), musculoskeletal, or vascular disorder; drug use; trauma; or ingestion of toxins. At times, such pain signals life-threatening complications.

Abdominal pain arises from the abdominopelvic viscera (in the abdominal organs) or the parietal peritoneum (outside the abdominal organs).[1] It may be acute or chronic and diffuse or localized. Visceral pain develops slowly into a deep, dull, aching pain that's poorly localized in the epigastric, periumbilical, or lower midabdominal (hypogastric) region. In contrast, parietal (peritoneal) pain produces a sharp, more intense, and well-localized discomfort.[1] Movement or coughing worsens this pain. (See *Abdominal pain: Types and locations.*)

Pain also may be referred to the abdomen from another site with the same or a similar nerve supply. This sharp, well-localized, referred pain is felt in skin or deeper tissues and may coexist with skin hyperesthesia and muscle hyperalgesia.

Mechanisms that produce abdominal pain include stretching or tension of the gut wall, traction on the peritoneum or mesentery, vigorous intestinal contraction, inflammation, ischemia, and sensory nerve irritation.

If the patient has sudden, severe abdominal pain, quickly take his vital signs and palpate pulses below the waist. Be alert for signs of hypovolemic shock, such as tachycardia and hypotension. Obtain I.V. access.

Emergency surgery may be needed if the patient has mottled skin below the waist and a pulsating epigastric mass or rebound tenderness and rigidity.

History and physical examination

If the patient has no life-threatening signs or symptoms, take his history. Ask him if he has had this type of pain before. Have him describe the pain. For example, is it dull, sharp, stabbing, or burning? Ask if anything relieves the pain or makes it worse. Ask the patient if the pain is constant or intermittent and when

the pain began. Constant, steady abdominal pain suggests organ perforation, ischemia, or inflammation or blood in the peritoneal cavity. Intermittent, cramping abdominal pain suggests the patient may have an obstruction of a hollow organ.

If pain is intermittent, find out the duration of a typical episode. In addition, ask where the pain is located and if it radiates to other areas.

Find out if movement, coughing, exertion, vomiting, eating, elimination, or walking worsens or relieves the pain. The patient may report abdominal pain as indigestion or gas pain, so have him describe the pain in detail.

Ask the patient if he has had recent abdominal trauma or a recent viral illness.[2] Also ask about a history of vascular, GI, GU, or reproductive disorders. Find out if there's any history of inherited diseases that could cause recurrent abdominal pain, such as sickle cell anemia or cystic fibrosis.[1] Ask a female patient the date of her last menses and if she has had changes in her menstrual pattern or dyspareunia. Ask about such habits as alcohol and drug use, caffeine consumption, and cigarette smoking.[1]

Also ask about appetite changes and the onset and frequency of nausea or vomiting. Find out about increased flatulence, constipation, diarrhea, and changes in stool consistency. When was the last bowel movement? Ask about urinary frequency, urgency, or pain. Is the urine cloudy or pink?

Perform a physical examination. Take the patient's vital signs, and assess skin turgor and mucous membranes. Inspect the abdomen for distention or visible peristaltic waves and, if indicated, measure abdominal girth.

Auscultate for bowel sounds, and characterize their motility. Percuss all quadrants, noting the percussion sounds. Palpate the entire abdomen for masses, rigidity, and tenderness. Check for costovertebral angle tenderness, abdominal tenderness with guarding, and rebound tenderness.

Medical causes

▶ *Abdominal aortic aneurysm (dissecting).* Initially, abdominal aortic aneurysm—a life-threatening disorder—may produce dull lower abdominal, lower back, or severe chest pain.

Abdominal pain: Types and locations

AFFECTED ORGAN	VISCERAL PAIN	PARIETAL PAIN	REFERRED PAIN
Stomach	Middle epigastrium	Middle epigastrium and left upper quadrant	Shoulders
Gallbladder	Middle epigastrium	Right upper quadrant	Right subscapular area
Pancreas	Middle epigastrium and left upper quadrant	Middle epigastrium and left upper quadrant	Back and left shoulder
Small intestine	Periumbilical area	Over affected site	Midback (rare)
Appendix	Periumbilical area	Right lower quadrant	Right lower quadrant
Proximal colon	Periumbilical area and right flank for ascending colon	Over affected site	Right lower quadrant and back (rare)
Distal colon	Hypogastrium and left flank for descending colon	Over affected site	Left lower quadrant and back (rare)
Ureters	Costovertebral angle	Over affected site	Groin; scrotum in men, labia in women (rare)
Ovaries, fallopian tubes, and uterus	Hypogastrium and groin	Over affected site	Inner thighs

In most cases, however, it produces constant upper abdominal pain, which may worsen when the patient lies down and may abate when he leans forward or sits up. Palpation may reveal an epigastric mass that pulsates before rupture but not after it.

Other findings may include mottled skin below the waist, absent femoral and pedal pulses, blood pressure that's lower in the legs than in the arms, mild to moderate abdominal tenderness with guarding, and abdominal rigidity. Signs of shock, such as tachycardia and tachypnea, may appear.

▶ *Abdominal cancer.* Abdominal pain usually occurs late in abdominal cancer. It may be accompanied by anorexia, weight loss, weakness, depression, an abdominal mass, and abdominal distention.

▶ *Abdominal trauma.* Generalized or localized abdominal pain occurs with ecchymoses on the abdomen; abdominal tenderness; vomiting; and, with hemorrhage into the peri-

toneal cavity, abdominal rigidity. Bowel sounds are decreased or absent. The patient may have signs of hypovolemic shock, such as hypotension and a rapid, thready pulse.

▶ *Adrenal crisis.* Severe abdominal pain appears early along with nausea, vomiting, dehydration, profound weakness, anorexia, and fever. Later signs include progressive loss of consciousness, hypotension, tachycardia, oliguria, cool and clammy skin, and increased motor activity, which may progress to delirium or seizures.

▶ *Anthrax, GI.* Anthrax is an acute infectious disease caused by the gram-positive, spore-forming bacterium *Bacillus anthracis.* Although the disease most commonly occurs in wild and domestic grazing animals, such as cattle, sheep, and goats, the spores can live in the soil for many years. The disease can occur in humans exposed to infected animals, tissue from infected animals, or biological agents. Most natural cases occur in agricultural regions worldwide. Anthrax may occur in cutaneous, inhaled, or GI forms.

GI anthrax is caused by eating contaminated meat from an infected animal. Initial signs and symptoms include anorexia, nausea, vomiting, and fever. Late signs and symptoms include abdominal pain, severe bloody diarrhea, and hematemesis.

▶ *Appendicitis.* Appendicitis is a life-threatening disorder in which pain initially occurs in the epigastric or umbilical region. Anorexia, nausea, and vomiting may develop. Pain localizes at McBurney's point in the right lower quadrant and is accompanied by abdominal rigidity, increasing tenderness (especially over McBurney's point), rebound tenderness, and retractive respirations. Later signs and symptoms include malaise, constipation (or diarrhea), low-grade fever, and tachycardia.

▶ *Cholecystitis.* When a patient is hospitalized with acute abdominal pain, the cause is acute cholecystitis about 3% to 9% of the time.[3] Severe pain in the right upper quadrant may arise suddenly or increase gradually over several hours, usually after meals. It may radiate to the right shoulder, chest, or back. Along with pain are anorexia, nausea, vomiting, fever, abdominal rigidity and tenderness, pallor, and diaphoresis. Murphy's sign (inspiratory arrest elicited when the examiner palpates the right upper quadrant as the patient takes a deep breath) is common.

▶ *Cholethiasis.* Patients may suffer sudden, severe, and paroxysmal pain in the right upper quadrant lasting several minutes to several hours. The pain may radiate to the epigastrium, back, or shoulder blades. The pain is accompanied by anorexia, nausea, vomiting (sometimes bilious), diaphoresis, restlessness, and abdominal tenderness with guarding over the gallbladder or biliary duct. The patient may also have intolerance of fatty food and frequent indigestion.

▶ *Cirrhosis.* Dull abdominal aching occurs early and is usually accompanied by anorexia, indigestion, nausea, vomiting, and constipation or diarrhea. Subsequent upper-right-quadrant pain worsens when the patient sits up or leans forward. Related signs and symptoms include fever, ascites, leg edema, weight gain, hepatomegaly, jaundice, severe pruritus, bleeding tendencies, palmar erythema, and spider angiomas. Gynecomastia and testicular atrophy also may be present.

▶ *Crohn's disease.* An acute attack causes severe cramping pain in the lower abdomen, typically preceded by weeks or months of milder cramping pain. Crohn's disease may also cause diarrhea, hyperactive bowel sounds, dehydration, weight loss, fever, abdominal tenderness with guarding, and possibly a palpable mass in a lower quadrant. Abdominal pain is commonly relieved by defecation. Milder chronic signs and symptoms include right-lower-quadrant pain with diarrhea, steatorrhea, and weight loss. Complications include perirectal or vaginal fistulas.

▶ *Cystitis.* Abdominal pain and tenderness usually occur in the suprapubic region. Related signs and symptoms include malaise, flank pain, low back pain, nausea, vomiting, urinary frequency and urgency, nocturia, dysuria, fever, and chills.

▶ *Diabetic ketoacidosis.* Rarely, severe, sharp, shooting, and girdling pain may persist for several days. Fruity breath odor, a weak and rapid pulse, Kussmaul's respirations, poor skin turgor, polyuria, polydipsia, nocturia, hypotension, decreased bowel sounds, and confusion also occur.

▶ *Diverticulitis.* Mild cases usually produce intermittent, diffuse left-lower-quadrant pain, which may be relieved by defecation or passage of flatus and worsened by eating. Other signs and symptoms include nausea, constipation or diarrhea, low-grade fever and, in many cases, a palpable abdominal mass that's usually tender, firm, and fixed. Rupture causes severe left-lower-quadrant pain, abdominal rigidity, and possibly signs and symptoms of sepsis and shock (high fever, chills, and hypotension).

▶ *Duodenal ulcer.* Localized abdominal pain—described as steady, gnawing, burning, aching, or hungerlike—may occur high in the midepigastrium, slightly off center, usually on the right. The pain usually doesn't radiate unless pancreatic penetration occurs. It typically begins 2 to 4 hours after a meal and may awaken the patient at night. Ingestion of food or antacids brings relief until the cycle starts again. Other symptoms include changes in bowel habits and heartburn or retrosternal burning.

▶ *Ectopic pregnancy.* Lower abdominal pain may be sharp, dull, or cramping and constant or intermittent in ectopic pregnancy, a potentially life-threatening disorder. Vaginal bleeding, nausea, and vomiting may occur along with urinary frequency, a tender adnexal mass, and a 1- to 2-month history of amenorrhea. Rupture of the fallopian tube produces sharp lower abdominal pain, which may radiate to the shoulders and neck and become extreme with cervical or adnexal palpation. Signs of shock (such as pallor, tachycardia, and hypotension) may also appear.

▶ *Endometriosis.* Constant, severe pain in the lower abdomen usually begins 5 to 7 days before the start of menses and may be aggravated by defecation. Depending on the location of the ectopic tissue, abdominal pain may be accompanied by abdominal tenderness, constipation, dysmenorrhea, dyspareunia, and deep sacral pain.

▶ Escherichia coli *O157:H7. E. coli* O157:H7 is an aerobic, gram-negative bacillus that causes food-borne illness. Most strains of *E. coli* are harmless and are part of the normal intestinal flora of healthy humans and animals. *E. coli* O157:H7, one of hundreds of strains of the bacterium, is capable of producing a powerful toxin and can cause severe illness. Eating undercooked beef or other foods contaminated with the bacterium causes the disease. Signs and symptoms include watery or bloody diarrhea, nausea, vomiting, fever, and abdominal cramps. In children younger than age 5 and the elderly, hemolytic uremic syndrome may develop and ultimately lead to acute renal failure.

▶ *Gastric ulcer.* Diffuse, gnawing, burning pain in the left upper quadrant or epigastric area commonly occurs 1 to 2 hours after meals and may be relieved by ingestion of food or antacids. Vague bloating and nausea after eating are common. Indigestion, weight change, anorexia, and episodes of GI bleeding also occur.

▶ *Gastritis.* With acute gastritis, the patient has rapid onset of abdominal pain that can range from mild epigastric discomfort to burning pain in the left upper quadrant. Other typical features include belching, fever, malaise, anorexia, nausea, bloody or coffee-ground vomitus, and melena. Significant bleeding is unusual unless the patient has hemorrhagic gastritis.

▶ *Gastroenteritis.* Cramping or colicky abdominal pain, which can be diffuse, originates in the left upper quadrant and radiates or migrates to the other quadrants, usually in a peristaltic manner. It's accompanied by diarrhea, hyperactive bowel sounds, headache, myalgia, nausea, and vomiting.

▶ *Heart failure.* Right-upper-quadrant pain commonly accompanies heart failure's hallmarks: jugular vein distention, dyspnea, tachycardia, and peripheral edema. Other findings include nausea, vomiting, ascites, productive cough, crackles, cool extremities, and cyanotic nail beds. Clinical signs are numerous and vary with the stage of the disease and amount of cardiovascular impairment.

▶ *Hepatic abscess.* Steady, severe abdominal pain in the right upper quadrant or midepigastrium commonly accompanies hepatic abscess—a rare disorder—but right-upper-quadrant tenderness is the most important finding. Other signs and symptoms are anorexia, diarrhea, nausea, fever, diaphoresis, elevated right hemidiaphragm and, rarely, vomiting.

▶ *Hepatic amebiasis.* Rare in the United States, hepatic amebiasis causes relatively severe right-upper-quadrant pain and tenderness over the liver and possibly the right shoulder. Accompanying signs and symptoms include fever, weakness, weight loss, chills, diaphoresis, and jaundiced or brownish skin.

▶ *Hepatitis.* Liver enlargement from any type of hepatitis causes discomfort or dull pain and tenderness in the right upper quadrant. Related signs and symptoms may include dark urine, clay-colored stools, nausea, vomiting, anorexia, jaundice, malaise, and pruritus.

▶ *Herpes zoster.* Herpes zoster of the thoracic, lumbar, or sacral nerves can cause localized abdominal and chest pain in the areas served by these nerves. Pain, tenderness, and fever can precede or accompany erythematous papules, which rapidly evolve into grouped vesicles.

▶ *Intestinal obstruction.* Short episodes of intense, colicky, cramping pain alternate with pain-free intervals in intestinal obstruction, a life-threatening disorder. Other signs and symptoms may include abdominal distention, tenderness, and guarding; visible peristaltic waves; high-pitched, tinkling, or hyperactive bowel sounds proximal to the obstruction and hypoactive or absent sounds distally; obstipation; and pain-induced agitation. In jejunal and duodenal obstruction, nausea and bilious vomiting occur early. In distal small- or large-bowel obstruction, nausea and vomiting are commonly feculent. Complete obstruction produces absent bowel sounds. Late-stage obstruction produces signs of hypovolemic shock, such as hypotension and tachycardia.

▶ *Irritable bowel syndrome.* Lower abdominal cramping or pain is aggravated by ingestion of coarse or raw foods and may be alleviated by defecation or passage of flatus. Related findings include abdominal tenderness, diurnal diarrhea alternating with constipation or normal bowel function, and small stools with visible mucus. Dyspepsia, nausea, and abdominal distention with a feeling of incomplete evacuation may also occur. Stress, anxiety, and emotional lability intensify the symptoms.

▶ *Listeriosis.* Listeriosis is a serious infection caused by eating food contaminated with the bacterium *Listeria monocytogenes*. This illness mainly affects pregnant women, neonates, and those with weakened immune systems. Signs and symptoms include fever, myalgia, abdominal pain, nausea, vomiting, and diarrhea. If the infection spreads to the nervous system, it may cause meningitis, characterized by fever, headache, nuchal rigidity, and altered level of consciousness (LOC). Listeriosis infection during pregnancy may lead to premature delivery, infection of the neonate, or stillbirth.

▶ *Mesenteric artery ischemia.* Always suspect mesenteric artery ischemia in patients older than age 50 with chronic heart failure, cardiac arrhythmias, cardiovascular infarct, or hypotension who develop sudden, severe abdominal pain after 2 to 3 days of colicky periumbilical pain and diarrhea. Initially, the abdomen is soft and tender with decreased bowel sounds. Related findings include vomiting, anorexia, alternating periods of diarrhea and constipation and, in late stages, extreme abdominal tenderness with rigidity, tachycardia, tachypnea, absent bowel sounds, and cool, clammy skin.

▶ *Myocardial infarction (MI).* In MI—a life-threatening disorder—substernal chest pain may radiate to the abdomen. Related signs and symptoms include weakness, diaphoresis, nausea, vomiting, anxiety, syncope, jugular vein distention, and dyspnea.

▶ *Norovirus infection.* Abdominal pain or cramping is common in norovirus infection. Transmitted by the fecal-oral route and highly contagious, these viruses may produce gastroenteritis, acute-onset vomiting, nausea, and diarrhea. Less common symptoms include low-grade fever, headache, chills, muscle aches, and generalized fatigue. People who are otherwise healthy usually recover in 24 to 60 hours without lasting effects. (See *Norovirus transmission*.)

▶ *Ovarian cyst.* Torsion or hemorrhage causes pain and tenderness in the right or left lower quadrant. Sharp and severe if the patient suddenly stands or stoops, the pain becomes brief and intermittent if the torsion self-corrects or dull and diffuse after several hours if it doesn't. Pain is accompanied by a slight fever, mild nausea and vomiting, abdominal tenderness, a palpable abdominal mass, and possibly amenorrhea. Abdominal distention may occur if the cyst is large. Peritoneal irritation, or rupture and ensuing peritonitis, causes high fever and severe nausea and vomiting.

▶ *Pancreatitis.* Abdominal pain is the chief symptom of acute pancreatitis.[2] Life-threatening acute pancreatitis produces fulminating, continuous upper abdominal pain that may radiate to both flanks and to the back. To relieve this pain, the patient may bend forward, draw his knees to his chest, or move about restlessly. Early findings include abdominal tenderness, nausea, vomiting, fever, pallor, tachycardia and, in some patients, abdominal rigidity, rebound tenderness, and hypoactive bowel sounds. Turner's sign (ecchymosis of the abdomen or flank) or Cullen's sign (a bluish tinge around the umbilicus) signals hemorrhagic pancreatitis. Jaundice may occur as inflammation subsides.

Chronic pancreatitis produces severe left-upper-quadrant or epigastric pain that radiates to the back. Abdominal tenderness, a midepigastric mass, jaundice, fever, and

Norovirus transmission

Norovirus infection has become the leading cause of nonbacterial gastroenteritis worldwide and causes about 23 million cases each year in the United States.[4] These infections have spread from the community into hospitals, nursing homes, and other health care settings.[5] More than ever, it's important for health care professionals to understand norovirus transmission and how to prevent it.

A CLOSER LOOK AT NOROVIRUS
Noroviruses, of the family *Caliciviridae*, are highly contagious viruses once known as "Norwalk-like" viruses. There are at least five genogroups of norovirus; groups I, II, and IV cause infections in humans. These strains are in turn divided into more than 30 groups based on their genetic makeup. For exempla, viral strain GII.4 is an aggressive norovirus that has caused outbreaks across Europe and the United States.

Noroviruses are transmitted mainly via the fecal-oral route through consumption of food or water contaminated with infectious feces. They also may spread through direct person-to-person contact and by vectors. Noroviruses are stable and can survive a long time on surfaces despite exposure to heat or cold; oral contact with contaminated surfaces can lead to infection. Noroviruses may also be transmitted via inhalation of aerosolized viral particles produced when an infected person vomits.

EDUCATION AND PREVENTION
Although norovirus infection typically is short-lived, with symptoms lasting only 12 to 72 hours, it may pose dangers, especially for those whose health is already compromised. Education of patients and health care workers is necessary for preventing the spread of the virus and should include these points:[4]
● Maintain strict hand-washing.
● Wash linens soiled with infectious feces or vomit promptly in hot water.
● Clean contaminated surfaces with a bleach solution.
● Use contact precautions for patients who could be infected. Droplet precautions may be needed if the patient is vomiting.
● Report clusters of infection to public health agencies to help identify outbreaks and promote the need for preventive measures.

splenomegaly may occur. Steatorrhea, weight loss, maldigestion, and diabetes mellitus are common.

▶ *Pelvic inflammatory disease.* Pain in the right or left lower quadrant ranges from vague discomfort worsened by movement to deep, severe, and progressive pain. Sometimes, metrorrhagia precedes or accompanies the onset of pain. Extreme pain accompanies cervical or adnexal palpation. Related findings include abdominal tenderness, a palpable abdominal or pelvic mass, fever, occasional chills, nausea, vomiting, discomfort on urination, and abnormal vaginal bleeding or a purulent vaginal discharge.

▶ *Perforated ulcer.* In a life-threatening perforated ulcer, sudden, severe, and prostrating epigastric pain may radiate through the abdomen to the back or right shoulder. Other signs and symptoms include boardlike abdominal rigidity, tenderness with guarding,

generalized rebound tenderness, absent bowel sounds, grunting and shallow respirations and, in many cases, fever, tachycardia, hypotension, and syncope.

▶ *Peritonitis.* In this life-threatening disorder, sudden and severe pain can be diffuse or localized in the area of the underlying disorder; movement worsens the pain. The degree of abdominal tenderness usually varies according to the extent of disease. Typical findings include fever; chills; nausea; vomiting; hypoactive or absent bowel sounds; abdominal tenderness, distention, and rigidity; rebound tenderness and guarding; hyperalgesia; tachycardia; hypotension; tachypnea; and positive psoas and obturator signs.

▶ *Pleurisy.* Pleurisy may produce upper abdominal or costal margin pain referred from the chest. Characteristic sharp, stabbing chest pain increases with inspiration and movement. Many patients have a pleural friction rub and rapid, shallow breathing; some have a low-grade fever.

▶ *Pneumonia.* Lower-lobe pneumonia can cause pleuritic chest pain and referred, severe upper abdominal pain, tenderness, and rigidity that diminish with inspiration. It can also cause fever, shaking chills, achiness, headache, blood-tinged or rusty sputum, dyspnea, and a dry, hacking cough. Accompanying signs include crackles, egophony, decreased breath sounds, and dullness on percussion.

▶ *Pneumothorax.* Pneumothorax is a potentially life-threatening disorder that can cause referred pain from the chest to the upper abdomen and costal margin. Characteristic chest pain arises suddenly and worsens with deep inspiration or movement. Other signs and symptoms include anxiety, dyspnea, cyanosis, decreased or absent breath sounds over the affected area, tachypnea, and tachycardia. Watch for asymmetrical chest movement on inspiration.

▶ *Prostatitis.* The patient may report vague abdominal pain or discomfort in the lower abdomen, groin, perineum, or rectum. Other findings include dysuria, urinary frequency and urgency, fever, chills, low back pain, myalgia, arthralgia, and nocturia. Chronic prostatitis may cause scrotal pain, penile pain, and pain on ejaculation.

▶ *Pyelonephritis (acute).* Progressive lower quadrant pain in one or both sides, flank pain, and costovertebral angle tenderness characterize pyelonephritis. Pain may radiate to the lower midabdomen or the groin. Other signs and symptoms include abdominal and back tenderness, high fever, shaking chills, nausea, vomiting, and urinary frequency and urgency.

▶ *Renal calculi.* Depending on their location, calculi may cause severe abdominal or back pain. However, the classic symptom is severe, colicky pain that travels from the costovertebral angle to the flank, suprapubic region, and external genitalia. The pain may be excruciating or dull and constant and may be accompanied by agitation, nausea, vomiting, abdominal distention, fever, chills, hypertension, and urinary urgency with hematuria and dysuria.

▶ *Sickle cell crisis.* Sudden, severe abdominal pain may accompany chest, back, hand, or foot pain. Related signs and symptoms include weakness, aching joints, dyspnea, and scleral jaundice.

▶ *Smallpox (variola major).* Worldwide eradication of smallpox was achieved in 1980; the United States and Russia have the only known storage sites for the virus, which is considered a possible agent of biological warfare. Initial signs and symptoms include high fever, malaise, prostration, severe headache, backache, and abdominal pain. A maculopapular rash develops on the oral mucosa, pharynx, face, and forearms and then spreads to the trunk and legs. Within 2 days, the rash becomes vesicular and later pustular. The lesions develop at the same time, appear identical, and are more prominent on the face and limbs. The pustules are round, firm, and embedded in the skin. After 8 to 9 days, the pustules form a crust, which later separates from the skin, leaving a pitted scar. Death may result from encephalitis, extensive bleeding, or secondary infection.

▶ *Splenic infarction.* Fulminating pain in the left upper quadrant occurs with chest pain that may worsen on inspiration. Pain commonly radiates to the left shoulder with splinting of the left diaphragm, abdominal guarding and, occasionally, a splenic friction rub.

▶ *Systemic lupus erythematosus.* Generalized abdominal pain is unusual in this disease but may occur after meals. Nondeforming arthritis, photosensitivity, alopecia, mucous membrane ulcers, and butterfly rash are characteristic signs. Other common signs and symptoms include anorexia, vomiting, abdominal tenderness with guarding, abdominal distention after meals, fatigue, fever, and weight loss. Precordial chest pain and a pericardial rub also may occur.

▶ *Ulcerative colitis.* Ulcerative colitis may begin with vague abdominal discomfort that leads to cramping lower abdominal pain. As the disorder progresses, pain may become steady and diffuse, increasing with movement and coughing. The most common symptom—recurrent and possibly severe diarrhea with blood, pus, and mucus—may relieve the pain. The abdomen may feel soft and extremely tender. High-pitched, infrequent bowel sounds may accompany nausea, vomiting, anorexia, weight loss, and mild, intermittent fever.

▶ *Uremia.* Characterized by generalized or periumbilical pain that shifts and varies in intensity, uremia causes diverse GI signs and symptoms, such as nausea, vomiting, anorexia, and diarrhea. Other findings may include bleeding, abdominal tenderness that changes in location and intensity, visual disturbances, headache, decreased LOC, vertigo, and oliguria or anuria. Chest pain may occur secondary to pericardial effusion. Localized or diffuse pruritus is common.

Other causes

DRUG WATCH *Salicylates and nonsteroidal anti-inflammatory drugs may cause burning, gnawing pain in the left upper quadrant or epigastric area as well as nausea and vomiting.*

▶ *Insect toxins.* Generalized, cramping abdominal pain usually occurs with low-grade fever, nausea, vomiting, abdominal rigidity, tremors, and burning sensations in the hands or feet.

Special considerations

Help the patient find a comfortable position to ease his distress. Try placing him in a supine position with his head flat on the table, arms at his sides, and knees slightly flexed to relax the abdominal muscles. Monitor him closely because abdominal pain can signal a life-threatening disorder. Especially important indications include tachycardia, hypotension, clammy skin, abdominal rigidity, rebound tenderness, a change in the location or intensity of pain, or sudden relief from the pain.

Withhold analgesics because they may mask symptoms. Also withhold food and fluids because surgery may be needed. Prepare for I.V. infusion and insertion of a nasogastric or other intestinal tube. Peritoneal lavage or abdominal paracentesis may be needed.

You may have to prepare the patient for a diagnostic procedure, such as a pelvic and rectal examination; blood, urine, and stool tests; X-rays; barium studies; ultrasonography; endoscopy; and biopsy.

Pediatric pointers

Because children commonly have trouble describing abdominal pain, pay close attention to nonverbal clues, such as wincing, lethargy, or unusual positioning (such as a side-lying position with knees flexed to the abdomen). Observing the child while he coughs, walks, or climbs may offer some diagnostic clues. Also, remember that a parent's description of the child's complaints is a subjective interpretation of what the parent believes is wrong.

Abdominal pain in children may signal a more serious disorder or a disorder that produces different signs and symptoms than in adults. For example, appendicitis is more likely to result in rupture and death in children, and vomiting may be its only other sign. Acute pyelonephritis may cause abdominal pain, vomiting, and diarrhea, but not the classic urologic signs found in adults. Peptic ulcer, which is becoming increasingly common in teenagers, causes nocturnal pain and colic that may not be relieved by food, unlike peptic ulcer in adults.

Remember, too, that a child's complaint of abdominal pain may be functional, or psychosomatic, in nature. Rather than an organic cause, this type of abdominal pain probably relates to psychological disturbances, such as family or school stressors or behavioral or personality disorders.[1]

In children younger than age 5, abdominal pain commonly results from colic (which affects 10% to 20% of infants in the first month after birth and may cause screaming, drawing the knees up toward the chest, and the appearance of severe pain); pyloric stenosis; intussusception; and poison ingestion.[1] School-age children commonly have recurrent abdominal pain, which occurs in multiple episodes over at least 3 months.[1] This pain may have organic causes or be functional. Common causes of abdominal pain in adolescents include appendicitis and inflammatory bowel disease (ulcerative colitis or Crohn's disease).[1] In sexually active adolescent girls with pelvic or lower abdominal pain, also consider pelvic inflammatory disease or ectopic pregnancy.[1]

Geriatric pointers

Advanced age may decrease the effects acute abdominal disease. Pain may be less severe, fever less pronounced, and signs of peritoneal inflammation reduced or absent. These changes leave the elderly patient at greater risk of late diagnosis.[1]

The aging process increases the risk of certain diseases that commonly produce abdominal pain, such as biliary tract disease, diverticulitis, bowel obstruction, mesenteric artery ischemia, abdominal aortic aneurysm, and malignancies.[1]

Patient counseling

Teach the patient how to use positioning to help alleviate discomfort. Explain what to expect from diagnostic testing, which may include pelvic and rectal examinations, X-rays, computed tomography scans, barium studies, and collection of blood, urine, and stool samples. Ultrasonography, endoscopy, and biopsy also may be performed. If surgery is needed, provide preoperative teaching.

REFERENCES

1. Miller, S.K. and Alpert, P.T. "Assessment and Differential Diagnosis of Abdominal Pain." *The Nurse Practitioner* 31(7):38-47, July 2006.
2. Holcomb, S.S. "Stopping the Destruction of Acute Pancreatitis." *Nursing* 37(6):42-47, June 2007.
3. Baltimore, J.J. and Davidson, J. "Caring For A Patient With Acute Cholecystitis." *Nursing* 37(3):64hn1-64hn4, March 2007.
4. Estes, M.K., Prasad, B.V.V., and Atmar, R.L. "Noroviruses Everywhere: Has Something Changed?" *Current Opinions in Infectious Diseases* 19(5):467-74, October 2006.
5. Coffman, S. "Bugs Among Us." *Nursing Management* 38(10):33-40, October 2007.

● AMNESIA

A mnesia—a disturbance in or loss of memory—may be classified as partial or complete and as anterograde or retrograde. Anterograde amnesia denotes memory loss for events that occurred after the onset of the causative trauma or disease; retrograde amnesia, for events that occurred before the onset. Depending on the cause, amnesia may arise suddenly or slowly and may be temporary or permanent.

Organic (or true) amnesia results from temporal lobe dysfunction, and it characteristically spares patches of memory. A common symptom in patients with seizures or head trauma, organic amnesia also may be an early indicator of Alzheimer's disease. Those with mental retardation, schizophrenia, or human immunodeficiency virus infection or acquired immunodeficiency syndrome, and those who abuse alcohol or drugs, are also at risk for memory disturbances.[1] Hysterical amnesia has a psychogenic origin and characteristically causes complete memory loss. Treatment-induced amnesia is usually transient.

History and physical examination

Because the patient often isn't aware of his amnesia, you'll usually need help in gathering information from his family or friends. Throughout your assessment, notice the patient's general appearance, behavior, mood, and train of thought. Ask when the amnesia first appeared and what types of things the patient can't remember. Can he learn new information? How long does he remember it? Does the amnesia involve a recent or a remote period?

Test the patient's recent memory by asking him to identify and repeat three items. Retest him after 3 minutes. Test his intermediate memory by asking, "Who was the president before this one?" and "What was the last type of car you bought?" Test remote memory with such questions as "How old are you?" and "Where were you born?"

Take the patient's vital signs and assess his level of consciousness (LOC). Check his pupils. They should be equal in size and should constrict quickly when exposed to direct light. Also, assess extraocular movement. Test motor function by having the patient move his arms and legs through their range of motion. Evaluate sensory function with pinpricks.

Medical causes

▶ *Alzheimer's disease.* Alzheimer's disease usually begins with retrograde amnesia, which progresses slowly over many months or years to include anterograde amnesia and, eventually, severe and permanent memory loss. Related findings include agitation, inability to concentrate, disregard for personal hygiene, confusion, irritability, and emotional lability. Later signs include aphasia, dementia, incontinence, and muscle rigidity.

▶ *Cerebral hypoxia.* After recovery from hypoxia (brought on by such conditions as carbon monoxide poisoning or acute respiratory failure), the patient may have total amnesia for the event along with sensory disturbances such as numbness and tingling.

▶ *Head trauma.* Depending on the severity of trauma, amnesia may last minutes, hours, or longer. Usually, the patient has brief retrograde and longer anterograde amnesia as well as persistent amnesia about the traumatic event. Severe head trauma can cause permanent amnesia or difficulty retaining recent memories. Related findings may include altered respirations and LOC; headache; dizziness; confusion; visual disturbances, such as blurred or double vision; and motor and sensory disturbances, such as hemiparesis and paresthesia, on the side of the body opposite the injury.

▶ *Herpes simplex encephalitis.* Recovery from herpes simplex encephalitis commonly leaves the patient with severe and possibly permanent amnesia. Related findings include evidence of meningeal irritation, such as headache, fever, and altered LOC; seizures; and various motor and sensory disturbances, such as paresis, numbness, and tingling.

▶ *Hysteria.* Hysterical amnesia, a complete and long-lasting memory loss, begins and ends abruptly and is typically accompanied by confusion.

▶ *Seizures.* In temporal lobe seizures, amnesia occurs suddenly and lasts for several seconds to minutes. The patient may recall an aura or nothing at all. An irritable focus on the left side of the brain primarily causes amnesia for verbal memories, whereas an irritable focus on the right side of the brain causes graphic and nonverbal amnesia. Related signs and symptoms may include decreased LOC during the seizure, confusion, abnormal mouth movements, and visual, olfactory, and auditory hallucinations.

▶ *Vertebrobasilar circulatory disorders.* Vertebrobasilar ischemia, infarction, embolus, or hemorrhage may cause complete amnesia that begins abruptly, lasts for several hours, and ends abruptly. Related findings include dizziness, decreased LOC, ataxia, blurred or double vision, vertigo, nausea, and vomiting.

▶ *Wernicke-Korsakoff syndrome.* Retrograde and anterograde amnesia can become permanent without treatment in Wernicke-Korsakoff syndrome. Other signs and symptoms include apathy, an inability to concentrate or put events into sequence, and confabulation to fill memory gaps. The syndrome also may cause diplopia, decreased LOC, headache, ataxia, and symptoms of peripheral neuropathy such as numbness and tingling.

Other causes

DRUG WATCH *Anterograde amnesia may be caused by general anesthetics, especially fentanyl, halothane, and isoflurane; barbiturates, most commonly pentobarbital; and certain benzodiazepines, especially triazolam.*

▶ *Electroconvulsive therapy.* Sudden onset of retrograde or anterograde amnesia occurs with electroconvulsive therapy. Typically, the amnesia lasts several minutes to several hours, but severe, prolonged amnesia occurs with frequent treatments over a long period.

▶ *Temporal lobe surgery.* Usually performed on only one lobe, this surgery causes brief, mild amnesia. However, removal of both lobes results in permanent amnesia.

Special considerations

Prepare the patient for diagnostic tests, such as computed tomography scan, magnetic resonance imaging, electroencephalography, or cerebral angiography.

Provide reality orientation for the patient with retrograde amnesia, and encourage his family to help by supplying familiar photos, objects, and music.

If the patient has severe amnesia, consider his basic needs, such as safety, elimination, and nutrition. If needed, arrange for placement in an extended-care facility.

Pediatric pointers

A child who has amnesia during seizures may be mistakenly labeled as learning disabled. To prevent this mislabeling, stress the importance of following the prescribed drug schedule, and discuss ways that the child, his parents, and his teachers can cope with amnesia.

Patient counseling

Adjust your patient-teaching techniques for the patient with anterograde amnesia because he can't acquire new information. Include his family in teaching sessions. In addition, write down all instructions—particularly drug dosages and schedules—so the patient won't have to rely on his memory.

Encourage the patient and his family to develop memory aids, such as lists and maps, to help him through periods of memory loss.[2]

REFERENCES

1. Pereira, A.P.A. "Assessment of Memory in Rehabilitation Counseling." *Journal of Rehabilitation* 73(2):15-25, April/May 2007.
2. Uko-Ekpenyong, G. "What You Should Know About Electroconvulsive Therapy." *Nursing* 37(8):56hn1–56hn4, August 2007.

ANOREXIA

Anorexia, a lack of appetite despite a physiologic need for food, is a common symptom of GI and endocrine disorders and is characteristic of certain severe psychological disturbances, such as anorexia nervosa. It also can result from such factors as anxiety, chronic pain, poor oral hygiene, increased body temperature due to hot weather or fever, and changes in taste or smell that normally accompany aging. Anorexia also can result from drug therapy or abuse. Short-term anorexia rarely jeopardizes health, but chronic anorexia can lead to life-threatening malnutrition.

History and physical examination

Take the patient's vital signs and weight and height. Ask about weight history, including previous minimum and maximum weights.[1]

Ask about involuntary weight loss of more than 10 lb (4.5 kg) in the last six months.[1,2] Explore dietary habits. Ask what foods he likes and dislikes and why. The patient may identify tastes and smells that nauseate him and cause loss of appetite. Ask about dental problems that interfere with chewing, including periodontal disease and poorly fitting dentures.[2] Ask if he has difficulty or pain when swallowing or if he vomits or has diarrhea after meals. Ask the patient how often and intensely he exercises.

Check for a history of stomach or bowel disorders, which can interfere with the ability to digest, absorb, or metabolize nutrients. Find out about changes in bowel habits. Ask about alcohol use and drug use and dosage.

If the medical history doesn't reveal an organic basis for anorexia, consider psychological factors. Ask the patient if he knows what's causing his decreased appetite. Situational factors—such as a death in the family or problems at school or at work—can lead to depression and subsequent loss of appetite. Be alert for signs of malnutrition, consistent refusal of food, and a 7% to 10% loss of body weight in the preceding month. (See *Is your patient malnourished?*)

Medical causes

▶ *Acquired immunodeficiency syndrome (AIDS).* An infection or Kaposi's sarcoma affecting the GI or respiratory tract may lead to anorexia in a patient with AIDS. Other findings include fatigue, afternoon fevers, night sweats, diarrhea, cough, bleeding, lymphadenopathy, oral thrush, gingivitis, and skin disorders, including persistent herpes zoster and recurrent herpes simplex, herpes labialis, or herpes genitalis.

▶ *Adrenocortical hypofunction.* In adrenocortical hypofunction, anorexia may begin slowly and subtly, causing gradual weight loss. Other common signs and symptoms include nausea and vomiting, abdominal pain, diarrhea, weakness, fatigue, malaise, vitiligo, bronze-colored skin, and purple striae on the breasts, abdomen, shoulders, and hips.

▶ *Alcoholism.* Chronic anorexia commonly accompanies alcoholism, eventually leading to malnutrition. Other findings include signs of liver damage (jaundice, spider angiomas, as-

Is your patient malnourished?

When assessing a patient with anorexia, check for these common signs of malnutrition.

Hair	• Dull, dry, thin, fine, straight, and easily plucked • Areas of lighter or darker spots and hair loss
Face	• Generalized swelling • Dark areas on cheeks and under eyes • Lumpy or flaky skin around the nose and mouth • Enlarged parotid glands
Eyes	• Dull appearance • Dry and either pale or red membranes • Triangular, shiny gray spots on conjunctivae • Red and fissured eyelid corners • Bloodshot ring around cornea
Lips	• Red and swollen, especially at corners
Tongue	• Swollen, purple, and raw-looking • Sores or abnormal papillae
Teeth	• Missing or emerging abnormally • Visible cavities or dark spots • Spongy, bleeding gums
Neck	• Swollen thyroid gland
Skin	• Dry, flaky, swollen, and dark, with lighter or darker spots, some resembling bruises • Tight and drawn, with poor skin turgor
Nails	• Spoon-shaped • Brittle • Ridged
Musculoskeletal system	• Muscle wasting • Knock-kneed or bowlegged • Bumps on ribs • Swollen joints • Musculoskeletal hemorrhages
Cardiovascular system	• Heart rate above 100 beats/minute • Arrhythmias • Elevated blood pressure
Abdomen	• Enlarged liver and spleen
Reproductive system	• Decreased libido • Amenorrhea

(continued)

Is your patient malnourished? *(continued)*

Nervous system	• Irritability, confusion
	• Paresthesia in hands and feet
	• Loss of proprioception
	• Decreased ankle and knee reflexes

cites, edema), paresthesia, tremors, increased blood pressure, bruising, GI bleeding, and abdominal pain.

▶ *Anorexia nervosa.* Chronic anorexia nervosa is an eating disorder that begins insidiously and eventually leads to life-threatening malnutrition, as evidenced by skeletal muscle atrophy, loss of fatty tissue, constipation, amenorrhea, dry and blotchy or sallow skin, alopecia, sleep disturbances, distorted self-image, anhedonia, and decreased libido. Paradoxically, many patients have extreme restlessness and vigor and may exercise avidly; many also have complicated food preparation and eating rituals.

▶ *Appendicitis.* Anorexia closely follows the abrupt onset of generalized or localized epigastric pain, nausea, and vomiting. It can continue as pain localizes in the right lower quadrant (McBurney's point) and other signs and symptoms—abdominal rigidity, rebound tenderness, constipation or diarrhea, slight fever, and tachycardia—appear.

▶ *Cancer.* Chronic anorexia may be accompanied by weight loss, weakness, apathy, and cachexia; it commonly results from chemotherapy drugs.

▶ *Chronic renal failure.* Chronic anorexia is common and develops insidiously in chronic renal failure. It's accompanied by changes in all body systems, such as nausea, vomiting, mouth ulcers, ammonia breath odor, metallic taste, GI bleeding, constipation or diarrhea, drowsiness, confusion, tremors, pallor, dry and scaly skin, pruritus, alopecia, purpuric lesions, and edema.

▶ *Cirrhosis.* Anorexia occurs early in cirrhosis and may be accompanied by weakness, nausea, vomiting, constipation or diarrhea, and dull abdominal pain. It continues after these early signs and symptoms subside and is

accompanied by lethargy, slurred speech, bleeding tendencies, ascites, severe pruritus, dry skin, poor skin turgor, hepatomegaly, fetor hepaticus, jaundice, edema of the legs, gynecomastia, and right-upper-quadrant pain.

▶ *Crohn's disease.* Chronic anorexia causes marked weight loss in Crohn's disease. Related signs vary according to the site and extent of the lesion but may include diarrhea, abdominal pain, fever, abdominal mass, weakness, perianal or vaginal fistulas and, rarely, clubbing of the fingers. Acute inflammatory signs and symptoms—right-lower-quadrant pain, cramping, tenderness, flatulence, fever, nausea, diarrhea (including nocturnal), and bloody stools—mimic those of appendicitis.

▶ *Depressive syndrome.* Anorexia reflects anhedonia in depressive syndrome. Other signs and symptoms include poor concentration, indecisiveness, delusions, menstrual irregularities, decreased libido, insomnia or hypersomnia, fatigue, mood swings, poor self-image, and gradual social withdrawal.

▶ *Gastritis.* In acute gastritis, anorexia may have a sudden onset. The patient may have postprandial epigastric distress with nausea, vomiting (often with hematemesis), fever, belching, hiccups, and malaise.

▶ *Hepatitis.* In viral hepatitis (hepatitis A, B, C, or D), anorexia begins in the preicteric phase and is accompanied by fatigue, malaise, headache, arthralgia, myalgia, photophobia, nausea and vomiting, mild fever, hepatomegaly, and lymphadenopathy. It may continue throughout the icteric phase along with mild weight loss, dark urine, clay-colored stools, jaundice, right-upper-quadrant pain and, possibly, irritability and severe pruritus.

Signs and symptoms of nonviral hepatitis usually resemble those of viral hepatitis but may vary, depending on the cause and the extent of liver damage.

▶ *Hypopituitarism.* Anorexia usually develops slowly in hypopituitarism, which usually begins with hypergonadism. Additional signs and symptoms vary with the disorder's severity and the number and type of deficient hormones. They may include amenorrhea; decreased libido; lethargy; cold intolerance; pale, thin, and dry skin; dry, brittle hair; and decreased temperature, blood pressure, and pulse rate.

▶ *Hypothyroidism.* Anorexia is common and usually insidious in patients with thyroid hormone deficiency. Vague early findings typically include fatigue, forgetfulness, cold intolerance, unexplained weight gain, and constipation. Subsequent findings include decreased mental stability; dry, flaky, and inelastic skin; edema of the face, hands, and feet; ptosis; hoarseness; thick, brittle nails; coarse, broken hair; and signs of decreased cardiac output such as bradycardia. Other common findings include abdominal distention, menstrual irregularities, decreased libido, ataxia, intention tremor, nystagmus, dull facial expression, and slow reflex relaxation time.

▶ *Ketoacidosis.* Anorexia usually arises gradually in ketoacidosis and is accompanied by dry, flushed skin; fruity breath odor; polydipsia; polyuria and nocturia; hypotension; weak, rapid pulse; dry mouth; abdominal pain; and vomiting.

▶ *Pernicious anemia.* In pernicious anemia, insidious anorexia may cause considerable weight loss. Related findings include the classic triad of burning tongue, general weakness, and numbness and tingling in the limbs; alternating constipation and diarrhea; abdominal pain; nausea and vomiting; bleeding gums; ataxia; positive Babinski's and Romberg's signs; diplopia and blurred vision; irritability, headache, malaise, and fatigue.

Other causes

DRUG WATCH *Anorexia may result from the use of amphetamines, chemotherapy drugs, sympathomimetics such as ephedrine, and some antibiotics. It also may signal digoxin toxicity. Anorexia also may occur during the early stages of aceta-* *minophen toxicity, along with nausea, vomiting, pallor, and lethargy.*[3]

▶ *Radiation therapy.* Radiation treatments can cause anorexia, possibly as the result of metabolic disturbances.

▶ *Total parenteral nutrition.* Maintenance of blood glucose levels by I.V. therapy may cause anorexia.

Special considerations

Because the causes of anorexia are diverse, diagnostic procedures may include thyroid function studies, endoscopy, upper GI series, gallbladder series, barium enema, liver and kidney function tests, hormone assays, computed tomography scans, ultrasonography, and blood studies to assess nutritional status. If physical causes of anorexia are ruled out, a psychiatric consultation may be needed.

Take a 24-hour diet history daily. The patient may exaggerate his food intake (common in patients with anorexia nervosa), so you'll need to maintain strict calorie and nutrient counts for the patient's meals. In severe malnutrition, provide supplemental nutritional support, such as total parenteral nutrition or oral nutritional supplements.

Because anorexia and poor nutrition increase susceptibility to infection, monitor the patient's vital signs and white blood cell count and closely observe any wounds.

Pediatric pointers

In children, many illnesses can cause anorexia, and it usually resolves promptly. However, be alert for subtle signs of anorexia nervosa in preadolescent and adolescent patients; evidence may include decreased heart rate and blood pressure, constipation, amenorrhea, thin and brittle nails, alopecia, wasted appearance, and lethargy.[4]

Patient counseling

Instruct the patient to eat high-calorie snacks or small, frequent meals to promote adequate protein and calorie intake. Urge the patient's family to supply his favorite foods to help stimulate his appetite.

REFERENCES

1. DiMaria-Ghaili, R.A. and Amella, E. "Nutrition in Older Adults: Intervention and Assess-

ment Can Help Curb the Growing Threat of Malnutrition. *AJN* 105(3):40-50, March 2005.

2. Martin, C.T., Kayser-Jones, J., Stotts, N.A., Porter, C., and Froelicher, E.S. "Risk for Low Weight In Community-Dwelling, Older Adults." *Clinical Nurse Specialist* 21(4):203-211, July/August 2007.

3. Smith, D.H. "Managing Acute Acetaminophen Toxicity," *Nursing* 37(1): 58–63, January 2007.

4. Hockenberry, M.J. and Wilson, D. (Eds.) *Wong's Nursing Care of Infants and Children*, 8th ed. St. Louis: Mosby, 2007.

● ANURIA

Anuria is clinically defined as urine output of less than 100 ml in 24 hours.[1] It indicates either urinary tract obstruction or acute renal failure. (See *Major causes of acute renal failure*.) Fortunately, anuria is rare; even with renal failure, the kidneys usually produce at least 75 ml of urine daily.

Because urine output is easily measured, anuria rarely goes undetected. However, without immediate treatment, it can rapidly cause uremia and other complications of urine retention.

If your patient has anuria, you'll need to find out whether urine is being formed and then intervene appropriately. Prepare to catheterize the patient to relieve lower urinary tract obstruction and to check for residual urine. If the patient has an obstruction, it may hinder catheter insertion, and the urine may be cloudy and foul smelling. If you collect more than 75 ml of urine, suspect lower urinary tract obstruction; if you collect less than 75 ml, suspect renal dysfunction or obstruction higher in the urinary tract.

History and physical examination

Take the patient's vital signs, and obtain a complete history. First ask about any changes in his voiding pattern. Determine the amount of fluid he normally consumes each day, the amount of fluid he consumed in the last 24 to 48 hours, and the time and amount of his last urination. Review his medical history, noting especially previous kidney disease, urinary

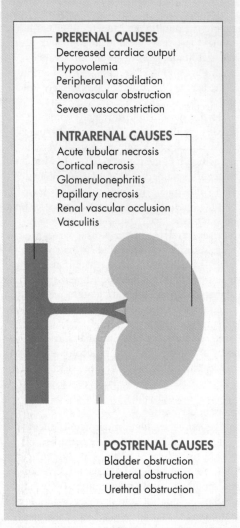

Major causes of acute renal failure

PRERENAL CAUSES
Decreased cardiac output
Hypovolemia
Peripheral vasodilation
Renovascular obstruction
Severe vasoconstriction

INTRARENAL CAUSES
Acute tubular necrosis
Cortical necrosis
Glomerulonephritis
Papillary necrosis
Renal vascular occlusion
Vasculitis

POSTRENAL CAUSES
Bladder obstruction
Ureteral obstruction
Urethral obstruction

tract obstruction or infection, prostate enlargement, renal calculi, neurogenic bladder, or congenital abnormalities. Ask about the patient's drug regimen, noting drugs that may be nephrotoxic or that may warrant renal dosing.[2] Ask if the patient has had unexplained weight gain, which may reflect the body's inability to excrete fluids effectively.[3] Ask about any abdominal, renal, or urinary tract surgery.

Inspect and palpate the abdomen for asymmetry, distention, or bulging. Inspect the flank area for edema or erythema, and percuss and palpate the bladder. Palpate the kidneys both anteriorly and posteriorly, and percuss them at the costovertebral angle. Auscultate over the renal arteries, listening for bruits.

Medical causes

▶ *Acute tubular necrosis.* Oliguria (occasionally anuria) is a common finding in acute tubular necrosis. It precedes the onset of diuresis, which is heralded by polyuria. Related findings reflect the underlying cause and may include signs and symptoms of hyperkalemia (muscle weakness, cardiac arrhythmias), uremia (anorexia, nausea, vomiting, confusion, lethargy, twitching, seizures, pruritus, uremic frost, and Kussmaul's respirations), and heart failure (edema, jugular vein distention, crackles, and dyspnea).
▶ *Cortical necrosis (bilateral).* Cortical necrosis is characterized by a sudden change from oliguria to anuria along with gross hematuria, flank pain, and fever.
▶ *Glomerulonephritis (acute).* The patient may have anuria or oliguria. Related effects include mild fever, malaise, flank pain, gross hematuria, facial and generalized edema, elevated blood pressure, headache, nausea, vomiting, abdominal pain, and signs and symptoms of pulmonary congestion (crackles, dyspnea).
▶ *Hemolytic-uremic syndrome.* Anuria typically occurs in the initial stages of hemolytic-uremic syndrome and may last 1 to 10 days. The patient may have vomiting, diarrhea, abdominal pain, hematemesis, melena, purpura, fever, elevated blood pressure, hepatomegaly, ecchymoses, edema, hematuria, and pallor. He may also show signs of upper respiratory tract infection.
▶ *Papillary necrosis (acute).* Bilateral papillary necrosis produces anuria or oliguria as well as flank pain, costovertebral angle tenderness, renal colic, abdominal pain and rigidity, fever, vomiting, decreased bowel sounds, hematuria, and pyuria.
▶ *Renal artery occlusion (bilateral).* The patient may have anuria or severe oliguria, commonly accompanied by severe, continuous upper abdominal and flank pain, nausea and

vomiting, decreased bowel sounds, fever up to 102° F (38.9° C), and diastolic hypertension.
▶ *Renal vein occlusion (bilateral).* Renal vein occlusion occasionally causes anuria; more typical effects include acute low back pain, fever, flank tenderness, and hematuria. Development of pulmonary emboli—a common complication—produces sudden dyspnea, pleuritic pain, tachypnea, tachycardia, crackles, pleural friction rub, and possibly hemoptysis.
▶ *Urinary tract obstruction.* Severe obstruction can produce acute and sometimes total anuria alternating with or preceded by burning and pain on urination, overflow incontinence or dribbling, increased urinary frequency and nocturia, voiding of small amounts, or altered urine stream. Related findings include bladder distention, pain, and a sensation of fullness in the lower abdomen and groin, upper abdominal and flank pain, nausea and vomiting, and signs of secondary infection, such as fever, chills, malaise, and cloudy, foul-smelling urine.
▶ *Vasculitis.* Vasculitis occasionally produces anuria. More typical findings include malaise, myalgia, polyarthralgia, fever, elevated blood pressure, hematuria, proteinuria, arrhythmias, pallor, and possibly skin lesions, urticaria, and purpura.

Other causes

▶ *Diagnostic tests.* Contrast media used in radiographic studies can cause nephrotoxicity, producing oliguria and, rarely, anuria.

DRUG WATCH *Many classes of drugs can cause anuria or, more commonly, oliguria through their nephrotoxic effects. Antibiotics, especially the aminoglycosides, are the most common nephrotoxins. Anesthetics, heavy metals, ethyl alcohol, and organic solvents also may be nephrotoxic. Adrenergics and anticholinergics may cause urine retention by affecting the nerves and muscles of micturition.*

Special considerations

If catheterization doesn't start urine flow, prepare the patient for diagnostic studies—such as ultrasonography, cystoscopy, retrograde pyelography, and renal scan—to detect any obstruction higher in the urinary tract. If these tests reveal an obstruction, prepare him for immediate surgery to remove the obstruction and insert a nephrostomy or ureterostomy tube to drain the urine. If these tests fail to reveal an obstruction, prepare the patient for further kidney function studies.

Carefully monitor the patient's vital signs and intake and output, saving urine for inspection as appropriate. Restrict the daily fluid allowance to 600 ml more than the previous day's total urine output. Restrict foods and juices high in potassium and sodium, and make sure the patient maintains a balanced diet with controlled protein levels. Provide low-sodium hard candy to help decrease thirst. Record fluid intake and output, and weigh the patient daily.

Pediatric pointers

In neonates, anuria is defined as the absence of urine output for 24 hours. It can be classified as primary or secondary. Primary anuria results from bilateral renal agenesis, aplasia, or multicystic dysplasia. Secondary anuria, related to edema or dehydration, results from renal ischemia, renal vein thrombosis, or congenital anomalies of the genitourinary tract. Anuria in children commonly results from loss of renal function.

Geriatric pointers

In elderly patients, anuria is a gradually occurring sign of underlying pathology. Hospitalized or bedridden elderly patients may be unable to generate the pressure needed to void if they remain in a supine position.

Patient counseling

Explain all tests and procedures to the patient. Depending on the cause of anuria, review the disorder's early warning signs and symptoms. If the patient needs surgery, withhold food and fluids. Review drugs that may worsen renal function.

REFERENCES

1. Jilinski, S.L., Perkins, R.M., Yuan, C.M., and DeZee, K.J. "Anuria and Acute Renal Failure Caused by Renal Artery Occlusion." *Hospital Physician* 42(7):43-46, July 2006.
2. Small, K.R. and McMullen, M. "When Clear Becomes Cloudy: A Review of Acute Tubular Necrosis, A Form of Renal Failure," *AJN* 105(1):72AA-72GG, January 2005.
3. Ward, K. "Kidneys, Don't Fail Me Now!" *Nursing Made Incredibly Easy!* 3(2):18-26, March/April 2005.

ANXIETY

Anxiety is the most common psychiatric symptom and can result in significant impairment.[1] A subjective reaction to a real or imagined threat, anxiety is a nonspecific feeling of uneasiness or dread. It may be mild, moderate, or severe. Mild anxiety may cause slight physical or psychological discomfort. Severe anxiety may be incapacitating or even life-threatening.

Everyone feels anxiety from time to time. It's a normal response to actual danger, prompting the body (through stimulation of the sympathetic and parasympathetic nervous systems) to purposeful action. It's also a normal response to physical and emotional stress, which can be produced by virtually any illness. In addition, anxiety can be caused or worsened by many nonpathologic factors, including lack of sleep, poor diet, and excessive intake of caffeine or other stimulants. However, excessive unprecipitated anxiety or anxiety that persists despite removal of the stressor may indicate an underlying psychological problem.[2] (See *Comparing common anxiety disorders*.)

History and physical examination

If the patient displays acute, severe anxiety, quickly take his vital signs and determine his chief complaint; this will serve as a guide for how to proceed. For example, if the patient's anxiety occurs with chest pain and shortness of breath, you might suspect myocardial infarction and act accordingly. While examining the patient, try to keep him calm. Suggest relaxation techniques, and talk to him in a reassuring, soothing voice. Uncontrolled anxiety can alter vital signs and worsen the causative disorder.

If the patient shows mild or moderate anxiety, ask about its duration. Is the anxiety constant or sporadic? Did he notice what started

Comparing common anxiety disorders

Question: *What is the prevalence of the four most common anxiety disorders— generalized anxiety disorder, panic disorder, social anxiety disorder, and post-traumatic stress disorder (PTSD)—in primary care? How do these disorders compare in terms of functional impairment, health care use, and co-morbid depressive and somatic symptoms? How effective is a brief measure in screening for each disorder?*

Research: Results from a large primary care–based anxiety study were analyzed to answer the above questions. The sample consisted of 965 clinical patients who completed a self-report questionnaire, which included the Generalized Anxiety Disorder (GAD)-7 scale; questions about demographic information; the Medical Outcomes Study Short Form-20, which measures functional status; the 10-item anxiety subscale from the Hopkins Symptom Checklist; the PHQ-8 depression scale; a three-item version of the social phobia Inventory; the five-item PHQ panic module; and the PHQ-15 somatic symptom scale. The questionnaire also asked about global assessments of anxiety, depression, and pain, and the numbers of physician visits and disability days the patient incurred over the previous 3 months. Structured psychiatric interviews were then performed by telephone by two mental health professionals who were blinded to the results of the questionnaire.

Conclusion: Analysis and statistical comparisons of the data revealed that PTSD was present in 8.6% of patients, GAD in 7.6% of patients, panic disorder in 6.8% of patients, and social anxiety in 6.2% of patients. Of the 188 patients with at least 1 anxiety disorder, 124 had 1 disorder, 42 had 2 disorders, 14 had 3 disorders, and 8 had all 4 disorders. Each patient with an anxiety disorder also had the presence

of moderate levels of depressive and somatic symptoms. It's important to note that 42% of these patients weren't receiving any form of treatment for an anxiety disorder.

Each anxiety disorder was strongly associated with impaired functioning. Compared with 4% of patients with no anxiety disorder, 32% to 43% of patients with anxiety disorders reported that anxiety made it "very difficult or extremely difficult" to work, take care of things at home, or get along with others.

Application: The increased frequency of anxiety disorders in patients with chronic medical conditions demonstrates the need for assessing this symptom in all patients. Practitioners in primary care offices and clinics should consider the use of a screening questionnaire or tool. Treatment of anxiety or depressive disorders can increase function and somatic symptoms. Become educated about treatment options, including pharmacologic therapies and evidence-based psychotherapies. Reassure patients that treatments are available and provide emotional support as indicated.

Source: Kroenke, K., Spitzer, R. L., Williams, J. B. W., Monahan, P. O., & Löwe, B. "Anxiety Disorders in Primary Care: Prevalence, Impairment, Comorbidity, and Detection." *Annals of Internal Medicine,* 146(5):317-325, 2007.

the anxiety? Find out if it's made worse by stress, lack of sleep, or excessive caffeine intake and alleviated by rest, tranquilizers, or exercise.

Obtain a complete medical history, especially noting drug use. Then perform a physical examination, focusing on any complaints that may trigger or be aggravated by anxiety.

If the patient's anxiety isn't accompanied by significant physical signs, suspect a psychological cause. Determine the patient's level of consciousness (LOC) and observe his behavior. If appropriate, refer the patient for psychiatric evaluation.

Medical causes

▶ *Acute respiratory distress syndrome.* Acute anxiety occurs along with tachycardia, mental sluggishness and, in severe cases, hypotension. Respiratory signs and symptoms include dyspnea, tachypnea, intercostal and suprasternal retractions, crackles, and rhonchi.

▶ *Anaphylactic shock.* Acute anxiety is usually the first sign of anaphylactic shock. It's accompanied by urticaria, angioedema, pruritus, and shortness of breath. Soon, other signs and symptoms develop: light-headedness, hypotension, tachycardia, nasal congestion, sneezing, wheezing, dyspnea, barking cough, abdominal cramps, vomiting, diarrhea, and urinary urgency and incontinence.

▶ *Angina pectoris.* Acute anxiety may either precede or follow an attack of angina pectoris. An attack produces sharp and crushing substernal or anterior chest pain that may radiate to the back, neck, arms, or jaw. The pain may be relieved by nitroglycerin or rest, which eases anxiety.

▶ *Asthma.* In allergic asthma attacks, acute anxiety occurs with dyspnea, wheezing, productive cough, accessory muscle use, hyperresonant lung fields, diminished breath sounds, coarse crackles, cyanosis, tachycardia, and diaphoresis.

▶ *Autonomic hyperreflexia.* The earliest signs of autonomic hyperreflexia may be acute anxiety accompanied by a severe headache and dramatic hypertension. Pallor and motor and sensory deficits occur below the level of the lesion; flushing occurs above it.

▶ *Cardiogenic shock.* Acute anxiety is accompanied by cool, pale, clammy skin; tachycardia; weak, thready pulse; tachypnea; ventricular gallop; crackles; jugular vein distention; decreased urine output; hypotension; narrowing pulse pressure; and peripheral edema.

▶ *Chronic obstructive pulmonary disease (COPD).* Acute anxiety, exertional dyspnea, cough, wheezing, crackles, hyperresonant lung fields, tachypnea, and accessory muscle use characterize COPD.

▶ *Heart failure.* In heart failure, acute anxiety is commonly the first symptom of inadequate oxygenation. Related findings include restlessness, shortness of breath, tachypnea, decreased LOC, edema, crackles, ventricular gallop, hypotension, diaphoresis, and cyanosis. In the long term, anxiety may result from the difficulty of managing heart failure symptoms at home.[3]

▶ *Hyperthyroidism.* Acute anxiety may be an early sign of hyperthyroidism. Classic signs and symptoms include heat intolerance, weight loss despite increased appetite, nervousness, tremor, palpitations, diaphoresis, an enlarged thyroid, and diarrhea. Exophthalmos also may occur.

▶ *Hyperventilation syndrome.* Hyperventilation syndrome produces acute anxiety, pallor, circumoral and peripheral paresthesia and, occasionally, carpopedal spasms.

▶ *Hypochondriasis.* Mild to moderate chronic anxiety occurs in hypochondriasis. The patient focuses more on the belief that he has a serious disease rather than on the actual symptoms. Difficulty swallowing, back pain, light-headedness, and upset stomach are common complaints. The patient tends to "doctor hop" and isn't reassured by favorable physical examinations and laboratory test results.

▶ *Hypoglycemia.* Anxiety resulting from hypoglycemia is usually mild to moderate and accompanied by hunger, mild headache, palpitations, blurred vision, weakness, and diaphoresis.

▶ *Mitral valve prolapse.* Panic may occur in patients with this valvular disorder, also known as *click-murmur syndrome* because its hallmark is a midsystolic click, followed by an apical systolic murmur. Mitral valve prolapse also may cause paroxysmal palpitations accompanied by sharp, stabbing, or aching precordial pain.

▶ *Mood disorder.* Anxiety may be the patient's chief complaint in the depressive or manic form of mood disorder. In the depressive form, chronic anxiety of varying severity occurs along with dysphoria; anger; insomnia or hypersomnia; decreased libido, interest, energy, and concentration; appetite disturbance; multiple somatic complaints; and suicidal thoughts. In the manic form, the patient's chief complaint may be a reduced need for sleep, hyperactivity, increased energy, rapid or pressured speech and, in severe cases, paranoid ideas and other psychotic symptoms.

▶ *Myocardial infarction (MI).* Anxiety occurs in 70% to 80% of patients recovering from an acute cardiac event.[4] In a life-threatening MI, acute anxiety commonly occurs with persistent, crushing substernal pain that may radiate to the left arm, jaw, neck, or shoulder blades. MI may be accompanied by shortness of breath, nausea, vomiting, diaphoresis, and cool, pale skin.

▶ *Obsessive-compulsive disorder.* Chronic anxiety occurs in obsessive-compulsive disorder, which is marked by recurrent, unshakable thoughts or impulses to perform ritualistic acts. The patient recognizes these acts as irrational but is unable to control them. Anxiety builds if he can't perform these acts and diminishes after he does.

▶ *Pheochromocytoma.* Acute, severe anxiety accompanies pheochromocytoma's cardinal sign: persistent or paroxysmal hypertension. Other common findings include tachycardia, diaphoresis, orthostatic hypotension, tachypnea, flushing, severe headache, palpitations, nausea, vomiting, epigastric pain, and paresthesia.

▶ *Phobias.* In phobias, chronic anxiety accompanies persistent fear of an object, an activity, or a situation that results in a compelling desire to avoid it. The patient recognizes the fear as irrational but can't suppress it.

▶ *Pneumonia.* Acute anxiety may occur in pneumonia because of hypoxemia. Other findings include productive cough, pleuritic chest pain, fever, chills, crackles, diminished breath sounds, and hyperresonant lung fields.

▶ *Pneumothorax.* Acute anxiety and profound respiratory distress occur in moderate to severe pneumothorax. Other findings include sharp pleuritic pain, coughing, shortness of breath, cyanosis, asymmetrical chest expansion, pallor, jugular vein distention, and a weak, rapid pulse.

▶ *Postconcussion syndrome.* Postconcussion syndrome may produce chronic anxiety or periodic attacks of acute anxiety. The anxiety usually is most pronounced in situations demanding attention, judgment, or comprehension. Related findings include irritability, insomnia, dizziness, and mild headache.

▶ *Posttraumatic stress disorder.* Posttraumatic stress disorder may occur after an extremely traumatic event. It produces chronic anxiety of varying severity and is accompanied by intrusive, vivid memories and thoughts of the traumatic event. The patient also relives the event in dreams and nightmares. Insomnia, depression, and feelings of numbness and detachment are common.

▶ *Pulmonary edema.* In pulmonary edema, acute anxiety occurs with dyspnea, orthopnea, cough with frothy sputum, tachycardia, tachypnea, crackles, ventricular gallop, hypotension, and thready pulse. The patient's skin may be cool, clammy, and cyanotic.

▶ *Pulmonary embolism.* Acute anxiety is usually accompanied by dyspnea, tachypnea, chest pain, tachycardia, blood-tinged sputum, and low-grade fever.

▶ *Rabies.* Anxiety signals the beginning of the acute phase of rabies. This rare disorder is characterized by painful laryngeal spasms, trouble swallowing, and hydrophobia.

▶ *Somatoform disorder.* Somatoform disorder, which usually begins in young adulthood, is characterized by anxiety and multiple somatic complaints that can't be explained physiologically. The symptoms aren't produced intentionally but are severe enough to significantly impair functioning. Pain disorder, conversion disorder, and hypochondriasis are examples of somatoform disorder.

Other causes

DRUG WATCH *Many drugs cause anxiety, especially sympathomimetics and CNS stimulants. In addition, many antidepressants may cause paradoxical anxiety.*

Special considerations

Supportive care can help relieve anxiety in many cases. Provide a calm, quiet atmosphere and make the patient comfortable. Encourage him to express his feelings and concerns freely. If it helps, take a short walk with him while you're talking. Anxiety-reducing measures, such as distraction, relaxation techniques, and biofeedback, may also be helpful.

Behavioral therapy, exposure therapy, cognitive therapy, cognitive-behavioral therapy, psychodynamic therapy, and group therapy are all techniques useful in reducing anxiety. Many are combined with drug therapy to treat more severe anxiety.[2]

Pediatric pointers

Anxiety in children usually results from painful physical illness or inadequate oxygenation. Its autonomic signs tend to be more common and dramatic than in adults. Individual and family cognitive behavioral therapy can be helpful in treating children with anxiety disorders.[5]

Geriatric pointers

Changes in an elderly patient's routine may provoke anxiety or agitation.

Patient counseling

Teach the patient to recognize early symptoms of anxiety so he can use relaxation techniques such as breathing exercises to minimize or prevent it.[1] Instruct him to avoid caffeine, cigarettes, and alcohol, which are known to increase anxiety.[1] Teach the patient about his medications, including proper dosages, how they work, and any adverse effects.

REFERENCES

1. Murphy, K. "Anxious Moments: Understanding Common Anxiety Disorders." *LPN* 3(2):26-33, March/April 2007.
2. Murphy, K. "Anxiety: When Is It Too Much?" *Nursing Made Incredibly Easy!* 3(5):22-31, September/October 2005.
3. Anderson, J.H. "Nursing Presence In A Community Heart Failure Program." *The Nurse Practitioner* 32(10):14-21, October 2007.
4. Moser, D.K. "'The Rust of Life:' Impact of Anxiety on Cardiac Patients." *American Journal of Critical Care* 16(4):361-9, July 2007.
5. Wood, J.J., Piacentini, J.C., Southam-Gerow, M., Chu, B.C., Sigman, M. "Family Cognitive Behavioral Therapy for Child Anxiety Disorders." *Journal of the American Academy of Child and Adolescent Psychiatry* 45(3):314-321, March 2006.

● APHASIA

Aphasia (dysphagia) is impaired expression or comprehension of written or spoken language and reflects disease or injury in the brain's language centers. (See *Where language originates.*) Depending on its severity, aphasia may slightly impede communication or may make it impossible. It can be classified as Broca's, Wernicke's, anomic, or global aphasia. Anomic aphasia eventually resolves in more than 50% of patients, but global aphasia is usually irreversible. (See *Identifying types of aphasia,* page 32.)

Quickly look for signs and symptoms of increased intracranial pressure (ICP), such as pupillary changes, decreased level of consciousness (LOC), vomiting, seizures, bradycardia, widening pulse pressure, and irregular respirations. If you detect signs of increased ICP, give mannitol I.V. to decrease cerebral edema. In addition, make sure that emergency resuscitation equipment is readily available to support respiratory and cardiac function, if necessary. You may have to prepare the patient for emergency surgery.

History and physical examination

If the patient has no signs of increased ICP, or if his aphasia has developed gradually, perform a thorough neurologic examination, starting with the patient's history. You'll probably need to obtain this history from the patient's family or companion because of the patient's impairment. Ask if the patient has a history of headaches, hypertension, seizure disorders, or drug use. Also ask about the patient's ability to communicate and perform routine activities before he developed aphasia.

Check for obvious signs of neurologic deficit, such as ptosis or fluid leakage from the nose and ears. Take the patient's vital signs, and assess his level of consciousness (LOC). Be aware, though, that the patient's verbal responses may be unreliable, making LOC assessment difficult. Also, recognize that dysarthria (impaired articulation from weakness or paralysis of muscles needed for speech) or speech apraxia (inability to voluntarily control the muscles of speech) may accompany aphasia, so speak slowly and distinctly, and give the patient ample time to respond. Assess the patient's pupillary response, eye movements, and motor function, especially his mouth and tongue movement, swallowing ability, and spontaneous movements and gestures. To best assess motor function, first demonstrate the motions and then have the patient imitate them.

Where language originates

Aphasia reflects damage to one or more of the brain's primary language centers, which, in most people, are located in the left hemisphere. *Broca's area* lies next to the region of the motor cortex that controls the muscles of speech. *Wernicke's area* is the center of auditory, visual, and language comprehension. It lies between *Heschl's gyrus*, the primary receiver of auditory stimuli, and the *angular gyrus*, a "way station" between the brain's auditory and visual regions. Connecting Wernicke's and Broca's areas is a large nerve bundle, the *arcuate fasciculus*, which allows repetition of speech.

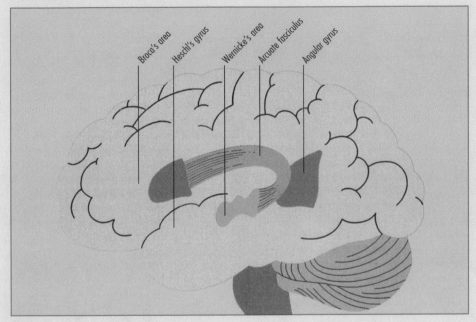

Medical causes

▶ *Alzheimer's disease.* Alzheimer's disease is characterized by aphasia, apraxia, and agnosia.[1] In this degenerative disease, anomic aphasia may begin insidiously and then progress to severe global aphasia. Related effects include behavioral changes, loss of memory, poor judgment, restlessness, myoclonus, and muscle rigidity. Incontinence is usually a late sign.

▶ *Brain abscess.* A brain abscess may cause any type of aphasia. It usually develops insidiously and may be accompanied by hemiparesis, ataxia, facial weakness, and signs of increased ICP.

▶ *Brain tumor.* A brain tumor may cause any type of aphasia. As the tumor enlarges, other aphasia types may occur along with behavioral changes, memory loss, motor weakness, seizures, auditory hallucinations, visual field deficits, and increased ICP.

▶ *Creutzfeldt-Jakob disease.* This disease is a rapidly progressive dementia accompanied by neurologic signs and symptoms, such as myoclonic jerking, ataxia, aphasia, visual disturbances, and paralysis. It typically affects adults ages 40 to 65.

▶ *Encephalitis.* Encephalitis usually produces transient aphasia. Early signs and symptoms include fever, headache, and vomiting. Seizures, confusion, stupor or coma, hemiparesis, asymmetrical deep tendon reflexes, positive Babinski's reflex, ataxia, myoclonus,

Identifying types of aphasia

TYPE	LOCATION OF LESION	SIGNS AND SYMPTOMS
Anomic aphasia	Temporal-parietal area; may extend to angular gyrus, but sometimes poorly localized	The patient's understanding of written and spoken language is relatively unimpaired. His speech, although fluent, lacks meaningful content. Word-finding difficulty and circumlocution are characteristic. Rarely, the patient also has paraphasias.
Broca's aphasia (expressive aphasia)	Broca's area; usually in third frontal convolution of the left hemisphere	The patient's understanding of written and spoken language is relatively spared, but speech is nonfluent, with word-finding difficulty, jargon, paraphasias, limited vocabulary, and simple sentence construction. The patient can't repeat words and phrases. If Wernicke's area is intact, he recognizes speech errors and shows frustration. Hemiparesis is common.
Global aphasia	Broca's and Wernicke's areas	The patient's receptive and expressive ability is profoundly impaired. He can't repeat words or phrases and can't follow directions. His occasional speech is marked by paraphasias or jargon.
Wernicke's aphasia (receptive aphasia)	Wernicke's area; usually in posterior or superior temporal lobe	The patient has trouble understanding written and spoken language. He can't repeat words or phrases and can't follow directions. His speech is fluent but may be rapid and rambling, with paraphasias. He has trouble naming objects (anomia) and is unaware of speech errors.

nystagmus, ocular palsies, and facial weakness may accompany aphasia.

▶ *Head trauma.* Severe head trauma may cause any type of aphasia. It typically occurs suddenly and may be transient or permanent, depending on the extent of brain damage. Related signs and symptoms include blurred or double vision, headache, pallor, diaphoresis, numbness and paresis, cerebrospinal otorrhea or rhinorrhea, altered respirations, tachycardia, disorientation, behavioral changes, and signs of increased ICP.

▶ *Seizures.* Seizures and the postictal state may cause transient aphasia if the seizures involve the language centers.

▶ *Stroke.* About 25% of stroke patients have some form of aphasia.[2,3] Stroke may produce Wernicke's, Broca's, or global aphasia. Related findings include decreased LOC, right-sided hemiparesis, homonymous hemianopia, paresthesia, and loss of sensation. (These signs and symptoms may appear on the left side if the right hemisphere contains the language centers.)

▶ *Transient ischemic attack (TIA).* TIA can produce any type of aphasia, which occurs suddenly and resolves within 24 hours of the attack. Related signs and symptoms include transient hemiparesis, hemianopia, and paresthesia (all usually right-sided) as well as dizziness and confusion.

Special considerations

Immediately after aphasia develops, the patient may become confused or disoriented. Help to restore a sense of reality by frequently telling him what has happened, where he is and why, and what the date is. Carefully explain diagnostic tests, such as skull X-rays, computed tomography scan or magnetic resonance imaging, angiography, and electroencephalogram. Later, expect periods of depression as the patient recognizes his disability.

Help the patient communicate by providing a relaxed, accepting environment with a minimum of distracting stimuli. Don't be surprised if the patient has sudden outbursts of profanity. This common behavior usually reflects intense frustration with his impairment. Deal with such outbursts as gently as possible to minimize embarrassment.

When you speak to the patient, don't assume that he understands you. He may simply be interpreting subtle clues to meaning, such as social context, facial expressions, and gestures. To help avoid misunderstanding, use nonverbal techniques, speak to him in simple phrases, and use demonstration to clarify your verbal directions.

Remember that aphasia is a language disorder, not an emotional or auditory one, so speak to the patient in a normal tone of voice. Make sure he has necessary aids, such as eyeglasses or dentures, to facilitate communication. Refer the patient to a speech pathologist early to help him cope with his aphasia.

Pediatric pointers

Recognize that the term *childhood aphasia* is sometimes mistakenly applied to children who fail to develop normal language skills but who aren't considered mentally retarded or developmentally delayed. *Aphasia* refers solely to loss of previously developed communication skills.

Brain damage associated with aphasia in children most commonly follows anoxia—the result of near drowning or airway obstruction.

Patient counseling

Encourage the patient to use hand gestures or drawing to facilitate communication.[2] Encourage the patient and his family to focus on his remaining abilities.[2] Explain the related effects of aphasia to the patient and his family, such as possible depression.[3]

REFERENCES

1. Byrd, C. "Normal Pressure Hydrocephalus: Dementia's Hidden Cause." *The Nurse Practitioner* 31(7):28-35, July 2006.
2. Baldwin, K.M. "Stroke: It's A Knock Out Punch." *Nursing Made Incredibly Easy!* 4(2):10-23, March/April 2006.
3. Rombough, R.E., Howse, E.L., and Bartfay, W.J. "Caregiver Strain and Caregiver Burden of Primary Caregivers of Stroke Survivors With and Without Aphasia." *Rehabilitation Nursing* 31(5):199-209, September/October 2006.

● APNEA

A pnea, the cessation of spontaneous respiration, is occasionally temporary and self-limiting, as in Cheyne-Stokes and Biot's respirations. In most cases, though, it's a life-threatening emergency that requires immediate intervention to prevent death. (See *Post-surgical monitoring with capnography,* page 34.)

Apnea usually results from one or more of six pathophysiologic mechanisms, each of which has numerous causes. Its most common causes include trauma, cardiac arrest, neurologic disease, aspiration of a foreign object, bronchospasm, and drug overdose. (See *Causes of apnea,* page 35.)

If you detect apnea, first establish and maintain a patent airway. Place the patient in a supine position, and open his airway using the head-tilt, chin-lift technique. (Caution: If the patient has or may have a head or neck injury, use the jaw-thrust technique to avoid hyperextending the neck.) Next, quickly look, listen, and feel for spontaneous respiration; if

EVIDENCE-BASED PRACTICE

Post-surgical monitoring with capnography

Question: *Is capnography a good way to measure at-risk surgical patients?*

Research: A patient being treated with opioids for pain after surgery must be assessed regularly for sedation level and respiratory depression. Patients are typically monitored by direct observation and pulse oximetry. In capnography, a nasal cannula is used to administer supplemental oxygen. The device also measures respiration, including end-tidal carbon dioxide (CO_2), apneic events, and respiratory rate.

In the study cited, 54 opioid-naïve patients—who were admitted for orthopedic surgery and met inclusion criteria—were enrolled. For inclusion the patient had to be older than 18 years of age, have a physician's order for opioid analgesia, was breathing spontaneously, was not diagnosed with obstructive sleep apnea (OSA), was not using a continuous positive airway pressure (CPAP) device, and was able to report pain intensity using a 0 to 10 scale. Also, patients had to meet one of the following criteria: body mass index of 30 or more, history of snoring, history in the post-anesthesia care unit (PACU) of one episode of a respiratory rate less than ten, or basal dosage of I.V. opioid or continuous-release oral opioid.

Patients were randomized into the control group or the capnography group. The control group was monitored every 4 hours by spot-check pulse oximetry, direct observation, and auscultation. The capnography group was monitored solely by capnography.

Conclusion: Respiratory depression was detected at a significantly higher rate in the control group. A total of 146 episodes were detected during the 36 hours on the general nursing unit: 140 in the capnography group and 6 in the control group. Seventeen patients accounted for all of the episodes: 15 in the capnography group and 2 in the control group. Of the last four inclusion criteria, only an event of a respiratory rate less than 10 breaths per minute in the PACU was a strong predictive indicator of subsequent episodes of respiratory depression on the general care unit.

Application: Consider capnographic monitoring for all post-surgical patients at high risk for respiratory depression, particularly those who have an event in the PACU. Be aware that capnography is also useful for identifying pauses in breathing during sleep, which is a risk factor for OSA. Attend appropriate inservices and become educated on the device used where you work. Educate patients about the benefits of capnography and assist patients with activities of daily living when capnography is in place.

Source: Hutchison, R. & Rodriguez, L. "Capnography and Respiratory Depression." *American Journal of Nursing* 108(2):35-39, 2008.

---

it's absent, begin artificial ventilation until it occurs or until mechanical ventilation can be started.

Because apnea may result from (or may cause) cardiac arrest, assess the patient's carotid pulse immediately after you've established a patent airway. Or, if the patient is an infant or small child, assess the brachial pulse instead. If you can't palpate a pulse, begin cardiac compression.

History and physical examination

When the patient's respiratory and cardiac status is stable, investigate the underlying cause of apnea. Ask him (or, if he's unable to answer, anyone who witnessed the episode) about the onset of apnea and events immediately preceding it. The cause may become readily apparent, as in trauma.

Take a patient history, especially noting reports of headache, chest pain, muscle weakness, sore throat, or dyspnea. Ask about a history of respiratory, cardiac, or neurologic disease and about allergies and drug use.

Causes of apnea

Many disorders may cause apnea, as shown here.

AIRWAY OBSTRUCTION
- Asthma
- Bronchospasm
- Chronic bronchitis
- Chronic obstructive pulmonary disease
- Foreign body aspiration
- Hemothorax or pneumothorax
- Mucus plug
- Obstruction by tongue or tumor
- Obstructive sleep apnea
- Secretion retention
- Tracheal or bronchial rupture

BRAIN STEM DYSFUNCTION
- Brain abscess
- Brain stem injury
- Brain tumor
- Central nervous system depressants
- Central sleep apnea
- Cerebral hemorrhage
- Cerebral infarction
- Encephalitis
- Head trauma
- Increased intracranial pressure
- Medullary or pontine hemorrhage or infarction
- Meningitis
- Transtentorial herniation

NEUROMUSCULAR FAILURE
- Amyotrophic lateral sclerosis
- Botulism
- Diphtheria
- Guillain-Barré syndrome
- Myasthenia gravis
- Phrenic nerve paralysis
- Rupture of the diaphragm
- Spinal cord injury

PARENCHYMATOUS DISEASE
- Acute respiratory distress syndrome
- Diffuse pneumonia
- Emphysema
- Near drowning
- Pulmonary edema
- Pulmonary fibrosis
- Secretion retention

PLEURAL PRESSURE GRADIENT DISRUPTION
- Flail chest
- Open chest wounds

PULMONARY CAPILLARY PERFUSION DECREASE
- Arrhythmias
- Cardiac arrest
- Myocardial infarction
- Pulmonary embolism
- Pulmonary hypertension
- Shock

If sleep apnea is suspected, ask the patient about a history of loud snoring, feeling tired upon awakening, and daytime drowsiness. Find out if he has been observed holding his breath or gasping during sleep.[1]

Inspect the head, face, neck, and trunk for soft-tissue injury, hemorrhage, or skeletal deformity. Don't overlook obvious clues, such as oral and nasal secretions (reflecting fluid-filled airways and alveoli) or facial soot and singed nasal hair (suggesting thermal injury to the tracheobronchial tree).

Auscultate over all lung lobes for adventitious breath sounds, particularly crackles and rhonchi, and percuss the lung fields for in-creased dullness or hyperresonance. Move on to the heart, auscultating for murmurs, pericardial friction rub, and arrhythmias. Check for cyanosis, pallor, jugular vein distention, and edema. If appropriate, perform a neurologic assessment. Evaluate level of consciousness, orientation, and mental status; test cranial nerve and motor function, sensation, and reflexes in all limbs.

Medical causes
▶ *Airway obstruction.* Occlusion or compression of the trachea, central airways, or smaller airways can cause sudden apnea by blocking

the patient's airflow and producing acute respiratory failure.

▶ *Brain stem dysfunction.* Primary or secondary brain stem dysfunction can cause apnea by destroying the brain stem's ability to initiate respirations. Apnea may arise suddenly (as in trauma, hemorrhage, or infarction) or gradually (as in degenerative disease or tumor). Apnea may be preceded by decreased LOC and various motor and sensory deficits.

▶ *Neuromuscular failure.* Trauma or disease can disrupt the mechanics of respiration, causing sudden or gradual apnea. Related findings include diaphragmatic or intercostal muscle paralysis from injury, or respiratory weakness or paralysis from acute or degenerative disease.

▶ *Parenchymatous lung disease.* An accumulation of fluid in the alveoli produces apnea by interfering with pulmonary gas exchange and producing acute respiratory failure. Apnea may arise suddenly, as in near drowning and acute pulmonary edema, or gradually, as in emphysema. Apnea also may be preceded by crackles and labored respirations with accessory muscle use.

▶ *Pleural pressure gradient disruption.* Conversion of normal negative pleural air pressure to positive pressure by chest wall injuries (such as flail chest) causes lung collapse, producing respiratory distress and, if untreated, apnea. Related signs include an asymmetrical chest wall and asymmetrical or paradoxical respirations.

▶ *Pulmonary capillary perfusion decrease.* Apnea can stem from obstructed pulmonary circulation, most commonly due to heart failure or lack of circulatory patency. It occurs suddenly in cardiac arrest, massive pulmonary embolism, and most cases of severe shock; it occurs progressively in septic shock and pulmonary hypertension. Related findings include hypotension, tachycardia, and edema.

Other causes

DRUG WATCH *CNS depressants may cause hypoventilation and apnea. Opioids may cause respiratory depression. Carefully monitor patients receiving I.V. morphine, especially with repeated doses or delivery by patient-controlled analgesia. Benzodiazepines may cause respiratory depres-*

sion and apnea when given I.V. with other CNS depressants to elderly or acutely ill patients.

Neuromuscular blockers—such as curariform drugs and anticholinesterases—may produce sudden apnea from respiratory muscle paralysis.

▶ *Sleep-related apnea.* These repetitive apneas affect about 18 million adults in the United States and occur during sleep from obstructed airflow (most common) or brain stem dysfunction.[1] Other signs and symptoms include loud snoring, restless sleep, and daytime drowsiness.

Special considerations
Closely monitor the apneic patient's cardiac and respiratory status to prevent further apneic episodes.

Pediatric pointers
Premature neonates are especially susceptible to periodic apneic episodes because of CNS immaturity; this type of apnea is known as apnea of prematurity. It involves a pause of greater than 20 seconds between breaths.[2] Apnea in neonates can be differentiated from periodic breathing by the length of time of the pause. A pause of less than 20 seconds between breaths is called periodic breathing. If apnea progresses without self-recovery or intervention, it may progress to bradycardia and oxygen desaturation, and it also may cause hypoxia, hypercarbia, and hypotension. Tactile stimulation is the most common intervention for an apneic event in progress.[2] More severe episodes may require positive pressure ventilation and oxygen delivery. Other treatments may include caffeine and use of continuous positive airway pressure via nasal prongs, nasal mask, or nasal canula. Other common causes of apnea in infants include sepsis, intraventricular and subarachnoid hemorrhage, seizures, bronchiolitis, and sudden infant death syndrome.

In toddlers and older children, the primary cause of apnea is acute airway obstruction from aspiration of foreign objects. Obstructive sleep apnea occurs in 2% of all children, most commonly between ages 2 and 6.[3] Other causes include acute epiglottitis, croup, asthma, and systemic disorders, such as muscular dystrophy and cystic fibrosis.

Geriatric pointers

In elderly patients, increased sensitivity to analgesics, sedative-hypnotics, or any combination of these drugs may produce apnea, even with normal dosage ranges.

Patient counseling

Educate the patient about safety measures related to aspiration of drugs. Encourage cardiopulmonary resuscitation training for all adolescents and adults. If the patient has sleep apnea, teach him about various treatment options, as well as lifestyle changes that may reduce the condition, such as diet and exercise to promote weight loss, elevating the head of his bed, avoiding alcohol before bedtime, and practicing good sleep hygiene.[1]

REFERENCES

1. Dugan, M. "A Tale of Sleep Apnea." *Nursing Made Incredibly Easy!* 5(3):28-37, May/June 2007.
2. Stokowski, L. "A Primer on Apnea of Prematurity." *Advances in Neonatal Care* 5(3):155-170, June 2005.
3. Ward, T. "Caring for Children with Sleep Problems." *Journal of Pediatric Nursing* 22(4):283-296, August 2007.

ATAXIA

Classified as cerebellar or sensory, ataxia refers to incoordination and irregularity of voluntary, purposeful movements. *Cerebellar ataxia* results from disease of the cerebellum and its pathways to and from the cerebral cortex, brain stem, and spinal cord. It causes gait, trunk, limb, and possibly speech disorders. *Sensory ataxia* results from impaired position sense (proprioception) due to interruption of afferent nerve fibers in the peripheral nerves, posterior roots, posterior columns of the spinal cord, or medial lemnisci or, occasionally, from a lesion in both parietal lobes. It causes gait disorders. (See *Identifying ataxia*.)

Ataxia occurs in acute and chronic forms. Acute ataxia may result from stroke, hemor-

Identifying ataxia

Ataxia may be observed in the patient's speech, in the movements of his trunk and limbs, or in his gait.

In *speech ataxia*, a form of dysarthria, the patient typically speaks slowly and stresses words and syllables that usually aren't stressed. Speech content is unaffected.

In *truncal ataxia*, a disturbance in equilibrium, the patient can't sit or stand without falling, and his head and trunk may bob and sway (titubation). If he can walk, his gait is reeling.

In *limb ataxia*, the patient loses the ability to gauge distance, speed, and power of movement, resulting in poorly controlled, variable, and inaccurate voluntary movements. He may move too quickly or too slowly, or his movements may break down into component parts, giving him the appearance of a puppet or a robot. Other effects include a coarse, irregular tremor in purposeful movement (but not at rest) and reduced muscle tone.

In *gait ataxia*, the patient's gait is wide based, unsteady, and irregular.

In *cerebellar ataxia*, the patient may stagger or lurch in zigzag fashion, turn with extreme difficulty, and lose his balance when his feet are together.

In *sensory ataxia*, the patient moves abruptly and stomps or taps his feet. This occurs because he throws his feet forward and outward, and then brings them down first on the heels and then on the toes. The patient also fixes his eyes on the ground, watching his steps; if he can't watch his steps, staggering worsens. When he stands with his feet together, he sways or loses balance.

rhage, or a large tumor in the posterior fossa. In this life-threatening condition, the cerebellum may herniate downward through the foramen magnum behind the cervical spinal cord, or upward through the tentorium on the cerebral hemispheres. Herniation also may compress the brain stem. Acute ataxia also may result from drug toxicity or poisoning. Chronic ataxia can be progressive and may result from acute disease. It also can occur in metabolic and chronic degenerative neurologic disease.

If ataxic movements develop suddenly, examine the patient for signs of increased intracranial pressure and impending herniation. Determine his level of consciousness (LOC), and be alert for pupillary changes, motor weakness or paralysis, neck stiffness or pain, and vomiting. Check vital signs, especially respirations; abnormal respiratory patterns may lead quickly to respiratory arrest. Elevate the head of the bed. Have emergency resuscitation equipment readily available. Prepare the patient for a computed tomography scan or surgery.

History and physical examination

If the patient isn't in distress, review his history. Ask about multiple sclerosis, diabetes, CNS infection, neoplastic disease, previous stroke, and a family history of ataxia. Also ask about chronic alcohol abuse or prolonged exposure to industrial toxins such as mercury. Find out if the ataxia developed suddenly or gradually.

If needed, perform Romberg's test to help distinguish between cerebellar and sensory ataxia. Tell the patient to stand with his feet together and his arms at his sides. Note his posture and balance, first with his eyes open and then with them closed. Test results may indicate normal posture and balance (minimal swaying), cerebellar ataxia (swaying and inability to maintain balance with eyes open or closed), or sensory ataxia (increased swaying and inability to maintain balance with eyes closed). Stand close to the patient during this test to prevent his falling.

If you test for gait and limb ataxia, be aware that motor weakness may mimic ataxic movements, so check motor strength, too. Gait ataxia may be severe, even when limb ataxia is minimal. Ask the patient with gait ataxia if he tends to fall to one side and if he falls more at night. With truncal ataxia, remember that the patient's inability to walk or stand, combined with the absence of other signs while he's lying down, may give the impression of hysteria or drug or alcohol intoxication.

Medical causes

▶ *Cerebellar abscess.* Cerebellar abscess commonly causes limb ataxia on the same side as the lesion as well as gait and truncal ataxia. Typically, the initial symptom is headache localized behind the ear or in the occipital region, followed by oculomotor palsy, fever, vomiting, altered LOC, and coma.

▶ *Cerebellar hemorrhage.* Cerebellar hemorrhage is a life-threatening disorder in which ataxia is usually acute but transient. Unilateral or bilateral ataxia affects the trunk, gait, or limbs. The patient initially has repeated vomiting, an occipital headache, vertigo, oculomotor palsy, dysphagia, and dysarthria. Later signs, such as decreased LOC or coma, signal impending herniation.

▶ *Cranial trauma.* Cranial trauma rarely produces ataxia, but when it does, the ataxia is usually unilateral; bilateral ataxia suggests traumatic hemorrhage. Related signs and symptoms include vomiting, headache, decreased LOC, irritability, and focal neurologic defects. If the cerebral hemispheres are also affected, focal or generalized seizures may occur.

▶ *Creutzfeldt-Jakob disease.* This disease is a rapidly progressive dementia accompanied by neurologic signs and symptoms, such as myoclonic jerking, ataxia, aphasia, visual disturbances, and paralysis. It typically affects adults ages 40 to 65.

▶ *Diabetic neuropathy.* Peripheral nerve damage from diabetes mellitus may cause sensory ataxia, limb pain, slight leg weakness, skin changes, and bowel and bladder dysfunction.

▶ *Diphtheria.* Within 4 to 8 weeks of the onset of symptoms, a life-threatening neuropathy can produce sensory ataxia. Diphtheria may be accompanied by fever, paresthesia, and paralysis of the limbs and possibly the respiratory muscles.

▶ *Encephalomyelitis.* This complication of measles, smallpox, chickenpox, rubella, or rabies or smallpox vaccines may damage cerebrospinal white matter. Rarely, it's accompanied by cerebellar ataxia. Other signs and symptoms include headache, fever, vomiting, altered LOC, paralysis, seizures, oculomotor palsy, and pupillary changes.

▶ *Friedreich's ataxia.* This progressive familial disorder affects the spinal cord and cerebellum. It causes gait ataxia, followed by truncal, limb, and speech ataxia. Other signs and symptoms include pes cavus, kyphoscoliosis, cranial nerve palsy, and motor and sensory deficits. A positive Babinski's reflex may appear.

▶ *Guillain-Barré syndrome.* This syndrome usually begins with a mild viral infection, followed by peripheral nerve involvement and, rarely, sensory ataxia. It also may cause ascending paralysis and respiratory distress.

▶ *Hepatocerebral degeneration.* Some patients who survive hepatic coma are left with residual neurologic defects, including mild cerebellar ataxia with a wide-based, unsteady gait. Ataxia may be accompanied by altered LOC, dysarthria, rhythmic arm tremors, and choreoathetosis of the face, neck, and shoulders.

▶ *Hyperthermia.* Cerebellar ataxia occurs if the patient survives the coma and seizures characteristic of the acute phase of hyperthermia. Subsequent findings include spastic paralysis, dementia, and slowly resolving confusion.

▶ *Metastatic cancer.* Cancer that metastasizes to the cerebellum may cause gait ataxia accompanied by headache, dizziness, nystagmus, decreased LOC, nausea, and vomiting.

▶ *Multiple sclerosis.* Nystagmus and cerebellar ataxia commonly occur in this disorder, but they aren't always accompanied by limb weakness and spasticity. The patient also may have speech ataxia (especially scanning) as well as sensory ataxia from spinal cord involvement. During remissions, ataxia may subside or even disappear. During exacerbations, it may reappear, worsen, or even become permanent. It also causes optic neuritis, optic atrophy, numbness and weakness, diplopia, dizziness, and bladder dysfunction.

▶ *Olivopontocerebellar atrophy.* This disorder produces gait ataxia and, later, limb and speech ataxia. Rarely, it produces an intention tremor. It's accompanied by choreiform movements, dysphagia, and loss of sphincter tone.

▶ *Polyarteritis nodosa.* Acute or subacute polyarteritis may cause sensory ataxia, abdominal and limb pain, hematuria, fever, and elevated blood pressure.

▶ *Polyneuropathy.* Carcinomatous and myelomatous polyneuropathy may occur be-

fore detection of the primary tumor in cancer, multiple myeloma, or Hodgkin's disease. Signs and symptoms include ataxia, severe motor weakness, muscle atrophy, and sensory loss in the limbs. Pain and skin changes also may occur.

▶ *Porphyria.* Porphyria affects the sensory and, more commonly, the motor nerves, possibly leading to ataxia. It also causes abdominal pain, mental disturbances, vomiting, headache, focal neurologic defects, altered LOC, generalized seizures, and skin lesions.

▶ *Posterior fossa tumor.* Gait, truncal, or limb ataxia is an early sign and may worsen as the tumor enlarges. It's accompanied by vomiting, headache, papilledema, vertigo, oculomotor palsy, decreased LOC, and motor and sensory impairment on the same side as the lesion.

▶ *Spinocerebellar ataxia.* In spinocerebellar ataxia, the patient may initially experience fatigue, followed by stiff-legged gait ataxia. Eventually, limb ataxia, dysarthria, static tremor, nystagmus, cramps, paresthesia, and sensory deficits occur.

▶ *Stroke.* In a stroke, occlusions in the vertebrobasilar arteries halt blood flow, causing infarction in the medulla, pons, or cerebellum that may lead to ataxia. Ataxia may occur at the onset of the stroke and remain as a residual deficit. Worsening ataxia during the acute phase may indicate extension of the stroke or severe swelling. Ataxia may be accompanied by unilateral or bilateral motor weakness, altered LOC, sensory loss, vertigo, nausea, vomiting, oculomotor palsy, and dysphagia.

▶ *Syringomyelia.* Syringomyelia is a chronic degenerative disorder that may cause a mixed spastic-ataxic gait. It's associated with loss of pain and temperature sensation (but preservation of touch sensation), skin changes, amyotrophy, and thoracic scoliosis.

▶ *Wernicke's encephalopathy.* Wernicke's encephalopathy produces three classic symptoms: confusion, ataxia, and nystagmus.[1] The result of a thiamine deficiency, it produces gait ataxia and, rarely, intention tremor or speech ataxia. With severe ataxia, the patient may be unable to stand or walk. Ataxia decreases with thiamine therapy. Related signs and symptoms include nystagmus, diplopia, ocular palsies, confusion, tachycardia, exertional dyspnea, and orthostatic hypotension.

Other causes

DRUG WATCH *Toxic levels of anticonvulsants, especially phenytoin, may result in gait ataxia. Toxic levels of anticholinergics and tricyclic antidepressants may also result in ataxia. Aminoglutethimide causes ataxia in about 10% of patients; however, this effect usually disappears 4 to 6 weeks after therapy stops.*

▶ *Poisoning.* Chronic arsenic poisoning may cause sensory ataxia along with headache, seizures, altered LOC, motor deficits, and muscle aching. Chronic mercury poisoning causes gait ataxia and limb ataxia, principally of the arms. Chronic mercury poisoning also causes tremors of the extremities, tongue, and lips; mental confusion; mood changes; and dysarthria.

Special considerations

Assess the patient's neurologic status often. Then focus on helping the patient adapt to his condition. Promote rehabilitation goals and help ensure the patient's safety. For example, instruct a patient with sensory ataxia to move slowly, especially when turning or getting up from a chair. Provide a cane or walker for extra support. Ask the patient's family to check his home for hazards, such as uneven surfaces or the absence of handrails on stairs. If appropriate, refer the patient with progressive disease for counseling.

Pediatric pointers

In children, ataxia occurs in acute and chronic forms and results from congenital or acquired disease. Acute ataxia may stem from febrile infection, brain tumors, mumps, and other disorders. Chronic ataxia may stem from Gaucher's disease, Refsum's disease, and other inborn errors of metabolism.

When assessing a child for ataxia, consider his level of motor skills and emotional state. Your examination may be limited to observing the child in spontaneous activity and carefully questioning his parents about changes in his motor activity, such as increased unsteadiness or falling. If you suspect ataxia, refer the

child for a neurologic evaluation to rule out a brain tumor.

Geriatric pointers

Because the aging process can affect balance and reflexes, mild ataxia may not be from disease. However, the patient should be evaluated for a medical cause before attributing ataxia to normal aging.[2]

Patient counseling

Instruct the patient with sensory ataxia to move slowly, especially when turning or rising from a chair. Provide a cane or walker for extra support. Ask the patient's family to assess his home for safety hazards, such as uneven surfaces or the absence of handrails on stairs. Refer the patient for home care nursing and rehabilitative services as ordered.

REFERENCES

1. "Heading Off Neuro Problems." *Nursing* 37(6):26-27, June 2007.
2. Neal-Boylan, L. "Health Assessment of the Very Old Person at Home." *Home Healthcare Nurse. The Journal for the Home Care and Hospice Professional* 25(6):388-398, June 2007.

B

BABINSKI'S REFLEX

Babinski's reflex, or *extensor plantar reflex*—dorsiflexion of the great toe with extension and fanning of the other toes—is an abnormal reflex elicited by stroking the lateral aspect of the sole of the foot.[1] (See *How to elicit Babinski's reflex,* page 42.) In some patients, this reflex can be triggered by noxious stimuli, such as pain, noise, or even bumping of the bed. An indicator of upper motor neuron disease, Babinski's reflex may occur unilaterally or bilaterally and may be temporary or permanent.[1] A temporary Babinski's reflex commonly occurs during the postictal phase of a seizure, whereas a permanent Babinski's reflex occurs with corticospinal damage. A positive Babinski's reflex is normal in neonates and in infants up to age 12 months.[2]

History and physical examination

After eliciting a positive Babinski's reflex, evaluate the patient for other neurologic signs. Assess muscle strength in each limb by having the patient push or pull against your resistance. Passively flex and extend the limb to assess muscle tone. Intermittent resistance to flexion and extension indicates spasticity, and a lack of resistance indicates flaccidity.

Next, check for evidence of incoordination by asking the patient to perform a repetitive activity. Test deep tendon reflexes (DTRs) in the elbow, antecubital area, wrist, knee, and ankle by striking the tendon with a reflex hammer. An exaggerated muscle response indicates hyperactive DTRs; little or no muscle response indicates hypoactivity.

Then evaluate pain sensation and proprioception in the feet. As you move the patient's toes up and down, ask him to identify the direction in which the toes have been moved without looking at his feet.

Medical causes

▶ *Amyotropihc lateral sclerosis (ALS).* In this progressive motor neuron disorder, bilateral Babinski's reflex may occur with hyperactive DTRs and spasticity. Typically, ALS produces fasciculations, muscle atrophy, and weakness. Incoordination makes activities of daily living difficult to perform. Related signs and symptoms include impaired speech; difficulty chewing, swallowing, and breathing; urinary frequency and urgency; and, occasionally, choking and excessive drooling. Although mental status remains intact, the patient's poor prognosis may cause periodic depression. Progressive bulbar palsy involves the brain stem and may cause episodes of crying or inappropriate laughter.

▶ *Brain tumor.* A brain tumor in corticospinal tract may produce Babinski's reflex, hyperactive DTRs (unilateral or bilateral), spasticity, seizures, cranial nerve dysfunction, hemiparesis or hemiplegia, decreased pain sensation, unsteady gait, incoordination, headache, emotional lability, and decreased level of consciousness (LOC).

▶ *Familial spastic paraparesis.* Bilateral Babinski's reflex may occur with hyperactive DTRs, progressive spasticity, ataxia, and weakness.

How to elicit Babinski's reflex

To check for Babinski's reflex, stroke the lateral aspect of the sole of the patient's foot with your thumbnail or other moderately sharp object. Normally, this elicits flexion of all toes (a negative Babinski's reflex), as shown in the top illustration. In a positive Babinski's reflex, the great toe dorsiflexes and the other toes fan out, as shown at bottom.

NORMAL TOE FLEXION

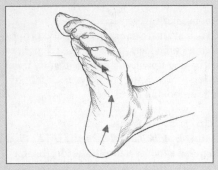

POSITIVE BABINSKI'S REFLEX

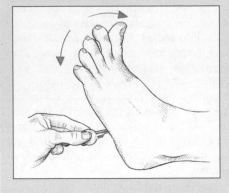

▶ *Friedreich's ataxia.* This familial disorder may produce bilateral Babinski's reflex. it also causes high-arched feet, hypoactive DTRs, hypotonia, ataxia, head tremor, weakness, and paresthesia.

▶ *Head trauma.* Unilateral or bilateral Babinski's reflex may result from primary corticospinal damage or secondary injury with increased intracranial pressure. Hyperactive DTRs and spasticity commonly occur with Babinski's reflex, possibly with weakness and incoordination. Other signs and symptoms vary with the type of head trauma and include headache, vomiting, behavior changes, altered vital signs, and decreased LOC with abnormal pupillary size and response to light.

▶ *Hepatic encephalopathy.* Babinski's reflex occurs late in hepatic encephalopathy when the patient slips into a coma. It's accompanied by hyperactive DTRs and fetor hepaticus.

▶ *Meningitis.* Bilateral Babinski's reflex commonly follows fever, chills, and malaise and is accompanied by nausea and vomiting. As meningitis progresses, it also causes decreased LOC, nuchal rigidity, positive Brudzinski's and Kernig's signs, hyperactive DTRs, and opisthotonos. Other signs and symptoms include irritability, photophobia, diplopia, delirium, and deep stupor that may progress to coma.

▶ *Multiple sclerosis (MS).* In most patients with MS—a demyelinating disorder—bilateral Babinski's reflex eventually follows initial signs and symptoms of paresthesia, nystagmus, and blurred or double vision. Related signs and symptoms include scanning speech (clipped speech with some pauses between syllables), dysphagia, intention tremor, weakness, incoordination, spasticity, gait ataxia, seizures, paraparesis or paraplegia, bladder incontinence, and emotional lability. Loss of pain and temperature sensation and proprioception occur occasionally.

▶ *Pernicious anemia.* Bilateral Babinski's reflex occurs in pernicious anemia when vitamin B_{12} deficiency affects the central nervous system.[3] Anemia may eventually cause widespread GI, neurologic, and cardiovascular effects. GI signs and symptoms include nausea, vomiting, anorexia, weight loss, flatulence, diarrhea, and constipation. Gingival bleeding and a sore, inflamed tongue may make eating painful and intensify anorexia. The lips, gums, and tongue appear markedly pale. Jaundice may cause pale to bright yellow skin.

Neurologic signs and symptoms include neuritis, weakness, peripheral paresthesia, disturbed position sense, incoordination, ataxia, positive Romberg's sign, light-headedness, bowel and bladder incontinence, and altered vision (diplopia, blurred vision), taste, and hearing (tinnitus). Pernicious anemia also may produce irritability, poor memory, headache, depression, impotence, and delirium.

Cardiovascular signs and symptoms include palpitations, wide pulse pressure, dyspnea, orthopnea, and tachycardia.

▶ *Rabies.* Bilateral Babinski's reflex—possibly elicited by nonspecific noxious stimuli alone—appears in the excitation phase of rabies. This phase occurs 2 to 10 days after the onset of prodromal signs and symptoms, such as fever, malaise, and irritability (which occur 30 to 40 days after a bite from an infected animal). Rabies is characterized by marked restlessness and extremely painful pharyngeal muscle spasms. Difficulty swallowing causes excessive drooling and hydrophobia in about 50% of affected patients. Seizures and hyperactive DTRs also may occur.

▶ *Spinal cord injury.* In an acute injury, spinal shock temporarily erases all reflexes. As shock resolves, Babinski's reflex occurs—unilaterally when the injury affects only one side of the spinal cord (Brown-Séquard syndrome) and bilaterally when the injury affects both sides. Rather than signaling the return of neurologic function, this reflex confirms corticospinal damage. It's accompanied by hyperactive DTRs, spasticity, and variable or total loss of pain and temperature sensation, proprioception, and motor function. Horner's syndrome, marked by unilateral ptosis, pupillary constriction, and facial anhidrosis, may occur in a lower cervical cord injury.

▶ *Spinal cord tumor.* Bilateral Babinski's reflex occurs with variable loss of pain and temperature sensation, proprioception, and motor function. Spasticity, hyperactive DTRs, absent abdominal reflexes, and incontinence also occur. Diffuse pain may occur at the level of the tumor.

▶ *Spinal paralytic piliomyelitis.* Unilateral or bilateral Babinski's reflex occurs 5 to 7 days after the onset of fever. It's accompanied by progressive weakness, paresthesia, muscle tenderness, spasticity, irritability and, later, atrophy. Resistance to neck flexion is characteristic, as are Hoyne's, Kernig's, and Brudzinski's signs.

▶ *Spinal tuberculosis.* This disorder may produce bilateral Babinski's reflex accompanied by variable loss of pain and temperature sensation, proprioception, and motor function.

It also causes spasticity, hyperactive DTRs, bladder incontinence, and absent abdominal reflexes.

▶ *Stroke.* Babinski's reflex varies with the site of the stroke. A stroke involving the cerebrum produces unilateral Babinski's reflex with hemiplegia or hemiparesis, unilateral hyperactive DTRs, hemianopsia, and aphasia. A stroke involving the brain stem produces bilateral Babinski's reflex accompanied by bilateral weakness or paralysis, bilateral hyperactive DTRs, cranial nerve dysfunction, incoordination, and unsteady gait. Generalized signs and symptoms of stroke include headache, vomiting, fever, disorientation, nuchal rigidity, seizures, and coma.

▶ *Syringomyelia.* In syringomyelia, bilateral Babinski's reflex occurs with muscle atrophy and weakness that may progress to paralysis. It's accompanied by spasticity, ataxia and, occasionally, deep pain. DTRs may be hypoactive or hyperactive. Cranial nerve dysfunction, such as dysphagia and dysarthria, commonly appears late in the disorder.

Special considerations

Babinski's reflex usually occurs with incoordination, weakness, and spasticity, all of which increase the patient's risk of injury. To prevent injury, help the patient with activities and keep his environment free from obstructions.

Pediatric pointers

Babinski's reflex occurs normally in infants up to age 12 months, reflecting immaturity of the corticospinal tract.[2] After age 1, Babinski's reflex is pathologic and may result from hydrocephalus or any of the causes commonly seen in adults.

Patient counseling

Prepare the patient as needed for diagnostic tests, which may include computed tomography scaningn or magnetic resonance imaging of the brain or spine, angiography or myelography, and possibly a lumbar puncture to clarify or confirm the cause of Babinski's reflex.

REFERENCES

1. Riggio, S. and Jagoda, A. "What You Forgot About the Neurologic Exam, Part 2: Move-

ment, Reflexes, Sensation, Balance." *Consultant* 45(1):53-58, January 2005.

2. Hockenberry, M.J. and Wilson, D. (Eds.) *Wong's Nursing Care of Infants and Children.* 8th ed. St. Louis: Mosby, 2007.

3. Holcomb, S.S. "Recognizing and Managing Anemia." *The Nurse Practitioner* 30(12):16-31, December 2005.

BACK PAIN

Back pain affects about 50% to 80% of all adults.[1,2,3] In fact, it's the second leading reason—after the common cold—for visits to primary care providers.[2] Although this symptom may herald a spondylogenic disorder, it also may stem from a genitourinary, GI, cardiovascular, or neoplastic disorder. Postural imbalance in pregnancy also may cause back pain.

The onset, location, and distribution of pain and its response to activity and rest provide important clues about the cause. Pain may be acute or chronic and constant or intermittent. It may remain localized in the back or radiate along the spine or down one or both legs. It may be worsened by activity—usually, bending, stooping, or lifting—and alleviated by rest, or it may be unaffected by either.

Intrinsic back pain results from muscle spasm, nerve root irritation, fracture, or a combination of these mechanisms. It usually occurs in the lower back, or lumbosacral area. Back pain also may be referred from the abdomen or flank, possibly signaling a life-threatening perforated ulcer, acute pancreatitis, or dissecting abdominal aortic aneurysm.

If the patient reports acute, severe back pain, quickly take his vital signs; then perform a rapid evaluation to rule out life-threatening causes. Ask him when the pain began. Can he relate it to any causes? For example, did the pain occur after eating? After falling on the ice? Have the patient describe the pain. Is it burning, stabbing, throbbing, or aching? Is it constant or intermittent? Does it radiate to the buttocks or legs? Does he have leg weakness? Does the pain seem to originate in the abdomen and radiate to the back? Has he had a pain like this before? What makes it better

or worse? Is it affected by activity or rest? Is it worse in the morning or evening? Does it wake him up? Typically, visceral-referred back pain is unaffected by activity and rest. In contrast, spondylogenic-referred back pain worsens with activity and improves with rest. Pain of neoplastic origin is usually relieved by walking and worsens at night.

If the patient describes deep lumbar pain unaffected by activity, palpate for a pulsating epigastric mass. If this sign is present, suspect dissecting abdominal aortic aneurysm. Withhold food and fluid in anticipation of emergency surgery. Prepare for I.V. fluid replacement and oxygen administration.

If the patient describes severe epigastric pain that radiates through the abdomen to the back, assess him for absent bowel sounds and for abdominal rigidity and tenderness. If these occur, suspect a perforated ulcer or acute pancreatitis. Start an I.V. line for fluids and drugs, give oxygen, insert a nasogastric tube, and withhold food.

History and physical examination

If life-threatening causes of back pain are ruled out, continue with a complete history and physical examination. Be aware of the patient's expressions of pain as you do so. Ask if the pain affects his ability to walk or use steps, or if it affects his sleep, diet, or relationships.[1] Obtain a medical history, including past injuries and illnesses, and a family history. Ask about diet and alcohol intake. Also, take a drug history, including past and present prescription and over-the-counter drugs. Use of an expanded pain assessment tool, such as the Owestry Brief Pain Inventory, may be helpful for patients with chronic low back pain.[1]

Next, perform a thorough physical examination. Observe skin color, especially in the legs, and palpate skin temperature. Palpate femoral, popliteal, posterior tibial, and pedal pulses. Ask about unusual sensations in the legs, such as numbness and tingling. Observe the patient's posture if pain doesn't prohibit standing. Does he stand erect or tend to lean toward one side? Observe the level of the shoulders and pelvis and the curvature of the back. Ask the patient to bend forward, backward, and from side to side while you palpate for paravertebral muscle spasms. Note rotation of the spine on the trunk. Palpate the dorsolumbar spine for point tenderness. Then ask the patient to walk—first on his heels, then on his toes; protect him from falling as he does so. Weakness may reflect a muscular disorder or spinal nerve root irritation. Place the patient in a sitting position to evaluate and compare patellar tendon (knee), Achilles tendon, and Babinski's reflexes. Evaluate the strength of the extensor hallucis longus by asking the patient to hold up his big toe against resistance. Measure leg length and hamstring and quadriceps muscles bilaterally. Note a difference of more than ⅜″ (1 cm) in muscle size, especially in the calf.

To reproduce leg and back pain, place the patient in a supine position on the examining table. Grasp his heel and slowly lift his leg. If he feels pain, note its exact location and the angle between the table and his leg when it occurs. Repeat this maneuver with the opposite leg. Pain along the sciatic nerve may indicate disk herniation or sciatica. Also, note the range of motion of the hip and knee.

Palpate the flanks and percuss with the fingertips or perform fist percussion to elicit costovertebral angle tenderness.

Medical causes

▶ *Abdominal aortic aneurysm (dissecting).* Life-threatening dissection of an abdominal aortic aneurysm may initially cause low back pain or dull abdominal pain, but it usually produces constant upper abdominal pain. A pulsating abdominal mass may be palpated in the epigastrium; after rupture, though, it no longer pulsates. Aneurysm dissection can also cause mottled skin below the waist, absent femoral and pedal pulses, blood pressure that's lower in the legs than in the arms, mild to moderate tenderness with guarding, and abdominal rigidity. Signs of shock (such as cool, clammy skin) appear if blood loss is significant.
▶ *Ankylosing spondylitis.* Ankylosing spondylitis is a chronic, progressive disorder that causes sacroiliac pain, which radiates up the spine and is aggravated by lateral pressure on the pelvis. The pain is usually most severe in the morning or after a period of inactivity

and isn't relieved by rest. Abnormal rigidity of the lumbar spine with forward flexion is also characteristic. This disorder can cause local tenderness, fatigue, fever, anorexia, weight loss, and occasionally iritis.
▶ *Appendicitis.* Appendicitis is a life-threatening disorder in which a vague and dull discomfort in the epigastric or umbilical region migrates to McBurney's point in the right lower quadrant. In retrocecal appendicitis, pain may also radiate to the back. The shift in pain is preceded by anorexia and nausea and is accompanied by fever, occasional vomiting, abdominal tenderness (especially over McBurney's point), and rebound tenderness. Some patients also have painful urinary urgency.
▶ *Cholecystitis.* Cholecystitis produces severe pain in the right upper quadrant of the abdomen that may radiate to the right shoulder, chest, or back. The pain may arise suddenly or may increase gradually over several hours; many patients have a history of similar pain after a high-fat meal. Accompanying signs and symptoms include anorexia, fever, nausea, vomiting, right-upper-quadrant tenderness, abdominal rigidity, pallor, and sweating.
▶ *Chordoma.* A slowly developing malignant tumor, chordoma causes persistent pain in the lower back, sacrum, and coccyx. As the tumor expands, pain may be accompanied by constipation and bowel or bladder incontinence.
▶ *Endometriosis.* Endometriosis causes deep sacral pain and severe cramping pain in the lower abdomen. The pain worsens just before or during menstruation and may be aggravated by defecation. It's accompanied by constipation, abdominal tenderness, dysmenorrhea, and dyspareunia.
▶ *Intervertebral disk rupture.* The patient will have gradual or sudden low back pain with or without leg pain (sciatica), rarely leg pain alone. Pain usually begins in the back and radiates to the buttocks and leg. The pain is worsened by activity, coughing, and sneezing and is eased by rest. It's accompanied by paresthesia (most commonly, numbness or tingling in the lower leg and foot), paravertebral muscle spasm, and decreased reflexes on the affected side. This disorder also affects posture and gait. The patient's spine is slightly

flexed and he leans toward the painful side. He walks slowly and rises from a sitting to a standing position with extreme difficulty.

▶ *Lumbosacral sprain.* Lumbosacral sprain, the most common cause of mechanical low back pain, causes localized aching pain and tenderness with muscle spasm on lateral motion.[3] The recumbent patient typically flexes his knees and hips to help ease pain. Flexion of the spine and movement intensify the pain, whereas rest helps relieve it.

▶ *Metastatic tumors.* Metastatic tumors commonly spread to the spine, causing low back pain in at least 25% of patients. Typically, the pain begins abruptly, is accompanied by cramping muscle pain (usually worse at night), and isn't relieved by rest.

▶ *Myeloma.* Back pain caused by myeloma—a primary malignant tumor—usually begins abruptly and worsens with exercise. It may be accompanied by arthritic signs and symptoms, such as achiness, joint swelling, and tenderness. Other signs and symptoms include fever, malaise, peripheral paresthesia, and weight loss.

▶ *Pancreatitis (acute).* Pancreatitis is a life-threatening disorder that usually produces fulminating, continuous upper abdominal pain that may radiate to both flanks and to the back. To relieve this pain, the patient may bend forward, draw his knees to his chest, or move about restlessly.

Early signs and symptoms include abdominal tenderness, nausea, vomiting, fever, pallor, and tachycardia; some patients have abdominal guarding and rigidity, rebound tenderness, and hypoactive bowel sounds. Jaundice may be a late sign. Occurring as inflammation subsides, Turner's sign (ecchymosis of the abdomen or flank) or Cullen's sign (bluish discoloration of skin around the umbilicus and in both flanks) signals hemorrhagic pancreatitis.

▶ *Perforated ulcer.* In some patients, perforation of a duodenal or gastric ulcer causes sudden, prostrating epigastric pain that may radiate throughout the abdomen and to the back. This life-threatening disorder also causes boardlike abdominal rigidity, tenderness with guarding, generalized rebound tenderness, absence of bowel sounds, and grunting, shallow respirations. Other signs include fever, tachycardia, and hypotension.

▶ *Prostate cancer.* Chronic aching back pain may be the only symptom of prostate cancer. This disorder also may cause hematuria and decreased urine stream.

▶ *Pyelonephritis (acute).* Pyelonephritis produces progressive flank and lower abdominal pain accompanied by back pain or tenderness (especially over the costovertebral angle). Other signs and symptoms include high fever and chills, nausea and vomiting, flank and abdominal tenderness, and urinary frequency and urgency.

▶ *Reactive arthritis.* In some patients, sacroiliac pain is the first sign of reactive arthritis. it also causes conjunctivitis, urethritis, and arthritis.

▶ *Renal calculi.* The colicky pain of renal calculi usually results from irritation of the ureteral lining, which increases the frequency and force of peristaltic contractions. The pain travels from the costovertebral angle to the flank, suprapubic region, and external genitalia. It varies in intensity but may become excruciating if calculi travel down a ureter. Calculi in the renal pelvis and calyces may cause dull and constant flank pain. Renal calculi also cause nausea, vomiting, urinary urgency (if a calculus lodges near the bladder), hematuria, and agitation due to pain. Pain resolves or significantly decreases after calculi move to the bladder. Urge the patient to collect any expelled calculi for analysis.

▶ *Sacroiliac strain.* Sacroiliac strain causes sacroiliac pain that may radiate to the buttock, hip, and lateral aspect of the thigh. The pain is aggravated by weight bearing on the affected limb and by abduction with resistance of the leg. Other signs and symptoms include tenderness of the symphysis pubis and a limp or a gluteus medius or abductor lurch.

▶ *Smallpox (variola major).* Smallpox was eradicated worldwide in 1980 but could theoretically be used in biological warfare. The United States and Russia have the only known storage sites of the virus.[4] Initial signs and symptoms include high fever, malaise, prostration, severe headache, backache, and abdominal pain. A maculopapular rash develops on the oral mucosa, pharynx, face, and forearms and then spreads to the trunk and legs. Within 2 days, the rash becomes vesicular and later pustular. The lesions develop at the same time, appear identical, and are more prominent on the face and extremities. The pustules are round, firm, and deeply embedded in the skin. After 8 to 9 days, the pustules form a crust, which later separates from the skin, leaving a pitted scar. Death may result from encephalitis, extensive bleeding, or secondary infection.

▶ *Spinal neoplasm (benign).* Spinal neoplasm typically causes severe localized back pain and scoliosis.

▶ *Spinal stenosis.* Resembling a ruptured intervertebral disk, spinal stenosis produces back pain with or without sciatica, which commonly affects both legs. The pain may radiate to the toes and may progress to numbness or weakness unless the patient rests.

▶ *Spondylolisthesis.* A major structural disorder characterized by forward slippage of one vertebra onto another, spondylolisthesis may produce no symptoms or may cause low back pain with or without nerve root involvement. Other symptoms of nerve root involvement include paresthesia, buttock pain, and pain radiating down the leg. Palpation of the lumbar spine may reveal a "step-off" of the spinous process. Flexion of the spine may be limited.

▶ *Transverse process fracture.* This type of fracture causes severe localized back pain with muscle spasm and hematoma.

▶ *Vertebral compression fracture.* A vertebral compression fracture may be painless initially. Several weeks later, it causes back pain aggravated by weight bearing and local tenderness. Fracture of a thoracic vertebra may cause referred pain in the lumbar area.

▶ *Vertebral osteomyelitis.* Initially, vertebral osteomyelitis causes insidious back pain. As it progresses, the pain may become constant, more pronounced at night, and aggravated by spinal movement. Other signs and symptoms include vertebral and hamstring spasms, tenderness of the spinous processes, fever, and malaise.

▶ *Vertebral osteoporosis.* Vertebral osteoporosis causes chronic aching back pain that is aggravated by activity and somewhat relieved by rest. Tenderness also may occur.

Other causes
▶ *Neurologic tests.* Lumbar puncture and myelography can produce transient back pain.

Special considerations
Monitor the patient closely if back pain suggests a life-threatening cause. Be alert for increasing pain, altered neurovascular status in the legs, loss of bowel or bladder control, altered vital signs, sweating, and cyanosis.

Until a tentative diagnosis is made, withhold analgesics, which may mask symptoms. Also withhold food and fluids in case surgery is needed. Make the patient as comfortable as possible by raising the head of the bed and placing a pillow under his knees. Encourage relaxation techniques such as deep breathing. Prepare the patient for a rectal or pelvic examination. He also may need routine blood tests, urinalysis, computed tomography scan, appropriate biopsies, and X-rays of the chest, abdomen, and spine.

Fit the patient for a corset or lumbosacral support, but instruct him not to wear it in bed. He also may need heat or cold therapy, a backboard, a convoluted foam mattress, or pelvic traction. Explain these pain-relief measures to the patient. Teach the patient about alternatives to analgesic drug therapy, such as biofeedback and transcutaneous electrical nerve stimulation.

Be aware that back pain may be psychosomatic. Refer the patient to other professionals, such as a physical therapist, an occupational therapist, or a psychologist, if indicated.

Pediatric pointers
Children may have trouble describing back pain, so be alert for nonverbal clues, such as wincing or refusing to walk. Closely observe the family dynamics during history taking for clues of child abuse.

Back pain in children may stem from intervertebral disk inflammation (diskitis), neoplasms, idiopathic juvenile osteoporosis, and spondylolisthesis. Heavy backpacks may be a common cause of back pain in children; however, recommendations for weight limitations haven't yet been devised.[5] Disk herniation typically doesn't cause back pain. Scoliosis, a common disorder in adolescents, rarely causes back pain.

Geriatric pointers

The aging process leads to osteoporosis and cartilage erosion between vertebrae, resulting in compression fractures that press on nerve roots and cause back pain.[1] Suspect metastatic cancer—especially of the prostate, colon, or breast—in older patients with a recent onset of back pain that usually isn't relieved by rest and worsens at night.

Patient counseling

If the patient has chronic back pain, reinforce instructions about bed rest, analgesics, anti-inflammatories, and exercise. Exercise helps strengthen muscles in the lower back. Encourage the patient to try yoga, which can safely and effectively reduce moderate chronic back pain.[6] Also, suggest that he take daily warm baths to help relieve pain. Help the patient recognize the need to make lifestyle changes, such as losing weight or correcting poor posture. Advise patients with acute back pain secondary to a musculoskeletal problem to continue their daily activities as tolerated, rather than staying on total bed rest.

REFERENCES

1. D'Arcy, Y. "Treatment Strategies for Low Back Pain Relief." *The Nurse Practitioner* 31(4):16-25, April 2006.
2. Ijzelenberg, W. and Burdorf, A. "Risk Factors for Musculoskeletal Symptoms and Ensuing Healthcare use and Sick Leave." *Spine* 30(13):1550-1556, July 2005.
3. Kinkade, S. "Evaluation and Treatment of Acute Low Back Pain." *American Family Physician* 75(8):1181-1189.
4. Centers for Disease Control and Prevention. "What You Should Know About A Smallpox Outbreak." Department of Health and Human Services, Centers for Disease Control and Prevention. 2004. Available at http://emergency.cdc.gov/agent/smallpox/basics/outbreak.asp.
5. Staggs, D.L., Early, S.D., D'Ambra, P., Tolo, V.T., and Kay, R.M. "Back Pain and Backpacks in School Children." *Journal of Pediatric Orthopedics* 26(3):358-363, May/June 2006.
6. Cain, J. "Gentle Yoga Effective for Chronic Low Back Pain: It Can Offer Relief of Moderate Pain." *AJN* 106(3):22, March 2006.

● BLADDER DISTENTION

Bladder distention—abnormal enlargement of the bladder—results from an inability to excrete urine, which then accumulates in the bladder. Distention can be caused by a mechanical or anatomic obstruction, a neuromuscular disorder, or the use of certain drugs. Relatively common in all ages and both sexes, it's most common in older men with prostate disorders that cause urine retention.

Distention usually develops gradually, but it occasionally has a sudden onset. Gradual distention usually causes no symptoms until stretching of the bladder produces discomfort. Acute distention produces suprapubic fullness, pressure, and pain. If severe distention isn't corrected promptly by catheterization or massage, the bladder rises within the abdomen, its walls become thin, and renal function can be impaired.

Bladder distention is aggravated by the intake of caffeine, alcohol, large quantities of fluid, and diuretics.

If the patient has severe distention, insert an indwelling urinary catheter to help relieve discomfort and prevent bladder rupture. If more than 700 ml is emptied from the bladder, compressed blood vessels dilate, which may make the patient feel faint. Typically, the indwelling urinary catheter is clamped for 30 to 60 minutes to permit vessel compensation.

History and physical examination

If distention isn't severe, start by reviewing the patient's voiding patterns. Find out the time and amount of the patient's last voiding and the amount of fluid consumed since then. Ask if he has difficulty urinating. Does he use Valsalva's or Credé's maneuver to start urinating? Does he urinate with urgency or without warning? Is urination painful or irritating? Ask about the force and continuity of his urine stream and whether he feels that his bladder is empty after voiding.

Explore the patient's history of urinary tract obstruction or infections; venereal disease; neurologic, intestinal, or pelvic surgery; lower abdominal or urinary tract trauma; and systemic or neurologic disorders. Ask about his drug history, including his use of over-the-counter drugs.

Take the patient's vital signs, and percuss and palpate the abdomen and bladder. If the bladder contains 150 ml or more of urine, you may be able to palpate or percuss it above the symphysis pubis.[1] If the bladder is empty, it can't be palpated through the abdominal wall. Inspect the urethral meatus, and measure its diameter. Describe the appearance and amount of any discharge. Finally, test for perineal sensation and anal sphincter tone; in male patients, digitally examine the prostate gland.

Medical causes

▶ *Benign prostatic hyperplasia (BPH)*. In BPH, bladder distention develops gradually as the prostate enlarges. Occasionally, its onset is acute. Initially, the patient has urinary hesitancy, straining, and frequency; reduced force of and inability to stop the urine stream; nocturia; and postvoiding dribbling. As the disorder progresses, it produces prostate enlargement, sensations of suprapubic fullness and incomplete bladder emptying, perineal pain, constipation, and hematuria.

▶ *Bladder calculi*. Bladder calculi may produce bladder distention, but pain is usually the only symptom. The pain is usually referred to the tip of the penis, the vulvar area, the lower back, or the heel. It worsens during walking or exercise and abates when the patient lies down. It's usually most severe when micturition stops. The pain may be accompanied by urinary frequency and urgency, terminal hematuria, and dysuria.

▶ *Bladder cancer*. By blocking the urethral orifice, neoplasms can cause bladder distention. Other signs and symptoms include hematuria (most common sign); urinary frequency and urgency; nocturia; dysuria; pyuria; pain in the bladder, rectum, pelvis, flank, back, or legs; vomiting; diarrhea; and sleeplessness. A mass may be palpable on bimanual examination.

▶ *Multiple sclerosis*. In this neuromuscular disorder, urine retention and bladder distention result from interruption of upper motor neuron control of the bladder. Other signs and symptoms include optic neuritis, paresthesia, impaired position and vibratory senses, diplopia, nystagmus, dizziness, abnormal reflexes, dysarthria, muscle weakness, emotional lability, Lhermitte's sign (transient, electric-like shocks that spread down the body when the head is flexed), Babinski's sign, and ataxia.

▶ *Prostate cancer*. In prostate cancer, obstruction of urine flow eventually causes bladder distention. Usual signs and symptoms include dysuria, urinary frequency and urgency, nocturia, weight loss, fatigue, perineal pain, constipation, and induration of the prostate or a rigid, irregular prostate on digital rectal examination. In some patients, urine retention and bladder distention are the only signs.

▶ *Prostatitis*. In acute prostatitis, bladder distention occurs rapidly along with perineal discomfort and a sensation of suprapubic fullness. Other signs and symptoms include perineal pain; tense, boggy, tender, and warm enlarged prostate; decreased libido; impotence; decreased force of the urine stream; dysuria; hematuria; and urinary frequency and urgency. Additional signs and symptoms include fatigue, malaise, myalgia, fever, chills, nausea, and vomiting.

Bladder distention is rare in chronic prostatitis, which may be accompanied by perineal discomfort, a sensation of suprapubic fullness, prostatic tenderness, decreased libido, urinary frequency and urgency, dysuria, pyuria, hematuria, persistent urethral discharge, ejaculatory pain, and dull pain radiating to the lower back, buttocks, penis, or perineum.

▶ *Spinal neoplasms*. Disrupting upper neuron control of the bladder, spinal neoplasms cause neurogenic bladder and resultant distention. Other signs and symptoms include a sense of pelvic fullness, continuous overflow dribbling, back pain that often mimics sciatica pain, constipation, tender vertebral processes, sensory deficits, and muscle weakness, flaccidity, and atrophy. Signs and symptoms of urinary tract infection (dysuria, urinary frequency and urgency, nocturia, tenesmus, hematuria, and weakness) may also occur.

▶ *Urethral calculi.* In urethral calculi, urethral obstruction leads to interrupted urine flow and bladder distention. The obstruction causes pain radiating to the penis or vulva and referred to the perineum or rectum. It may also produce a palpable stone and urethral discharge.

▶ *Urethral stricture.* Urethral stricture results in urine retention and bladder distention with chronic urethral discharge (most common sign), urinary frequency (also common), dysuria, urgency, decreased force and diameter of the urine stream, and pyuria. Urinoma and urosepsis may also develop.

Other causes

▶ *Catheterization.* Using an indwelling urinary catheter can result in urine retention and bladder distention. While the catheter is in place, inadequate drainage due to kinked tubing or an occluded lumen may lead to urine retention. In addition, a misplaced urinary catheter or irritation due to catheter removal may cause edema, thereby blocking urine outflow.

DRUG WATCH *Parasympatholytics, anticholinergics, ganglionic blockers, sedatives, anesthetics, and opioids can produce urine retention and bladder distention.*

Special considerations

Monitor the patient's vital signs and the extent of bladder distention. Encourage the patient to change positions to alleviate discomfort. Provide an analgesic if needed.

Noninvasive ultrasound scanning using a bladder scanner calculates and displays the volume of urine in the bladder. This device is useful in evaluating a distended bladder and in deciding when catheterization may be needed.[2]

Prepare the patient for diagnostic tests (such as endoscopy and radiologic studies) to determine the cause of bladder distention. You may need to prepare him for surgery if interventions don't relieve bladder distention and obstruction prevents catheterization.

Pediatric pointers

Look for urine retention and bladder distention in any infant who doesn't void normal amounts. Normally, infants produce about 30 to 60 ml of urine daily in the first 48 hours after birth and about 300 ml of urine daily during the next week.[3] In boys, posterior urethral valves, meatal stenosis, phimosis, spinal cord anomalies, bladder diverticula, and other congenital defects may cause urinary obstruction and resultant bladder distention.

Patient counseling

If the patient doesn't need immediate urinary catheterization, provide privacy and suggest that he assume the normal voiding position. Teach him to perform Valsalva's maneuver, or gently perform Credé's maneuver. You can also stroke or intermittently apply ice to the inner thigh, or help him relax in a warm tub or sitz bath. Use the power of suggestion to stimulate voiding. For example, run water in the sink, pour warm water over his perineum, place his hands in warm water, or play tapes of aquatic sounds.

REFERENCES

1. Newman, D.K. "Assessment of the Patient with an Overactive Bladder." *Journal of Wound, Ostomy, and Continence Nursing* 32(3S)Supplement 1:S5-S10, May/June 2005.
2. Patraca, K. "Measure Bladder Volume Without Catheterization." *Nursing* 35(4):46-47, April 2005.
3. Hockenberry, M.J. and Wilson, D. (Eds.) *Wong's Nursing Care of Infants and Children.* 8th ed. St. Louis: Mosby, 2007.

BLOOD PRESSURE DECREASE

Low blood pressure (hypotension) refers to inadequate intravascular pressure to perfuse the body's tissues and maintain oxygen requirements.[1] Although commonly linked to shock, this sign also may result from cardiovascular, respiratory, neurologic, or metabolic disorders. Hypoperfusion states especially affect the kidneys, brain, and heart, and may lead to renal failure, change in level of consciousness (LOC), or myocardial ischemia. Low blood pressure also may be caused by certain diagnostic tests—most commonly those using contrast media—and the use of certain drugs. It may stem from stress or a change of position—specifically, rising abruptly from a supine or sitting position to a standing position (orthostatic hypotension).

Normal blood pressure varies considerably; what qualifies as low blood pressure for one person may be normal for another. Consequently, every blood pressure reading must be compared against the patient's baseline. Typically, a reading below 90/60 mm Hg, or a drop of 30 mm Hg from the baseline, is considered low blood pressure.

Low blood pressure can result from an expanded intravascular space (as in severe infections, allergic reactions, or adrenal insufficiency), reduced intravascular volume (as in dehydration and hemorrhage), or decreased cardiac output (as in impaired cardiac muscle contractility). Because the body's pressure-regulating mechanisms are complex and interrelated, a combination of these factors usually contributes to low blood pressure.

If the patient's systolic pressure is less than 80 mm Hg, or 30 mm Hg below his baseline, suspect shock immediately. Quickly evaluate the patient for a decreased LOC. Check his apical pulse for tachycardia and respirations for tachypnea. Also, inspect the patient for cool, clammy skin. Then start an I.V. line using a large-bore needle to replace fluids and blood or to deliver drugs. Rapidly infuse Ringer's lactate or normal saline solution to increase intravascular circulation and cardiac preload.[2] Prepare to give oxygen with mechanical ventilation if needed. Monitor the patient's intake and output, and insert an indwelling urinary catheter for the accurate measurement of urine. The patient may also need a central venous line or a pulmonary artery catheter to facilitate monitoring of fluid status. Prepare for cardiac monitoring to evaluate cardiac rhythm. Be ready to insert a nasogastric tube to prevent aspiration in the comatose patient. Throughout emergency interventions, keep the patient's spinal column immobile until spinal cord trauma is ruled out.

History and physical examination

If the patient is conscious, ask him about his symptoms. Does he feel unusually weak or fatigued? Has he had nausea, vomiting, or dark or bloody stools? Is his vision blurred? Gait unsteady? Does he have palpitations, chest or abdominal pain, or difficulty breathing? Has he had episodes of dizziness or fainting? Do these episodes occur when he stands up suddenly? If so, take the patient's blood pressure while he's lying down, sitting, and then standing and compare readings.[3,4] A blood pressure decrease of at least 20 mm Hg systolic or 10 mm Hg diastolic within 3 minutes of standing up suggests orthostatic hypotension.[3,4] (See *Ensuring accurate blood pressure measurement*, page 52.)

Next, continue with a physical examination. Inspect the skin for pallor, sweating, and clamminess. Palpate peripheral pulses. Note a paradoxical pulse—an accentuated fall in systolic pressure during inspiration—which suggests pericardial tamponade. Then auscultate for abnormal heart sounds (gallops, murmurs), rate (bradycardia, tachycardia), or rhythm. Auscultate the lungs for abnormal breath sounds (diminished sounds, crackles, wheezing), rate (bradypnea, tachypnea), or rhythm (agonal or Cheyne-Stokes respirations). Look for signs of hemorrhage, including visible bleeding, palpable masses, bruising, and tenderness. Assess the patient for abdominal rigidity and rebound tenderness; auscultate for abnormal bowel sounds. Also, carefully assess the patient for possible sources of infection such as open wounds.

Medical causes

▶ *Adrenal insufficiency (acute).* Orthostatic hypotension is characteristic in acute adrenal insufficiency and is accompanied by fatigue, weakness, nausea, vomiting, abdominal discomfort, weight loss, fever, and tachycardia. The patient may also have hyperpigmentation of fingers, nails, nipples, scars, and body folds; pale, cool, clammy skin; restlessness; decreased urine output; tachypnea; and coma.

▶ *Alcohol toxicity.* Low blood pressure occurs infrequently in alcohol toxicity; more common signs and symptoms include a distinct alcohol breath odor, tachycardia, bradypnea, hypothermia, decreased LOC, seizures, staggering gait, nausea, vomiting, diuresis, and slow, stertorous breathing.

Ensuring accurate blood pressure measurement

To keep your blood pressure readings as accurate as possible, take steps to avoid the common pitfalls described here.

- *Wrong-sized cuff.* Select a cuff of appropriate size for the patient. This ensures that adequate pressure is applied to compress the brachial artery during cuff inflation. A cuff bladder that's too narrow will yield a false-high reading; one that's too wide, a false-low reading. The cuff bladder width should be about 40% of the circumference of the midpoint of the limb; bladder length should be twice the width. If the arm circumference is less than 13″ (33 cm), select a regular-sized cuff; if it's between 13″ and 16″ (33 to 40.5 cm), a large-sized cuff; if it's more than 16″, a thigh cuff. Pediatric cuffs are also available.
- *Improper application.* Make sure you apply the cuff correctly, as shown in this illustration.

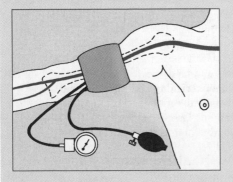

- *Slow cuff deflation.* This error causes venous congestion in the limb and a flase-high blood pressure reading. Don't deflate the cuff more slowly than 2 mm Hg/heartbeat.
- *Cuff wrapped too loosely.* When the cuff is too loose, its effective width is reduced, giving you a false-high reading. Tighten the cuff appropriately.
- *Mercury column not read at eye level.* Read the mercury column at eye level. If the column is below eye level, you may record a false-low reading; if it's above eye level, a false-high reading.
- *Tilted mercury column.* Keep the mercury column in a vertical position to avoid a false-high reading.
- *Poorly timed measurement.* Don't take the patient's blood pressure if he seems anxious or has just eaten or ambulated; you'll get a false-high reading.
- *Incorrect arm position.* Keep the patient's arm level with his heart to avoid a false-low reading.
- *Cuff overinflation.* Don't overinflate the cuff because you'll get a false-high reading in addition to causing venospasm or pain.
- *Failure to notice an auscultatory gap.* In an auscultatory gap, the sound fades out for 10 to 15 mm Hg and then returns. To avoid missing the top Korotkoff sound, estimate systolic pressure by palpation first. Then inflate the cuff rapidly—at 2 to 3 mm Hg/second—to about 30 mm Hg above the palpable systolic pressure.
- *Inaudibility of feeble sounds.* Before reinflating the cuff, have the patient raise his arm to reduce venous pressure and amplify low-volume sounds. After inflating the cuff, lower the patient's arm; then deflate the cuff and listen. Or, with the patient's arm positioned at heart level, inflate the cuff and have the patient make a fist. Have him rapidly open and close his hand 10 times before you start deflating the cuff; then listen. Be sure to document that the blood pressure reading was augmented.

▶ *Anaphylactic shock.* Following exposure to an allergen, such as penicillin or insect venom, a dramatic fall in blood pressure and narrowed pulse pressure signal this severe allergic reaction. Initially, anaphylactic shock causes anxiety, restlessness, a feeling of doom, intense itching (especially of the hands and feet), and a pounding headache. Later, it may also produce weakness, sweating, nasal congestion, coughing, difficulty breathing, nausea, abdominal cramps, involuntary defecation, seizures, flushing, urinary incontinence, tachycardia, and change or loss of voice due to laryngeal edema.

▶ *Anthrax, inhalation.* Anthrax is an acute infectious disease that's caused by the gram-positive, spore-forming bacterium *Bacillus anthracis*. Although the disease most commonly occurs in wild and domestic grazing animals, such as cattle, sheep, and goats, the spores can live in the soil for many years. The disease can occur in humans exposed to infected animals, tissue from infected animals, or biological agents. Most natural cases occur in agricultural regions worldwide. Anthrax may occur in cutaneous, inhalation, or GI forms.

Inhalation anthrax is caused by inhalation of aerosolized spores. Initial signs and symptoms are flulike and include fever, chills, weakness, cough, and chest pain. The disease generally occurs in two stages with a period of recovery after the initial signs and symptoms. The second stage develops abruptly with rapid deterioration marked by fever, dyspnea, stridor, and hypotension generally leading to death within 24 hours. Radiologic findings include mediastinitis and symmetrical mediastinal widening.

▶ *Cardiac arrhythmias.* In an arrhythmia, blood pressure may fluctuate between normal and low readings. Dizziness, chest pain, difficulty breathing, light-headedness, weakness, fatigue, and palpitations may also occur. Auscultation typically reveals an irregular rhythm and a pulse rate greater than 100 beats/minute or less than 60 beats/minute.

▶ *Cardiac contusion.* In a cardiac contusion, low blood pressure occurs along with tachycardia and, at times, anginal pain and dyspnea.

▶ *Cardiac tamponade.* An accentuated fall in systolic pressure (more than 10 mm Hg) during inspiration, known as *paradoxical pulse,* is characteristic in patients with cardiac tamponade. This disorder also causes restlessness, cyanosis, tachycardia, jugular vein distention, muffled heart sounds, dyspnea, and Kussmaul's sign (increased venous distention with inspiration).

▶ *Cardiogenic shock.* In cardiogenic shock, pump impairment or failure renders the heart unable to adequately perfuse organs and tissues.[5] Accompanying low blood pressure are tachycardia, narrowed pulse pressure, diminished Korotkoff sounds, peripheral cyanosis, and pale, cool, clammy skin. Cardiogenic shock also causes restlessness and anxiety, which may progress to disorientation and confusion. Other signs and symptoms include angina, dyspnea, jugular vein distention, oliguria, ventricular gallop, tachypnea, and weak, rapid pulse.

▶ *Cholera.* Cholera is an acute infection caused by the bacterium *Vibrio cholerae* that may be mild with uncomplicated diarrhea or severe and life-threatening. Cholera is spread by ingestion of contaminated water or food, especially shellfish. Signs include abrupt watery diarrhea and vomiting. Severe water and electrolyte loss leads to thirst, weakness, muscle cramps, decreased skin turgor, oliguria, tachycardia, and hypotension. Without treatment, death can occur within hours.

▶ *Diabetic ketoacidosis.* Hypovolemia triggered by osmotic diuresis in hyperglycemia is responsible for the low blood pressure associated with diabetic ketoacidosis, which is usually present in patients with type 1 diabetes mellitus. It also commonly produces polydipsia, polyuria, polyphagia, dehydration, weight loss, abdominal pain, nausea, vomiting, breath with fruity odor, Kussmaul's respirations, tachycardia, seizures, confusion, and stupor that may progress to coma.

▶ *Heart failure.* In heart failure, blood pressure may fluctuate between normal and low readings, but a precipitous drop in blood pressure may signal cardiogenic shock. Other signs and symptoms of heart failure include exertional dyspnea, dyspnea of abrupt or gradual onset, paroxysmal nocturnal dyspnea or difficulty breathing in the supine position (orthopnea), fatigue, weight gain, pallor or cyanosis, sweating, and anxiety. Auscultation reveals ventricular gallop, tachycardia, bilateral crackles, and tachypnea. Dependent edema, jugular vein distention, increased capillary refill time, and hepatomegaly may also occur.

▶ *Hyperosmolar hyperglycemic nonketotic syndrome (HHNS).* HHNS, which is common in persons with type 2 diabetes mellitus, decreases blood pressure—at times dramatically, if the patient loses significant fluid from diuresis due to severe hyperglycemia and hyperosmolarity. It also produces dry mouth, poor skin turgor, tachycardia, confusion progressing to coma and, occasionally, generalized tonic-clonic seizures.

▶ *Hypovolemic shock*. Hypovolemic shock is characterized by a decrease in circulating blood volume, usually from acute blood loss.[5] Accompanying it are diminished Korotkoff sounds, narrowed pulse pressure, and rapid, weak, and irregular pulse. Peripheral vasoconstriction causes cyanosis of the extremities and pale, cool, clammy skin. Other signs and symptoms include oliguria, confusion, disorientation, restlessness, and anxiety.

▶ *Hypoxemia*. Initially, blood pressure may be normal or slightly elevated, but as hypoxemia becomes more pronounced blood pressure drops. The patient also may have tachycardia, tachypnea, dyspnea, confusion, and stupor that may progress to coma.

▶ *Myocardial infarction*. In this life-threatening disorder, blood pressure may be low or high. However, a precipitous drop in blood pressure may signal cardiogenic shock. Other signs and symptoms include chest pain that may radiate to the jaw, shoulder, arm, or epigastrium; dyspnea; anxiety; nausea or vomiting; sweating; and cool, pale, or cyanotic skin. Auscultation may reveal an atrial gallop, a murmur and, occasionally, an irregular pulse.

▶ *Neurogenic shock*. The result of sympathetic denervation due to cervical injury or anesthesia, neurogenic shock produces low blood pressure and bradycardia. However, the patient's skin remains warm and dry because of cutaneous vasodilation and sweat gland denervation. Depending on the cause of shock, motor weakness of the limbs or diaphragm may also occur.

▶ *Pulmonary embolism*. Pulmonary embolism causes sudden, sharp chest pain and dyspnea accompanied by cough and, occasionally, low-grade fever. Low blood pressure occurs with narrowed pulse pressure and diminished Korotkoff sounds. Other signs include tachycardia, tachypnea, paradoxical pulse, jugular vein distention, and hemoptysis.

▶ *Septic shock*. Initially, septic shock produces fever and chills. Low blood pressure, tachycardia, and tachypnea may also develop early, but the patient's skin remains warm. Later, low blood pressure becomes increasingly severe—with systolic pressure less than 80 mm Hg, or 30 mm Hg less than the base-

line—and is accompanied by narrowed pulse pressure. Other late signs and symptoms include pale skin, cyanotic extremities, apprehension, thirst, oliguria, and coma.

▶ *Vasovagal syncope*. Vasovagal syncope is a transient loss or near-loss of consciousness that's characterized by low blood pressure, pallor, cold sweats, nausea, palpitations or bradycardia, and weakness following stressful, painful, or claustrophobic experiences.

Other causes

▶ *Diagnostic tests*. These include the gastric acid stimulation test using histamine and X-ray studies using contrast media. The latter may trigger an allergic reaction, which causes low blood pressure.

DRUG WATCH *Calcium channel blockers, diuretics, vasodilators, alpha blockers, beta blockers, general anesthetics, opioid analgesics, monoamine oxidase inhibitors, anxiolytics (such as benzodiazepines), tranquilizers, and most I.V. antiarrhythmics (especially bretylium tosylate) can cause low blood pressure.*

Special considerations

Check the patient's vital signs often to determine if low blood pressure is constant or intermittent. If blood pressure is extremely low, an arterial catheter may be inserted to allow close monitoring of pressures. Or, a Doppler flowmeter may be used.

While Trendelenburg positioning to treat acute hypotension has been widely utilized, recent research could not strongly support this practice, and found that its risks (increased intracranial pressure, impaired lung expansion) might outweigh its benefits. Further research is needed to determine the safety and efficacy of this intervention.[1]

Place the patient on bed rest. Keep the side rails of the bed up. If the patient is ambulatory, assist him as needed. To avoid falls, don't leave a dizzy patient unattended when he's sitting or walking.

Prepare the patient for laboratory tests, which may include urinalysis, routine blood studies, an electrocardiogram, and chest, cervical, and abdominal X-rays.

Normal pediatric blood pressure

AGE	NORMAL SYSTOLIC PRESSURE	NORMAL DIASTOLIC PRESSURE
Birth to 3 months	40 to 80 mm Hg	Not detectable
3 months to 1 year	80 to 100 mm Hg	Not detectable
1 to 4 years	80 to 110 mm Hg	60 mm Hg
4 to 12 years	80 to 120 mm Hg	60 to 70 mm Hg

Pediatric pointers

Blood pressure is normally lower in children than in adults. (See *Normal pediatric blood pressure.*)

Because children are prone to accidents, suspect trauma or shock first as a possible cause of low blood pressure. Remember that low blood pressure typically doesn't accompany head injury in adults because intracranial hemorrhage is insufficient to cause hypovolemia. However, it does accompany head injury in infants and young children; their expandable cranial vaults allow significant blood loss into the cranial space, resulting in hypovolemia.

Another common cause of low blood pressure in children is dehydration, which may result from persistent (as little as 24 hours) diarrhea and vomiting, decreased oral intake, and diabetic ketoacidosis.[6]

Geriatric pointers

In elderly patients, low blood pressure commonly results from the use of multiple drugs with this potential adverse effect, a problem that needs to be addressed. Orthostatic hypotension due to autonomic dysfunction is another common cause.

Patient counseling

If the patient has orthostatic hypotension, instruct him to stand up slowly from a sitting or lying position. Advise patients with vasovagal syncope to avoid situations that trigger the episodes. Evaluate the patient's need for a cane or walker. Explain all procedures and tests.

REFERENCES

1. Shammas, A. and Clark, A.P. "Trendelenburg Positioning to treat Acute Hypotension: Helpful or Harmful?" *Clinical Nurse Specialist* 21(4):181-187, July/August 2007.
2. Cottingham, C. "Resuscitation of Traumatic Shock: A Hemodynamic Review." *AACN Advanced Critical Care* 17(3):317-326, July/September 2006.
3. "The Ups and Downs of Orthostatic Hypotension." *Nursing Made Incredibly Easy!* 3(3):46-49, May/June 2005.
4. Rushing, J. "Assessing for Orthostatic Hypotension." *Nursing* 35(1):30, January 2005.
5. Kelley, D.M. "Hypovolemic Shock: An Overview." *Critical Care Nursing Quarterly* 28(1):2-21, January/March 2005.
6. Hockenberry, M.J. and Wilson, D. (Eds.) *Wong's Nursing Care of Infants and Children.* 8th ed. St. Louis: Mosby, 2007.

BLOOD PRESSURE INCREASE

Hypertension is defined as an intermittent or sustained increase in blood pressure exceeding 140/90 mm Hg.[1] This condition affects more men than women and twice as many Blacks as Whites. (See *Hypertension reduction in Black patients,* page 56.) By itself, this common sign is easily ignored by the patient; after all, he can't see or

Hypertension reduction in Black patients

Question: *What is the effect of usual care (UC) plus blood pressure (BP) tele-monitoring (TM) on BP reduction in Black patients with hypertension?*

Research: High blood pressure among Black patients is a growing problem. In this random-ized, controlled trial, comparisons were made of UC only to UC plus BP and TM to determine which leads to a greater reduction in BP. Black patients were recruited for the study through free BP screenings in the community. Partici-pants were screened three times to confirm the presence of uncontrolled BP and to determine eligibility for the study. A block-stratified ran-domization was done to ensure equal numbers of participants taking antihypertensive medica-tions in the control group and in the treatment group. The TM group had 194 participants and the UC group had 193 participants.

Subjects in the treatment group received UC plus nurse-managed TM. Telemonitoring in-volved patients self-monitoring their BP at home and then transmitting readings via telephone. The intervention nurse delivered the device, taught subjects how to use it, set up and demonstrated the system, had patients practice using it, and answered questions. Subjects were asked to measure their BP three times per week in the morning before taking antihyper-tensives. After reports were transmitted, the nurse telephoned each subject and provided telecounseling.

Conclusion: Over the 12 months, the nurse-managed TM group showed clinically and sta-tistically significant reductions in systolic BP (13 mm Hg). A decrease in the diastolic BP of 6.3 mm Hg was clinically, but not statistically, significant. Maintained over time, such actions could improve outcomes for Black patients with hypertension.

Application: Recognize the effect of nurse con-tact on patient compliance and desire to modify lifestyle. Educate patients about BP monitoring and ways to improve health. Teach patients about high BP and its complications. Tell pa-tients that by controlling high BP, drug regimens may be avoided or minimized, thereby reduc-ing risk of medication side effects.

Source: Artinian, N. T., Flack, J. M., Nord-strom, C. K., Hockman, E. M., Washington, O. G. M., Jen, K. C., and Fathy, M. "Effects of Nurse-Managed Telemonitoring on Blood Pressure at 12-Month Follow-Up Among Urban African Americans." *Nursing Research* 56(5):312-322, 2007.

feel it. However, its causes can be life threat-ening.

Elevated blood pressure may develop sud-denly or gradually. A sudden, severe rise in pressure (exceeding 180/110 mm Hg) may in-dicate life-threatening hypertensive crisis. However, even a less dramatic rise may be equally significant if it heralds a dissecting aortic aneurysm, increased intracranial pres-sure, myocardial infarction, eclampsia, or thy-rotoxicosis.

Usually associated with essential hyperten-sion, elevated blood pressure also may result from a renal or endocrine disorder, a treat-ment that affects fluid status (such as dialy-sis), or from the use of certain drugs. Inges-tion of large amounts of certain foods, such as black licorice and cheddar cheese, may tem-porarily elevate blood pressure. (See *Patho-physiology of elevated blood pressure.*)

Sometimes, elevated blood pressure may simply reflect inaccurate blood pressure meas-urement. (See *Ensuring accurate blood pres-sure measurement,* page 52.) However, careful measurement alone doesn't ensure a clinically useful reading. To be useful, each blood pres-sure reading must be compared with the pa-tient's baseline. In some cases, serial readings may be necessary to establish elevated blood pressure.

Pathophysiology of elevated blood pressure

Blood pressure—the force exerted on vessels by blood as it flows through them—varies with cardiac output, peripheral resistance, and blood volume. A brief review of its regulating mechanisms—nervous system control, capillary fluid shifts, kidney excretion, and hormonal changes—will help you understand how elevated blood pressure develops.

● Nervous system control involves the sympathetic system, chiefly baroreceptors and chemoreceptors. This system promotes moderate vasoconstriction to maintain normal blood pressure. When it responds inappropriately, increased vasoconstriction enhances peripheral resistance, resulting in elevated blood pressure.

● Capillary fluid shifts regulate blood volume by responding to arterial pressure. Increased pressure forces fluid into the interstitial space; decreased pressure allows it to be drawn back into the arteries by osmosis. However, this fluid shift may take several hours to adjust blood pressure.

● Kidney excretion also helps regulate blood volume by increasing or decreasing urine formation. Normally, an arterial pressure of about 60 mm Hg maintains urine output. When pressure drops below this reading, urine formation ceases, thereby increasing blood volume. Conversely, when arterial pressure exceeds this reading, urine formation increases, thereby reducing blood volume. Like capillary fluid shifts, this mechanism may take several hours to adjust blood pressure.

● Hormonal changes reflect stimulation of the renin-angiotensin-aldosterone system of the kidney in response to low arterial pressure. This system causes vasoconstriction, which increases arterial pressure, and stimulates aldosterone release, which regulates sodium retention—a key determinant of blood volume.

Elevated blood pressure signals the breakdown or inappropriate response of these pressure-regulating mechanisms. Its signs and symptoms concentrate in the target organs and tissues illustrated below.

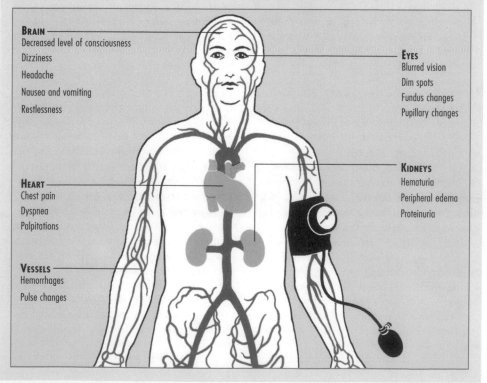

BRAIN
Decreased level of consciousness

Dizziness

Headache

Nausea and vomiting

Restlessness

EYES
Blurred vision

Dim spots

Fundus changes

Pupillary changes

HEART
Chest pain

Dyspnea

Palpitations

KIDNEYS
Hematuria

Peripheral edema

Proteinuria

VESSELS
Hemorrhages

Pulse changes

Managing elevated blood pressure

Elevated blood pressure can signal a life-threatening disorder. If pressure exceeds 180/110 mm Hg, the patient may be in hypertensive crisis and need prompt treatment. Maintain a patent airway in case the patient vomits, and take seizure precautions. Prepare to give an I.V. antihypertensive and diuretic. You'll also need to insert an indwelling urinary catheter to accurately monitor urine output.

If the patient's blood pressure elevation is less severe, continue to rule out other life-threatening causes. If the patient is pregnant, suspect preeclampsia or eclampsia. Place her on bed rest, and insert an I.V. line. Give magnesium sulfate (to decrease neuromuscular irritability) and an antihypertensive. Monitor vital signs closely for 24 hours. If diastolic blood pressure continues to exceed 100 mm Hg despite drug therapy, you may need to prepare the patient for induced labor and delivery or for cesarean delivery. Offer emotional support if she faces a premature birth.

If the patient isn't pregnant, quickly look for equally obvious clues. Assess the patient for exophthalmos and an enlarged thyroid gland. If these signs are present, ask about a history of hyperthyroidism. Then look for other signs and symptoms, including tachycardia, widened pulse pressure, palpitations, severe weakness, diarrhea, fever exceeding 100° F (37.8° C), and nervousness. Prepare to give an antithyroid drug orally or by nasogastric tube, if needed. Also, evaluate fluid status; look for signs of dehydration, such as poor skin turgor. Prepare for I.V. fluid replacement and temperature control using a cooling blanket, if needed.

If the patient shows signs of increased intracranial pressure (such as decreased level of consciousness and fixed or dilated pupils), ask him or a family member about recent head trauma. Then check for an increased respiratory rate and bradycardia. Maintain a patent airway in case the patient vomits. In addition, take seizure precautions, and prepare to give an I.V. diuretic. Insert an indwelling urinary catheter, and monitor intake and output. Check vital signs every 15 minutes until stable.

If the patient has absent or weak peripheral pulses, ask about chest pressure or pain, which suggests a dissecting aortic aneurysm. Enforce bed rest until a diagnosis has been established. As appropriate, give the patient an I.V. antihypertensive or prepare him for surgery.

History and physical examination

If you detect sharply elevated blood pressure, quickly rule out possible life-threatening causes. (See *Managing elevated blood pressure*.)

After ruling out life-threatening causes, complete a more leisurely history and physical examination. Determine if the patient has a history of cardiovascular or cerebrovascular disease, diabetes, or renal disease. Ask about a family history of high blood pressure—a likely finding in patients with essential hypertension, pheochromocytoma, or polycystic kidney disease. Then ask about its onset. Did high blood pressure appear abruptly? Ask the patient's age. Sudden onset of high blood pressure in middle-aged or elderly patients suggests renovascular stenosis. Although essential hypertension may begin in childhood, it typically isn't diagnosed until near age 35.

Pheochromocytoma and primary aldosteronism usually occur between ages 40 and 60. If you suspect either, check for orthostatic hypotension. Take the patient's blood pressure with him supine, sitting, and then standing. Normally, systolic pressure falls and diastolic pressure rises on standing; in orthostatic hypotension, both pressures fall.

Note headache, palpitations, blurred vision, and sweating. Ask about wine-colored urine and decreased urine output; these signs suggest glomerulonephritis, which can cause elevated blood pressure.

Obtain a drug history, including past and present prescription and over-the-counter drugs (especially decongestants) as well as herbal preparations. If the patient is already taking an antihypertensive, determine how well he complies with the regimen. Ask about his perception of elevated blood pressure.

How serious does he believe it is? Does he expect drug therapy to help? Explore psychosocial or environmental factors that may impact blood pressure control.

Follow up the history with a thorough physical examination. Using a funduscope, check for intraocular hemorrhage, exudate, and papilledema, which characterize severe hypertension. Perform a thorough cardiovascular assessment. Check for carotid bruits and jugular vein distention. Assess skin color, temperature, and turgor. Palpate peripheral pulses. Auscultate for abnormal heart sounds (gallops, louder second sound, murmurs), rate (bradycardia, tachycardia), or rhythm. Then auscultate for abnormal breath sounds (crackles, wheezing), rate (bradypnea, tachypnea), or rhythm.

Palpate the abdomen for tenderness, masses, or liver enlargement. Auscultate for abdominal bruits. Renal artery stenosis produces bruits over the upper abdomen or in the costovertebral angles. Easily palpable, enlarged kidneys and a large, tender liver suggest polycystic kidney disease. Obtain a urine specimen to check for microscopic hematuria.

Medical causes

▶ *Aldosteronism (primary).* In aldosteronism, elevated diastolic pressure may be accompanied by orthostatic hypotension. Other findings include constipation, muscle weakness, polyuria, polydipsia, and personality changes.
▶ *Anemia.* Accompanying elevated systolic pressure in anemia are pulsations in the capillary beds, bounding pulse, tachycardia, systolic ejection murmur, pale mucous membranes and, in patients with sickle cell anemia, ventricular gallop and crackles.
▶ *Aortic aneurysm (dissecting).* Initially, aortic aneurysm—a life-threatening disorder—causes a sudden rise in systolic pressure (which may be the precipitating event), but no change in diastolic pressure. However, this increase is brief. The body's ability to compensate fails, resulting in hypotension.

Other signs and symptoms vary, depending on the type of aortic aneurysm. An abdominal aneurysm may cause persistent abdominal and back pain, weakness, sweating, tachycardia, dyspnea, a pulsating abdominal mass, restlessness, confusion, and cool, clammy skin. A thoracic aneurysm may cause a ripping or tearing sensation in the chest, which may radiate to the neck, shoulders, lower back, or abdomen; pallor; syncope; blindness; loss of consciousness; sweating; dyspnea; tachycardia; cyanosis; leg weakness; murmur; and absent radial and femoral pulses.
▶ *Atherosclerosis.* In atherosclerosis, systolic pressure rises while diastolic pressure commonly remains normal or slightly elevated. The patient may show no other signs, or he may have a weak pulse, flushed skin, tachycardia, angina, and claudication.
▶ *Cushing's syndrome.* Twice as common in women as in men, Cushing's syndrome causes elevated blood pressure and widened pulse pressure, as well as truncal obesity, moon face, and other cushingoid signs. It's usually caused by corticosteroid use.
▶ *Hypertension.* Essential hypertension develops insidiously and is characterized by a gradual increase in blood pressure from decade to decade. Except for this high blood pressure, the patient may be asymptomatic or (rarely) may complain of suboccipital headache, lightheadedness, tinnitus, and fatigue.

In malignant hypertension, diastolic pressure abruptly rises above 120 mm Hg, and systolic pressure may exceed 200 mm Hg. Typically, the patient has pulmonary edema marked by jugular vein distention, dyspnea, tachypnea, tachycardia, and a cough with pink, frothy sputum. Other characteristic signs and symptoms include severe headache, confusion, blurred vision, tinnitus, epistaxis, muscle twitching, chest pain, nausea, and vomiting.
▶ *Increased intracranial pressure (ICP).* Increased ICP causes an increased respiratory rate initially, followed by increased systolic pressure and widened pulse pressure. Increased ICP affects heart rate last, causing bradycardia (Cushing's reflex). Other signs and symptoms include headache, projectile vomiting, decreased level of consciousness, and fixed or dilated pupils.
▶ *Metabolic syndrome.* Blood pressure that exceeds 135/85 mm Hg is one of the conditions associated with metabolic syndrome (previously called *syndrome X*). Other conditions that define this syndrome are obesity, abnormal cholesterol level, and high blood in-

sulin level. People with these traits are at significantly greater risk of heart disease, stroke, peripheral vascular disease, and type 2 diabetes. Factors contributing to these conditions include physical inactivity, excessive weight gain, and genetic predisposition. Self-care measures, such as exercising, following a heart-healthy diet, and not smoking, often combined with medical therapy, are essential treatments.

▶ *Myocardial infarction (MI).* MI is a life-threatening disorder that may cause high or low blood pressure. The most common symptom is crushing chest pain that may radiate to the jaw, shoulder, arm, or epigastrium. Other findings include dyspnea, anxiety, nausea, vomiting, weakness, diaphoresis, atrial gallop, and murmurs.

▶ *Pheochromocytoma.* Paroxysmal or sustained elevated blood pressure characterizes pheochromocytoma and may be accompanied by orthostatic hypotension. Other signs and symptoms include anxiety, diaphoresis, palpitations, tremors, pallor, nausea, weight loss, and headache.

▶ *Polycystic kidney disease.* Elevated blood pressure is typically preceded by flank pain. Other signs and symptoms include enlarged kidneys, an enlarged and tender liver, and intermittent gross hematuria.

▶ *Preeclampsia and eclampsia.* Potentially life threatening to mother and fetus, preeclampsia and eclampsia are defined by a blood pressure of 140/90 mm Hg or more if the woman had normal blood pressure readings before 20 weeks gestation.[2] If the woman's blood pressure is less than 140/90 mm Hg but has increased 30 mm Hg above her baseline systolic or 15 mm Hg above her baseline diastolic pressure, monitor her closely for these disorders.[2] Other findings include generalized edema, sudden weight gain of 3 lb (1.4 kg) or more weekly during the second or third trimester, severe frontal headache, blurred or double vision, decreased urine output, proteinuria, midabdominal pain, neuromuscular irritability, nausea, and possibly seizures (eclampsia).

▶ *Renovascular stenosis.* Renovascular stenosis produces abruptly elevated systolic and diastolic pressures. Other characteristic signs and symptoms include bruits over the upper abdomen or in the costovertebral angles, hematuria, and acute flank pain.

▶ *Thyrotoxicosis.* Accompanying the elevated systolic pressure associated with thyrotoxicosis—a potentially life-threatening disorder— are widened pulse pressure, tachycardia, bounding pulse, pulsations in the capillary nail beds, palpitations, weight loss, exophthalmos, an enlarged thyroid gland, weakness, diarrhea, fever over 100° F (37.8° C), and warm, moist skin. The patient may appear nervous and emotionally unstable, displaying occasional outbursts or even psychotic behavior. Heat intolerance, exertional dyspnea and, in females, decreased or absent menses may also occur.

Other causes

DRUG WATCH *CNS stimulants (such as amphetamines), sympathomimetics, corticosteroids, nonsteroidal anti-inflammatory drugs, hormonal contraceptives, monoamine oxidase inhibitors, and over-the-counter cold remedies can increase blood pressure.*

▶ *Herbal products.* Ephedra (banned by the Food and Drug Administration), ginseng, and licorice may cause hypertension or arrhythmias. St. John's wort may increase blood pressure, especially when taken with substances that antagonize hypericin, such as amphetamines, cold and hay fever drugs, nasal decongestants, pickled foods, beer, coffee, wine, and chocolate.

▶ *Illicit drugs.* Cocaine abuse may raise blood pressure.

Special considerations

If routine screening detects elevated blood pressure, stress to the patient the need for follow-up diagnostic tests. Then prepare him for routine blood tests and urinalysis. Depending on the suspected cause of the increased blood pressure, radiographic studies, especially of the kidneys, may be needed.

If the patient has essential hypertension, explain the importance of long-term control of elevated blood pressure and the purpose, dosage, schedule, route, and adverse effects of prescribed antihypertensives. Reassure him that there are other drugs he can take if the one he's taking isn't effective or causes intolerable adverse reactions. Encourage him to report adverse reactions; the drug dosage or schedule may simply need adjustment.

Be aware that the patient may have elevated blood pressure only when in the physician's office (known as "white-coat hypertension"). In such cases, 24-hour blood pressure monitoring is indicated to confirm elevated readings in other settings. In addition, other risk factors for coronary artery disease, such as smoking and elevated cholesterol levels, need to be addressed.

Hypertension has been reported to be two to three times more common in women taking hormonal contraceptives than those not taking them. Women age 35 and older who smoke cigarettes should be strongly encouraged to stop smoking; if they continue, they should be discouraged from using hormonal contraceptives.

Pediatric pointers
Normally, blood pressure is lower in children than in adults, an essential point to recognize when assessing a child for elevated blood pressure. (See *Normal pediatric blood pressure,* page 55.) Hypertension in children is defined as a systolic or diastolic blood pressure greater than the 95th percentile for gender, age, and height.[3,4]

Elevated blood pressure in children may result from essential hypertension, congenital renal abnormalities, renovascular stenosis, chronic pyelonephritis, coarctation of the aorta, patent ductus arteriosus, anemia, glomerulonephritis, adrenogenital syndrome, or neuroblastoma.[4] The risk of hypertension in children increases with body mass index (BMI); about 30% of children with a BMI greater than the 95th percentile are hypertensive.[3] Treatment typically starts with drug therapy. Surgery may follow in patients with patent ductus arteriosus, coarctation of the aorta, neuroblastoma, and some cases of renovascular stenosis. Diuretics and antibiotics are used to treat glomerulonephritis and chronic pyelonephritis; hormonal therapy, to treat adrenogenital syndrome.

Geriatric pointers
Atherosclerosis commonly produces isolated systolic hypertension in elderly patients.

Treatment is warranted to prevent long-term complications.

Patient counseling
The Joint National Committee on Prevention, Detection, Evaluation, and Treatment of High Blood Pressure recommends lifestyle changes in addition to drugs to reduce hypertension, such as weight loss; regular exercise; a low-fat, low-salt diet with plenty of fruits and vegetables; moderate alcohol consumption; and smoking cessation.[5]

Teach the patient how to monitor his blood pressure so he can evaluate the effectiveness of drug therapy and lifestyle changes.[6] Have him record blood pressure readings and symptoms, and ask him to share this information on his return visits.[6]

REFERENCES
1. Sauerbeck, L. "Primary Stroke Prevention." *AJN American Journal of Nursing* 106(11):40-49, November 2006.
2. Gardner, J. "Managing Preeclampsia Buys Time for a Safe Delivery." *Nursing* 35(3):50-52, March 2005.
3. Suresh, S., Mahajan, P., and Kamat, D. "Emergency Management of Pediatric Hypertension." *Clinical Pediatrics* 44(9):739-745, November/December 2005.
4. Rowan, S., Adrogues, H., Mathur, A., and Kamat, D. "Pediatric Hypertension: A Review for the Primary Care Provider." *Clinical Pediatrics* 44(4):289-296, May 2005.
5. Chobanian, A.V., et al. "The Seventh Report of the Joint National Committee on Prevention, Detection, Evaluation, and Treatment of High Blood Pressure: The JNC 7 Report." *JAMA* 289(19):2560-2572, 2003.
6. Phillips-Edwards, A., Collins-Smith, R., Del Rio, G.C., brown, C., Wu, L., and Singh, H. "'ALLHAT' and Innovations in Nursing." *AJN* 107(5):72C-72H, May 2007.

BOWEL SOUNDS, ABSENT

If you hear no bowel sounds (silent abdomen) after listening through a stethoscope for at least 5 minutes in each abdominal quadrant, your patient has absent bowel sounds. (See *Are bowel sounds really absent?* page 62.) Bowel sounds cease when

Are bowel sounds really absent?

Before concluding that your patient has absent bowel sounds, ask yourself these three questions:

1. *Did you use the diaphragm of your stethoscope to auscultate for the bowel sounds?*
   The diaphragm detects high-frequency sounds, such as bowel sounds, whereas the bell detects low-frequency sounds, such as a vascular bruit or a venous hum.
2. *Did you listen in the same spot for at least 5 minutes for the presence of bowel sounds?*
   Normally, bowel sounds occur every 5 to 15 seconds, but the duration of a single sound may be less than 1 second.
3. *Did you listen for bowel sounds in all quadrants?*
   Bowel sounds may be absent in one quadrant but present in another.

mechanical or vascular obstruction or neurogenic inhibition halts peristalsis. When peristalsis stops, gas (from bowel contents) and fluid (secreted from the intestinal walls) accumulate and distend the lumen, leading to life-threatening complications (such as perforation, peritonitis, and sepsis) or hypovolemic shock.

Simple mechanical obstruction, resulting from adhesions, hernia, or tumor, causes loss of fluids and electrolytes and induces dehydration. Vascular obstruction cuts off circulation to the intestinal walls, leading to ischemia, necrosis, and shock. Neurogenic inhibition, affecting innervation of the intestinal wall, may result from infection, bowel distention, or trauma. It may also follow mechanical or vascular obstruction or a metabolic imbalance such as hypokalemia.

Abrupt cessation of bowel sounds, when accompanied by abdominal pain, rigidity, and distention, signals a life-threatening crisis requiring immediate intervention. Absent bowel sounds following a period of hyperactive sounds are equally ominous and may indicate strangulation of a mechanically obstructed bowel.

If you fail to detect bowel sounds and the patient reports sudden, severe abdominal pain and cramping or exhibits severe abdominal distention, prepare to insert a nasogastric (NG) or intestinal tube to suction lumen contents and decompress the bowel. Administer I.V. fluids and electrolytes to offset any dehydration and imbalances caused by the dysfunctioning bowel.

Because the patient may need surgery to relieve an obstruction, withhold oral intake. Take the patient's vital signs, and be alert for signs of shock, such as hypotension, tachycardia, and cool, clammy skin. Measure abdominal girth as a baseline for gauging subsequent changes.

History and physical examination

If the patient's condition permits, proceed with a brief history. Start with abdominal pain: When did it begin? Has it gotten worse? Where does he feel it? Ask about bloating and flatulence. Find out if the patient has had diarrhea or has passed pencil-thin stools—possible signs of a developing luminal obstruction. The patient may have had no bowel movements at all—a possible sign of complete obstruction or paralytic ileus.

Ask about conditions that commonly lead to mechanical obstruction, such as abdominal tumors, hernias, and adhesions from past abdominal surgery. Determine if the patient was involved in an accident—even a seemingly minor one, such as falling off a stepladder—that may have caused vascular clots. Check for a history of acute pancreatitis, diverticulitis, or gynecologic infection, which may have led to intra-abdominal infection and bowel dysfunction. Be sure to ask about previous toxic conditions, such as uremia, and about spinal cord injury, which can lead to paralytic ileus.

If the patient's pain isn't severe or accompanied by other life-threatening signs or symptoms, obtain a detailed medical and surgical history and perform a complete physical examination followed by an abdominal assessment and a pelvic examination.

Start your assessment by inspecting abdominal contour. Stoop at the recumbent patient's side and then at the foot of his bed to detect localized or generalized distention. Auscultate all four quadrants. Percuss and palpate the abdomen gently. Listen for dullness over fluid-filled areas and tympany over pockets of gas. Palpate, noting any tenderness or the presence of any masses.

Medical causes

▶ *Mechanical intestinal obstruction, complete.* Absent bowel sounds follow a period of hyperactive bowel sounds in complete mechanical intestinal obstruction—a potentially life-threatening disorder. This silence accompanies acute, colicky abdominal pain that arises in the quadrant of obstruction and may radiate to the flank or lumbar regions. Other signs and symptoms include abdominal distention and bloating, constipation, and nausea and vomiting (the higher the blockage, the earlier and more severe the vomiting). In late stages, signs of shock may occur with fever, rebound tenderness, and abdominal rigidity.
▶ *Mesenteric artery occlusion.* In this life-threatening disorder, bowel sounds disappear after a brief period of hyperactive sounds. Sudden, severe midepigastric or periumbilical pain occurs next, followed by abdominal distention, bruits, vomiting, constipation, and signs of shock. Fever is common. Abdominal rigidity may appear later.
▶ *Paralytic (adynamic) ileus.* The cardinal sign of paralytic ileus is reduced or absent bowel sounds.[1] In addition to abdominal distention, other signs and symptoms of paralytic ileus include generalized discomfort and constipation or passage of small, liquid stools. If paralytic ileus follows acute abdominal infection, the patient also may have fever and abdominal pain.

Other causes

▶ *Abdominal surgery.* Bowel sounds are normally absent after abdominal surgery—the result of anesthetic use and surgical manipulation. Auscultating for the return of bowel sounds postoperatively has been the traditional method of assessing the return of gastric motility. However, recent research suggests that alternate methods, such as first passage of flatus, first postoperative bowel movement, and return of appetite, are also accurate measures of restored gastric motility.[2]

Special considerations

After you've inserted an NG or intestinal tube, raise the head of the patient's bed at least 30 degrees, and turn the patient to facilitate passage of the tube through the GI tract. (Remember not to tape an intestinal tube to the patient's face.) Ensure tube patency by checking for drainage and properly functioning suction devices, and irrigate accordingly.

Continue to give I.V. fluids and electrolytes. The patient may need X-rays and further blood work to determine the cause of absent bowel sounds.

After mechanical obstruction and intra-abdominal sepsis have been ruled out as the cause of absent bowel sounds, give the patient drugs to control pain and stimulate peristalsis.

Pediatric pointers

Absent bowel sounds in children may result from Hirschsprung's disease or intussusception, both of which can lead to life-threatening obstruction.

Geriatric pointers

Older patients with a bowel obstruction that doesn't respond to decompression should be considered for early surgical intervention to avoid the risk of bowel infarct.

Patient counseling

Explain all procedures and tests to the patient.

REFERENCES
1. Nettina, S.M. (Ed.) *Lippincott Manual of Nursing Practice.* 8th ed. Philadelphia: Lippincott Williams & Wilkins, 2005.
2. Madsen, D., Sebolt, T., Cullen, L., Folkedahl, B., Mueller, T., Richardson, C., and Titler, M. "Listening to Bowel Sounds: An Evidence-Based Practice Project." *AJN* 105(12):40-49, December 2005.

BOWEL SOUNDS, HYPERACTIVE

Sometimes audible without a stethoscope, hyperactive bowel sounds reflect increased intestinal motility (peristalsis). They're commonly characterized as rapid, rushing, gurgling waves. (See *Characteristics of bowel sounds*.) They may stem from life-threatening bowel obstruction or GI hemorrhage or from GI infection, inflammatory bowel disease (which usually follows a chronic course), food allergies, or stress.

After detecting hyperactive bowel sounds, quickly check vital signs and ask the patient about other symptoms, such as abdominal pain, vomiting, and diarrhea. If he reports cramping abdominal pain or vomiting, continue to auscultate for bowel sounds. If bowel sounds stop abruptly, suspect complete bowel obstruction. Prepare to assist with GI suction and decompression and to give I.V. fluids and electrolytes, and prepare the patient for surgery.

If the patient has diarrhea, record its frequency, amount, color, and consistency. If you detect excessive watery diarrhea or bleeding, prepare to give an antidiarrheal, I.V. fluids and electrolytes and, possibly, blood transfusions.

History and physical examination

If you've ruled out life-threatening conditions, obtain a detailed medical and surgical history. Ask the patient if he has had a hernia or abdominal surgery because these may cause mechanical intestinal obstruction. Does he have a history of inflammatory bowel disease? Also, ask about recent episodes of gastroenteritis among family members, friends, or coworkers. If the patient has traveled recently, even within the United States, was he aware of any endemic illnesses?

In addition, determine whether stress may have contributed to the patient's problem. Ask about food allergies and recent ingestion of unusual foods or fluids. Check for fever, which suggests infection. Having already auscultated, now gently inspect, percuss, and palpate the abdomen.

Characteristics of bowel sounds

The sounds of swallowed air and fluid moving through the GI tract are known as bowel sounds. These sounds usually occur every 5 to 15 seconds, but their frequency may be irregular. For example, bowel sounds are normally more active just before and after a meal. They may last less than 1 second or up to several seconds.

● Normal bowel sounds can be characterized as murmuring, gurgling, or tinkling.
● Hyperactive bowel sounds can be characterized as loud, gurgling, splashing, and rushing; they're higher pitched and occur more often than normal sounds.
● Hypoactive bowel sounds are softer or lower in tone and occur less frequently than normal sounds.

Medical causes

▶ *Crohn's disease.* Hyperactive bowel sounds usually arise insidiously in Crohn's disease. Other signs and symptoms include diarrhea, cramping abdominal pain that may be relieved by defecation, anorexia, low-grade fever, abdominal distention and tenderness and, in many cases, a fixed mass in the right lower quadrant. Perianal and vaginal lesions are common. Muscle wasting, weight loss, and signs of dehydration may occur as Crohn's disease progresses.

▶ *Food hypersensitivity.* Malabsorption—typically lactose intolerance—may cause hyperactive bowel sounds. Other signs and symptoms include diarrhea, bloating, and, possibly, nausea and vomiting, angioedema, and urticaria.

▶ *Gastroenteritis.* Hyperactive bowel sounds follow sudden nausea and vomiting and accompany "explosive" diarrhea. Abdominal cramping or pain is common, often after a peristaltic wave. Fever may occur, depending on the causative organism.

▶ *GI hemorrhage.* Hyperactive bowel sounds provide the most immediate indication of persistent upper GI bleeding. Other findings include hematemesis, coffee-ground vomitus, abdominal distention, bloody diarrhea, rectal passage of bright red clots and jellylike material or melena, and pain during bleeding. Decreased urine output, tachycardia, and hypotension accompany blood loss.[1]

▶ *Mechanical intestinal obstruction.* Hyperactive bowel sounds occur with cramping abdominal pain every few minutes in patients with mechanical intestinal obstruction—a potentially life-threatening disorder. Bowel sounds may later become hypoactive and then disappear. Nausea and vomiting occur earlier and with greater severity in small-bowel obstruction than in large-bowel obstruction. In complete bowel obstruction, hyperactive sounds are also accompanied by abdominal distention and constipation, although the part of the bowel distal to the obstruction may continue to empty for up to 3 days.

▶ *Ulcerative colitis (acute).* Hyperactive bowel sounds arise abruptly in patients with ulcerative colitis and are accompanied by bloody diarrhea, anorexia, abdominal pain, nausea and vomiting, fever, and tenesmus. Weight loss, arthralgia, and arthritis may occur.

Special considerations

Prepare the patient for diagnostic tests, which may include endoscopy to view a suspected lesion, barium X-rays, or stool analysis.

Pediatric pointers

Hyperactive bowel sounds in children usually result from gastroenteritis, erratic eating habits, excessive ingestion of certain foods (such as unripened fruit), or food allergy.

Patient counseling

Explain prescribed dietary changes to the patient. These may range from complete food and fluid restrictions to a liquid or bland diet. Because stress often precipitates or aggravates bowel hyperactivity, teach the patient relaxation techniques such as deep breathing. Encourage rest and restrict the patient's physical activity.

REFERENCES

1. Krumberger, J. "How to Manage An Acute Upper GI Bleed." *RN* 68(3):34-40, March 2005.

BRADYCARDIA

Bradycardia refers to a heart rate of less than 60 beats/minute.[1] It occurs normally in young adults, trained athletes, and elderly people as well as during sleep. It's also a normal response to vagal stimulation caused by coughing, vomiting, or straining during defecation. When bradycardia results from these causes, the heart rate rarely drops below 40 beats/minute. However, when it results from pathologic causes (such as cardiovascular disorders), the heart rate may be slower.

By itself, bradycardia is a nonspecific sign. However, together with such symptoms as chest pain, dizziness, syncope, and shortness of breath, it can signal a life-threatening disorder. (See *Differential diagnosis in bradycardia,* pages 66 and 67.)

Depending on the accompanying signs and symptoms, the patient with bradycardia may require immediate emergency care. For symptomatic bradycardia, atropine I.V. may be ordered, a transcutaneous pacemaker may be required, and full cardiorespiratory arrest may occur.[2]

History and physical examination

After detecting bradycardia, check for related signs of life-threatening disorders. (See *Managing severe bradycardia,* page 68.) If bradycardia isn't accompanied by untoward signs, ask the patient if he or a family member has a history of a slow pulse rate because this may be inherited. Also, find out if he has an underlying metabolic disorder, such as hypothyroidism, which can lead to bradycardia. Ask which drugs he's taking and if he's complying with the prescribed schedule and dosage. Monitor vital signs, temperature, pulse rate, respirations, blood pressure, and oxygen saturation.

Medical causes

▶ *Cardiac arrhythmias.* Depending on the type of arrhythmia and the patient's tolerance of it, bradycardia may be transient or sustained and benign or life-threatening. Related

Differential diagnosis in bradycardia

To help determine the origin of your patient's bradycardia and, in turn, the appropriate treatment and follow-up, perform a focused physical examination (vital signs; thyroid status; cardiovascular, neurologic, and pulmonary systems) and consider these possible causes.

POSSIBLE CAUSE	SIGNS AND SYMPTOMS	DIAGNOSIS	TREATMENT AND FOLLOW-UP
Cardiac arrhythmia	• Bradycardia (transient or sustained) • Hypotension • Palpitations • Dizziness or syncope • Nausea • Weakness or fatigue • Pallor	• Laboratory tests (arterial blood gas analysis, complete blood count, cardiac enzymes, electrolytes, glucose) • Electrocardiogram (ECG) • 24-hour Holter monitoring	• Medication (antiarrhythmic, vagolytic) • Pacemaker *Follow-up:* Referral to cardiologist
Cardiomyopathy	• Bradycardia (transient or sustained) • Dizziness or syncope • Edema • Jugular vein distention • Fatigue • Orthopnea • Dyspnea • Peripheral cyanosis • Chest pain	• Drug screen • Electrolytes • Imaging studies (chest X-ray, echocardiogram) • ECG • Cardiac catheterization	• Medication (antiarrhythmics, diuretics, angiotensin-converting enzyme inhibitors) • Oxygen therapy • Limited activity • Low-fat, low-salt diet *Follow-up:* Referral to cardiologist
Cervical spine injury	• Bradycardia (transient or sustained) • Hypotension • Hypothermia • Slowed peristalsis • Leg paralysis • Partial arm paralysis	• History of trauma • Imaging studies (computed tomography [CT] scan, magnetic resonance imaging [MRI]) of spine	• Spine stabilization • Corticosteroids *Follow-up:* Transfer to spinal injury center
Hypothermia	• Temperature below 89.6° F (32° C) • Shivering • Peripheral cyanosis • Muscle rigidity • Bradypnea • Confusion and stupor	• Temperature • ECG	• Establishment of ABCs (airway, breathing, circulation) • Temperature monitoring • Warm I.V. fluids, warming blanket • Treatment of underlying cause (if physiologic) *Follow-up:* Return visit 2 weeks after hospitalization
Hypothyroidism	• Fatigue • Constipation • Weight gain • Cold sensitivity	• Thyroid studies • ECG	• Thyroid hormone replacement

Differential diagnosis in bradycardia *(continued)*

POSSIBLE CAUSE	SIGNS AND SYMPTOMS	DIAGNOSIS	TREATMENT AND FOLLOW-UP
Hypothyroidism *(continued)*	• Cool, dry, thick skin • Sparse, dry hair • Alopecia • Facial swelling • Periorbital edema • Thick, brittle nails • Neck swelling • Goiter		*Follow-up:* Return visits every 4 to 6 weeks until thyroid-stimulating hormone level is normal; then every 6 months
Intracranial hypertension	• Bradypnea or tachypnea • Widened pulse pressure • Persistent headache • Projectile vomiting • Fixed, unequal, or dilated pupils • Decreased level of consciousness	• Imaging studies (CT scan, MRI)	• Treatment of underlying cause • Medication (osmotic diuretics, barbiturates) • Ventilatory support *Follow-up:* Referral to neurologist or neurosurgeon
Myocardial infarction	• Chest, back, or abdominal pain • Shortness of breath • Cough • Dizziness • Nausea and vomiting • Diaphoresis • Anxiety	• Laboratory tests (lactate dehydrogenase, isoenzymes, troponin I and T) • Imaging studies (angiography, echocardiogram) • ECG • Cardiac catheterization	• Medication (aspirin, nitrates, analgesics, thrombolytics, anticoagulants, beta-adrenergic blockers, vasopressors) • Oxygen therapy • Angioplasty • Coronary artery bypass graft *Follow-up:* Referral to cardiologist; return visit 3 to 6 weeks after hospitalization, then every 3 months

findings include hypotension, palpitations, dizziness, weakness, syncope, and fatigue.

▶ *Cardiomyopathy.* Cardiomyopathy is a potentially life-threatening disorder that may cause transient or sustained bradycardia. Other findings include dizziness, syncope, edema, fatigue, jugular vein distention, orthopnea, dyspnea, and peripheral cyanosis.

▶ *Cervical spinal injury.* Bradycardia may be transient or sustained, depending on the severity of the injury. Its onset coincides with sympathetic denervation. Other signs and symptoms include hypotension, decreased body temperature, slowed peristalsis, leg paralysis, and partial arm and respiratory muscle paralysis.

▶ *Hypothermia.* Bradycardia usually appears when the core temperature drops below 89.6° F (32° C). It's accompanied by shivering, peripheral cyanosis, muscle rigidity, bradypnea, and confusion leading to stupor.

▶ *Hypothyroidism.* Hypothyroidism causes severe bradycardia in addition to fatigue, constipation, unexplained weight gain, and sensi-

Managing severe bradycardia

Bradycardia can signal prolonged exposure to cold; head or neck trauma; or a life-threatening disorder when accompanied by pain, shortness of breath, dizziness, syncope, or other symptoms. In such patients, quickly take vital signs. Connect the patient to a cardiac monitor, and insert an I.V. line. Depending on the cause of bradycardia, you'll need to administer fluids, atropine, steroids, or thyroid medication. If indicated, insert an indwelling urinary catheter. Intubation, mechanical ventilation, or placement of a pacemaker may be necessary if the patient's respiratory rate falls.

If appropriate, perform a focused evaluation to help locate the cause of bradycardia. For example, ask about pain. Viselike pressure or crushing or burning chest pain that radiates to the arms, back, or jaw may indicate an acute myocardial infarction (MI); a severe headache may indicate increased intracranial pressure. Also ask about nausea, vomiting, or shortness of breath—signs and symptoms associated with an acute MI and cardiomyopathy. Observe the patient for peripheral cyanosis, edema, or jugular vein distention, which may indicate cardiomyopathy. Look for a thyroidectomy scar because severe bradycardia may result from hypothyroidism caused by failure to take thyroid hormone replacements.

If the cause of bradycardia is evident, provide supportive care. For example, keep the hypothermic patient warm by applying blankets, and monitor his core temperature until it reaches 99° F (37.2° C); stabilize the head and neck of a trauma patient until cervical spinal injury is ruled out.

---

tivity to cold. Related signs include cool, dry, thick skin; sparse, dry hair; facial swelling; periorbital edema; thick, brittle nails; and confusion leading to stupor.

▶ *Increased intracranial pressure (ICP).* Bradycardia occurs as a late sign of increased ICP along with rapid respiratory rate, elevated systolic pressure, decreased diastolic pressure, and widened pulse pressure. Other signs and symptoms include persistent headache, projectile vomiting, decreased level of consciousness (LOC), and fixed, unequal, and possibly dilated pupils.

▶ *Myocardial infarction (MI).* Sinus bradycardia is the most common arrhythmia associated with an acute MI. Accompanying signs and symptoms of an MI include an aching, burning, or viselike pressure in the chest that may radiate to the jaw, shoulder, arm, back, or epigastric area; nausea and vomiting; cool, clammy, and pale or cyanotic skin; anxiety; and dyspnea. Blood pressure may be elevated or depressed. Auscultation may reveal abnormal heart sounds.

Other causes
▶ *Diagnostic tests.* Cardiac catheterization and electrophysiologic studies can induce temporary bradycardia.

DRUG WATCH *Beta blockers, some calcium channel blockers, cardiac glycosides, topical miotics (such as pilocarpine), protamine, quinidine and other antiarrhythmics, and sympatholytics may cause transient bradycardia. Failure to take prescribed thyroid replacement hormone may cause bradycardia.*

▶ *Invasive treatments.* Suctioning can induce hypoxia and vagal stimulation, causing bradycardia. Cardiac surgery can cause edema or damage to conduction tissues, causing bradycardia.

Special considerations
Monitor vital signs often. Be especially alert for changes in cardiac rhythm, respiratory rate, and LOC. Aso, prepare the patient for laboratory tests, which can include complete blood count; cardiac enzyme, serum electrolyte, blood glucose, blood urea nitrogen, arterial blood gas, and blood drug levels; thyroid function tests; and a 12-lead electrocar-

diogram. If appropriate, prepare the patient for 24-hour Holter monitoring.

Pediatric pointers

Heart rates are normally higher in children than in adults. Fetal bradycardia—a heart rate less than 120 beats/minute—may occur during prolonged labor or as a complication of delivery, as from compression of the umbilical cord, partial abruptio placentae, and placenta previa. Intermittent bradycardia, sometimes accompanied by apnea, commonly occurs in premature infants.[3] Bradycardia rarely occurs in full-term infants or children. However, it can result from congenital heart defects, acute glomerulonephritis, and transient or complete heart block associated with cardiac catheterization or cardiac surgery.

Geriatric pointers

Sinus node dysfunction is the most common bradyarrhythmia in the elderly. Patients with this disorder may cite fatigue, exercise intolerance, dizziness, or syncope as their chief complaint. If the patient is asymptomatic, no intervention is needed. Symptomatic patients, however, require careful scrutiny of their drug therapy. Beta blockers, verapamil, diazepam, sympatholytics, antihypertensives, and some antiarrhythmics have been implicated; symptoms may clear when these drugs are discontinued. Pacing is usually indicated in patients with symptomatic bradycardia lacking a correctable cause.

Patient counseling

Explain all tests and procedures to the patient and his family. Explain the need for cardiac monitoring and common alarms that may be heard. Teach the patient and his family how to take a radial pulse.

REFERENCES
1. Plummer, B.J. "ECG Challenge: How Strip Savvy Are You?" *AJN* 107(6):72A-72C, June 2007.
2. Fugate, J. "Pharmacologic Management of Cardiac Emergencies." *Journal of Infusion Nursing* 29(3):147-150, May/June 2006.
3. Stokowski, L. "A Primer on Apnea of Prematurity." *Advances in Neonatal Care* 5(3):155-170, June 2005.

BRADYPNEA

Commonly preceding life-threatening apnea or respiratory arrest, bradypnea is a pattern of regular respirations with a rate of fewer than 10 breaths/minute. This sign may result from neurologic or metabolic disorders or a drug overdose, all of which depress the brain's respiratory control centers. (See *Understanding how the nervous system controls breathing,* page 70.)

Depending on the degree of central nervous system (CNS) depression, a patient with severe bradypnea may require constant stimulation to breathe. If the patient seems excessively sleepy, try to arouse him by shaking him and instructing him to breathe. Quickly take the patient's vital signs, and monitor pulse oximetry. Assess his neurologic status by checking pupil size and reactions and by evaluating his level of consciousness (LOC) and his ability to move his limbs.

Connect the patient to an apnea monitor, keep emergency airway equipment available, and be prepared to assist with intubation and mechanical ventilation if spontaneous respirations cease. To prevent aspiration, position the patient on his side or keep his head 30 degrees higher than the rest of the body, and clear his airway with suction.

History and physical examination

Obtain a brief history from the patient, if possible, or from whoever accompanied him to your facility. Ask if he's having a drug overdose and, if so, try to determine which drugs he took, how much, when, and by what route. Check his arms for needle marks, indicating possible drug abuse. You may need to give I.V. naloxone, an opioid antagonist.

If you rule out a drug overdose, ask about chronic illnesses, such as diabetes and renal failure. Check for a medical identification bracelet or card that identifies an underlying condition. Also ask whether the patient has a history of head trauma, brain tumor, neurologic infection, or stroke.

Medical causes

▶ *Diabetic ketoacidosis.* Bradypnea occurs late in patients with severe, uncontrolled hy-

Understanding how the nervous system controls breathing

Stimulation from external sources and from higher brain centers acts on respiratory centers in the pons and medulla. These centers, in turn, send impulses to the various parts of the respiratory system to alter respiratory patterns.

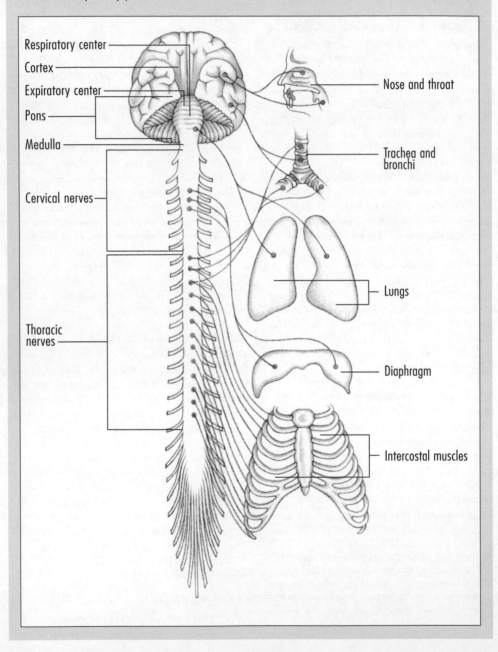

Respiratory center

Cortex

Expiratory center

Pons

Medulla

Cervical nerves

Thoracic nerves

Nose and throat

Trachea and bronchi

Lungs

Diaphragm

Intercostal muscles

perglycemia. Patients with severe ketoacidosis may experience Kussmaul's respirations. Other signs and symptoms include decreased LOC, fatigue, weakness, fruity breath odor, and oliguria.

▶ *Hepatic failure.* Occurring in end-stage hepatic failure, bradypnea may be accompanied by coma, hyperactive reflexes, asterixis, a positive Babinski's reflex, fetor hepaticus, and other signs.

▶ *Hypothermia.* Untreated hypothermia can cause severe bradypnea and bradycardia. Related signs and symptoms include shivering, decreased level of consciousness, and arrhythmias.[1]

▶ *Increased intracranial pressure (ICP).* A late sign of increased ICP—a life-threatening condition—bradypnea is preceded by decreased LOC, deteriorating motor function, and fixed, dilated pupils. The triad of bradypnea, bradycardia, and hypertension is a classic sign of brain ischemia or infarction.[2]

▶ *Renal failure.* Occurring in end-stage renal failure, bradypnea may be accompanied by seizures, decreased LOC, GI bleeding, hypotension or hypertension, uremic frost, and diverse other signs.

▶ *Respiratory failure.* Bradypnea occurs in end-stage respiratory failure along with cyanosis, diminished breath sounds, tachycardia, mildly increased blood pressure, and decreased LOC.

Other causes

DRUG WATCH *An overdose of an opioid analgesic or, less commonly, a sedative, barbiturate, phenothiazine, or another CNS depressant can cause bradypnea. Use of any of these drugs with alcohol can also cause bradypnea.*

Special considerations

Because a patient with bradypnea may develop apnea, check his respiratory status frequently and be prepared to give ventilatory support if needed. Don't leave the patient unattended, especially if his LOC is decreased. Keep his bed in the lowest position and raise the side rails. Obtain blood for arterial blood gas analysis, electrolyte studies, and possibly a drug screen. Ready the patient for chest X-

Respiratory rates in children

This graph shows normal respiratory rates in children, which are higher than normal rates in adults. Accordingly, bradypnea in children is defined according to age.

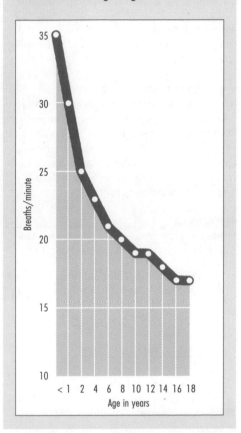

rays and possibly a computed tomography scan of the head.

Give prescribed drugs and oxygen. Avoid giving the patient a CNS depressant because it can worsen bradypnea. Similarly, give oxygen judiciously to a patient with chronic carbon dioxide retention, which may occur in chronic obstructive pulmonary disease, because excess oxygen therapy can have a negative effect.

When dealing with slow breathing in hospitalized patients, always review all drugs and dosages given during the last 24 hours.

Pediatric pointers

Because respiratory rates are normally higher in children than in adults, bradypnea in children is defined according to age. (See *Respiratory rates in children,* page 71.)

Geriatric pointers

When giving drugs to elderly patients, keep in mind that they have a higher risk of bradypnea from drug toxicity. That's because many of them take several drugs or have other conditions that predispose them to it. Warn older patients about this potentially life-threatening complication.

Patient counseling

Alert patients who regularly take an opioid—for example, those with advanced cancer or sickle cell anemia—that bradypnea is a serious complication, and teach them to recognize early signs of toxicity, such as nausea and vomiting. Also, try to identify patients who may be abusing these drugs.

REFERENCES

1. Day, M.P. "Hypothermia: A Hazard for All Seasons." *Nursing* 36(12):44-47, December 2006.
2. "Don't Let Your Head Explode Over Increased ICP." *Nursing Made Incredibly Easy!* 5(2):21-25, March/April 2007.

● BREAST DIMPLING

Breast dimpling—the puckering or retraction of skin on the breast—results from abnormal attachment of the skin to underlying tissue. It suggests an inflammatory or malignant mass beneath the skin surface and usually represents a late sign of breast cancer; benign lesions usually don't produce this effect. Dimpling usually affects women older than age 40, but it also occasionally affects men.

Because breast dimpling occurs over a mass or an induration, the patient usually discovers other signs before becoming aware of the dimpling. A thorough breast examination may reveal dimpling and alert the patient and nurse to a breast problem.

History and physical examination

Obtain a medical, reproductive, and family history, noting factors that increase the patient's risk of breast cancer. Also obtain a pregnancy history because women who haven't had a full-term pregnancy before age 30 have a higher risk of breast cancer. Has the patient's mother or sister had breast cancer? Has the patient had a previous malignancy, especially cancer in the other breast? Ask about the patient's dietary habits because a high-fat diet predisposes women to breast cancer.

Ask the patient if she has noticed any changes in the shape of her breast. Is any area painful or tender, and is the pain cyclic? If she's breast-feeding, has she recently experienced high fever, chills, malaise, muscle aches, fatigue, or other flulike signs or symptoms? Can she remember sustaining any trauma to the breast?

Carefully inspect the dimpled area. Is it swollen, red, or warm to the touch? Do you see bruises or contusions? Ask the patient to tense her pectoral muscles by pressing her hips with both hands or by raising her hands over her head. Does the puckering increase? Gently pull the skin upward toward the clavicle. Is the dimpling exaggerated?

Observe the breast for nipple retraction. Do both nipples point in the same direction? Is either nipple flattened or inverted? Does the patient report nipple discharge? If so, ask her to describe its color and character. Observe the contour of both breasts. Are they symmetrical?

Examine both breasts with the patient supine, sitting, and then leaning forward. Does the skin move freely over both breasts? If you can palpate a lump, describe its size, location, consistency, mobility, and delineation. What relation does the lump have to the breast dimpling? Gently mold the breast skin around the lump. Is the dimpling exaggerated? Also examine breast and axillary lymph nodes, noting any enlargement.

Medical causes

▶ *Breast abscess.* Breast dimpling sometimes accompanies a chronic breast abscess. Other findings include a firm, irregular, nontender lump and signs of nipple retraction, such as deviation, inversion, or flattening. Axillary lymph nodes may be enlarged.

▶ *Breast cancer.* Breast dimpling is an important but somewhat late sign of breast cancer. A neoplasm that causes dimpling is usually close to the skin and at least 1 cm in diameter. It feels irregularly shaped and fixed to underlying tissue, and it's usually painless. Other signs of breast cancer include peau d'orange, changes in breast symmetry or size, nipple retraction, and a unilateral, spontaneous, nonmilky nipple discharge that's serous or bloody. (A bloody nipple discharge in the presence of a lump is a classic sign of breast cancer.) Axillary lymph nodes may be enlarged. Pain may be present but isn't a reliable symptom of breast cancer. A breast ulcer may appear as a late sign.

▶ *Fat necrosis.* Breast dimpling due to fat necrosis follows inflammation and trauma to the fatty tissue of the breast (although the patient usually can't remember such trauma). Tenderness, erythema, bruising, and contusions may occur. Other findings include a firm, irregular, fixed mass and skin retraction signs, such as skin dimpling and nipple retraction. Fat necrosis is difficult to differentiate from breast cancer.

▶ *Mastitis.* Breast dimpling may signal bacterial mastitis, which usually results from duct obstruction and milk stasis during lactation. Heat, erythema, swelling, induration, pain, and tenderness usually accompany mastitis. Dimpling is more likely to occur with diffuse induration than with a single hard mass. The skin on the breast may feel fixed to underlying tissue. Other possible findings include nipple retraction, nipple cracks, a purulent discharge, and enlarged axillary lymph nodes. Flulike signs and symptoms (such as fever, malaise, fatigue, and aching) are common.

▶ *Sarcoidosis.* Sarcoidosis of the breast, a rare disorder, can be mistaken for breast cancer because it can cause skin dimpling as well as a peau d'orange appearance.[1]

Special considerations

Remember that any breast problem can arouse fears of mutilation, loss of sexuality, and death. Allow the patient to express her feelings. Carefully document the location of breast dimpling by placing a diagram of the patient's breasts in the medical record.[2]

Pediatric pointers

Because breast cancer, the most likely cause of dimpling, is extremely rare in children, consider trauma as a likely cause. As in adults, breast dimpling may occur in adolescents when trauma leads to fatty tissue necrosis.

Patient counseling

Provide a clear explanation of diagnostic tests that may be ordered, such as mammography, thermography, ultrasonography, cytology of nipple discharge, and biopsy. Discuss breast self-examination, and provide follow-up teaching when the patient expresses a readiness to learn. If a breast-feeding patient has mastitis, advise her to pump her breasts to prevent further milk stasis, to discard the milk, and to substitute formula until the breast infection responds adequately to antibiotic therapy.

REFERENCES

1. Yamamoto, D.S. and Viale, P.H. "Does Every Breast Lump Need to Be Worked Up Despite Previous Diagnosis?" *Clinical Journal of Oncology Nursing* 10(6):821-823, December 2006.
2. Barron, M. and Fishel, R. "Talk to Your Patients About Breast Disease." *The Nurse Practitioner* 32(10):22-32, October 2007.

● BREAST WITH FRUITY ODOR

Fruity breath odor results from respiratory elimination of excess acetone. This sign characteristically occurs in ketoacidosis, a potentially life-threatening condition that requires immediate treatment to prevent severe dehydration, irreversible coma, and death. Diabetic ketoacidosis may cause more than 100,000 hospital admissions in the U.S., and it has a mortality rate of 8% to 33%.[1]

Ketoacidosis results from the excessive catabolism of fats for cellular energy in the absence of usable carbohydrates. This process begins when insulin levels are insufficient to transport glucose into the cells, as in diabetes mellitus, or when glucose is unavailable and hepatic glycogen stores are depleted, as in low-carbohydrate diets and malnutrition. Lacking glucose, the cells burn fat faster than enzymes can handle the ketones, the acidic end products. As a result, the ketones (acetone, beta-hydroxybutyric acid, and acetoacetic acid) accumulate in the blood and urine. To compensate for increased acidity, Kussmaul's respirations expel carbon dioxide with enough acetone to flavor the breath. Eventually, this compensatory mechanism fails, producing ketoacidosis.

When you detect fruity breath odor, check for Kussmaul's respirations and assess the patient's level of consciousness (LOC). Take vital signs and check skin turgor. Be alert for fruity breath odor that accompanies rapid, deep respirations; stupor; and poor skin turgor. Try to obtain a brief history, noting especially diabetes mellitus, nutritional problems such as anorexia nervosa, and fad diets with few or no carbohydrates. Ensure a patent airway; oxygen therapy, an oral airway, or intubation may be needed.[1] Obtain venous and arterial blood samples for complete blood count and glucose, electrolyte, acetone, and arterial blood gas (ABG) levels. Also obtain a urine specimen to test for glucose and acetone. Administer I.V. fluids and electrolytes to maintain hydration and electrolyte balance, and give regular insulin to patients with diabetic ketoacidosis to reduce blood glucose levels. Potassium replacement may be needed because osmotic diuresis depletes potassium.[1]

If the patient is obtunded, you'll need to insert endotracheal and nasogastric (NG) tubes. Suction as needed. Insert an indwelling urinary catheter, and monitor intake and output. Insert central venous pressure and arterial lines to monitor the patient's fluid status and blood pressure. Connect the patient to a cardiac monitor, monitor vital signs and neurologic status, and draw blood hourly to check glucose, electrolyte, acetone, and ABG levels.

History and physical examination

If the patient isn't in severe distress, obtain a thorough history. Ask about the onset and duration of fruity breath odor. Also ask about any changes in breathing pattern, increased thirst, frequent urination, weight loss, fatigue,

and abdominal pain. Ask the female patient if she has had candidal vaginitis or vaginal secretions with itching. If the patient has a history of diabetes mellitus, ask about stress, infections, and noncompliance with therapy—the most common causes of ketoacidosis in known diabetics. If the patient may have anorexia nervosa, obtain a dietary and weight history.

Medical causes

▶ *Anorexia nervosa.* Severe weight loss from anorexia nervosa may produce fruity breath odor, usually with nausea, constipation, and cold intolerance. Induced vomiting may cause dental enamel erosion and scars or calluses in the dorsum of the hand.

▶ *Ketoacidosis.* Fruity breath odor accompanies alcoholic ketoacidosis, which is usually seen in poorly nourished alcoholics with a history of vomiting, abdominal pain, and only minimal food intake over several days. Kussmaul's respirations begin abruptly and accompany dehydration, abdominal pain and distention, and absent bowel sounds. Blood glucose levels are normal or slightly decreased.

In diabetic ketoacidosis, fruity breath odor commonly acompanies the development of ketoacidosis over 1 to 2 days. Other findings include polydipsia, polyuria, nocturia, weak and rapid pulse, hunger, weight loss, weakness, fatigue, nausea, vomiting, and abdominal pain. Eventually, Kussmaul's respirations, orthostatic hypotension, dehydration, tachycardia, confusion, and stupor occur. Signs and symptoms may lead to coma.

Starvation ketoacidosis is a potentially life-threatening disorder that has a gradual onset. Besides fruity breath odor, typical findings include signs of cachexia and dehydration, decreased LOC, bradycardia, and a history of anorexia nervosa.

Other causes

DRUG WATCH *Any drug known to cause metabolic acidosis, such as nitroprusside and salicylates, can result in fruity breath odor.*

▶ *Low-carbohydrate diets.* Diets that promote little or no carbohydrate intake may cause ketoacidosis and the resulting fruity breath odor.

Special considerations

Provide emotional support for the patient and his family. Explain tests and treatments clearly. When the patient is more alert and his condition stabilizes, remove the NG tube and start him on an appropriate diet. Switch his insulin from the I.V. to the subcutaneous route.

Pediatric pointers

Fruity breath odor in an infant or a child usually stems from uncontrolled diabetes mellitus and signals the onset of diabetic ketoacidosis.[2] Ketoacidosis develops rapidly in this age-group because of their low glycogen reserves and is the leading cause of death in children with type 1 diabetes mellitus.[2] As a result, prompt administration of insulin and correction of fluid and electrolyte imbalance are necessary to prevent shock and death.

Patient counseling

Patient teaching and referrals should be based on the underlying cause. For example, teach the patient with uncontrolled diabetes mellitus to recognize the signs of hyperglycemia and to wear a medical identification bracelet. Provide detailed medication teaching as well as home glucose monitoring instructions.[1] Refer the patient with starvation ketoacidosis to a psychologist or a support group, and recognize the need for possible long-term follow-up.

REFERENCES
1. Brenner, Z. "Management of Hyperglycemic Emergencies." *AACN Clinical Issues: Advanced Practice in Acute and Critical Care* 17(1):56-65, January/March 2006.
2. Steinmann, R. "Pediatric Diabetic Ketoacidosis." *AJN* 107(3):72CC-72KK, March 2007.

BRUDZINSKI'S SIGN

A positive Brudzinski's sign (flexion of the hips and knees in response to passive flexion of the neck) signals meningeal irritation.[1] Passive flexion of the neck stretches the nerve roots, causing pain and involuntary flexion of the knees and hips.

Brudzinski's sign is a common and important early indicator of life-threatening meningitis and subarachnoid hemorrhage. It can be elicited in children and adults, although more reliable indicators of meningeal irritation exist for infants.

Testing for Brudzinski's sign isn't part of a routine physical examination unless meningeal irritation is suspected. (See *Testing for Brudzinski's sign,* page 76.)

If the patient is alert, ask him about headache, neck pain, nausea, and vision disturbances (blurred or double vision and photophobia)—all indications of increased intracranial pressure (ICP). Next, observe the patient for signs and symptoms of increased ICP, such as an altered level of consciousness (LOC), pupillary changes, bradycardia, widened pulse pressure, irregular respiratory patterns (Cheyne-Stokes or Kussmaul's respirations), vomiting, and moderate fever.

Keep artificial airways, intubation equipment, a handheld resuscitation bag, and suction equipment on hand because the patient's condition may suddenly deteriorate. Elevate the head of his bed 30 to 60 degrees to promote venous drainage. Administer an osmotic diuretic, such as mannitol, to reduce cerebral edema.

Be alert for further increases in ICP. You may have to provide mechanical ventilation and administer a barbiturate and additional doses of a diuretic. Also, cerebrospinal fluid (CSF) may have to be drained.

History and physical examination

Continue your neurologic examination by evaluating the patient's cranial nerve function and noting any motor or sensory deficits. Be sure to look for Kernig's sign (resistance to knee extension after flexion of the hip), a further indication of meningeal irritation. Also look for signs of central nervous system infection, such as fever and nuchal rigidity.

Ask the patient—or his family, if necessary—about a history of hypertension, spinal arthritis, or recent head trauma. Also ask about dental work and abscessed teeth (a pos-

Testing for Brudzinski's sign

Here's how to test for Brudzinski's sign when you suspect meningeal irritation:

With the patient in a supine position, place your hands behind her neck and lift her head toward her chest.

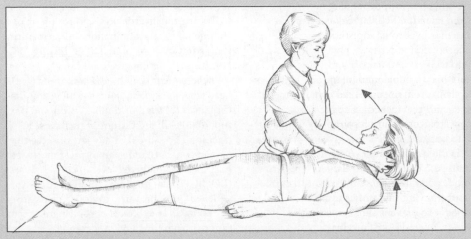

If your patient has meningeal irritation, she'll flex her hips and knees in response to the passive neck flexion.

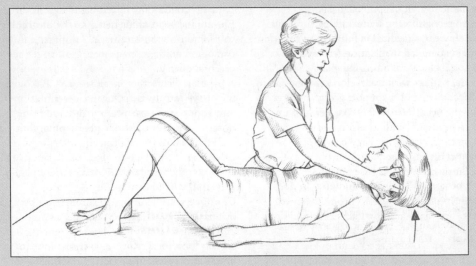

sible cause of meningitis), open-head injury, endocarditis, and I.V. drug abuse. Ask about the sudden onset of headaches, which may be associated with subarachnoid hemorrhage.

Medical causes

▶ *Arthritis.* A positive Brudzinski's sign occasionally can be elicited in patients with severe spinal arthritis. The patient also may report back pain (especially after weight bearing) and limited mobility.

▶ *Meningitis.* A positive Brudzinski's sign usually can be elicited 24 hours after the onset of meningitis, a life-threatening disorder. Other findings may include headache, a positive Kernig's sign, nuchal rigidity, irritability or restlessness, deep stupor or coma, vertigo, fever (high or low, depending on the severity of the infection), chills, malaise, hyperalgesia, muscular hypotonia, opisthotonos, symmetrical deep tendon reflexes, papilledema, ocular and facial palsies, nausea and vomiting, photophobia, diplopia, and unequal, sluggish pupils. As ICP rises, arterial hypertension, bradycardia, widened pulse pressure, Cheyne-Stokes or Kussmaul's respirations, and coma may develop.

▶ *Subarachnoid hemorrhage.* A positive Brudzinski's sign may be elicited in subarachnoid hemorrhage, a life-threatening disorder.[2] Accompanying signs and symptoms include sudden onset of a severe headache, nuchal rigidity, altered LOC, dizziness, photophobia, cranial nerve palsies (as evidenced by ptosis, pupil dilation, and limited extraocular muscle movement), nausea and vomiting, fever, and a positive Kernig's sign. Focal signs—such as hemiparesis, vision disturbances, and aphasia—may also occur. As ICP rises, arterial hypertension, bradycardia, widened pulse pressure, Cheyne-Stokes or Kussmaul's respirations, and coma may develop.

Special considerations

Many patients with a positive Brudzinski's sign are critically ill. They need constant ICP monitoring and frequent neurologic checks in addition to intensive assessment and monitoring of vital signs, intake and output, and cardiorespiratory status. To promote patient comfort, maintain low lights and minimal noise and elevate the head of the bed. The patient usually won't receive an opioid analgesic because it may mask signs of increased ICP.

Pediatric pointers

Brudzinski's sign may not be a useful indicator of meningeal irritation in infants until age 12 to 18 months.[3] Be alert for signs such as bulging fontanels, a high-pitched cry, fretfulness, seizures, vomiting, and poor feeding that indicate meningitis in this young population.

Patient counseling

Prepare the patient for diagnostic tests. These may include blood, urine, and sputum cultures to identify bacteria; lumbar puncture to assess CSF and relieve pressure; and computed tomography scan, magnetic resonance imaging, cerebral angiography, or spinal X-rays to locate a hemorrhage.

REFERENCES
1. Lawes, R. "Uncovering the Layers of Meningitis and Encephalitis." *Nursing Made Incredibly Easy!* 5(4):26-35, July/August 2007.
2. Reddy, L.C.S. "Heads Up on Cerebral Bleeds." *Nursing* 36(5) ED Insider:4-9, Spring 2006.
3. Hockenberry, M.J. and Wilson, D. (Eds.) *Wong's Nursing Care of Infants and Children.* 8th ed. St. Louis: Mosby, 2007.

● BRUITS

Commonly an indicator of life- or limb-threatening vascular disease, bruits are swishing sounds caused by turbulent blood flow. They're characterized by location, duration, intensity, pitch, and time of onset in the cardiac cycle. Loud bruits produce intense vibration and a palpable thrill. A thrill, however, doesn't provide any further clue to the causative disorder or its severity.

Bruits are most significant when heard over the abdominal aorta; the renal, carotid, femoral, popliteal, or subclavian artery; or the thyroid gland. (See *Preventing false bruits,* page 78.) They're also significant when heard consistently despite changes in patient position and when heard during diastole.

History and physical examination

If you detect bruits over the abdominal aorta, check for a pulsating mass or a bluish discoloration around the umbilicus (Cullen's sign). Either of these signs—or severe, tearing pain in the abdomen, flank, or lower back—may signal life-threatening dissection of an aortic aneurysm. Also check peripheral pulses, comparing intensity in the upper and lower limbs.

Preventing false bruits

Auscultating bruits accurately requires practice and skill. These sounds typically stem from arterial luminal narrowing or arterial dilation, but they can also result from excessive pressure applied to the stethoscope's bell during auscultation. This pressure compresses the artery, creating turbulent blood flow and a false bruit.

To prevent false bruits, place the bell lightly on the patient's skin. Also, if you're auscultating for a popliteal bruit, help the patient to a supine position, place your hand behind his ankle, and lift his leg slightly before placing the bell behind the knee.

NORMAL BLOOD FLOW, NO BRUIT

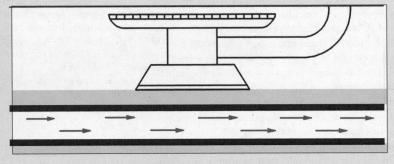

TURBULENT BLOOD FLOW AND RESULTANT BRUIT CAUSED BY ANEURYSM

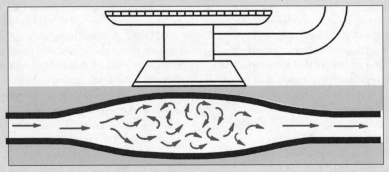

TURBULENT BLOOD FLOW AND FALSE BRUIT CAUSED BY COMPRESSION OF ARTERY

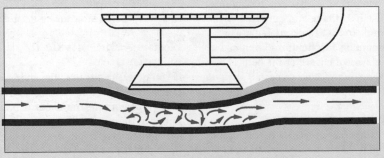

If you suspect dissection, monitor the patient's vital signs continuously, and withhold food and fluids until a definitive diagnosis is made. Watch for signs and symptoms of hypovolemic shock, such as thirst; hypotension; tachycardia; weak, thready pulse; tachypnea; altered level of consciousness (LOC); mottled knees and elbows; and cool, clammy skin.

If you detect bruits over the thyroid gland, ask the patient if he has a history of hyperthyroidism or signs and symptoms of it, such as nervousness, tremors, weight loss, palpitations, heat intolerance, and (in females) amenorrhea. Watch for signs and symptoms of life-threatening thyroid storm, such as tremor, restlessness, diarrhea, abdominal pain, and hepatomegaly.

If you detect carotid artery bruits, be alert for signs and symptoms of a transient ischemic attack (TIA), including dizziness, diplopia, slurred speech, flashing lights, and syncope. These findings may indicate an impending stroke. Be sure to evaluate the patient frequently for changes in LOC and muscle function.

If you detect bruits over the femoral, popliteal, or subclavian artery, watch for signs and symptoms of decreased or absent peripheral circulation—edema, weakness, and paresthesia. Ask the patient if he has a history of intermittent claudication. Frequently check distal pulses and skin color and temperature. Pallor, coolness, or the sudden absence of a pulse may indicate a threat to the affected limb.

If you detect a bruit, be sure to check for further vascular damage and perform a thorough cardiac assessment.

Medical causes

▶ *Abdominal aortic aneurysm.* A pulsating periumbilical mass accompanied by a systolic bruit over the aorta characterizes an abdominal aortic aneurysm. Other signs and symptoms include a rigid, tender abdomen; mottled skin; diminished peripheral pulses; and claudication. Sharp, tearing pain in the abdomen, flank, or lower back signals imminent dissection.

▶ *Abdominal aortic atherosclerosis.* Loud systolic bruits in the epigastric and midabdominal areas are common in this disorder.

They may be accompanied by leg pain, weakness, numbness, paresthesia, or paralysis or by decreased or absent femoral, popliteal, or pedal pulses. Abdominal pain is rare.

▶ *Anemia.* Increased cardiac output in anemia causes increased blood flow. In patients with severe anemia, short systolic bruits may be heard over both carotid arteries and may be accompanied by headache, fatigue, dizziness, pallor, jaundice, palpitations, mild tachycardia, dyspnea, nausea, anorexia, and glossitis.

▶ *Carotid artery stenosis.* Systolic bruits heard over one or both carotid arteries may be the only sign of this disorder.[1] However, dizziness, vertigo, headache, syncope, aphasia, dysarthria, sudden vision loss, hemiparesis, or hemiparalysis signals TIA and may herald a stroke.

▶ *Carotid cavernous fistula.* Continuous bruits heard over the eyeballs and temples are characteristic, as are vision disturbances and protruding, pulsating eyeballs.

▶ *Peripheral arteriovenous fistula.* A rough, continuous bruit with systolic accentuation may be heard over the fistula; a palpable thrill is also common.

▶ *Peripheral vascular disease.* Peripheral vascular disease characteristically produces bruits over the femoral artery and other arteries in the legs. It can also cause diminished or absent femoral, popliteal, or pedal pulses; intermittent claudication; numbness, weakness, pain, and cramping in the legs, feet, and hips; and cool, shiny skin and hair loss on the affected extremity. It also predisposes the patient to lower extremity ulcers that heal with difficulty.

▶ *Renal artery stenosis.* Systolic bruits are commonly heard over the abdominal midline and flank on the affected side. Hypertension commonly accompanies stenosis. Headache, palpitations, tachycardia, anxiety, dizziness, retinopathy, hematuria, and mental sluggishness may also appear.

▶ *Subclavian steal syndrome.* In subclavian steal syndrome, systolic bruits may be heard over one or both subclavian arteries as a result of narrowing of the arterial lumen. They may be accompanied by decreased blood pressure and claudication in the affected arm, hemiparesis, vision disturbances, vertigo, and dysarthria.

▶ *Thyrotoxicosis.* A systolic bruit is commonly heard over the thyroid gland. Accompanying signs and symptoms appear in all body systems, but the most characteristic ones include thyroid enlargement, fatigue, nervousness, tachycardia, heat intolerance, sweating, tremor, diarrhea, and weight loss despite increased appetite. Exophthalmos may also be present.

Special considerations

Because bruits can signal a life-threatening vascular disorder, frequently check the patient's vital signs and auscultate over the affected arteries. Be especially alert for bruits that become louder or develop a diastolic component.

As needed, administer prescribed drugs, such as a vasodilator, an anticoagulant, an antiplatelet drug, or an antihypertensive. Prepare the patient for diagnostic tests, such as blood studies, radiography, an electrocardiogram, cardiac catheterization, and ultrasonography.

Pediatric pointers

Bruits are common in young children but are usually of little significance; for example, cranial bruits are normal until age 4. However, certain bruits may be significant. Because birthmarks commonly accompany congenital arteriovenous fistulas, carefully auscultate for bruits in a child with port-wine spots or cavernous or diffuse hemangiomas.

Geriatric pointers

Elderly people with atherosclerosis may develop bruits over several arteries. Those related to carotid artery stenosis are particularly important because of the increased risk of stroke.[2] Close follow-up is mandatory as well as prompt surgical referral when indicated.

Patient counseling

Instruct the patient to inform the practitioner if he develops dizziness, pain, or any symptom that suggests a stroke because this may indicate a worsening of his condition.

REFERENCES
1. Neal-Boylan, L. "Health Assessment of the Very Old Person at Home." *Home Healthcare Nurse: The Journal for the Home Care and Hospice Professional* 25(6):388-398, June 2007.
2. Mauk, K. "Heeding TIAs: Stroke's Early Warning System." *Nursing* 36(5):20-21, May 2006.

CHEST EXPANSION, ASYMMETRICAL

Asymmetrical chest expansion is the uneven extension of portions of the chest wall during inspiration. Normally, the thorax expands uniformly upward and outward and then contracts downward and inward. When this process is disrupted, breathing becomes uncoordinated, resulting in asymmetrical chest expansion.

Asymmetrical chest expansion may develop suddenly or gradually and may affect one or both sides of the chest wall. It may occur as delayed expiration (chest lag), as abnormal movement during inspiration (for example, intercostal retractions, paradoxical movement, or chest–abdomen asynchrony), or as unilateral absence of movement. This sign usually results from pleural disorders, such as life-threatening hemothorax or tension pneumothorax. (See *Recognizing life-threatening causes of asymmetrical chest expansion*, page 82.) However, it also may result from a musculoskeletal or urologic disorder, airway obstruction, or trauma. Regardless of the underlying cause, asymmetrical chest expansion produces rapid and shallow or deep respirations that increase the work of breathing.

If you detect asymmetrical chest expansion, first consider traumatic injury to the patient's ribs or sternum, which can cause flail chest, a life-threatening emergency characterized by paradoxical chest movement. Quickly take the patient's vital signs and look for signs of acute respiratory distress: rapid and shallow respirations, tachycardia, and cyanosis. Position the patient with the injured side down, and use tape or rolled towels to temporarily splint the unstable flail segment.[1] Don't use sandbags; their weight may further hamper the patient's respiratory efforts.[1]

Depending on the severity of respiratory distress, give oxygen by nasal cannula, mask, or mechanical ventilator. Insert an I.V. line for fluid replacement and delivery of analgesics. Avoid giving excessive IV fluids, which could worsen edema at the site of lung injury.[1] Draw a blood sample for arterial blood gas analysis, and connect the patient to a cardiac monitor.

Although asymmetrical chest expansion may result from hemothorax, tension pneumothorax, bronchial obstruction, and other life-threatening causes, it isn't a cardinal sign of these disorders. Because any form of asymmetrical chest expansion can compromise the patient's respiratory status, don't leave the patient unattended, and be alert for signs of respiratory distress.

History and physical examination

If you don't suspect flail chest and if the patient isn't in acute respiratory distress, obtain a brief history. Asymmetrical chest expansion commonly results from mechanical airflow obstruction, so find out if the patient has dyspnea or pain during breathing. If so, does he feel short of breath constantly or intermittently? Does the pain worsen the feeling of breathlessness? Does repositioning, coughing, or any other activity relieve or worsen the dyspnea or pain? Is the pain more noticeable

Recognizing life-threatening causes of asymmetrical chest expansion

Asymmetrical chest expansion can result from several life-threatening disorders. Two common caus-es—bronchial obstruction and flail chest—produce distinctive chest wall movements that provide important clues about the underlying disorder.

In *bronchial obstruction,* only the unaffected portion of the chest wall expands during inspiration. Intercostal bulging during expiration may indicate that air is trapped in the chest.

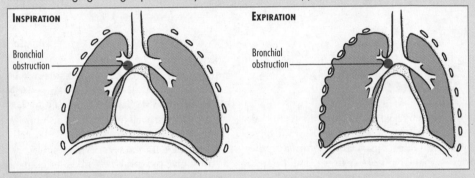

In *flail* chest—a disruption of the thorax from multiple rib fractures—the unstable portion of the chest wall collapses inward during inspiration and balloons outward during expiration.

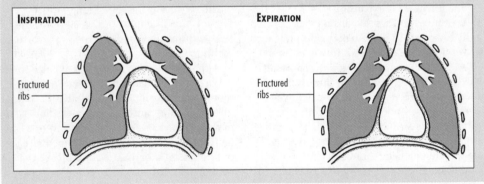

during inspiration or expiration? Can he inhale deeply?

Ask if the patient has a history of pulmonary or systemic illness, such as frequent upper respiratory tract infections, asthma, tuberculosis, pneumonia, or cancer. Has he had thoracic surgery? (This typically produces asymmetrical chest expansion on the affected side.) Also, ask about blunt or penetrating chest trauma, which may have caused pulmonary injury. Obtain an occupational history to find out if the patient may have inhaled toxic fumes or aspirated a toxic substance.

Next, perform a physical examination. Begin by gently palpating the trachea for midline positioning. (Deviation of the trachea usually indicates an acute problem requiring immediate intervention.) Then examine the posterior chest wall for areas of tenderness or deformity. To evaluate the extent of asymmetrical chest expansion, place your hands—fingers together and thumbs abducted toward the spine—flat on both sections of the lower posterior chest wall. Position your thumbs at the 10th rib, and grasp the lateral rib cage with your hands. As the patient inhales, note the uneven separation of your thumbs, and gauge the distance between them. Then repeat this technique on the upper posterior chest wall. Next, use the ulnar surface of your hand to palpate for vocal or tactile fremitus on both sides of the chest. To check for vocal fremitus, ask the patient to repeat "99" as you proceed. Note any asymmetrical vibrations and areas of enhanced, diminished, or absent fremitus. Then percuss and auscultate to detect air and fluid in the lungs and pleural spaces. Finally, auscultate all lung fields for normal and adventitious breath sounds. Examine the anterior chest wall using the same assessment techniques.

Medical causes

▶ *Bronchial obstruction.* Life-threatening loss of airway patency may occur gradually or suddenly in bronchial obstruction. Typically, lack of chest movement indicates complete obstruction; chest lag signals partial obstruction. If air is trapped in the chest, you may detect intercostal bulging during expiration and hyperresonance on percussion. You also may note dyspnea, accessory muscle use, decreased or absent breath sounds, and suprasternal, substernal, or intercostal retractions.

▶ *Flail chest.* In this life-threatening injury to the ribs or sternum, the unstable portion of the chest wall collapses inward during inspiration and balloons outward during expiration (paradoxical movement). Flail chest usually results from traumatic injury.[2] The patient may have ecchymoses, severe localized pain, or other signs of traumatic injury to the chest wall. He also may have rapid, shallow respirations, tachycardia, and cyanosis.

▶ *Hemothorax.* Hemothorax is life-threatening bleeding into the pleural space that causes chest lag during inspiration. It occurs in about 25% of patients with chest trauma.[1] Other findings include signs of traumatic chest injury, stabbing pain at the injury site, anxiety, dullness on percussion, tachypnea, tachycardia, and hypoxemia. If hypovolemia occurs, you'll note signs of shock, such as hypotension and rapid, weak pulse.

▶ *Kyphoscoliosis.* Abnormal curvature of the thoracic spine in the anteroposterior direction (kyphosis) and the lateral direction (scoliosis) gradually compresses one lung and distends the other. This decreases chest wall movement on the compressed-lung side and expands the intercostal muscles during inspiration on the opposite side. It can also produce ineffective coughing, dyspnea, back pain, and fatigue.

▶ *Myasthenia gravis.* Progressive loss of ventilatory muscle function produces chest–abdomen asynchrony during inspiration (known as *abdominal paradox*), which can lead to acute respiratory distress. Typically, shallow respirations and increased muscle weakness cause severe dyspnea, tachypnea and, possibly, apnea.

▶ *Phrenic nerve dysfunction.* In this disorder, the paralyzed hemidiaphragm fails to contract downward, causing asynchrony of the thorax and upper abdomen on the affected side during inspiration (abdominal paradox). Its onset may be sudden, as in trauma, or gradual, as in infection or spinal cord disease. If the patient has underlying pulmonary dysfunction that contributes to hyperventilation, his inability to breathe deeply or to cough effectively may cause atelectasis of the affected lung.

▶ *Pleural effusion.* Chest lag at end-inspiration occurs gradually in this life-threatening accumulation of fluid, blood, or pus in the pleural space. Usually, some combination of dyspnea, tachypnea, and tachycardia precedes chest lag; the patient also may have pleuritic pain that worsens with coughing or deep breathing. The area of the effusion is delineated by dullness on percussion and by egophony, bronchophony, whispered pectoriloquy, decreased or absent breath sounds, and decreased tactile fremitus. The patient may have a fever if infection caused the effusion.

▶ *Pneumonia.* Depending on whether fluid consolidation in the lungs develops unilaterally or bilaterally, asymmetrical chest expansion occurs as inspiratory chest lag or as chest–abdomen asynchrony. The patient typically has fever, chills, tachycardia, tachypnea, and dyspnea along with crackles, rhonchi, and chest pain that worsens during deep breathing. He also may be fatigued and anorexic and have a productive cough with rust-colored sputum.

▶ *Pneumothorax.* Trapped air in the pleural space can cause chest lag at end-inspiration. This life-threatening condition also causes sudden, stabbing chest pain that may radiate to the arms, face, back, or abdomen and dyspnea unrelated to the severity of chest pain. Other findings include tachypnea, decreased tactile fremitus, tympany on percussion, decreased or absent breath sounds over the trapped air, tachycardia, restlessness, and anxiety.

Tension pneumothorax produces the same signs and symptoms as pneumothorax, but they're much more severe. A tension pneumothorax rapidly compresses the heart and great vessels, causing cyanosis, hypotension, tachycardia, restlessness, and anxiety. The patient also may develop subcutaneous crepitation of the upper trunk, neck, and face. Mediastinal and tracheal deviation away from the affected side are classic signs.[1] Auscultation of a crunching sound over the precordium with each heartbeat indicates pneumomediastinum.

▶ *Poliomyelitis.* Although rare in the U.S., polio still exists in third world and developing countries. In this disorder, paralysis of the chest wall muscles and diaphragm produces chest–abdomen asynchrony (abdominal paradox), fever, muscle pain, and weakness. Other findings include decreased reflex response in the affected muscles and impaired swallowing and speaking.

▶ *Pulmonary embolism.* This acute, life-threatening disorder causes chest lag; sudden, stabbing chest pain; and tachycardia. The patient usually has severe dyspnea, blood-tinged sputum, pleural friction rub, and acute anxiety.

Other causes

▶ *Treatments.* Asymmetrical chest expansion can result from pneumonectomy and surgical removal of several ribs. Chest lag or the absence of chest movement also may result from intubation of a mainstem bronchus, a serious complication typically caused by incorrect insertion of an endotracheal tube or movement of the tube while it's in the trachea.

Special considerations

If you're caring for an intubated patient, regularly auscultate breath sounds in the lung peripheries to help detect a misplaced tube. If this occurs, prepare the patient for a chest X-ray to allow rapid repositioning of the tube. Maintain the ventilator settings and alarms, as ordered. Because asymmetrical chest expansion increases the work of breathing, supplemental oxygen is usually given during acute events. Assess the patient's respiratory status often.

If the patient has a chest tube in place, change dressings around the insertion site as needed. Be careful not to reposition or dislodge the tube. If the tube dislodges, place a petroleum gauze dressing over the opening immediately to prevent rapid lung collapse. Monitor the patient for chest tube–related complications, including bleeding, infection, and subcutaneous emphysema.[3]

Pediatric pointers

Children are at greater risk than adults for inadvertent intubation of a mainstem bronchus (especially the left bronchus). Their breath sounds usually are referred from one lung to the other because of the small size of the thoracic cage, so use chest wall expansion as an indicator of correct tube position in children. Children also develop asymmetrical chest expansion, paradoxical breathing, and retractions with acute respiratory illnesses, such as bronchiolitis, asthma, and croup. Children are less likely than adults to have a flail chest injury because of the increased compliance of their thoracic cage.[2]

Congenital abnormalities, such as cerebral palsy and diaphragmatic hernia, also can cause asymmetrical chest expansion. In cerebral palsy, asymmetrical facial muscles usually accompany chest–abdomen asynchrony. In a life-threatening diaphragmatic hernia, asymmetrical expansion usually occurs on the left side of the chest.

Geriatric pointers

Asymmetrical chest expansion may be more difficult to detect in elderly patients because of the structural deformities of aging.

Patient counseling

Explain all procedures and tests, especially if the patient is intubated. Teach the patient and his family early signs of infection.

REFERENCES

1. Yamamoto, L., Schroeder, C., Morley, D., and Beliveau, C. "Thoracic Trauma: The Deadly Dozen." *Critical Care Nursing Quarterly* 28(1):22-40, January/March 2005.
2. Gipson, C. and Tobias, J. "Flail Chest in a Neonate Resulting from Nonaccidental Trauma." *Southern Medical Journal* 99(5):536-538, May 2006.
3. Coughlin, A. and Parchinsky, C. "Go With The Flow of Chest Tube Therapy." *Nursing* 36(3):36-41, March 2006.

CHEST PAIN

Chest pain is one of the most common symptoms and also one of the most difficult to diagnose.[1] An important indicator of several acute and life-threatening cardiopulmonary and GI disorders, chest pain also may result from a musculoskeletal or hematologic disorder, anxiety, or drug therapy. It usually results from disorders that affect thoracic or abdominal organs—the heart, pleurae, lungs, esophagus, rib cage, gallbladder, pancreas, or stomach.

Chest pain may arise suddenly or gradually, and its cause may be difficult to ascertain initially. Pain may radiate to the arms, neck, jaw, or back. It may be steady or intermittent and mild or acute. It may range in character from a sharp, shooting sensation to a feeling of heaviness, fullness, or even indigestion. It may be provoked or aggravated by stress, anxiety, exertion, deep breathing, or eating certain foods. Keep in mind that some groups, such as women, older adults, and patients with diabetes, may be less likely to have chest pain and more likely to have dyspnea, nausea, vomiting, diaphoresis, or unexplained fatigue.[1,2]

Ask the patient when his chest pain began. Did it develop suddenly or gradually? Is it more severe or frequent now than when it first started? Does anything relieve the pain? Does anything aggravate it? Ask the patient about related symptoms. Sudden, severe chest pain requires prompt evaluation and treatment because it may herald a life-threatening disorder. (See *Managing severe chest pain*, page 86.)

History and physical examination

The key to a proper diagnosis is a thorough, detailed history.[1] If the chest pain isn't severe, proceed with the history. Ask if the patient feels diffuse pain or can point to the painful area. Sometimes a patient won't perceive the sensation he's feeling as pain, so ask whether he has any discomfort radiating to his neck, jaw, arms, or back. If he does, ask him to describe it. Is it a dull, aching, pressurelike sensation? A sharp, stabbing, knifelike pain? Does he feel it on the surface or deep inside? On a scale of 0 to 10, with 0 being no pain and 10 being the worst pain possible, how does he rate his pain?[3] Find out whether it's constant or intermittent. If it's intermittent, how long does it last? Ask if movement, exertion, breathing, position changes, or eating certain foods worsens or helps relieve the pain. Does anything in particular seem to bring it on? Ask if the patient has other symptoms, such as dyspnea, nausea, vomiting, palpitations, anxiety, light-headedness, or syncope.[1]

Review the patient's history for cardiac or pulmonary disease, chest trauma, intestinal disease, or sickle cell anemia. Find out which drugs he's taking, if any, and ask about recent dosage or schedule changes.

Take the patient's vital signs, noting tachypnea, fever, tachycardia, oxygen saturation, paradoxical pulse, and hypertension or hypotension. Also, look for jugular vein distention and peripheral edema. Observe the patient's breathing pattern, and inspect his chest for asymmetrical expansion. Auscultate his lungs for pleural friction rub, crackles, rhonchi, wheezing, and diminished or absent breath sounds. Next, auscultate for murmurs, clicks, gallops, and pericardial friction rub. Palpate for lifts, heaves, thrills, gallops, tactile fremitus, and abdominal masses or tenderness.

Medical causes

▶ *Acute coronary syndromes.* Unstable angina and acute myocardial infarction (MI), including ST-segment elevation MI (STEMI) and non–ST-segment elevation MI (NSTEMI), are each classified as an acute coronary syn-

Managing severe chest pain

Sudden, severe chest pain may result from one of several life-threatening disorders. Your evaluation and interventions will vary, depending on the location and character of the pain. This flowchart will help you establish priorities for managing this emergency successfully.

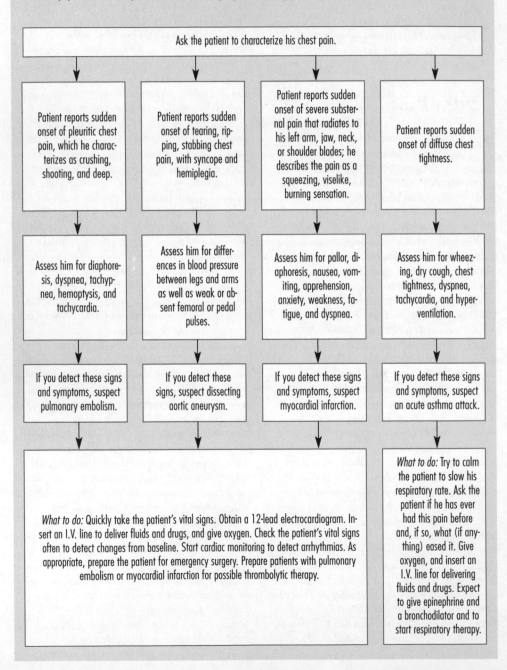

Ask the patient to characterize his chest pain.

Patient reports sudden onset of pleuritic chest pain, which he characterizes as crushing, shooting, and deep.

Patient reports sudden onset of tearing, ripping, stabbing chest pain, with syncope and hemiplegia.

Patient reports sudden onset of severe substernal pain that radiates to his left arm, jaw, neck, or shoulder blades; he describes the pain as a squeezing, viselike, burning sensation.

Patient reports sudden onset of diffuse chest tightness.

Assess him for diaphoresis, dyspnea, tachypnea, hemoptysis, and tachycardia.

Assess him for differences in blood pressure between legs and arms as well as weak or absent femoral or pedal pulses.

Assess him for pallor, diaphoresis, nausea, vomiting, apprehension, anxiety, weakness, fatigue, and dyspnea.

Assess him for wheezing, dry cough, chest tightness, dyspnea, tachycardia, and hyperventilation.

If you detect these signs and symptoms, suspect pulmonary embolism.

If you detect these signs, suspect dissecting aortic aneurysm.

If you detect these signs and symptoms, suspect myocardial infarction.

If you detect these signs and symptoms, suspect an acute asthma attack.

What to do: Quickly take the patient's vital signs. Obtain a 12-lead electrocardiogram. Insert an I.V. line to deliver fluids and drugs, and give oxygen. Check the patient's vital signs often to detect changes from baseline. Start cardiac monitoring to detect arrhythmias. As appropriate, prepare the patient for emergency surgery. Prepare patients with pulmonary embolism or myocardial infarction for possible thrombolytic therapy.

What to do: Try to calm the patient to slow his respiratory rate. Ask the patient if he has ever had this pain before and, if so, what (if anything) eased it. Give oxygen, and insert an I.V. line for delivering fluids and drugs. Expect to give epinephrine and a bronchodilator and to start respiratory therapy.

drome (ACS).[4] Signs and symptoms of ACS are caused by myocardial ischemia.

Patients may describe the resulting chest pain as a burning, squeezing, and crushing tightness in the substernal or precordial chest that may radiate to the left arm or shoulder blade, the neck, or the jaw.[4] This pain usually lasts longer than 15 minutes. Other signs and symptoms may include light-headedness, fainting, sweating, nausea, shortness of breath, or anxiety. However, up to 43% of patients may have atypical chest pain, especially women, elderly patients, and patients with diabetes.[2] Atypical chest pain may appear as discomfort between the shoulder blades, palpitations, a feeling of fullness in the neck, nausea, abdominal discomfort, dizziness, unexplained fatigue, and exhaustion or shortness of breath.

▶ *Angina pectoris.* A patient with angina pectoris may have tightness or pressure in the chest that he describes as pain or a sensation of indigestion or expansion. The pain usually occurs in the retrosternal region over a palm-sized or larger area. It may radiate to the neck, jaw, and arms, particularly to the inner aspect of the left arm. Angina tends to start gradually, build to a maximum, and then subside slowly. Provoked by exertion, emotional stress, or a heavy meal, the pain typically lasts 2 to 10 minutes (usually no longer than 20 minutes). Other findings include dyspnea, nausea, vomiting, tachycardia, dizziness, diaphoresis, belching, and palpitations. You may hear an atrial gallop (a fourth heart sound [S_4]) or a murmur during an anginal episode.

In Prinzmetal's angina, which results from vasospasm of coronary vessels, chest pain typically occurs when the patient is at rest—or it may awaken him. Other findings may include dyspnea, nausea, vomiting, dizziness, and palpitations. During an attack, you may hear an atrial gallop.

▶ *Anthrax (inhalation).* This acute infectious disease is caused by the gram-positive, spore-forming bacterium *Bacillus anthracis.* Although the disease is most common in wild and domestic grazing animals, such as cattle, sheep, and goats, spores can live in the soil for many years. The disease can occur in humans exposed to infected animals, tissue from infected animals, or intentional spread as a biological weapon. Most natural cases occur in agricultural regions worldwide. Anthrax may occur in cutaneous, inhalation, or GI forms.

Inhalation anthrax results from inhaling aerosolized spores. Initial flulike signs and symptoms include fever, chills, weakness, cough, and chest pain. The disease typically occurs in two stages, with a period of recovery after the initial signs and symptoms. The second stage develops abruptly and causes rapid deterioration marked by fever, dyspnea, stridor, and hypotension; death typically results within 24 hours. Radiologic findings include mediastinitis and symmetrical mediastinal widening.

▶ *Anxiety.* Acute anxiety—commonly known as a panic attack—can produce intermittent, sharp, stabbing pain, typically behind the left breast. This pain isn't related to exertion and lasts only a few seconds, but the patient may have a precordial ache or a sensation of heaviness that lasts for hours or days. Other signs and symptoms include precordial tenderness, palpitations, fatigue, headache, insomnia, breathlessness, nausea, vomiting, diarrhea, and tremors. Panic attacks may be linked with agoraphobia—fear of leaving home or being in open places with other people.

▶ *Aortic aneurysm (dissecting).* In this life-threatening disorder, chest pain usually begins suddenly and is most severe at its onset. The patient describes an excruciating tearing, ripping, stabbing pain. Dissection of the ascending aorta may cause anterior chest and neck pain; dissection of the descending aorta typically causes back pain.[5] The patient also may have abdominal tenderness, a palpable abdominal mass, tachycardia, murmurs, syncope, blindness, loss of consciousness, weakness or transient paralysis of the arms or legs, a systolic bruit, systemic hypotension, asymmetrical brachial pulses, lower blood pressure in the legs than in the arms, and weak or absent femoral or pedal pulses. His skin will be pale, cool, diaphoretic, and mottled below the waist. Capillary refill time is increased in the toes, and palpation reveals decreased pulsation in one or both carotid arteries.

▶ *Asthma.* In a life-threatening asthma attack, diffuse and painful chest tightness arises suddenly along with a dry cough and mild wheezing, which progress to a productive cough, audible wheezing, and severe dyspnea. Related respiratory findings include rhonchi, crackles, prolonged expirations, intercostal and supraclavicular retractions on inspiration, accessory muscle use, flaring nostrils, and tachypnea. The patient also may have anxiety, tachycardia, diaphoresis, flushing, and cyanosis.

▶ *Blast lung injury.* Caused by a percussive shock wave after an explosion, blast lung injury can cause severe chest pain and possibly tearing, contusion, edema, and hemorrhage of the lungs. Worldwide terrorist activity has increased the occurrence of this condition, which also may cause dyspnea, hemoptysis, wheezing, and cyanosis. Chest X-rays, arterial blood gas measurements, and computed tomography scans are common diagnostic tools. Although no definitive guidelines exist for caring for those with blast lung injury, treatment is based on the nature of the explosion, the environment in which it occurred, and any chemical or biological agents involved.

▶ *Blastomycosis.* Besides pleuritic chest pain, this disorder initially produces signs and symptoms like those of a viral upper respiratory tract infection: a dry, hacking, or productive cough (and sometimes hemoptysis), fever, chills, anorexia, weight loss, fatigue, night sweats, and malaise.

▶ *Bronchitis.* In its acute form, this disorder produces burning chest pain or a sensation of substernal tightness. It also produces a cough, initially dry but later productive, that worsens the chest pain. Other findings include a low-grade fever, chills, sore throat, tachycardia, muscle and back pain, rhonchi, crackles, and wheezing. Severe bronchitis causes a fever of 101° to 102° F (38.3° to 38.9° C) and possibly bronchospasm with increased coughing and wheezing.

▶ *Cardiomyopathy.* In hypertrophic cardiomyopathy, angina-like chest pain may occur with dyspnea, a cough, dizziness, syncope, gallops, murmurs, and palpitations.

▶ *Cholecystitis.* This disorder typically produces abrupt epigastric or right-upper-quadrant pain, which may be sharp or intensely aching. Steady or intermittent pain may radiate to the back or the right shoulder. Other findings commonly include nausea,

vomiting, fever, diaphoresis, and chills. Palpation of the right upper quadrant may reveal an abdominal mass, rigidity, distention, or tenderness. Murphy's sign—inspiratory arrest when you palpate the right upper quadrant as the patient takes a deep breath—also may occur.

▶ *Coccidioidomycosis.* In this disorder, pleuritic chest pain occurs with a dry or slightly productive cough. Other effects include fever, rhonchi, wheezing, occasional chills, sore throat, backache, headache, malaise, marked weakness, anorexia, and a macular rash.

▶ *Costochondritis.* Pain and tenderness occur at the costochondral junctions, especially at the second costicartilage. The pain usually can be elicited by palpating the inflamed joint.

▶ *Distention of colon's splenic flexure.* Central chest pain may radiate to the left arm in patients with this disorder. The pain may be relieved by defecation or the passage of flatus.

▶ *Esophageal spasm.* Substernal chest pain may last up to an hour and may radiate to the neck, jaw, arms, or back. It commonly mimics the squeezing or dull sensation of angina. Other signs and symptoms include dysphagia for solid foods, bradycardia, and nodal rhythm.

▶ *Herpes zoster (shingles).* The pain of preeruptive herpes zoster may mimic that of myocardial infarction (MI). Initially, the pain is sharp, shooting, and unilateral. About 4 to 5 days after its onset, small, red, nodular lesions erupt on the painful areas—usually the thorax, arms, and legs—and the chest pain becomes burning. Other findings include fever, malaise, pruritus, and paresthesia or hyperesthesia of the affected areas.

▶ *Hiatal hernia.* Typically, this disorder produces an angina-like sternal burning (heartburn), ache, or pressure that may radiate to the left shoulder and arm. The discomfort commonly occurs after a meal when the patient bends over or lies down. Other findings include a bitter taste and pain while eating or drinking, especially spicy foods and hot drinks.

▶ *Interstitial lung disease.* As this disease advances, the patient may develop pleuritic chest pain with progressive dyspnea, cellophane-type crackles, a nonproductive cough, fatigue, weight loss, decreased exercise tolerance, clubbing, and cyanosis.

▶ *Legionnaires' disease.* This disorder produces pleuritic chest pain, malaise, headache, and possibly diarrhea, anorexia, diffuse myalgia, and general weakness. Within 12 to 24 hours, the patient suddenly develops a high fever and chills, and an initially nonproductive cough progresses to a productive cough with mucoid and then mucopurulent sputum and possibly hemoptysis. Patients also may have flushed skin, mild diaphoresis, prostration, nausea and vomiting, mild temporary amnesia, confusion, dyspnea, crackles, tachypnea, and tachycardia.

▶ *Lung abscess.* Pleuritic chest pain develops insidiously along with a pleural friction rub and a cough that produces copious amounts of purulent, foul-smelling, blood-tinged sputum. The affected side is dull on percussion, and decreased breath sounds and crackles may be heard. The patient also has diaphoresis, anorexia, weight loss, fever, chills, fatigue, weakness, dyspnea, and clubbing.

▶ *Lung cancer.* The chest pain from lung cancer is commonly described as an intermittent aching deep in the chest. If the tumor metastasizes to the ribs or vertebrae, the pain becomes localized, continuous, and gnawing. Other findings include a cough (sometimes blood-tinged), wheezing, dyspnea, fatigue, anorexia, weight loss, and fever.

▶ *Mediastinitis.* This disorder produces severe retrosternal chest pain that radiates to the epigastrium, back, or shoulder and may worsen with breathing, coughing, or sneezing. Other signs and symptoms include chills, fever, and dysphagia.

▶ *Mitral valve prolapse.* Most patients with mitral valve prolapse are asymptomatic, but some may have sharp, stabbing precordial chest pain or precordial ache. The pain can last for seconds or hours and may mimic the pain of ischemic heart disease. The characteristic sign of mitral prolapse is a midsystolic click followed by a systolic murmur at the apex. The patient may have cardiac awareness, migraine headache, dizziness, weakness, episodic severe fatigue, dyspnea, tachycardia, mood swings, and palpitations.

▶ *Muscle strain.* Strained chest, arm, or shoulder muscles may cause a superficial and continuous ache or pulling sensation in the chest. Lifting, pulling, or pushing heavy objects may aggravate this discomfort. With acute muscle strain, the patient may have fatigue, weakness, and rapid swelling of the affected area.

▶ *Nocardiosis.* This disorder causes pleuritic chest pain with a cough that produces thick, tenacious, purulent or mucopurulent, and possibly blood-tinged sputum. Nocardiosis also may cause fever, night sweats, anorexia, malaise, weight loss, and diminished or absent breath sounds.

▶ *Pancreatitis.* Acute pancreatitis usually causes intense epigastric pain that radiates to the back and worsens when the patient is in a supine position. Nausea, vomiting, fever, abdominal tenderness and rigidity, diminished bowel sounds, and crackles at the lung bases also may occur. A patient with severe pancreatitis may be extremely restless and have mottled skin, tachycardia, and cold, sweaty limbs. Fulminant pancreatitis causes massive hemorrhage, shock, and coma.

▶ *Peptic ulcer.* In this disorder, sharp and burning pain usually arises in the epigastric region. The pain typically arises hours after food intake, commonly during the night. It lasts longer than angina-like pain and is relieved by food or an antacid. Other findings include nausea, vomiting (sometimes with blood), melena, and epigastric tenderness.

▶ *Pericarditis.* This disorder produces precordial or retrosternal pain that's aggravated by deep breathing, coughing, position changes, and occasionally by swallowing. The pain is commonly sharp or cutting and radiates to the shoulder and neck. Associated signs and symptoms include pericardial friction rub, fever, tachycardia, and dyspnea. Pericarditis usually follows a viral illness, but several other causes should be considered.

▶ *Plague.* Caused by *Yersinia pestis,* plague is one of the most virulent and, if untreated, most lethal bacterial infections. Most cases are sporadic, but the potential for epidemic spread still exists. Clinical forms include bubonic (the most common), septicemic, and pneumonic plagues. The bubonic form is transmitted to people from the bite of infected fleas. Signs and symptoms include fever, chills, and swollen, inflamed, and tender lymph nodes near the site of the fleabite. Septicemic plague may develop as a complication of untreated bubonic or pneumonic plague and occurs when the plague bacteria enter the bloodstream and multiply. The pneumonic form can be contracted by inhaling respiratory droplets from an infected person or inhaling the organism that has been dispersed in the air through biological warfare. The onset is usually sudden with chills, fever, headache, and myalgia. Pulmonary signs and symptoms include a productive cough, chest pain, tachypnea, dyspnea, hemoptysis, increasing respiratory distress, and cardiopulmonary insufficiency.

▶ *Pleurisy.* The sharp, even knifelike chest pain of pleurisy arises abruptly and reaches maximum intensity within a few hours. The pain is usually unilateral and located in the lower and lateral aspects of the chest. Deep breathing, coughing, or thoracic movement characteristically aggravates it. Auscultation over the painful area may reveal decreased breath sounds, inspiratory crackles, and a pleural friction rub. Dyspnea, rapid and shallow breathing, cyanosis, fever, and fatigue also may occur.

▶ *Pneumonia.* This disorder produces pleuritic chest pain that increases with deep inspiration and is accompanied by shaking chills and fever. The patient has a dry cough that later becomes productive. Other signs and symptoms include crackles, rhonchi, tachycardia, tachypnea, myalgia, fatigue, headache, dyspnea, abdominal pain, anorexia, cyanosis, decreased breath sounds, and diaphoresis.

▶ *Pneumothorax.* Spontaneous pneumothorax, a life-threatening disorder, causes sudden severe, sharp chest pain that increases with chest movement; it's typically unilateral and rarely localized. When the pain is centrally located and radiates to the neck, it may mimic that of an MI. After the pain's onset, dyspnea and cyanosis progressively worsen. Breath sounds are decreased or absent on the affected side with hyperresonance or tympany, subcutaneous crepitation, and decreased vocal fremitus. Asymmetrical chest expansion, accessory muscle use, a nonproductive cough, tachypnea, tachycardia, anxiety, and restlessness also occur.

▶ *Psittacosis.* This disorder may produce pleuritic chest pain on rare occasions. It typically begins abruptly with chills, fever, headache, myalgia, epistaxis, and prostration.

▶ *Pulmonary actinomycosis.* This disorder causes pleuritic chest pain with a cough that's initially dry but later produces purulent sputum. The patient also may have hemoptysis, fever, weight loss, fatigue, weakness, dyspnea, and night sweats. Multiple sinuses may extend through the chest wall and drain externally.

▶ *Pulmonary embolism.* After dyspnea, pleuritic chest pain is the most common symptom of this disorder.[6] This intense angina-like or pleuritic pain is aggravated by deep breathing and thoracic movement. Other findings include tachycardia, tachypnea, cough (nonproductive or producing blood-tinged sputum), low-grade fever, restlessness, diaphoresis, crackles, pleural friction rub, diffuse wheezing, dullness on percussion, signs of circulatory collapse (weak, rapid pulse; hypotension), paradoxical pulse, signs of cerebral ischemia (transient unconsciousness, coma, seizures), signs of hypoxia (restlessness) and, particularly in the elderly, hemiplegia and other focal neurologic deficits. Less common signs include massive hemoptysis, chest splinting, and leg edema. A patient with a large embolus may have cyanosis and distended neck veins.

▶ *Pulmonary hypertension (primary).* Angina-like pain develops late in this disorder, usually on exertion. The precordial pain may radiate to the neck but doesn't usually radiate to the arms. Other signs and symptoms typically include exertional dyspnea, fatigue, syncope, weakness, cough, and hemoptysis.

▶ *Q fever.* Q fever is a rickettsial disease caused by *Coxiella burnetii,* an organism found in cattle, sheep, and goats. Human infection usually results from exposure to contaminated milk, urine, feces, or other fluids from infected animals, but it also may result from inhaling contaminated barnyard dust. *C. burnetii* is highly infectious and theoretically could be used in biological warfare. Signs and symptoms include fever, chills, severe headache, malaise, chest pain, nausea, vomiting, and diarrhea. The fever may last up to 2 weeks. In severe cases, the patient may develop hepatitis or pneumonia.

▶ *Rib fracture.* The chest pain caused by fractured ribs is usually sharp, severe, and aggravated by inspiration, coughing, or pressure on the affected area. Besides shallow, splinted respirations, dyspnea, and cough, the patient will have slight edema at the fracture site.

▶ *Sickle cell crisis.* The chest pain of sickle cell crisis typically has a bizarre distribution. It may start as a vague pain, commonly in the back, hands, or feet. As the pain worsens, it becomes generalized or localized to the abdomen or chest, causing severe pleuritic pain. The presence of chest pain and trouble breathing requires prompt intervention. The patient also may have abdominal distention and rigidity, dyspnea, fever, and jaundice.

▶ *Thoracic outlet syndrome.* Often causing paresthesia along the ulnar distribution of the arm, this syndrome can be confused with angina, especially when it affects the left arm. The patient usually has angina-like pain after lifting his arms above his head, working with his hands above his shoulders, or lifting a weight. The pain disappears as soon as he lowers his arms. Other signs and symptoms include pale skin and a difference in blood pressure between arms.

▶ *Tuberculosis.* Pleuritic chest pain and fine crackles occur after coughing in a patient with tuberculosis. Other signs and symptoms include night sweats, anorexia, weight loss, fever, malaise, dyspnea, easy fatigability, mild to severe productive cough, occasional hemoptysis, dullness on percussion, increased tactile fremitus, and amphoric breath sounds.

▶ *Tularemia.* Also known as *rabbit fever,* this infectious disease is caused by the gram-negative, non–spore-forming bacterium *Francisella tularensis.* This organism is found in wild animals, water, and moist soil, typically in rural areas. It's transmitted to humans through being bitten by an infected insect or tick, handling infected animal carcasses, drinking contaminated water, or inhaling the bacterium. Its use as an airborne agent for biological warfare is theoretically possible. Signs and symptoms after inhalation of the organism include the abrupt onset of fever, chills headache, generalized myalgia, a nonproductive cough, dyspnea, pleuritic chest pain, and empyema.

Other causes

▶ *Chinese restaurant syndrome.* This benign condition—a reaction to excessive ingestion of monosodium glutamate, a common additive in Chinese foods—mimics the signs of an acute MI. The patient may have retrosternal burning, ache, or pressure; a burning sensation over his arms, legs, and face; a sensation of facial pressure; headache; shortness of breath; and tachycardia.

DRUG WATCH *If the patient has coronary artery disease, abrupt withdrawal of a beta blocker can cause rebound angina, especially if he took large doses for a long time.*

Special considerations

As needed, prepare the patient for cardiopulmonary studies, such as an electrocardiogram and a lung scan. Perform a venipuncture to collect a serum sample for cardiac enzyme and other studies. Assess the cardiovascular system often, and interpret changes in cardiac rhythm. Patients who come to the emergency department with chest pain and those in the early stages of ACS should have continuous ST-segment monitoring, a specialized type of ECG monitoring that allows early detection of ischemic events.[7,8] (See *Decreasing LOS of patients with chest pain,* page 92.) Be prepared for emergency procedures.

Pediatric pointers

Even children old enough to talk may have trouble describing chest pain, so be alert for nonverbal clues, such as restlessness, grimacing, or holding the painful area. Ask the child to point to the painful area and then to where the pain goes (to find out if it's radiating). Determine the pain's severity by asking the parents if the pain interferes with the child's normal activities and behavior.

Geriatric pointers

Because older patients have a higher risk of life-threatening conditions (such as an MI, angina, and aortic dissection), you must evaluate chest pain carefully in these patients. Many elderly patients have atypical chest pain, such as dyspnea (most common), fatigue, and discomfort in the upper abdomen.[1] Additional atypical signs and symptoms in

Decreasing LOS of patients with chest pain

Question: *Is an emergency department observation unit (EDOBS) effective in decreasing length of stay (LOS) in patients presenting with unspecified chest pain?*

Research: While heart disease is a leading cause of death, only 20% of patients with chest pain are considered high-risk and require immediate intervention. Other patients, who are at intermediate risk, require observation and monitoring until a diagnosis is made. The cited study examined the benefits of an EDOBS unit, separate from the emergency department (ED), where this observation and monitoring could take place.

A retrospective chart review of 92 charts randomly selected by the medical records department of a large hospital system in the Detroit area was performed. Equal numbers of charts from before and after the establishment of the EDOBS were analyzed. Data collected included gender, age, race and ethnicity, time of ED registration, time of admission to the EDOBS (when applicable), hospital admission time, discharge time, diagnostic tests, laboratory results, final disposition, and discharge diagnosis. Patients older than age 18 presenting with chest pain and who had low risk factors for an acute coronary event were included.

In the EDOBS, an experienced emergency nurse practitioner (ENP) facilitated and coordinated care. A designated ED physician was assigned to be available for consultation. The responsibilities of the ENP included facilitating consults, reviewing diagnostic and laboratory results, and expediting hospital admission or discharge from the EDOBS.

Conclusion: The EDOBS group had a decrease in LOS by 2.7 days. For the inpatient group, the time from ED registration to the unit was 6.4 hours and the time from the unit to discharge was 80 hours. The EDOBS group had an ED registration time to unit of 3.5 hours and time from EDOBS to discharge was 16 hours.

Application: Teach ED staff and administrators about the benefits of EDOBS. Present research data, such as the information demonstrated by this study. Reassure patients with unspecified chest pain about the high quality of care in the EDOBS. Inform patients about the role of the ENP and cardiac monitoring and diagnostic measures that will occur in the EDOBS.

Source: Beck, L. A., Musial, F., & Barrett, C. L. "Using ED Observation Units to Decrease Length of Stay in Chest Pain Patients." *Advanced Emergency Journal* 29(2):140-144, 2007.

---

older adults include sweating, nausea, weakness, and confusion.[2]

Patient counseling

Explain the purpose and procedure of each diagnostic test to help reduce the patient's anxiety. Prepare him for cardiac catheterization or fibrinolytic therapy, as needed. Explain the purpose of any prescribed drugs, and make sure the patient understands the dosage, schedule, and possible adverse effects.

Teach patients with coronary artery disease about the typical features of cardiac ischemia as well as the symptoms that require prompt medical attention. Teach him how to use sublingual nitroglycerin, and urge him to seek medical attention if the pain lasts more than 20 minutes, fails to respond to nitroglycerin, or has a different pattern than his usual angina.

REFERENCES

1. Reigle, J. "Evaluating the Patient with Chest Pain: The Value of A Comprehensive History." *The Journal of Cardiovascular Nursing* 20(4): 226-231, July/August 2005.
2. Ryan, C.J., DeVon, H.A., and Zerwic, J.J. "Typical and Atypical Symptoms: Diagnosing Acute Coronary Syndromes Accurately." *AJN* 105(2):34-36, February 2005.

3. Pope, B.B. "What's Causing Your Patient's Chest Pain?" *Nursing* 36(Supplement): 21-24, Spring 2006.
4. DeVon, H.A., and Ryan, C.J. "Chest Pain and Associated Symptoms of Acute Coronary Syndromes. *The Journal of Cardiovascular Nursing* 20(4):232-238, July/August 2005.
5. Yee, C.A. "Aortic Dissection: The Tear that Kills." *Nursing* 37(Cardiac Insider):1-6, Spring 2007.
6. Charlebois, D. "Early Recognition of Pulmonary Embolism: The Key to Lowering Mortality." *The Journal of Cardiovascular Nursing* 20(4):254-259, July/August 2005.
7. Kumar, D.W. "Cardiac Monitoring: New Trends and Capabilities." *Nursing* 36(Cardiac Insider):7-10, Fall 2006.
8. Flanders, S. "ST-Segment Monitoring: Putting Standards Into Practice." *AACN Advanced Critical Care* 18(3):275-284, July/September 2007.

CHEYNE-STOKES RESPIRATIONS

The most common pattern of periodic breathing, Cheyne-Stokes respirations are characterized by a waxing and waning period of hyperpnea that alternates with a shorter period of apnea. This pattern can occur normally in patients with heart or lung disease, and it occurs in 30% to 40% of patients with heart failure.[1] Cheyne-Stokes respirations usually indicates increased intracranial pressure (ICP) from a deep cerebral or brain stem lesion, or a metabolic disturbance in the brain. (See *Recognizing Cheyne-Stokes respirations.*)

Cheyne-Stokes respirations may indicate a major change in the patient's condition—usually for the worse. For example, in a patient who has had head trauma or brain surgery, Cheyne-Stokes respirations may signal increasing ICP. Cheyne-Stokes respirations can occur normally in patients who live at high altitudes.

If you detect Cheyne-Stokes respirations in a patient with a history of head trauma, recent brain surgery, or another brain insult, quickly take his vital signs. Keep his head elevated 30 degrees, and perform a rapid neurologic examination to obtain baseline data. Reassess the patient's neurologic status often. If

Recognizing Cheyne-Stokes respirations

Cheyne-Stokes respirations are breaths that gradually become faster and deeper than normal, then slower, during a 30- to 170-second period. This pattern alternates with 20- to 60-second periods of apnea.

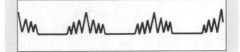

ICP continues to rise, you'll detect changes in the patient's level of consciousness (LOC), pupillary reactions, and ability to move his limbs. ICP monitoring is indicated.

Time the periods of hyperpnea and apnea for 3 to 4 minutes to assess respirations and obtain baseline data. Be alert for prolonged periods of apnea. Monitor pulse oximetry, and check blood pressure often; also check skin color to detect signs of hypoxemia. Maintain airway patency, and give oxygen as needed. If the patient's condition worsens, he'll need endotracheal intubation.

History and physical examination

If the patient's condition permits, obtain a brief history. Ask especially about drug use.

Medical causes

▶ *Adams-Stokes attacks.* Cheyne-Stokes respirations may follow an Adams-Stokes attack—a syncopal episode with atrioventricular block. The patient is hypotensive, with a heart rate between 20 and 50 beats/minute. He also may appear pale, shaking, and confused.

▶ *Heart failure.* Cheyne-Stokes respirations are linked to ventricular ectopy and increased mortality in patients with heart failure.[1,2] In left-sided heart failure, Cheyne-Stokes respirations may occur with exertional dyspnea and orthopnea. Related findings include fatigue, weakness, tachycardia, tachypnea, and crackles. The patient also may have a cough, typically nonproductive but occasionally producing clear or blood-tinged sputum.

▶ *Hypertensive encephalopathy.* In this life-threatening disorder, severe hypertension precedes Cheyne-Stokes respirations. The patient's LOC is decreased, and he may develop vomiting, seizures, severe headaches, vision disturbances (including transient blindness), and transient paralysis.

▶ *Increased ICP.* As ICP rises, Cheyne-Stokes is the first irregular respiratory pattern to occur. It's preceded by a decreased LOC and accompanied by hypertension, headache, vomiting, impaired or unequal motor movement, and vision disturbances (blurring, diplopia, photophobia, and pupillary changes). In late stages of increased ICP, bradycardia and widened pulse pressure occur.

▶ *Renal failure.* End-stage chronic renal failure may produce Cheyne-Stokes respirations, bleeding gums, oral lesions, ammonia breath odor, and marked changes in every body system.

Other causes

DRUG WATCH *Large doses of an opioid, a hypnotic, or a barbiturate can cause Cheyne-Stokes respirations.*

Special considerations

Obtain the patient's vital signs, noting respiratory rate and pattern. When evaluating Cheyne-Stokes respirations, be careful not to mistake periods of hypoventilation or decreased tidal volume for complete apnea.

Pediatric pointers

Cheyne-Stokes respirations rarely occur in children except during late heart failure.

Geriatric pointers

Cheyne-Stokes respirations can occur normally in elderly patients during sleep.

Patient counseling

Inform the patient or his family that sleep apnea and Cheyne-Stokes respirations have different causes and methods of treatment.

REFERENCES

1. Brack, T., Jubran, A., Laghi, F., and Tobin, M.J. "Fluctuations in End-Expiratory Lung Volume During Cheyne-Stokes Respiration." *American Journal of Respiratory and Critical Care Medicine* 171(12):1408-1413, June 2005.
2. Magin, A. and Spiegler, P. "Sleep and Heart Failure: Setting the Boundaries." *Clinical Pulmonary Medicine* 13(2):144-145, March 2006.

CHILLS

Chills, or *rigors,* are extreme, involuntary muscle contractions with characteristic paroxysms of shivering and teeth chattering. Commonly caused by an increased body temperature set by the hypothalamic thermostat, chills usually are accompanied by fever and tend to arise suddenly, heralding the onset of infection. Certain diseases, such as pneumococcal pneumonia, produce only a single, shaking chill. Other diseases, such as malaria, produce intermittent chills with recurring high fever. Still others produce continuous chills for up to 1 hour, precipitating a high fever. (See *Why chills accompany fever.*)

Chills also can result from lymphomas, blood transfusion reactions, and the use of certain drugs. Chills without fever are a normal response to exposure to cold. (See *Rare causes of chills.*)

History and physical examination

Ask the patient when the chills began and whether they're continuous or intermittent. Because fever commonly accompanies or follows chills, take his rectal temperature to obtain a baseline reading. Then check his temperature often to monitor fluctuations and determine his temperature curve. Typically, a localized infection produces a sudden onset of shaking chills, sweats, and high fever, whereas a systemic infection produces intermittent chills with recurring episodes of high fever or continuous chills that may last up to 1 hour and cause a high fever.

Ask about related signs and symptoms, such as headache, malaise, fatigue, dysuria, diarrhea, confusion, abdominal pain, cough,

Why chills accompany fever

Fever usually occurs when exogenous pyrogens activate endogenous pyrogens to reset the body's thermostat to a higher level. At this higher thermostat setpoint, the body feels cold and responds through several compensatory mechanisms, including rhythmic muscle contractions, or chills. These muscle contractions generate body heat and help produce fever. This flowchart outlines the events that link chills to fever.

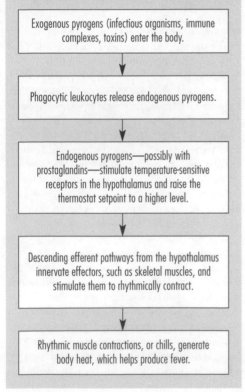

Exogenous pyrogens (infectious organisms, immune complexes, toxins) enter the body.

↓

Phagocytic leukocytes release endogenous pyrogens.

↓

Endogenous pyrogens—possibly with prostaglandins—stimulate temperature-sensitive receptors in the hypothalamus and raise the thermostat setpoint to a higher level.

↓

Descending efferent pathways from the hypothalamus innervate effectors, such as skeletal muscles, and stimulate them to rhythmically contract.

↓

Rhythmic muscle contractions, or chills, generate body heat, which helps produce fever.

Rare causes of chills

Chills can result from disorders that are rare in the United States but may be fairly common worldwide. Remember to ask about recent foreign travel when you obtain a patient's history. Among the many rare disorders that produce chills are:
- brucellosis (undulant fever)
- dengue fever (breakbone fever)
- epidemic typhus (louse-borne typhus)
- leptospirosis
- lymphocytic choriomeningitis
- plague
- pulmonary tularemia
- rat bite fever
- relapsing fever.

sore throat, or nausea. Does the patient have any known allergies, an infection, or a recent history of an infectious disorder? Find out which drugs he's taking and whether any drug has improved or worsened his symptoms. Has he received any treatment that may predispose him to an infection (such as chemotherapy)? Ask about recent exposure to farm animals, guinea pigs, hamsters, dogs, and such birds as pigeons, parrots, and parakeets. Also ask about recent insect or animal bites, travel to foreign countries, and contact with persons who have an active infection.

Medical causes

▶ *Acquired immunodeficiency syndrome.* This commonly fatal disease is caused by infection with human immunodeficiency virus transmitted by blood or semen. The patient usually develops lymphadenopathy and also may experience fatigue, anorexia and weight loss, diarrhea, diaphoresis, skin disorders, and signs of upper respiratory tract infection. Opportunistic infections can cause serious disease in these patients.

▶ *Anthrax (inhalation).* This acute infectious disease is caused by the gram-positive, spore-forming bacterium *Bacillus anthracis*. Although the disease most commonly occurs in wild and domestic grazing animals, such as cattle, sheep, and goats, the spores can live in the soil for many years. The disease can occur in humans exposed to infected animals, tissue from infected animals, or biological agents. Most natural cases occur in agricultural regions worldwide. Anthrax may occur in cutaneous, inhalation, or GI forms.

Inhalation anthrax is caused by inhalation of aerosolized spores. Initial signs and symptoms are flulike and include fever, chills, weakness, cough, and chest pain. The disease generally occurs in two stages with a period of recovery after the initial signs and symptoms. The second stage develops abruptly, causing rapid deterioration marked by fever, dyspnea, stridor, and hypotension; death generally results within 24 hours. Radiologic findings include mediastinitis and symmetrical mediastinal widening.

▶ *Cholangitis*. Charcot's triad—chills with spiking fever, abdominal pain, and jaundice—characterizes sudden obstruction of the common bile duct. The patient may have associated pruritus, weakness, and fatigue.

▶ *Gram-negative bacteremia*. This infection causes sudden chills and fever, nausea, vomiting, diarrhea, and prostration.

▶ *Hemolytic anemia*. In acute hemolytic anemia, fulminating chills occur with fever and abdominal pain. The patient rapidly develops jaundice and hepatomegaly; he may develop splenomegaly.

▶ *Hepatic abscess*. This infection usually arises abruptly, with chills, fever, nausea, vomiting, diarrhea, anorexia, and severe upper abdominal tenderness and pain that may radiate to the right shoulder.

▶ *Hodgkin's disease*. The patient characteristically experiences several days or weeks of fever and chills alternating with periods of no fever and no chills. This disorder commonly produces regional lymphadenopathy that may progress to hepatosplenomegaly. Other findings include diaphoresis, fatigue, and pruritus.

▶ *Infective endocarditis*. This infection produces abrupt onset of intermittent shaking chills with fever. In addition to petechiae, the patient may have Janeway lesions on his hands and feet and Osler's nodes on his palms and soles. Associated findings include murmur, hematuria, eye hemorrhage, Roth's spots, and signs of heart failure (dyspnea, peripheral edema).

▶ *Influenza*. Initially, this disorder causes an abrupt onset of chills, high fever, malaise, headache, myalgia, and nonproductive cough. Some patients also may suddenly develop rhinitis, rhinorrhea, laryngitis, conjunctivitis, hoarseness, and sore throat. Chills typically subside after the first few days, but intermittent fever, weakness, and cough may persist for up to 1 week.

▶ *Legionnaires' disease*. Within 12 to 48 hours after the onset of this disease, the patient suddenly develops chills and a high fever. Prodromal signs and symptoms characteristically include malaise, headache, and possibly diarrhea, anorexia, diffuse myalgia, and general weakness. An initially nonproductive cough progresses to a productive cough with mucoid or mucopurulent sputum and possibly hemoptysis. Most patients also develop nausea and vomiting, confusion, mild temporary amnesia, pleuritic chest pain, dyspnea, tachypnea, crackles, tachycardia, and flushed and mildly diaphoretic skin.

▶ *Lung abscess*. In addition to chills, a lung abscess causes sweating, pleuritic chest pain, dyspnea, clubbing, weakness, headache, malaise, anorexia, weight loss, and a cough that produces large amounts of purulent, foul-smelling and, possibly, bloody sputum.

▶ *Lyme disease*. The bite of a tiny deer tick can transmit this infection, which causes a red macule or papule (erythema migrans) to develop at the bite site. It's accompanied by chills, fever, malaise, fatigue, lymphadenopathy, arthralgia, and rash. If untreated, Lyme disease may cause cranial neuritis with facial palsy, heart blocks, arthritis, and a characteristic sclerotic rash.

▶ *Lymphangitis*. Acute lymphangitis produces chills and other systemic signs and symptoms, such as fever, malaise, and headache. Its characteristic signs are red streaks radiating from a wound and cellulitis draining toward tender regional lymph nodes.

▶ *Lymphogranuloma venereum*. This disorder produces chills, fever, lymphadenopathy, headache, anorexia, myalgia, arthralgia, and weight loss. The primary genital lesion is a papule or small erosion that precedes lymphatic involvement and heals spontaneously within a few days.

▶ *Malaria*. Infection by one of several species of the parasite *Plasmodium* causes cycles of chills, fever, and sweating that last about 10 hours.[1] A cycle starts with chills lasting 1 to 2 hours. This is followed by a high fever lasting 3 to 4 hours and then 2 to 4 hours of profuse diaphoresis. These paroxysms occur every 48 to 72 hours with malaria caused by *P. malariae* and every 42 to 40 hours when caused by *P. vivax* or *P. ovale*. The patient also will have a headache, muscle pain, and possibly hepatosplenomegaly. In benign malaria, the paroxysms may be interspersed with well periods.

▶ *Miliary tuberculosis.* In the acute form of this disease, the patient has intermittent chills, high fever, and night sweats. Epididymal or testicular nodules and splenomegaly also may occur.

▶ *Monkeypox.* Many people infected with this rare virus have chills. Other common initial symptoms include fever, lymphadenopathy, sore throat, dyspnea, muscle aches, and rash. Although monkeypox occurs mainly in central and western Africa, it was confirmed in the United States in 2003 when several people contracted the virus from infected pet prairie dogs. Because the virus is similar to smallpox, the smallpox vaccine is sometimes used to protect people from monkeypox. No treatment is available.

▶ *Otitis media.* Acute suppurative otitis media produces chills with fever and severe deep, throbbing ear pain. The patient usually has mild conductive hearing loss and a bulging, hyperemic tympanic membrane. He also may have dizziness, nausea, and vomiting. When the tympanic membrane ruptures, pus drains out through the ear canal and the patient feels relief.

▶ *Pelvic inflammatory disease.* In this infection, chills and fever typically are accompanied by lower abdominal pain and tenderness; profuse, purulent vaginal discharge; or abnormal menstrual bleeding. The patient also may develop nausea and vomiting, an abdominal mass, and dysuria.

▶ *Plague.* Caused by *Yersinia pestis,* plague is one of the most virulent and, if untreated, lethal bacterial infections known. Most cases are sporadic, but the potential for epidemic spread still exists. Clinical forms include bubonic (the most common), septicemic, and pneumonic plagues. The bubonic form is transmitted to humans from the bite of infected fleas. Signs and symptoms include fever, chills, and swollen, inflamed, and tender lymph nodes near the site of the fleabite. Septicemic plague may develop as a complication of untreated bubonic or pneumonic plague and occurs when the plague bacteria enter the bloodstream and multiply. The pneumonic form can be contracted by inhaling respiratory droplets from an infected person or inhaling the organism that has been dispersed in the air through biological warfare. The onset is usually sudden with chills, fever, headache, and myalgia. Pulmonary signs and symptoms include a productive cough, chest pain, tachypnea, dyspnea, hemoptysis, increasing respiratory distress, and cardiopulmonary insufficiency.

▶ *Pneumonia.* A single shaking chill usually heralds the sudden onset of pneumococcal pneumonia; other pneumonias characteristically cause intermittent chills. In any type of pneumonia, related findings may include fever, productive cough with bloody sputum, pleuritic chest pain, dyspnea, tachypnea, and tachycardia. The patient may be cyanotic and diaphoretic, with bronchial breath sounds and crackles, rhonchi, increased tactile fremitus, and grunting respirations. He also may have achiness, anorexia, fatigue, and headache.

▶ *Psittacosis.* This disease typically begins with the sudden onset of chills, fever, headache, myalgia, epistaxis, and prostration. A dry, hacking cough occurs initially, progressing to pneumonia with a cough that produces small amounts of mucoid, blood-streaked sputum. The patient also has tachypnea, fine crackles, photophobia, abdominal distention and tenderness, nausea, vomiting, a faint macular rash and, rarely, chest pain.

▶ *Pyelonephritis.* In acute pyelonephritis, the patient develops chills, high fever, and possibly nausea and vomiting over several hours to days. He typically also has anorexia, fatigue, myalgia, flank pain, costovertebral angle tenderness, hematuria or cloudy urine, and urinary frequency, urgency, and burning.

▶ *Q fever.* Q fever is a rickettsial disease caused by *Coxiella burnetii,* an organism found in cattle, sheep, and goats. Human infection usually results from exposure to contaminated milk, urine, feces, or other fluids from infected animals, but it also may result from inhalation of contaminated barnyard dust. *C. burnetii* is highly infectious and is considered a possible airborne agent for biological warfare. Signs and symptoms include fever, chills, severe headache, malaise, chest pain, nausea, vomiting, and diarrhea. The fever may last up to 2 weeks. In severe cases, the patient may develop hepatitis or pneumonia.

▶ *Renal abscess*. This abscess initially produces sudden chills and fever. Later effects include flank pain, costovertebral angle tenderness, abdominal muscle spasm, and transient hematuria.

▶ *Rocky Mountain spotted fever*. This disorder begins suddenly with chills, fever, malaise, an excruciating headache, and muscle, bone, and joint pain. Typically, the patient's tongue is covered with a thick white coating that gradually turns brown. After 2 to 6 days of fever and occasional chills, a macular or maculopapular rash appears on the hands and feet and then becomes generalized; after a few days, the rash becomes petechial.

▶ *Sepsis, puerperal or postabortal*. Chills and high fever occur as early as 6 hours or as late as 10 days postpartum or postabortion. The patient also may have a purulent vaginal discharge, an enlarged and tender uterus, abdominal pain, backache and, possibly, nausea, vomiting, and diarrhea.

▶ *Septic arthritis*. Chills and fever accompany red, swollen, and painful joints.

▶ *Septic shock*. Initially, septic shock produces chills, fever and, possibly, nausea, vomiting, and diarrhea. The patient's skin is typically flushed, warm, and dry; his blood pressure is normal or slightly low; and he has tachycardia and tachypnea. As septic shock progresses, the patient's arms and legs become cool and cyanotic, and he has oliguria, thirst, anxiety, restlessness, confusion, and hypotension. Later, he develops cold and clammy skin, a rapid and thready pulse, severe hypotension, persistent oliguria or anuria, signs of respiratory failure, and coma.

▶ *Sinusitis*. In acute sinusitis, chills are accompanied by fever, headache, and pain, tenderness, and swelling over the affected sinuses. Maxillary sinusitis produces pain over the cheeks and upper teeth; ethmoid sinusitis, pain over the eyes; frontal sinusitis, pain over the eyebrows; and sphenoid sinusitis, pain behind the eyes. The primary indicator of sinusitis is nasal discharge, which is commonly bloody for 24 to 48 hours before gradually becoming purulent.

▶ *Snake bite*. Most pit viper bites that result in envenomization cause chills, typically with fever. Other systemic signs and symptoms include sweating, weakness, dizziness, fainting, hypotension, nausea, vomiting, diarrhea, and thirst. The area around the snake bite may be marked by immediate swelling and tenderness, pain, ecchymoses, petechiae, blebs, bloody discharge, and local necrosis. The patient may have trouble speaking, blurred vision, paralysis, bleeding tendencies, and signs of respiratory distress and shock.

▶ *Tularemia*. Also known as *rabbit fever,* this infectious disease is caused by the gram-negative, non–spore-forming bacterium *Francisella tularensis*. This organism is found in wild animals, water, and moist soil, typically in rural areas. People become infected through being bitten by an infected insect or tick, handling infected animal carcasses, drinking contaminated water, or inhaling the bacterium. Theoretically, the airborne organism could be used for biological warfare.[2] Signs and symptoms after inhalation of the organism include the abrupt onset of fever, chills, headache, generalized myalgia, a nonproductive cough, dyspnea, pleuritic chest pain, and empyema.

▶ *Typhoid fever*. This disorder may initially cause sudden chills and a sharply rising fever. More commonly, though, the patient's body temperature gradually increases for 5 to 7 days with accompanying chilliness or frank chills. Headache, abdominal discomfort, constipation, and demonstrable splenomegaly appear by the end of the first week. A characteristic rash called *rose spots* develops on the upper abdomen and anterior thorax during the second week but lasts only 2 to 3 days. Later, the patient may develop a dry cough, epistaxis, mental dullness or delirium, marked abdominal distention, significant weight loss, profound fatigue, and diarrhea. The heart rate may be unusually slow in relation to the high fever.

▶ *Typhus*. Typhus is a rickettsial disease transmitted to humans by fleas, mites, or body lice. Initial signs and symptoms include headache, myalgia, arthralgia, and malaise followed by an abrupt onset of chills, fever, nausea, and vomiting. A maculopapular rash may occur in some cases.

▶ *Violin spider bite.* This bite produces chills, fever, malaise, weakness, nausea, vomiting, and joint pain within 24 to 48 hours. The patient also may have a rash and delirium.

Other causes

DRUG WATCH *Amphotericin B may cause chills. Phenytoin also is a common cause of drug-induced fever that can produce chills. I.V. bleomycin and intermittent use of an oral antipyretic also can cause chills.*

▶ *I.V. therapy.* Infection at the I.V. insertion site (superficial phlebitis) can cause chills, high fever, and local redness, warmth, induration, and tenderness.

▶ *Transfusion reaction.* A hemolytic reaction is an acute emergency that can produce signs and symptoms as early as 5 minutes after starting the infusion, during the infusion, or immediately after the infusion.[3] Chills may be accompanied by fever, diaphoresis, flank pain, or a feeling of impending doom.

Special considerations

Check the patient's vital signs often, especially if his chills result from a known or suspected infection. Watch for signs of progressive septic shock, such as hypotension, tachycardia, and tachypnea. If appropriate, obtain samples of blood, sputum, or wound drainage for culturing to determine the causative organism. Give the appropriate antibiotic. Radiographic studies and serum and urine samples may be required.

If chills occur as a reaction to a blood transfusion, stop the transfusion immediately. Replace the I.V. set with new tubing, and infuse normal saline solution for hydration. Closely monitor the patient's vital signs and respiratory and cardiovascular status.[3]

Because chills are an involuntary response to an increased body temperature, blankets won't stop chills or shivering. Even so, keep his room temperature as steady as possible. Provide adequate hydration and nutrients, and give an antipyretic to help control fever. Irregular use of an antipyretic can trigger compensatory chills.

Pediatric pointers

Infants don't get chills because they have poorly developed shivering mechanisms. In addition, most classic febrile childhood infections, such as measles and mumps, don't typically produce chills. However, older children and teenagers may have chills with mycoplasma pneumonia and acute pyogenic osteomyelitis.

Geriatric pointers

As a person ages, lymphocytes known as helper T cells may lose their ability to function. Therefore, signs and symptoms typical of infection, such as chills or fever, might not be present in older adults.[4] Because infection may not be easily recognizable in this population, diagnosis may be delayed and treatment may be complicated.

Chills in an elderly patient usually indicate an underlying infection, such as a urinary tract infection, pneumonia (often with aspiration of gastric contents), diverticulitis, or skin breakdown in pressure areas. Also, consider an ischemic bowel in an elderly patient who has fever, chills, and abdominal pain.

Patient counseling

Advise the patient to take his temperature with a thermometer when he has chills and to document the exact readings and times. This will help reveal patterns that may point to a specific diagnosis.

REFERENCES

1. Hunter, A., Denman-Vitale, S., Garzon, L., Allen, P.J., and Schumann, L. "Global Infections: Recognition, Management, and Prevention." *The Nurse Practitioner* 32(2):34-41, February 2007.
2. Karwa, M., Currie, B., and Kvetan, V. "Bioterrorism: Preparing for the Impossible or Improbable." *Critical Care Medicine* 33(1):Supplement S75-S95, January 2005.
3. Kyles, D. "Is Your Patient Having a Transfusion Reaction?" *Nursing* 37(4):64hn1-64hn4, April 2007.
4. Durston, S. "Uncompromising Immunocompromised Patient Care." *Nursing Made Incredibly Easy!* 5(4):52-61, July/August 2007.

CHVOSTEK'S SIGN

Chvostek's sign is an abnormal spasm of the facial muscles that's elicited by lightly tapping the patient's facial nerve near his lower jaw. (See *Eliciting Chvostek's sign*.) This sign usually suggests hypocalcemia but can occur normally in about 25% of people. Typically, it precedes other signs of hypocalcemia and persists until the onset of tetany. It can't be elicited during tetany because of strong muscle contractions.

Normally, you'll only test for Chvostek's sign in patients with suspected hypocalcemia. However, because the parathyroid gland regulates calcium balance, Chvostek's sign also may be tested before neck surgery to obtain a baseline.

If your patient has Chvostek's sign, test for Trousseau's sign, a reliable indicator of hypocalcemia. Closely monitor the patient for signs of tetany, such as carpopedal spasms or circumoral or limb paresthesia.

Be prepared to act rapidly if a seizure occurs. Perform an electrocardiogram to check for hypocalcemic changes that increase the risk of arrhythmias. Place the patient on a cardiac monitor. Patients with severe hypocalcemia and seizures, tetany, or cardiac arrhythmias will need prompt infusion of calcium. During the infusion, monitor the patient closely for hypotension and bradycardia.[1]

History and physical examination

Obtain a brief history. Find out if the patient has had the parathyroid glands surgically removed or if he has a history of hypoparathyroidism, hypomagnesemia, or malabsorption disorder. Ask him or his family if they've noticed any mental changes, such as depression or slowed responses, which can accompany chronic hypocalcemia.

Medical causes

▶ *Hypocalcemia*. The degree of muscle spasm in Chvostek's sign reflects the patient's serum calcium level. Initially, hypocalcemia produces paresthesia in the fingers, toes, and circumoral area that progresses to muscle tension and carpopedal spasms. The patient also may complain of muscle weakness, fatigue, and

Eliciting Chvostek's sign

Begin by telling the patient to relax his face. Then stand directly in front of him and tap the facial nerve either just anterior to the earlobe and below the zygomatic arch or between the zygomatic arch and the corner of his mouth. A positive response varies from twitching of the lip at the corner of the mouth to spasm of all facial muscles, depending on the severity of hypocalcemia.

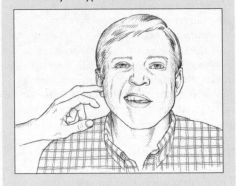

palpitations. Muscle twitching, hyperactive deep tendon reflexes, choreiform movements, and muscle cramps also may occur. A patient with chronic hypocalcemia may have mental status changes; diplopia; difficulty swallowing; abdominal cramps; dry, scaly skin; brittle nails; and thin, patchy scalp and eyebrow hair.

Other causes

▶ *Blood transfusion*. A massive transfusion can lower serum calcium levels and produce a positive Chvostek's sign.

Special considerations

Collect blood samples for serial calcium studies to evaluate the severity of hypocalcemia and the effectiveness of therapy, which includes oral or I.V. calcium supplements. Also, look for Chvostek's sign when evaluating a patient postoperatively.

Pediatric pointers

Because Chvostek's sign may occur in healthy infants, don't test for it to detect neonatal tetany.

Geriatric pointers

Always consider malabsorption and poor nutritional status in an elderly patient with Chvostek's sign and hypocalcemia.

Patient counseling

Inform patients who will be undergoing thyroidectomy or parathyroidectomy about the early signs and symptoms of hypocalcemia, such as numbness, tingling, and muscle cramps, and tell them to seek immediate medical attention if these occur.

REFERENCES

1. Avent, Y. "Managing Calcium Imbalance in Acute Care." *The Nurse Practitioner* 32(10):7-10, October 2007.

CLUBBING

A nonspecific sign of chronic, long-term pulmonary and cyanotic cardiovascular disorders, clubbing is the painless, usually bilateral increase in soft tissue around the terminal phalanges of the fingers or toes. (See *Rare causes of clubbing*.) It doesn't reflect changes in the underlying bone. As clubbing begins, the normal 160-degree angle between the nail and the nail base increases to about 180 degrees. As clubbing progresses, this angle widens and the base of the nail becomes visibly swollen. In late clubbing, the angle where the nail meets the now-convex nail base extends more than halfway up the nail.

History and physical examination

You'll probably detect clubbing while evaluating other signs of known pulmonary or cardiovascular disease. Therefore, review the patient's current plan of treatment because clubbing may resolve with correction of the underlying disorder. Also, evaluate the extent of clubbing in both the fingers and toes. (See *Checking for clubbed fingers*, page 102.)

Rare causes of clubbing

Clubbing typically is a sign of pulmonary or cardiovascular disease, but it also can result from certain hepatic and GI disorders, such as cirrhosis, Crohn's disease, and ulcerative colitis. Clubbing occurs only rarely in these disorders, however, so first check for more common signs and symptoms. For example, a patient with cirrhosis usually has right-upper-quadrant pain and hepatomegaly, a patient with Crohn's disease typically has abdominal cramping and tenderness, and a patient with ulcerative colitis may have diffuse abdominal pain and blood-streaked diarrhea.

Medical causes

▶ *Bronchiectasis.* Clubbing commonly occurs in the late stage of this disorder. Another classic sign is a cough producing copious, foul-smelling, and mucopurulent sputum. Hemoptysis and coarse crackles over the affected area during inspiration are also characteristic. The patient may complain of weight loss, fatigue, weakness, and exertional dyspnea. He also may have rhonchi, fever, malaise, and halitosis.

▶ *Bronchitis.* Clubbing may occur as a late sign in chronic bronchitis, but it doesn't reflect the severity of the disease. The patient has a chronic productive cough and may have barrel chest, dyspnea, wheezing, increased use of accessory muscles, cyanosis, tachypnea, crackles, scattered rhonchi, and prolonged expiration.

▶ *Emphysema.* Clubbing occurs late in this disease.[1] Emphysema also may cause anorexia, malaise, dyspnea, tachypnea, diminished breath sounds, peripheral cyanosis, pursed-lip breathing, accessory muscle use, barrel chest, and a productive cough.

▶ *Endocarditis.* In subacute infective endocarditis, clubbing may be accompanied by fever, anorexia, pallor, weakness, night sweats, fatigue, tachycardia, and weight loss. The patient also may develop arthralgia, petechiae, Osler's nodes, splinter hemorrhages,

Checking for clubbed fingers

To assess a patient for chronic tissue hypoxia, check his fingers for clubbing. Normally, the angle between the fingernail and the point where the nail enters the skin is about 160 degrees. Clubbing occurs when that angle increases to 180 degrees or more, as shown.

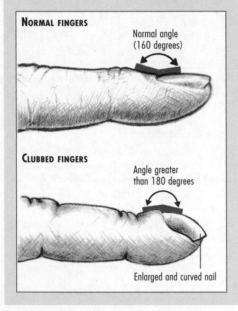

NORMAL FINGERS

Normal angle (160 degrees)

CLUBBED FINGERS

Angle greater than 180 degrees

Enlarged and curved nail

Janeway lesions, splenomegaly, and Roth's spots. Cardiac murmurs are usually present.

▶ *Heart failure.* Clubbing is a late sign of heart failure along with wheezing, dyspnea, and fatigue. Other findings include jugular vein distention, hepatomegaly, tachypnea, palpitations, dependent edema, unexplained weight gain, nausea, anorexia, chest tightness, slowed mental response, hypotension, diaphoresis, narrow pulse pressure, pallor, oliguria, a gallop rhythm (a third heart sound), and crackles on inspiration.

▶ *Interstitial fibrosis.* Clubbing occurs in almost all patients with advanced interstitial fibrosis. Typically, the patient also develops intermittent chest pain, dyspnea, crackles, fatigue, weight loss and, possibly, cyanosis.

▶ *Lung abscess.* Initially, this disorder produces clubbing, which may resolve with resolution of the abscess. It also can cause pleuritic chest pain, dyspnea, crackles, halitosis, and a productive cough with a large amount of purulent, foul-smelling, and commonly bloody sputum. The patient also may have weakness, fatigue, anorexia, headache, malaise, weight loss, and fever with chills. Auscultation may reveal decreased breath sounds.

▶ *Lung and pleural cancer.* Clubbing occurs commonly in these cancers. Other findings include hemoptysis, dyspnea, wheezing, chest pain, weight loss, anorexia, fatigue, and fever.

Special considerations

Don't mistake curved nails—a normal variation—for clubbing. In curved nails, the angle between the nail and its base remains normal.

Pediatric pointers

Clubbing usually occurs in children with certain congenital heart defects, and surgical correction of heart defects may reverse clubbing. Patients with cystic fibrosis may develop clubbing if chronic changes in the lungs impair gas exchange.[2] Clubbing is rare in patients with uncomplicated asthma.[3]

Geriatric pointers

Arthritic deformities of the fingers or toes may disguise clubbing in elderly patients.

Patient counseling

Inform the patient that clubbing doesn't always disappear, even if the cause has been resolved.

REFERENCES

1. Dahlin, C. "It Takes My Breath Away END-STAGE COPD: Part 1: A Case Study and An Overview of COPD." *Home Healthcare Nurse* 24(3):148-155, March 2006.
2. Gardner, J. "What You Need to Know About Cystic Fibrosis." *Nursing* 37(7):52-55, July 2007.
3. Conboy-Ellis, K. "Asthma Pathogenesis and Management." *The Nurse Practitioner* 31(11):24-37, November 2006.

CONSTIPATION

Constipation is defined as small, infrequent, or difficult bowel movements. Constipation (intermittent or chronic) affects about 12% to 19% of the population, and is common in women and adults over age 65.[1,2] Because normal bowel movements can vary in frequency and from person to person, constipation must be determined in relation to the patient's normal elimination pattern. Constipation may be a minor annoyance or, occasionally, a sign of a life-threatening disorder such as acute intestinal obstruction. Untreated, constipation can lead to headache, anorexia, and abdominal discomfort and can adversely affect the patient's lifestyle and well-being.

Constipation usually occurs when the urge to defecate is suppressed and the muscles associated with bowel movements remain contracted. Because the autonomic nervous system controls bowel movements—by sensing rectal distention from fecal contents and by stimulating the external sphincter—any factor that influences this system may cause bowel dysfunction. (See *How habits and stress cause constipation*.)

History and physical examination

Ask the patient to describe the frequency of his bowel movements and the size and consistency of his stools. How long has he had constipation? Acute constipation usually has an organic cause, such as an anal or rectal disor-

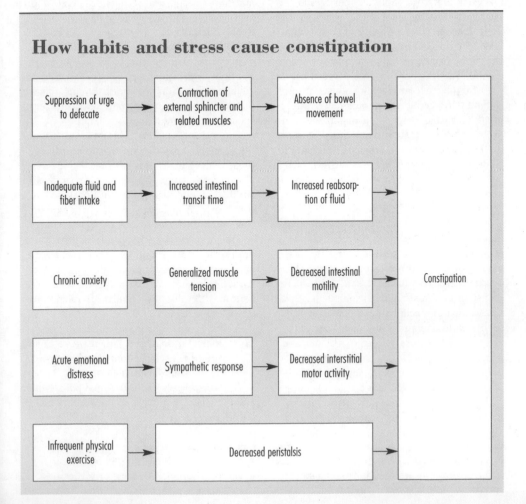

How habits and stress cause constipation

Suppression of urge to defecate	→ Contraction of external sphincter and related muscles	→ Absence of bowel movement	→
Inadequate fluid and fiber intake	→ Increased intestinal transit time	→ Increased reabsorption of fluid	→
Chronic anxiety	→ Generalized muscle tension	→ Decreased intestinal motility	→ Constipation
Acute emotional distress	→ Sympathetic response	→ Decreased interstitial motor activity	→
Infrequent physical exercise	→ Decreased peristalsis		→

der. In a patient older than age 45, a recent onset of constipation may be an early sign of colorectal cancer. Conversely, chronic constipation typically has a functional cause and may be related to stress. Also, find out if the patient ever notices blood in his stool.[2]

Does the patient have pain related to constipation? If so, when did he first notice the pain, and where is it located? Cramping abdominal pain and distention suggest obstipation—extreme, persistent constipation from intestinal tract obstruction. Ask the patient if defecation worsens or helps relieve the pain. Defecation usually worsens the pain, but in disorders such as irritable bowel syndrome, it may relieve it.

Ask the patient to describe a typical day's menu; estimate his daily fiber and fluid intake. Ask him, too, about any changes in eating habits, drug or alcohol use, or physical activity. Does he have a history of dehydration? Has he had recent emotional stress? Has constipation affected his family life or social contacts? Also, ask about his job. A sedentary or stressful job can contribute to constipation.

Find out whether the patient has a history of GI, rectoanal, neurologic, or metabolic disorders; abdominal surgery; or radiation therapy. Then ask about the drugs he's taking, including over-the-counter preparations, such as laxatives, mineral oil, stool softeners, and enemas.

Assess the patient's hydration status, noting signs of dehydration such as skin tenting, dry mucous membranes, sunken eyeballs, and rapid pulse.[1,3] Inspect the abdomen for distention or scars from previous surgery. Then auscultate for bowel sounds, and characterize their motility. Absent bowel sounds may indicate an ileus, especially if associated signs such as vomiting and abdominal distention are present.[1] Percuss all four quadrants, and gently palpate for abdominal tenderness, a palpable mass, and hepatomegaly. Next, examine the patient's rectum. Spread his buttocks to expose the anus, and inspect for inflammation, lesions, scars, fissures, and external hemorrhoids. Use a disposable glove and lubricant to palpate the anal sphincter for laxity or stricture. Also palpate for rectal masses and fecal impaction. Finally, obtain a stool specimen and test it for occult blood.

As you assess the patient, remember that constipation can result from several life-threatening disorders, such as acute intestinal obstruction and mesenteric artery ischemia, but it doesn't herald these conditions.

Medical causes

▶ *Anal fissure.* A crack or laceration in the lining of the anal wall can cause acute constipation, usually from the patient's fear of the severe tearing or burning pain that occurs with bowel movements. He may notice a few drops of blood streaking toilet tissue or his underwear.

▶ *Anorectal abscess.* In this disorder, constipation occurs with severe, throbbing, localized pain and tenderness at the abscess site. The patient also may have localized inflammation, swelling, and purulent drainage and may complain of fever and malaise.

▶ *Cirrhosis.* In the early stages of cirrhosis, the patient experiences constipation along with nausea and vomiting, and a dull pain in the right upper quadrant. Other early findings include indigestion, anorexia, fatigue, malaise, flatulence, hepatomegaly and, possibly, splenomegaly and diarrhea.

▶ *Diabetic neuropathy.* This type of neuropathy produces episodic constipation or diarrhea. Other signs and symptoms include dysphagia, orthostatic hypotension, syncope, and painless bladder distention with overflow incontinence. A male patient also may experience impotence and retrograde ejaculation.

▶ *Diverticulitis.* In this disorder, constipation or diarrhea occurs with left-lower-quadrant pain and tenderness and possibly a palpable, tender, firm, fixed abdominal mass. The patient may develop mild nausea, flatulence, or a low-grade fever.

▶ *Hemorrhoids.* Thrombosed hemorrhoids cause constipation as the patient tries to avoid the severe pain of defecation. The hemorrhoids may bleed during defecation.

▶ *Hepatic porphyria.* Abdominal pain, which may be severe, colicky, and localized or generalized, precedes constipation in hepatic porphyria. The patient also may have a fever, sinus tachycardia, labile hypertension, diaphoresis, severe vomiting, photophobia, urine retention, nervousness or restlessness, disorientation and, possibly, visual hallucinations. Deep tendon reflexes may be diminished or absent. Some patients have skin lesions causing itching, burning, erythema, altered pigmentation, and edema in areas exposed to light. Severe hepatic porphyria can produce delirium, coma, seizures, paraplegia, or complete flaccid quadriplegia.

▶ *Hypercalcemia.* In hypercalcemia, constipation usually is accompanied by anorexia, nausea, vomiting, polyuria, and polydipsia. The patient also may display arrhythmias, bone pain, muscle weakness and atrophy, hypoactive deep tendon reflexes, and personality changes.

▶ *Hypokalemia.* Hypokalemia can cause intestinal problems, such as constipation, decreased bowel sounds, and paralytic ileus. Other signs and symptoms may include skeletal muscle weakness and cramping, paresthesias, orthostatic hypotension, palpitations, a weak and irregular pulse, and arrhythmias.

▶ *Hypothyroidism.* Constipation occurs early and insidiously in patients with hypothyroidism; it may be accompanied by fatigue, sensitivity to cold, anorexia with weight gain, menorrhagia, decreased memory, hearing impairment, muscle cramps, and paresthesia.

▶ *Intestinal obstruction.* Constipation associated with this disorder varies in severity and onset, depending on the location and extent of the obstruction. In a partial obstruction, constipation may alternate with leakage of liquid stools. In a complete obstruction, obstipation may occur. Constipation can be the earliest sign of partial colon obstruction, but it usually occurs later if the level of the obstruction is more proximal. Associated findings include episodes of colicky abdominal pain, abdominal distention, nausea, and vomiting. The patient also may develop hyperactive bowel sounds, visible peristaltic waves, a palpable abdominal mass, and abdominal tenderness.

▶ *Irritable bowel syndrome.* This common syndrome usually produces chronic constipation, although some patients have intermittent watery diarrhea and others complain of alternating constipation and diarrhea. Stress may trigger nausea and abdominal distention and tenderness, but defecation usually relieves these signs and symptoms. (See *Stress and constipation in women with and without IBS,* page 106.) Many patients have an intense urge to defecate and feelings of incomplete evacuation. Typically, the stools are scybalous and contain visible mucus.

▶ *Mesenteric artery occlusion.* This life-threatening disorder produces sudden constipation with failure to expel stool or flatus. Initially, the abdomen is soft and nontender but soon severe abdominal pain, tenderness, vomiting, and anorexia occur. Later, the patient may develop abdominal guarding, rigidity, and distention; tachycardia; syncope; tachypnea; fever; and signs of shock, such as cool, clammy skin and hypotension. A bruit may be heard.

▶ *Multiple sclerosis (MS).* This disorder can produce constipation in addition to ocular disturbances, such as nystagmus, blurred vision, and diplopia; vertigo; and sensory disturbances. The patient also may have motor weakness, seizures, paralysis, muscle spasticity, gait ataxia, intention tremor, hyperreflexia, dysarthria, or dysphagia. MS can also produce urinary urgency, frequency, and incontinence as well as emotional instability. A male patient may experience impotence.

▶ *Spinal cord lesion.* Constipation may occur in this disorder along with urine retention, sexual dysfunction, pain, and possibly motor weakness, paralysis, or sensory impairment below the level of the lesion.

▶ *Tabes dorsalis.* In tabes dorsalis, constipation is accompanied by an ataxic gait; paresthesia; loss of sensation of body position, deep pain, and temperature; Charcot's joints; Argyll Robertson pupils; diminished deep tendon reflexes; and possibly impotence.

▶ *Ulcerative colitis.* Constipation may occur in patients with chronic ulcerative colitis, but bloody diarrhea with pus, mucus, or both is the hallmark of this disorder. Other signs and symptoms include cramping lower abdominal pain, tenesmus, anorexia, low-grade fever and, occasionally, nausea and vomiting. Bowel sounds may be hyperactive. Later, weight loss, weakness, and arthralgias occur.

▶ *Ulcerative proctitis.* This disorder produces acute constipation with tenesmus. The patient feels an intense urge to defecate but is unable to do so. Instead, he may eliminate mucus, pus, or blood.

EVIDENCE-BASED PRACTICE

Stress and constipation in women with and without IBS

Question: *What is the relationship of daily self-reported stress to gastrointestinal (GI) and psychological distress symptoms in women with irritable bowel syndrome (IBS) compared to women without IBS, and among subgroups of women with IBS?*

Research: IBS is a GI disorder characterized by abdominal discomfort or pain associated with constipation, diarrhea, or both constipation and diarrhea. Stress triggers or worsens the symptoms of IBS. The study cited examined the relationship of stress to abdominal discomfort symptoms, bowel pattern symptoms, and psychological distress across women, and in subgroups of women with IBS. The three subgroups were women with IBS-constipation (IBS-C), women with IBS-diarrhea (IBS-D), and women with IBS-alternating (IBS-A).

This report is a secondary analysis of data from two samples of women from previous studies. One hundred eighty-one women were divided into subgroups as follows: 52 with IBS-C, 67 with IBS-D, and 62 with IBS-A. These women were compared to a group of 48 women without IBS. The women completed a Daily Health Diary for 33 days, which asked questions and used scales to determine daily stress intensity; symptoms of abdominal discomfort (pain, bloating, and gas), bowel patterns (constipation and diarrhea), and psychological distress (anxiety and depression).

Conclusion: The research confirmed that women with IBS experience significantly more stress and greater psychological distress than women without IBS. Differences among the subtypes were not significant. Abdominal pain, bloating, and intestinal gas were correlated more strongly with stress than bowel pattern symptoms. Daily stress and GI symptoms were less when anxiety and depression were controlled in the analyses.

Application: Incorporate strategies to decrease stress in the care of women with IBS. Teach women stress management techniques and tell them that stress reduction can lessen psychological distress and GI symptoms. Assist with appropriate referrals and provide support as needed.

Source: Hertig, V. L., Cain, K. C., Jarrett, M. E., Burr, R. L., & Heitkemper, M. M. "Daily Stress and Gastrointestinal Symptoms in Women with Irritable Bowel Syndrome." *Nursing Research* 56(6):399-406, 2007.

Other causes

▶ *Diagnostic tests.* Constipation can result from the retention of barium given during certain GI studies.

DRUG WATCH *Many patients develop constipation when taking an opioid analgesic or other drug, such as a vinca alkaloid, a calcium channel blocker, an antacid containing aluminum or calcium, an anticholinergic, an iron supplement, or an antiparkinsonian drug.[1] Patients also may develop constipation from excessive use of laxatives or enemas.*

▶ *Surgery and radiation therapy.* Constipation can result from rectoanal surgery, which may traumatize nerves, and abdominal irradiation, which may cause intestinal stricture.

Special considerations

If the bowel has become impacted, enemas and oral laxatives may be necessary to remove the accumulation of stool. Repeated enemas may be needed to completely clear the bowel, especially if the patient hasn't had a bowel movement in a number of days.[1]

Pediatric pointers

Hirschsprung's disease and inadequate fluid intake are common causes of constipation in infants. The most common cause of constipation in infants greater than 1 month of age is functional; that is, it isn't caused by a disease or condition.[4] Functional constipation can occur if a child knowingly withholds the urge to defecate because of a previous history of painful bowel movements, a reluctance to stop playing for bathroom breaks, the lack of privacy in some school bathrooms, or the occurrence of stressful life events.

Geriatric pointers

The aging process can lead to a decrease in gastric motility, as well as impaired physical mobility.[5] Older age also is associated with an increased risk of dehydration from decreased thirst response, reduced kidney function, and decreased total body fluid.[3] Older adults also are more likely to have chronic illnesses and use medications. It isn't surprising, then, that for older adults, constipation is the most common bowel management problem.[5]

Patient counseling

Caution the patient not to strain during defecation to prevent injuring rectoanal tissue. Instruct him to avoid using laxatives or enemas. If he has been abusing these products, begin to wean him from them. Use a disposable glove and lubricant to remove impacted feces. (Check if an oil-retention enema can be given first to soften the fecal mass.)

As indicated, prepare the patient for diagnostic tests, such as proctosigmoidoscopy, colonoscopy, barium enema, plain abdominal films, and an upper GI series. If the patient is on bed rest, reposition him often, and help him perform active or passive exercises as indicated. Teach him abdominal toning exercises if his abdominal muscles are weak and relaxation techniques to help him reduce stress related to constipation.

Encourage the patient to comply with a bowel management program (a regimen of food, fluid, fiber, and activity), along with supplements and drugs to promote a regular elimination pattern.[1,2] Provide the patient with additional tips to prevent constipation, such as developing normal bowel and bathroom habits, and not resisting the urge to defecate.[6]

REFERENCES

1. Bisanz, A. "Chronic Constipation." *AJN* 107(4):72B-72H, April 2007.
2. Heitkemper, M. and Wolff, J. "Challenges in Chronic Constipation Management." *The Nurse Practitioner* 32(4):36-42, April 2007.
3. Mentes, J. "Oral Hydration in Older Adults: Greater Awareness is Needed in Preventing, Recognizing, and Treating Dehydration." *AJN* 106(6):40-49, June 2006.
4. "Evaluation and Treatment of Constipation in Infants and Children: Recommendations of the North American Society for Pediatric Gastroenterology, Hepatology, and Nutrition." *Journal of Pediatric Gastroenterology and Nutrition* 43(3):e1-e13, September 2006.
5. Mauk, K.L. "Preventing Constipation in Older Adults." *Nursing* 35(6):22-23, June 2005.
6. Amerine, E. and Keirsey, M. "How Should You Respond to Constipation?" *Nursing* 36(10):64hn1, 64hn2, 64hn4, October 2006.

COUGH, BARKING

Resonant, brassy, and harsh, a barking cough is part of a complex of signs and symptoms that characterize croup syndrome, a group of pediatric disorders marked by varying degrees of respiratory distress. Croup most commonly affects children ages 6 months to 36 months. Most cases result from parainfluenza virus infection.

A barking cough indicates edema of the larynx and surrounding tissue. Because children's airways are smaller in diameter than those of adults, edema can rapidly lead to airway occlusion, a life-threatening emergency.

Quickly evaluate the child's respiratory status. Then take his vital signs. Be particularly alert for tachycardia and signs of hypoxemia. Also, check for a decreased level of consciousness. Try to determine if the child was playing with a small object that he may have aspirated.

Check for cyanosis in the lips and nail beds. Observe the patient for sternal or intercostal retractions or nasal flaring. Next, note the depth and rate of his respirations; they may become increasingly shallow as respiratory distress increases. Observe the child's body position. Is he sitting up, leaning forward, and struggling to breathe? Observe his activity level and facial expression. As respiratory distress increases from airway edema, the child will become restless and have a frightened, wide-eyed expression. As air hunger continues, the child will become lethargic and difficult to arouse.

If the child shows signs of severe respiratory distress, try to calm him, maintain airway patency, and provide oxygen. Endotracheal intubation or a tracheotomy may be needed.

History and physical examination

Ask the child's parents when the barking cough began and what other signs and symptoms accompanied it. When did the child first appear to be ill? Has he had previous episodes of croup syndrome? Did his condition improve with exposure to cold air?

Spasmodic croup and epiglottiditis typically occur in the middle of the night. The child with spasmodic croup has no fever, but the child with epiglottiditis has a high fever of sudden onset. An upper respiratory tract infection typically is followed by laryngotracheobronchitis.

Medical causes

▶ *Aspiration of foreign body.* Partial obstruction of the upper airway first produces sudden hoarseness, then a barking cough and inspiratory stridor. Other effects of this life-threatening condition include gagging, tachycardia, dyspnea, decreased breath sounds, wheezing, and possibly cyanosis.

▶ *Epiglottiditis.* This life-threatening disorder has become less common since the use of influenza vaccines.[1] It occurs nocturnally, heralded by a barking cough and a high fever. The child is hoarse, dysphagic, dyspneic, and restless and appears extremely ill and panicky. The cough may progress to severe respiratory distress with sternal and intercostal retractions, nasal flaring, cyanosis, and tachycardia. The child will struggle to get sufficient air as epiglottic edema increases. Epiglottiditis is a true medical emergency.

▶ *Laryngotracheobronchitis (acute).* Also known as viral croup, this infection is most common in children ages 9 months to 18

months and usually occurs in the fall and early winter. It initially produces low to moderate fever, runny nose, poor appetite, and infrequent cough. When the infection descends into the laryngotracheal area, a barking cough, hoarseness, and inspiratory stridor occur.

As respiratory distress progresses, substernal and intercostal retractions occur along with tachycardia and shallow, rapid respirations. Sleeping in a dry room worsens these signs. The patient becomes restless, irritable, pale, and cyanotic.

▶ *Spasmodic croup.* Acute spasmodic croup always occurs at night with the abrupt onset of a barking cough that awakens the child.[2] Typically, he doesn't have a fever but may be hoarse, restless, and dyspneic. As his respiratory distress worsens, the child may have sternal and intercostal retractions, nasal flaring, tachycardia, cyanosis, and an anxious, frantic appearance. The signs typically subside within a few hours, but attacks tend to recur.

Special considerations

Don't try to inspect the throat of a child with a barking cough unless intubation equipment is available.[1] If the child isn't in severe respiratory distress, a lateral neck X-ray may be done to visualize epiglottal edema; however, a negative X-ray doesn't completely rule out epiglottal edema. A chest X-ray also may be done to rule out lower respiratory tract infection. Depending on the child's age and the degree of respiratory distress, oxygen may be given. Rapid-acting epinephrine and a steroid should be considered.

Be sure to closely monitor respiratory status and pulse oximetry.[3] Provide the child with periods of rest and minimal interruptions to conserve energy.[3] Maintain a calm, quiet environment and offer reassurance. Encourage the parents to stay with the child to help reduce stress.

Patient counseling

Teach parents how to evaluate and treat recurrent episodes of croup syndrome. For example, using a cool-air vaporizer may help relieve subsequent attacks. The child also may benefit from being brought outside (properly dressed) to breathe cold night air.[3]

REFERENCES

1. Chiocca, E.M. "Epiglottitis." *Nursing* 36(4):88, April 2006.
2. Cherry, J.D. "State of the Evidence for Standard-of-Care treatments for Croup: Are We Where We Need to Be?" *Pediatric Infectious Disease Journal. 2005 International Congress on Respiratory Viruses* 24(11)Supplement: S198-S202, November 2005.
3. Hockenberry, M.J. and Wilson, D. (Eds.) *Wong's Nursing Care of Infants and Children.* 8th ed. St. Louis: Mosby, 2007.

● COUGH, NONPRODUCTIVE

Anonproductive cough is a noisy, forceful expulsion of air from the lungs that doesn't yield sputum or blood. It's one of the most common complaints of patients with respiratory disorders.

Coughing is a necessary protective mechanism that clears airway passages. However, a nonproductive cough is ineffective and can cause damage, such as airway collapse or rupture of alveoli or blebs. A nonproductive cough that later becomes productive is a classic sign of progressive respiratory disease.

The cough reflex typically occurs when mechanical, chemical, thermal, inflammatory, or psychogenic stimuli activate cough receptors. (See *Reviewing the cough mechanism,* page 110.) However, external pressure—for example, from subdiaphragmatic irritation or a mediastinal tumor—can also induce it, as can voluntary expiration of air, which occasionally occurs as a nervous habit.

A nonproductive cough may occur in paroxysms and can worsen by becoming more frequent. An acute cough has a sudden onset and may be self-limiting; a cough that persists beyond 1 month is considered chronic and commonly results from cigarette smoking.

Someone with a chronic nonproductive cough may downplay or overlook it or accept it as normal. In fact, he generally won't seek medical attention unless he has other symptoms. A foreign body in a child's external auditory canal may result in a cough. Always examine the child's ears.

History and physical examination

Ask the patient when his cough began and whether any body position, time of day, or specific activity affects it. How does the cough sound—harsh, brassy, dry, or hacking? Try to determine if the cough is related to smoking or a chemical irritant. If the patient smokes or has smoked, note the number of packs smoked daily multiplied by years (pack-years). Next, ask about the frequency and intensity of the coughing. If he has any pain associated with coughing, breathing, or activity, when did it begin and where is it located?

Ask the patient about recent illness (especially a cardiovascular or pulmonary disorder), surgery, or trauma. Also ask about hypersensitivity to drugs, foods, pets, dust, or pollen. Find out which drugs the patient takes, if any, and ask about recent changes in schedule or dosages. Also ask about recent changes in his appetite, weight, exercise tolerance, or energy level; recent exposure to irritating fumes, chemicals, or smoke; and recent travel to foreign countries.

As you're taking his history, observe the patient's general appearance and manner: Is he agitated, restless, or lethargic; pale, diaphoretic, or flushed; anxious, confused, or nervous? Also, note whether he's cyanotic or has clubbed fingers or peripheral edema. Ask the patient at risk for TB—those born in another country, those in contact with acute TB, and those with high-risk behaviors—about possible TB exposure.

Next, perform a physical examination. Start by taking the patient's vital signs. Check the depth and rhythm of his respirations, and note wheezing or "crowing" noises that occur with breathing. Feel the patient's skin: Is it cold or warm; clammy or dry? Check his nose and mouth for congestion, inflammation, drainage, or signs of infection. Inspect his neck for distended veins and tracheal deviation, and palpate for masses or enlarged lymph nodes.

Examine his chest, observing its configuration and looking for abnormal chest wall motion. Do you note any retractions or use of accessory muscles? Percuss for dullness, tympany, or flatness. Auscultate for wheezing, crackles, rhonchi, pleural friction rub, and de-

Reviewing the cough mechanism

Cough receptors are thought to be located in the nose, sinuses, auditory canals, nasopharynx, larynx, trachea, bronchi, pleurae, diaphragm, and possibly the pericardium and GI tract. Once a cough receptor is stimulated, the vagus and glossopharyngeal nerves transmit the impulse to the cough center in the medulla. From there, the impulse is transmitted to the larynx and to the intercostal and abdominal muscles. Deep inspiration (1) is followed by closure of the glottis (2), relaxation of the diaphragm, and contraction of the abdominal and intercostal muscles. The resulting increased pressure in the lungs opens the glottis to release the forceful, noisy expiration known as a cough (3).

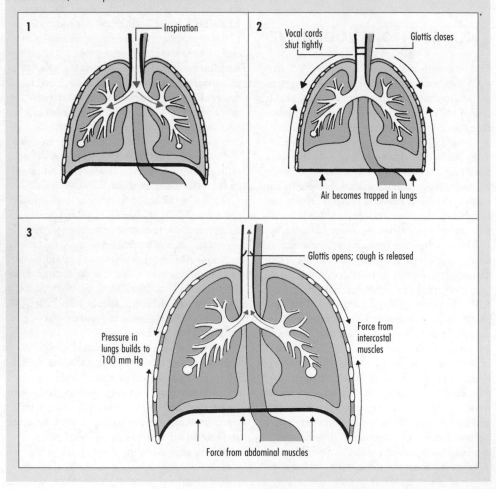

1 Inspiration

2 Vocal cords shut tightly   Glottis closes

Air becomes trapped in lungs

3 Glottis opens; cough is released

Pressure in lungs builds to 100 mm Hg

Force from intercostal muscles

Force from abdominal muscles

creased or absent breath sounds. Finally, examine his abdomen for distention, tenderness, or masses, and auscultate it for abnormal bowel sounds.

Medical causes

▶ *Airway occlusion.* Partial occlusion of the upper airway produces a sudden onset of dry, paroxysmal coughing. The patient exhibits gagging, wheezing, hoarseness, stridor, tachycardia, and decreased breath sounds.

▶ *Anthrax (inhalation).* This acute infectious disease is caused by the gram-positive, spore-forming bacterium *Bacillus anthracis.* Although the disease occurs most commonly in wild and domestic grazing animals, such as cattle, sheep, and goats, spores can live in the soil for many years. The disease can occur in humans exposed to infected animals, tissue from infected animals, or biological agents. Most natural cases occur in agricultural regions worldwide. Anthrax may occur in cutaneous, inhalation, or GI forms.

Inhalation anthrax results from inhaling aerosolized spores. Initial signs and symptoms are flulike and include fever, chills, weakness, cough, and chest pain. The disease typically occurs in two stages with a period of recovery after the initial signs and symptoms. The second stage develops abruptly and causes rapid deterioration marked by fever, dyspnea, stridor, and hypotension; death usually results within 24 hours. Radiologic findings include mediastinitis and symmetrical mediastinal widening.

▶ *Aortic aneurysm (thoracic).* This disorder causes a brassy cough with dyspnea, hoarseness, wheezing, and a substernal ache in the shoulders, lower back, or abdomen. The patient also may have facial or neck edema, jugular vein distention, dysphagia, prominent veins over his chest, stridor, and possibly paresthesia or neuralgia.

▶ *Asthma.* Asthma attacks commonly occur at night, starting with a nonproductive cough and mild wheezing and progressing to severe dyspnea, audible wheezing, chest tightness, and a cough that produces thick mucus. Other signs include apprehension, rhonchi, prolonged expirations, intercostal and supraclavicular retractions on inspiration, accessory muscle use, flaring nostrils, tachypnea, tachycardia, diaphoresis, and flushing or cyanosis.

▶ *Atelectasis.* As lung tissue deflates in atelectasis, it stimulates cough receptors, causing a nonproductive cough. The patient also may have pleuritic chest pain, anxiety, dyspnea, tachypnea, tachycardia, decreased breath sounds, cyanotic skin, and diaphoresis. His chest may be dull on percussion, and he may exhibit inspiratory lag, substernal or intercostal retractions, decreased vocal fremitus,

and tracheal deviation toward the affected side.

▶ *Avian influenza.* These potentially life-threatening viruses are spread to humans through infected poultry and surfaces contaminated with infected bird excretions. Infected people may initially have symptoms of conventional influenza, including a nonproductive cough, fever, sore throat, and muscle aches. The most virulent avian virus, influenza A (H5N1), may lead to severe and life-threatening complications, such as acute respiratory distress and pneumonia. To date, this strain of the virus hasn't been identified in the United States; however, an outbreak in Asia and Europe has caused worldwide concern that the virus may spread through both infected humans and birds. Treatment with two of the four FDA-approved antiviral drugs has proven effective with some virus strains, and a vaccine for humans against H5N1 was approved by the FDA in April 2007.

▶ *Bronchitis (chronic).* This disorder starts with a nonproductive, hacking cough that later becomes productive. Other findings include prolonged expiration, wheezing, dyspnea, accessory muscle use, barrel chest, cyanosis, tachypnea, crackles, and scattered rhonchi. Clubbing can occur in late stages.

▶ *Bronchogenic carcinoma.* The earliest indicators of this disease can be a chronic nonproductive cough, dyspnea, and vague chest pain. The patient also may be wheezing.

▶ *Common cold.* Most colds start with a nonproductive, hacking cough and progress to some mix of sneezing, rhinorrhea, nasal congestion, sore throat, headache, malaise, fatigue, myalgia, and arthralgia.

▶ *Esophageal achalasia.* In this disorder, regurgitation and aspiration produce a dry cough and, possibly, recurrent pulmonary infections and dysphagia.

▶ *Esophageal diverticula.* The patient with this disorder has a nocturnal nonproductive cough, regurgitation and aspiration, dyspepsia, and dysphagia. His neck may appear swollen and have a gurgling sound. He also may have halitosis and weight loss.

▶ *Esophageal occlusion.* This disorder is marked by sudden nonproductive coughing and gagging with a sensation of something

Preventing the spread of influenza

Influenza spreads when an infected person coughs or sneezes, sending respiratory droplets contaminated with the virus into the air. The droplets can then enter the upper respiratory tract of anyone within 3 feet of the infected patient. The virus also may be spread by contact with a contaminated surface, followed by contact with the eyes, nose, or mouth.

The influenza vaccine offers the best protection against influenza infection. The trivalent inactivated influenza vaccine is given by IM injection. The live, attenuated influenza vaccine is given by nasal spray. Antiviral drugs can inhibit viral replication (amantadine, rimantadine) and prevent release of viral particles (zanamivir, oseltamivir), but these drugs shouldn't take the place of an annual flu vaccination.

In addition to recommending flu vaccine, follow these guidelines to help curb the spread of this contagious illness:
- Follow strict hand hygiene.
- Assign patients with influenza to a private room. If this isn't possible, keep at least 3 feet between the patient and other patients, and keep the curtain drawn between patients.
- Use droplet precautions for at least 5 days.
- Have the patient wear a surgical mask if he needs to be transported outside of his room.
- Urge the patient to wash his hands often.
- Instruct the patient to cover his nose and mouth when coughing or sneezing. Coughing or sneezing into his elbow, upper arm, or a tissue will help prevent contamination of his hands. Tell the patient to dispose of used tissues promptly in a designated area.

stuck in the throat. Other findings include neck or chest pain and dysphagia.

▶ *Esophagitis with reflux.* This disorder commonly causes a nonproductive nocturnal cough due to regurgitation and aspiration. The patient also may have chest pain that mimics angina pectoris, heartburn that worsens if he lies down after eating, increased salivation, dysphagia, hematemesis, and melena.

▶ *Influenza.* This contagious viral infection, most common in late fall and winter, can cause a cough that produces little sputum; however, hemoptysis may result from strong, forceful coughing.[1] Other signs and symptoms include fever, chills, headache, rhinitis, myalgia, and fatigue. (See *Preventing the spread of influenza*.)

▶ Hantavirus *pulmonary syndrome.* A nonproductive cough is common in patients with this disorder, which is marked by noncardiogenic pulmonary edema. Other findings include headache, myalgia, fever, nausea, and vomiting.

▶ *Hodgkin's disease.* This disease may cause a crowing nonproductive cough. However, the earliest sign is usually painless swelling of one of the cervical lymph nodes or, occasionally, of the axillary, mediastinal, or inguinal

lymph nodes. Another early sign is pruritus. Other findings depend on the degree and location of systemic involvement and include dyspnea, dysphagia, hepatosplenomegaly, edema, jaundice, nerve pain, and hyperpigmentation.

▶ *Hypersensitivity pneumonitis.* In this disorder, an acute nonproductive cough, fever, dyspnea, and malaise usually occur 5 to 6 hours after exposure to an antigen.

▶ *Interstitial lung disease.* A patient with this disorder has a nonproductive cough and progressive dyspnea. He also may be cyanotic and have clubbing, fine crackles, fatigue, variable chest pain, and weight loss.

▶ *Laryngeal tumor.* A mild nonproductive cough, minor throat discomfort, and hoarseness are early signs of this disorder. Later, dysphagia, dyspnea, cervical lymphadenopathy, stridor, and earache may occur.

▶ *Laryngitis.* Acute laryngitis causes a nonproductive cough with localized pain (especially when the patient swallows or speaks) as well as fever and malaise. Hoarseness can range from mild to complete loss of voice.

▶ *Legionnaires' disease.* After a prodrome of malaise, headache and, possibly, diarrhea, anorexia, diffuse myalgia, and general weakness, legionnaires' disease causes a nonproductive cough that later produces mucoid, nonpurulent and, possibly, blood-tinged sputum.

▶ *Lung abscess.* This disorder typically begins with a nonproductive cough, weakness, dyspnea, and pleuritic chest pain. The patient also may exhibit diaphoresis, fever, headache, malaise, fatigue, crackles, decreased breath sounds, anorexia, and weight loss. Later, his cough produces large amounts of purulent, foul-smelling and, possibly, blood-tinged sputum.

▶ *Mediastinal tumor.* A large mediastinal tumor produces a nonproductive cough, dyspnea, and retrosternal pain. The patient also may develop stertorous respirations with suprasternal retraction on inspiration, hoarseness, dysphagia, tracheal shift or tug, jugular vein distention, and facial or neck edema.

▶ *Pericardial effusion.* The most common signs and symptoms of this disorder are dysphagia, fever, pleuritic chest pain, and pericardial friction rub. A severe nonproductive cough occurs rarely.

▶ *Pleural effusion.* A nonproductive cough, dyspnea, pleuritic chest pain, and decreased chest motion are characteristic of pleural effusion. Other findings include pleural friction rub, tachycardia, tachypnea, egophony, flatness on percussion, decreased or absent breath sounds, and decreased tactile fremitus.

▶ *Pneumonia.* Typical (bacterial) pneumonia usually starts with a nonproductive, hacking, painful cough that rapidly becomes productive. Other findings include shaking chills, headache, high fever, dyspnea, pleuritic chest pain, tachypnea, tachycardia, grunting respirations, nasal flaring, decreased breath sounds, fine crackles, rhonchi, and cyanosis. The patient's chest may be dull on percussion.

Atypical (non-bacterial) pneumonia causes a nonproductive, hacking cough and the gradual onset of malaise, headache, anorexia, and low-grade fever. Signs and symptoms usually are less severe than in bacterial pneumonia.[2]

Mycoplasma pneumoniae is the most common cause of atypical pneumonia.[2] In mycoplasmal pneumonia, a nonproductive cough develops 2 to 3 days after the onset of malaise, headache, and sore throat. The cough may be paroxysmal, causing substernal chest pain. The patient commonly has a fever but doesn't appear seriously ill.

▶ *Pneumothorax.* This life-threatening disorder causes a dry cough and signs of respiratory distress, such as severe dyspnea, tachycardia, tachypnea, and cyanosis. The patient experiences sudden, sharp chest pain that worsens with chest movement as well as subcutaneous crepitation, hyperresonance or tympany, decreased vocal fremitus, and decreased or absent breath sounds on the affected side.

▶ *Psittacosis.* In this disorder, an initially dry, hacking cough later produces small amounts of blood-streaked, mucoid sputum. Psittacosis may begin abruptly with chills, fever, headache, myalgia, and prostration. The patient also may have tachypnea, fine crackles, epistaxis and, rarely, chest pain.

▶ *Pulmonary edema.* This disorder initially causes a dry cough, exertional dyspnea, paroxysmal nocturnal dyspnea, orthopnea, tachycardia, tachypnea, dependent crackles, and ventricular gallop. If pulmonary edema is severe, the patient's respirations become more rapid and labored, with diffuse crackles and a cough that produces frothy, blood-streaked sputum.

▶ *Pulmonary embolism.* A life-threatening pulmonary embolism may suddenly produce a dry cough, dyspnea, and pleuritic or anginal chest pain. In most cases, though, the cough produces blood-tinged sputum. Tachycardia and low-grade fever are also common; less common signs and symptoms include massive hemoptysis, chest splinting, leg edema and, with a large embolus, cyanosis, syncope, and distended jugular veins. The patient also may have a pleural friction rub, diffuse wheezing, dullness on percussion, and decreased breath sounds.

▶ *Sarcoidosis.* In this disorder, a nonproductive cough is accompanied by dyspnea, substernal pain, and malaise. The patient also may develop fatigue, arthralgia, myalgia, weight loss, tachypnea, crackles, lymphadenopathy, hepatosplenomegaly, skin lesions, vision impairment, difficulty swallowing, and arrhythmias.

▶ *Severe acute respiratory syndrome (SARS).* SARS is an acute infectious disease of unknown etiology; however, a novel coronavirus has been implicated as a possible cause. Although most cases have been reported in Asia (China, Vietnam, Singapore, Thailand), cases have cropped up in Europe and North America. The incubation period is 2 to 7 days, and the illness generally begins with a fever (usually greater than 100.4° F [38° C]). Other symptoms include headache, malaise, a nonproductive cough, and dyspnea. The severity of the illness is highly variable, ranging from mild illness to pneumonia and, in some cases, progressing to respiratory failure and death.

▶ *Sinusitis (chronic).* This disorder can cause a chronic nonproductive cough due to postnasal drip. The patient's nasal mucosa may appear inflamed, and he may have nasal congestion and profuse drainage. Usually, his breath smells musty.

▶ *Tracheobronchitis (acute).* Initially, this disorder produces a dry cough that later becomes productive as secretions increase. Chills, sore throat, slight fever, muscle and back pain, and substernal tightness generally precede the cough's onset. Rhonchi and wheezing are usually heard. Severe illness causes a fever of 101° to 102° F (38.3° to 38.9° C) and possibly bronchospasm, severe wheezing, and increased coughing.

▶ *Tularemia.* Also known as *rabbit fever,* this infectious disease is caused by the gram-negative, non–spore-forming bacterium *Francisella tularensis.* This organism is found in wild animals, water, and moist soil, typically in rural areas. It's transmitted to humans through being bitten by an infected insect or tick, handling infected animal carcasses, drinking contaminated water, or inhaling the bacterium. It's considered a possible airborne agent for biological warfare. Signs and symptoms following inhalation of the organism include the abrupt onset of fever, chills, headache, generalized myalgia, a nonproductive cough, dyspnea, pleuritic chest pain, and empyema.

Other causes

▶ *Diagnostic tests.* Pulmonary function tests and bronchoscopy may stimulate cough receptors and trigger coughing.

DRUG WATCH *Certain drugs, such as angiotensin-converting enzyme inhibitors (the most common class that caus-*

es chronic cough), also may cause a nonproductive cough.[3]

▶ *Treatments.* Irritation of the carina during suctioning or deep endotracheal or tracheal tube placement can trigger a paroxysmal or hacking cough. Intermittent positive-pressure breathing or spirometry can also cause a nonproductive cough. Some inhalants, such as pentamidine, may stimulate coughing.

Special considerations

A nonproductive, paroxysmal cough may induce life-threatening bronchospasm. The patient may need a bronchodilator to relieve his bronchospasm and open his airways. A sedative may be needed to suppress the cough. Antitussives may be used to relieve cough in patients with chronic bronchitis, but they have little efficacy in relieving cough from upper airway infection.[4]

To relieve mucous membrane inflammation and dryness, humidify the air in the patient's room, or instruct him to use a humidifier at home. Make sure that the patient receives adequate fluids and nutrition.

Pediatric pointers

A nonproductive cough can be difficult to evaluate in infants and young children because it can't be voluntarily induced and must be observed.

A sudden onset of paroxysmal nonproductive coughing may indicate aspiration of a foreign body—a common danger in children, especially those between ages 6 months and 4 years. Nonproductive coughing can also result from several disorders that commonly affect infants and children. In asthma, a characteristic nonproductive "tight" cough can arise suddenly or insidiously as an attack begins. The cough usually becomes productive toward the end of the attack. In bacterial pneumonia, a nonproductive, hacking cough arises suddenly and becomes productive in 2 to 3 days. Acute bronchiolitis, which has a peak incidence at age 6, produces paroxysms of nonproductive coughing that become more frequent as the disease progresses. Acute otitis media, which is common in infants and young children because of their short eustachian tubes, also produces nonproductive coughing.

A child with measles typically has a slight nonproductive, hacking cough that increases in severity. The earliest sign of cystic fibrosis may be a nonproductive, paroxysmal cough from retained secretions. Life-threatening pertussis produces a cough that becomes paroxysmal with an inspiratory "whoop" or crowing sound. Airway hyperactivity causes a chronic nonproductive cough that increases with exercise or exposure to cold air. Psychogenic coughing may occur when a child is under stress, emotionally stimulated, or seeking attention.

Geriatric pointers
Always ask elderly patients about a nonproductive cough because it may be an indication of a serious acute or chronic illness.

Patient counseling
As indicated, prepare the patient for diagnostic tests, such as X-rays, a lung scan, bronchoscopy, and pulmonary function tests.

Explain to the patient why nonproductive coughs should be suppressed and productive coughs encouraged. Tell him to avoid using aerosols, powders, and other respiratory irritants—especially cigarettes. Urge the patient to use a respirator when exposed to airway irritants such as paint fumes and dust. Advise patients with chronic obstructive pulmonary disease to have an annual flu vaccination because it reduces the risk of serious illness and death in these patients by 50%.[5]

REFERENCES
1. Pruitt, B. "Fending Off InFLUenza." *Nursing* 37(10):44-46, October 2007.
2. Miskovich-Riddle, L. "CAP Management Guidelines." *The Nurse Practitioner* 31(1):43-53, January 2006.
3. Holcomb, S.S. "Understanding Chronic Cough." *The Nurse Practitioner* 32(11):9-11, November 2007.
4. Bolser, D.C. "Cough Suppressant and Pharmacologic Protussive Therapy. ACCP Evidence-Based Clinical Practice Guidelines." *Chest* 129(1 Suppl):238S-249S, January 2006.
5. Bruce, M.L. "COPD: Your Role In Early Detection." *The Nurse Practitioner* 32(11):24-33, November 2007.

COUGH, PRODUCTIVE

Productive coughing is the body's mechanism for clearing airway passages of accumulated secretions that normal mucociliary action doesn't remove. It's a sudden, forceful, noisy expulsion of air (from the lungs) that contains sputum or blood (or both). The sputum's color, consistency, and odor provide important clues about the patient's condition. A productive cough can occur as a single cough or as paroxysmal coughing, and it can be voluntarily induced but is usually a reflexive response to stimulation of the airway mucosa.

Usually caused by a cardiovascular or respiratory disorder, a productive cough commonly results from an acute or chronic infection that causes inflammation, edema, and increased mucus production in the airways. However, inhalation of antigenic or irritating substances or foreign bodies also can cause a productive cough. In fact, the most common cause of chronic productive coughing is cigarette smoking, which produces mucoid sputum ranging in color from clear to yellow to brown. This sign also can result from acquired immunodeficiency syndrome.

Many patients minimize or overlook a chronic productive cough or accept it as normal. Such patients may not seek medical attention until a related problem—such as dyspnea, hemoptysis, chest pain, weight loss, or recurrent respiratory tract infections—develops. The delay can have serious consequences because productive coughing may result from several life-threatening disorders and may lead to airway occlusion from excessive secretions.

A patient with a productive cough can develop acute respiratory distress from thick or excessive secretions, bronchospasm, or fatigue, so examine him before you take his history. Take vital signs and check the rate, depth, and rhythm of respirations. Keep his airway patent, and be prepared to provide supplemental oxygen if he becomes restless or confused, or if his respirations become shallow, irregular, rapid, or slow. Look for stridor, wheezing, choking, or gurgling. Be alert for nasal flaring and cyanosis.

A productive cough may signal a life-threatening disorder. For example, coughing with pulmonary edema produces thin, frothy, pink sputum, and coughing with an asthma attack produces thick, mucoid sputum.

History and physical examination

When the patient's condition permits, ask when the cough began and how much sputum he's coughing up each day. (Normally, the tracheobronchial tree produces up to 3 oz [89 ml] of sputum daily.) At what time of day does he cough up the most sputum? Is his sputum production affected by what or when he eats, his activities, or his environment? Ask him if he has noticed an increase in sputum production since his coughing began. This may result from external stimuli or from such internal causes as chronic bronchial infection or a lung abscess. Also ask about the color, odor, and consistency of the sputum. Blood-tinged or rust-colored sputum may result from trauma due to coughing or from an underlying condition, such as a pulmonary infection or a tumor. Foul-smelling sputum may result from an anaerobic infection, such as bronchitis or a lung abscess.

How does the cough sound? A hacking cough results from laryngeal involvement, whereas a "brassy" cough indicates major airway involvement. Does the patient feel any pain with his productive cough? If so, ask about its location and severity and whether it radiates to other areas. Does coughing, changing body position, or inspiration increase or help relieve his pain?

Next, ask the patient about his cigarette, drug, and alcohol use and whether his weight or appetite has changed. Find out if he has a history of asthma, allergies, or respiratory disorders, and ask about recent illnesses, surgery, or trauma. What drugs is he taking? Does he work around chemicals or respiratory irritants such as silicone?

Examine the patient's mouth and nose for congestion, drainage, or inflammation. Note his breath odor: Halitosis can be a sign of pulmonary infection. Inspect his neck for distended veins, and palpate it for tenderness, masses, and enlarged lymph nodes. Observe his chest for accessory muscle use, retractions, and uneven chest expansion, and percuss it for dullness, tympany, or flatness. Finally, auscultate for pleural friction rub and abnormal breath sounds, including rhonchi, crackles, or wheezing.

Medical causes

▶ *Actinomycosis.* This disorder starts with a cough that produces purulent sputum. Fever, weight loss, fatigue, weakness, dyspnea, night sweats, pleuritic chest pain, and hemoptysis also may occur.

▶ *Aspiration pneumonitis.* This disorder causes coughing that produces pink, frothy, possibly purulent sputum. The patient also has marked dyspnea, fever, tachypnea, tachycardia, wheezing, and cyanosis.

▶ *Asthma (acute).* A severe asthma attack, which can be life-threatening, may produce tenacious mucoid sputum and mucus plugs. Such an attack typically starts with a dry cough and mild wheezing, then progresses to severe dyspnea, audible wheezing, chest tightness, and a productive cough. Other findings include apprehension, prolonged expiration, intercostal and supraclavicular retraction on inspiration, accessory muscle use, rhonchi, crackles, flaring nostrils, tachypnea, tachycardia, diaphoresis, and flushing or cyanosis. Attacks commonly occur at night or during sleep.

▶ *Bronchiectasis.* The chronic cough in this disorder produces copious mucopurulent sputum that has characteristic layering (top, frothy; middle, clear; bottom, dense with purulent particles). The patient has halitosis: His sputum may smell foul or sickeningly sweet. Other findings include hemoptysis, persistent coarse crackles over the affected lung area, occasional wheezing, rhonchi, exertional dyspnea, weight loss, fatigue, malaise, weakness, recurrent fever, and late-stage finger clubbing.

▶ *Bronchitis (chronic).* The cough in chronic bronchitis may be nonproductive initially; eventually, however, it produces mucoid sputum that becomes purulent. Secondary infection can also cause mucopurulent sputum, which may become blood tinged and foul smelling. The cough, which may be paroxysmal during exercise, usually occurs when the patient is recumbent or rises from sleep.

The patient also has prolonged expiration, accessory muscle use, barrel chest, tachypnea, cyanosis, wheezing, exertional dyspnea, scattered rhonchi, coarse crackles (which can be caused by coughing), and late-stage clubbing.

▶ *Chemical pneumonitis.* This disorder causes a cough with purulent sputum. It also may cause dyspnea, wheezing, orthopnea, fever, malaise, crackles, laryngitis, rhinitis, and mucous membrane irritation of the conjunctivae, throat, and nose. Signs and symptoms may increase for 24 to 48 hours after exposure, then resolve; in severe pneumonitis, however, they may recur 2 to 5 weeks later.

▶ *Common cold.* The common cold may cause a productive cough with mucoid or mucopurulent sputum, but it usually starts with a dry, hacking cough, sore throat, sneezing, rhinorrhea, and nasal congestion. Headache, malaise, fatigue, myalgia, and arthralgia also may occur.

▶ *Emphysema.* This disorder causes a chronic productive cough with scant mucoid, translucent, grayish white sputum that can become mucopurulent. Patients with emphysema are typically thin and have the characteristic pink or red complexion ("pink puffer" appearance). They also may have increased accessory muscle use, tachypnea, grunting expirations through pursed lips, diminished breath sounds, exertional dyspnea, rhonchi, barrel chest, anorexia, and weight loss. Clubbing is a late sign.

▶ *Legionnaires' disease.* This disorder causes a cough that produces scant mucoid, nonpurulent and, possibly, blood-streaked sputum. Prodromal signs and symptoms typically include malaise, fatigue, weakness, anorexia, diffuse myalgia, and possibly diarrhea. Within 12 to 48 hours, the patient develops a dry cough and a sudden high fever with chills. Many patients also have pleuritic chest pain, headache, tachypnea, tachycardia, nausea, vomiting, dyspnea, crackles, mild temporary amnesia, disorientation, confusion, flushing, mild diaphoresis, and prostration.

▶ *Lung abscess (ruptured).* The cardinal sign of a ruptured lung abscess is a cough that produces copious amounts of purulent, foul-smelling and, possibly, blood-tinged sputum. A ruptured abscess can also cause diaphoresis, anorexia, clubbing, weight loss, weakness, fatigue, fever with chills, dyspnea, headache, malaise, pleuritic chest pain, halitosis, inspiratory crackles, and tubular or amphoric breath sounds. The patient's chest is dull on percussion on the affected side.

▶ *Lung cancer.* One of the earliest signs of bronchogenic carcinoma is a chronic cough that produces small amounts of purulent or mucopurulent, blood-streaked sputum. In a patient with bronchoalveolar cancer, however, coughing produces large amounts of frothy sputum. Other signs and symptoms of lung cancer include dyspnea, anorexia, fatigue, weight loss, chest pain, fever, diaphoresis, wheezing, and clubbing.

▶ *Nocardiosis.* This disorder causes a productive cough (with purulent, thick, tenacious, and possibly blood-tinged sputum) and fever that may last several months. Other findings include night sweats, pleuritic pain, anorexia, weight loss, malaise, fatigue, and diminished or absent breath sounds. The patient's chest is dull on percussion.

▶ *North American blastomycosis.* This chronic disorder may produce a dry hacking cough or a productive cough with bloody or purulent sputum. Other findings include pleuritic chest pain, fever, chills, anorexia, weight loss, malaise, fatigue, night sweats, cutaneous lesions (small, painless, nonpruritic macules or papules), and prostration.

▶ *Plague.* Caused by *Yersinia pestis,* plague is one of the most virulent and, if untreated, most lethal bacterial infections known. Most cases are sporadic, but the potential for epidemic spread still exists. Clinical forms include bubonic (the most common), septicemic, and pneumonic plagues. The bubonic form is transmitted to man from the bite of infected fleas. Signs and symptoms include fever, chills, and swollen, inflamed, and tender lymph nodes near the site of the fleabite. Septicemic plague may develop as a complication of untreated bubonic or pneumonic plague and occurs when plague bacteria enter the bloodstream and multiply. The pneumonic form can be contracted by inhaling respiratory droplets from an infected person or inhaling the organism that has been dispersed in the air through biological warfare. The onset is usually sudden with chills, fever, headache, and myalgia. Pulmonary signs and symptoms include a productive cough, chest pain, tachypnea, dyspnea, hemoptysis, increasing respiratory distress, and cardiopulmonary insufficiency.

▶ *Pneumonia.* Typical (bacterial) pneumonia initially produces a dry cough that becomes productive. Other signs and symptoms develop suddenly and include shaking chills, high fever, myalgia, headache, pleuritic chest pain that increases with chest movement, tachypnea, tachycardia, dyspnea, cyanosis, diaphoresis, decreased breath sounds, fine crackles, and rhonchi.

Streptococcus pneumoniae, which accounts for 40% to 70% of all cases of bacterial pneumonia, produces a cough with watery sputum that progresses to purulent, blood-tinged, or rust-colored.[1] *Haemophilus influenzae* causes a cough with purulent sputum.

Mycoplasmal pneumonia, a type of atypical or nonbacterial pneumonia, may cause a cough that produces scant blood-flecked sputum. In most cases, however, a nonproductive cough starts 2 to 3 days after the onset of malaise, headache, fever, and sore throat. Paroxysmal coughing causes substernal chest pain. Patients may develop crackles but generally don't appear seriously ill.

▶ *Psittacosis.* As this disorder progresses, the characteristic hacking cough, nonproductive at first, may later produce a small amount of mucoid, blood-streaked sputum. The infection may begin abruptly with chills, fever, headache, myalgia, and prostration. Other signs and symptoms include tachypnea, fine crackles, chest pain (rare), epistaxis, photophobia, abdominal distention and tenderness, nausea, vomiting, and a faint macular rash. Severe psittacosis may produce stupor, delirium, and coma.

▶ *Pulmonary coccidioidomycosis.* This disorder causes a nonproductive or slightly productive cough with fever, occasional chills, pleuritic chest pain, sore throat, headache, backache, malaise, marked weakness, anorexia, hemoptysis, and an itchy macular rash. Rhonchi and wheezing may be heard. The disease may spread to other areas, causing arthralgia, swelling of the knees and ankles, and erythema nodosum or erythema multiforme.

▶ *Pulmonary edema.* When severe, this life-threatening disorder causes a cough that produces frothy, blood-tinged sputum. Early signs and symptoms include exertional dyspnea, paroxysmal nocturnal dyspnea followed by orthopnea, and a cough that may be nonproductive initially. Fever, fatigue, tachycardia, tachypnea, dependent crackles, and ventricular gallop also may occur. As the patient's respirations become increasingly rapid and labored, he develops more diffuse crackles, productive cough, worsening tachycardia, and possibly arrhythmias. His skin becomes cold, clammy, and cyanotic; his blood pressure falls; and his pulse becomes thready.

▶ *Pulmonary embolism.* This life-threatening disorder causes a cough that may be nonproductive or may produce blood-tinged sputum. Usually, the first symptom of a pulmonary embolism is severe dyspnea, which may be accompanied by angina or pleuritic chest pain. The patient experiences marked anxiety, a low-grade fever, tachycardia, tachypnea, and diaphoresis. Less common signs include massive hemoptysis, chest splinting, leg edema and, in a large embolus, cyanosis, syncope, and distended jugular veins. The patient also may have a pleural friction rub, diffuse wheezing, crackles, chest dullness on percussion, decreased breath sounds, and signs of circulatory collapse.

▶ *Pulmonary tuberculosis.* This disorder causes a mild to severe productive cough along with some combination of hemoptysis, malaise, dyspnea, and pleuritic chest pain. Sputum may be scant and mucoid or copious and purulent. Typically, the patient has night sweats, easy fatigability, and weight loss. His breath sounds are amphoric. He may have chest dullness on percussion and, after coughing, increased tactile fremitus with crackles.

▶ *Silicosis.* A productive cough with mucopurulent sputum is the earliest sign of this disorder. The patient also has exertional dyspnea, tachypnea, weight loss, fatigue, general weakness, and recurrent respiratory infections. Auscultation reveals end-inspiratory, fine crackles at the lung bases.

▶ *Tracheobronchitis.* Inflammation initially causes a nonproductive cough followed by chills, sore throat, slight fever, muscle and back pain, and substernal tightness. As secretions increase, the cough produces mucoid, mucopurulent, or purulent sputum. The patient typically has rhonchi and wheezing; he also may develop crackles. Severe tracheobronchitis may cause a fever of 101° to 102° F (38.3° to 38.9° C) and bronchospasm.

Other causes

▶ *Diagnostic tests.* Bronchoscopy and pulmonary function tests may increase productive coughing.

DRUG WATCH *Angiotensin-converting enzyme inhibitors commonly cause a chronic cough.[2] Expectorants, such as ammonium chloride, guaifenesin, and potassium iodide, increase productive coughing.*

▶ *Respiratory therapy.* Intermittent positive-pressure breathing, nebulizer therapy, and incentive spirometry can help loosen secretions and cause or increase productive coughing.

Special considerations

Avoid taking measures to suppress a productive cough because retention of sputum may interfere with alveolar aeration or impair pulmonary resistance to infection. Expect to give a mucolytic and an expectorant, and increase the patient's intake of oral fluids to thin his secretions and increase their flow. In addition, you may give a bronchodilator to relieve bronchospasms and open airways. An antibiotic may be ordered to treat underlying infection.

Humidify the air around the patient; this will relieve mucous membrane inflammation and help loosen dried secretions. Provide pulmonary physiotherapy, such as postural drainage with vibration and percussion, to loosen secretions. Aerosol therapy may be necessary.

Provide the patient with uninterrupted rest periods. Keep him from using respiratory irritants. If he's confined to bed rest, change his position often to promote the drainage of secretions.

Prepare the patient for diagnostic tests, such as chest X-rays, bronchoscopy, a lung scan, and pulmonary function tests. Collect sputum specimens for culture and sensitivity testing.

Pediatric pointers

Because his airway is narrow, a child with a productive cough can quickly develop airway occlusion and respiratory distress from thick or excessive secretions. Causes of a productive cough in children include asthma, bronchiectasis, bronchitis, acute bronchiolitis, cystic fibrosis, and pertussis.

When caring for a child with a productive cough, expect to give an expectorant, but not a cough suppressant. To soothe inflamed mucous membranes and prevent drying of secretions, provide humidified air or oxygen. Remember, high humidity can induce bronchospasm in a hyperactive child or produce overhydration in an infant.

Geriatric pointers

Always ask elderly patients about a productive cough because this sign may indicate a serious acute or chronic illness. Elderly patients with pneumonia are less likely to present with a productive cough and fever than younger patients.[1] Tachypnea is a more likely finding.

Patient counseling

Encourage the patient not to smoke because doing so can aggravate his condition. Explain that quitting even after decades of smoking is helpful. Teach him how to breathe deeply, to cough effectively and, if appropriate, to splint his incision when he coughs. Tell him to sit or stand upright when coughing, if possible, to maximize chest expansion. Teach the patient and his family how to use chest percussion to loosen secretions.

Tell the patient to cover his mouth and nose with a tissue when he coughs and to dispose of contaminated tissues properly, to protect himself and others from the cough and secretions.[3] Be sure to provide a container for tissues and sputum. The patient could also cough or sneeze into his elbow or upper arm to avoid contaminating his hands.[3]

Advise patients with chronic obstructive pulmonary disease to have an annual flu vaccination because it reduces the risk of serious illness and death in these patients by 50%.[4]

REFERENCES

1. Miskovich-Riddle, L. "CAP Management Guidelines." *The Nurse Practitioner* 31(1):43-53, January 2006.
2. Holcomb, S.S. "Understanding Chronic Cough." *The Nurse Practitioner* 32(11):9-11, November 2007.
3. "Cold vs. Flu." *The Nurse Practitioner* 32(9):11-12, September 2007.
4. Bruce, M.L. "COPD: Your Role In Early Detection." *The Nurse Practitioner* 32(11):24-33, November 2007.

CRACKLES

A common finding in patients with certain cardiovascular and pulmonary disorders, crackles (also called *rales* or *crepitations*) are nonmusical clicking or rattling noises heard during auscultation of breath sounds. They usually occur during inspiration and recur constantly from one respiratory cycle to the next. They can be unilateral or bilateral and moist or dry. They're characterized by their pitch, loudness, location, persistence, and occurrence during the respiratory cycle.

Crackles indicate abnormal movement of air through airways narrowed by fluid, mucus, or pus.[1] They can be irregularly dispersed, as in pneumonia, or localized, as in bronchiectasis. (A few basilar crackles can be heard in normal lungs after prolonged shallow breathing. These normal crackles clear with a few deep breaths.) Crackles usually indicate the degree of an underlying illness. When crackles result from a generalized disorder, they usually occur in the less distended and more dependent areas of the lungs, such as the lung bases, when the patient is standing. Crackles caused by air passing through inflammatory exudate may not be audible if the involved portion of the lung isn't being ventilated because of shallow respirations. (See *How crackles occur.*)

Quickly take the patient's vital signs, and examine him for signs of respiratory distress or airway obstruction. Check the depth and rhythm of respirations. Is he struggling to breathe? Check for increased use of accessory muscles, chest wall motion, retractions, stri-

dor, or nasal flaring. Provide supplemental oxygen. Endotracheal intubation may be needed.

History and physical examination

If the patient also has a cough, ask when it began and if it's constant or intermittent. Find out what the cough sounds like and whether he's coughing up sputum or blood. If the cough is productive, determine the sputum's consistency, amount, odor, and color.

Ask the patient if he has any pain. If so, where is it located? When did he first notice it? Does it radiate to other areas? Also, ask the patient if movement, coughing, or breathing worsens or helps relieve his pain. Note the patient's position: Is he lying still or moving about restlessly?

Obtain a brief medical history. Does the patient have cancer or any known respiratory or cardiovascular problems? Ask about recent surgery, trauma, or illness. Does he smoke or drink alcohol? Is he experiencing hoarseness or difficulty swallowing? Find out what drugs he's taking. Also, ask about recent weight loss, anorexia, nausea, vomiting, fatigue, weakness, vertigo, and syncope. Has the patient been exposed to irritants, such as vapors, fumes, or smoke?

Next, perform a physical examination. Examine the patient's nose and mouth for signs of infection, such as inflammation or increased secretions. Note his breath odor: Halitosis could indicate pulmonary infection. Check his neck for masses, tenderness, swelling, lymphadenopathy, or venous distention.

Inspect the patient's chest for abnormal configuration or uneven expansion. Auscultate his lungs for abnormal, diminished, or absent breath sounds. Listen for a full inspiration and expiration at each auscultation point.[1] Listen to his heart for abnormal sounds, and check his hands and feet for edema or clubbing. Percuss for dullness, tympany, or flatness.

Medical causes

▶ *Acute respiratory distress syndrome.* This life-threatening disorder causes diffuse fine to coarse crackles that are usually heard in the

How crackles occur

Crackles occur when air passes through fluid-filled airways, causing collapsed alveoli to pop open as the airway pressure equalizes. They also can occur when membranes lining the chest cavity and the lungs become inflamed. These illustrations show a normal alveolus and two pathologic alveolar changes that cause crackles.

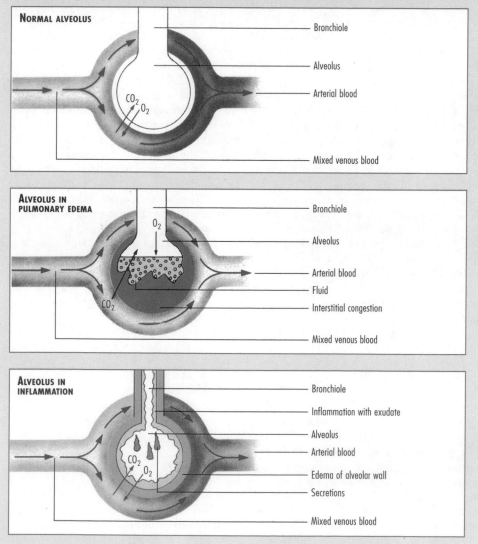

NORMAL ALVEOLUS
- Bronchiole
- Alveolus
- Arterial blood
- Mixed venous blood

CO_2 O_2

ALVEOLUS IN PULMONARY EDEMA
- Bronchiole
- Alveolus
- Arterial blood
- Fluid
- Interstitial congestion
- Mixed venous blood

O_2

CO_2

ALVEOLUS IN INFLAMMATION
- Bronchiole
- Inflammation with exudate
- Alveolus
- Arterial blood
- Edema of alveolar wall
- Secretions
- Mixed venous blood

CO_2 O_2

dependent portions of the lungs. It also produces cyanosis, nasal flaring, tachypnea, tachycardia, grunting respirations, rhonchi, dyspnea, anxiety, and decreased level of consciousness.

▶ *Asthma (acute).* A severe attack usually occurs at night or during sleep, causing dry, whistling crackles. An attack typically starts with a dry cough and mild wheezing and progresses to severe dyspnea, audible wheezing, chest tightness, and a productive cough. Other findings include apprehension, prolonged expirations, rhonchi, intercostal and supraclavicular retractions on inspiration, accessory muscle use, flaring nostrils, tachypnea, tachycardia, diaphoresis, and flushing or cyanosis.

▶ *Bronchiectasis.* In this disorder, persistent coarse crackles are heard over the affected area of the lung. They're accompanied by a chronic cough that produces copious amounts of mucopurulent sputum. Other characteristics include halitosis, occasional wheezing, exertional dyspnea, rhonchi, weight loss, fatigue, malaise, weakness, recurrent fever, and late-stage clubbing.

▶ *Bronchitis (chronic).* This disorder causes coarse crackles that are usually heard at the lung bases as well as prolonged expirations, wheezing, rhonchi, exertional dyspnea, tachypnea, and a persistent productive cough from increased bronchial secretions. Clubbing and cyanosis also may occur.

▶ *Chemical pneumonitis.* In acute chemical pneumonitis, diffuse fine to coarse, moist crackles accompany a productive cough with purulent sputum, dyspnea, wheezing, orthopnea, fever, malaise, and mucous membrane irritation. Signs and symptoms may worsen for 24 to 48 hours after exposure, then resolve; if severe, however, they may recur 2 to 5 weeks later.

▶ *Interstitial lung disease.* Velcro-like crackles can be heard over all lobes in this disorder.[2] As the disease progresses, a nonproductive cough, dyspnea, fatigue, weight loss, cyanosis, and pleuritic chest pain develop.

▶ *Legionnaires' disease.* This disorder causes diffuse moist crackles and a cough producing scant mucoid, nonpurulent and, possibly, blood-streaked sputum. Prodromal signs and symptoms usually include malaise, fatigue, weakness, anorexia, diffuse myalgia and, possibly, diarrhea. Within 12 to 48 hours, the patient develops a dry cough and a sudden high fever with chills. He also may have pleuritic chest pain, headache, dyspnea, tachypnea, tachycardia, nausea, vomiting, mild temporary amnesia, confusion, flushing, mild diaphoresis, and prostration.

▶ *Lung abscess.* This disorder produces fine to medium, moist inspiratory crackles. The onset is insidious; signs and symptoms include sweats, anorexia, weight loss, fever, fatigue, weakness, dyspnea, clubbing, pleuritic chest pain, pleural friction rub, and a cough producing copious amounts of foul-smelling, purulent and, possibly, blood-tinged sputum. The patient's breath sounds are hollow and tubular or amphoric; the affected side of his chest is dull on percussion.

▶ *Pneumonia.* Bacterial pneumonia produces diffuse fine crackles, sudden shaking chills, high fever, tachypnea, pleuritic chest pain, cyanosis, grunting respirations, nasal flaring, decreased breath sounds, myalgia, headache, tachycardia, dyspnea, cyanosis, diaphoresis, and rhonchi. The patient also has a dry cough that later becomes productive.

Mycoplasmal pneumonia produces medium to fine crackles with a nonproductive cough, malaise, sore throat, headache, and fever. The patient may have blood-flecked sputum. In viral pneumonia, diffuse crackles develop gradually and may be accompanied by a nonproductive cough, malaise, headache, anorexia, low-grade fever, and decreased breath sounds.

▶ *Postoperative atelectasis.* Late-inspiratory crackles are a sign of this condition, which affects 90% of patients to some extent who have had general anesthesia.[3] Other findings include tachypnea, tachycardia, and decreased breath sounds.

▶ *Psittacosis.* Diffuse fine crackles may be heard as this disorder progresses. Accompanying findings include a characteristic hacking, productive cough, chills, fever, headache, myalgia, and prostration. Other features include tachypnea, chest pain (rare), epistaxis, photophobia, abdominal distention and tenderness, nausea, vomiting, and a faint macular rash.

▶ *Pulmonary edema.* Moist, bubbling crackles on inspiration are one of the first signs of life-threatening pulmonary edema.[4] Other early findings include exertional dyspnea; paroxysmal nocturnal dyspnea, then orthopnea; and coughing, which may be initially nonproductive but later produces frothy, bloody sputum. Related clinical effects include tachycardia, tachypnea, and a ventricular gallop (a third heart sound [S_3]). As the patient's respirations become increasingly rapid and labored, he develops more diffuse crackles, worsening tachycardia, hypotension, a rapid and thready pulse, cyanosis, and cold, clammy skin.

▶ *Pulmonary embolism.* This life-threatening disorder can cause fine to coarse crackles and a cough that may be dry or may produce blood-tinged sputum. Usually, the first sign of pulmonary embolism is severe dyspnea, which may be accompanied by angina or pleuritic chest pain. The patient has marked anxiety, a low-grade fever, tachycardia, tachypnea, and diaphoresis. Less-common signs include massive hemoptysis, chest splinting, leg edema and, with a large embolus, cyanosis, syncope, and distended jugular veins. The patient also may have a pleural friction rub, diffuse wheezing, chest dullness on percussion, decreased breath sounds, and signs of circulatory collapse.

▶ *Pulmonary tuberculosis.* In this disorder, fine crackles occur after coughing along with some combination of hemoptysis, malaise, dyspnea, and pleuritic chest pain. Sputum may be scant and mucoid or copious and purulent. Typically, the patient is easily fatigued and experiences night sweats, weakness, and weight loss. His breath sounds are amphoric.

▶ *Sarcoidosis.* This disorder produces fine, bibasilar, end-inspiratory crackles and, rarely, wheezing. The patient doesn't have a fever but does have malaise, fatigue, weakness, weight loss, a cough, dyspnea, and tachypnea.

▶ *Silicosis.* This disorder produces fine end-inspiratory crackles heard at the lung bases. The earliest sign of silicosis is a productive cough with mucopurulent sputum. The patient also exhibits exertional dyspnea, tachypnea, weight loss, fatigue, general weakness, and recurrent respiratory tract infections.

▶ *Tracheobronchitis.* In its acute form, this disorder produces moist or coarse crackles along with a productive cough, rhonchi, wheezing, chills, sore throat, a slight fever, muscle and back pain, and substernal tightness. Severe tracheobronchitis may cause a moderate fever and bronchospasm.

Special considerations

To keep the patient's airway patent and facilitate his breathing, elevate the head of his bed. To liquefy thick secretions and relieve mucous membrane inflammation, administer fluids, humidified air, or oxygen. Diuretics may be needed if crackles result from cardiogenic pulmonary edema. Turn the patient every 1 to 2 hours, and encourage him to breathe deeply.

Plan daily uninterrupted rest periods to help the patient relax and sleep. Prepare the patient for diagnostic tests, such as chest X-rays, a lung scan, and sputum analysis.

Pediatric pointers

Preterm neonates are at high risk for respiratory distress syndrome, which can cause fine, inspiratory crackles bilaterally.[5] Crackles in an infant or a child may indicate a serious cardiovascular or respiratory disorder. Pneumonias produce sudden diffuse crackles in children. Esophageal atresia and tracheoesophageal fistula can cause bubbling, moist crackles due to aspiration of food or secretions into the lungs—especially in neonates. Pulmonary edema causes fine crackles at the base of the lungs, and bronchiectasis produces moist crackles. Cystic fibrosis produces widespread fine to coarse inspiratory crackles and wheezing in infants. Sickle cell anemia may produce crackles when it causes pulmonary infarction or infection.

Geriatric pointers

Crackles that clear after deep breathing may indicate mild basilar atelectasis. In elderly patients, auscultate lung bases before and after auscultating apices.

Patient counseling

Teach the patient how to cough effectively and splint incision areas if appropriate. Teach the patient how to use incentive spirometry preoperatively, and encourage him to use it postoperatively to help keep his lungs inflated and prevent pneumonia.[3] Encourage him to avoid smoking and using aerosols, powders, or other products that might irritate his airways.

REFERENCES

1. McCormick, M. "Every Breath you Take: Making Sense of Breath Sounds." *Nursing Made Incredibly Easy!* 5(1):7-11, January/February 2007.
2. Danoff, S.K., Terry, P.B., and Horton, M.R. "A Clinician's Guide to the Diagnosis and Treatment of Interstitial Lung Diseases." *Southern Medical Journal* 100(6):579-587, June 2007.

3. Pruitt, B. "Help Your Patient Combat Postoperative Atelectasis." *Nursing* 36(5):64hn1-64hn6, May 2006.
4. Bixby, M. "Turn Back the Tide of Cordiogenic Pulmonary Edema." *Nursing* 35(5):56-60, May 2005.
5. Hockenberry, M.J. and Wilson, D. (Eds.) *Wong's Nursing Care of Infants and Children,* 8th ed. St. Louis: Mosby, 2007.

● CYANOSIS

A bluish or bluish black discoloration of the skin and mucous membranes, cyanosis results from excessive concentration of unoxygenated hemoglobin in the blood. This common sign may develop abruptly or gradually. It can be classified as central or peripheral, although the two types may coexist.

Central cyanosis reflects inadequate oxygenation of systemic arterial blood caused by right-to-left cardiac shunting, pulmonary disease, or hematologic disorders. It may occur anywhere on the skin and also on the mucous membranes of the mouth, lips, and conjunctivae.

Peripheral cyanosis reflects sluggish peripheral circulation caused by vasoconstriction, reduced cardiac output, or vascular occlusion. It may be widespread or may affect only one extremity; however, it doesn't affect mucous membranes. Typically, peripheral cyanosis appears on exposed areas, such as the fingers, nail beds, feet, nose, and ears.

Although cyanosis is an important sign of cardiovascular and pulmonary disorders, it isn't always an accurate gauge of oxygenation. Several factors contribute to its development: hemoglobin concentration and oxygen saturation, cardiac output, and partial pressure of arterial oxygen (PaO_2). Cyanosis usually is undetectable until the oxygen saturation of hemoglobin falls below 80% to 85%.[1] Severe cyanosis is quite obvious, whereas mild cyanosis is more difficult to detect, even in natural bright light. In dark-skinned patients, cyanosis is most apparent in the mucous membranes and nail beds.

Transient, nonpathologic cyanosis may result from environmental factors. For example, peripheral cyanosis may result from cutaneous vasoconstriction after brief exposure to cold air or water, and central cyanosis may result from reduced PaO_2 at high altitudes.

If the patient has sudden, localized cyanosis and other signs of arterial occlusion, protect the affected limb from injury, but don't massage it. If you see central cyanosis stemming from a pulmonary disorder or shock, perform a rapid evaluation. Take immediate steps to maintain an airway, assist breathing, and monitor circulation.

History and physical examination

If cyanosis accompanies less acute conditions, perform a thorough examination. Begin with a history, focusing on cardiac, pulmonary, and hematologic disorders. Ask about previous surgery. Then begin the physical examination by taking vital signs. Inspect the skin and mucous membranes to determine the extent of cyanosis. Ask the patient when he first noticed the cyanosis. Does it subside and recur? Is it aggravated by cold, smoking, or stress? Is it alleviated by massage or rewarming? Check the skin for coolness, pallor, redness, pain, and ulceration. Also note clubbing.

Next, evaluate the patient's level of consciousness. Ask about headaches, dizziness, or blurred vision. Then test his motor strength. Ask about pain in the arms and legs (especially with walking) and about abnormal sensations, such as numbness, tingling, and coldness.

Ask about chest pain and its severity. Can the patient identify any aggravating or alleviating factors? Palpate peripheral pulses, and test capillary refill time. Also, check for edema. Auscultate heart rate and rhythm, especially noting gallops and murmurs. Also auscultate the abdominal aorta and femoral arteries to detect any bruits.

Does the patient have a cough? Is it productive? If so, have the patient describe the sputum. Evaluate respiratory rate and rhythm. Check for nasal flaring and use of accessory muscles. Ask about sleep apnea. Does the patient sleep with his head propped up on pillows? Inspect the patient for asymmetrical chest expansion or barrel chest. Percuss the lungs for dullness or hyperresonance, and auscultate for decreased or adventitious breath sounds.

Inspect the abdomen for ascites, and test for shifting dullness or a fluid wave. Percuss and palpate the abdomen for liver enlargement and tenderness. Also, ask about nausea, anorexia, and weight loss.

Medical causes

▶ *Arteriosclerotic occlusive disease (chronic).* In this disorder, peripheral cyanosis occurs in the legs whenever they're in a dependent position. Associated signs and symptoms include intermittent claudication and burning pain at rest, paresthesia, pallor, muscle atrophy, weak leg pulses, and impotence. Leg ulcers and gangrene are late signs.

▶ *Blast lung injury.* Cyanosis is a serious sign of blast lung injury. The impact of this condition on the lungs of affected individuals varies and may include tearing, contusion, edema, and hemorrhage. Other signs and symptoms may include chest pain, wheezing, hemoptysis, and dyspnea. Treatment for patients with blast lung injury typically involves high-flow oxygen, careful fluid management, possible intubation, and close observation in an intensive care setting.

▶ *Bronchiectasis.* This disorder produces chronic central cyanosis. Its classic sign, though, is a chronic productive cough with copious, foul-smelling, mucopurulent sputum or hemoptysis. Auscultation reveals rhonchi and coarse crackles during inspiration. Other signs and symptoms include dyspnea, recurrent fever and chills, weight loss, malaise, clubbing, and signs of anemia.

▶ *Buerger's disease.* In this disorder, exposure to cold initially causes the feet to become cold, cyanotic, and numb; later, they become red, hot, and tingly. Intermittent claudication of the instep, a characteristic sign, is aggravated by exercise and smoking and relieved by rest. Associated signs and symptoms include weak peripheral pulses and, in later stages, ulceration, muscle atrophy, and gangrene.

▶ *Chronic obstructive pulmonary disease (COPD).* Chronic central cyanosis occurs in advanced COPD and may be aggravated by exertion. Other signs and symptoms include exertional dyspnea, a productive cough with thick sputum, anorexia, weight loss, purse-lip breathing, tachypnea, and accessory muscle use. Examination reveals wheezing and hyperresonant lung fields. Barrel chest and clubbing are late signs. Tachycardia, diaphoresis, and flushing also may accompany COPD.

▶ *Deep vein thrombosis.* In this disorder, acute peripheral cyanosis in the affected limb is associated with tenderness, painful movement, edema, warmth, and prominent superficial veins. Homans' sign can also be elicited.

▶ *Heart failure.* Acute or chronic cyanosis may occur in patients with heart failure. It may be central, peripheral, or both and is typically a late sign. In left-sided heart failure, central cyanosis occurs with tachycardia, fatigue, dyspnea, cold intolerance, orthopnea, a cough, ventricular or atrial gallop, bibasilar crackles, and diffuse apical impulse. In right-sided heart failure, peripheral cyanosis occurs with fatigue, peripheral edema, ascites, jugular vein distention, and hepatomegaly.

▶ *Lung cancer.* This disease causes chronic central cyanosis accompanied by fever, weakness, anorexia, weight loss, dyspnea, chest pain, hemoptysis, and wheezing. Atelectasis causes mediastinal shift, decreased diaphragmatic excursion, asymmetrical chest expansion, a dull percussion note, and diminished breath sounds.

▶ *Peripheral arterial occlusion (acute).* This disorder produces acute cyanosis of one arm or leg or, occasionally, of both legs. The cyanosis is accompanied by sharp or aching pain that worsens when the patient moves. The affected extremity also exhibits paresthesia, weakness, and pale, cool skin. Examination reveals decreased or absent pulse and increased capillary refill time.

▶ *Pneumonia.* In pneumonia, acute central cyanosis is usually preceded by fever, shaking chills, a cough with purulent sputum, crackles, rhonchi, and pleuritic chest pain that's worsened by deep inspiration. Other signs and symptoms include tachycardia, dyspnea, tachypnea, diminished breath sounds, diaphoresis, myalgia, fatigue, headache, and anorexia.

▶ *Pneumothorax.* A cardinal sign of pneumothorax, acute central cyanosis is accompanied by dyspnea; sharp chest pain that's worsened by movement, deep breathing, and coughing; and asymmetrical chest wall expansion. The patient also may have rapid, shallow respirations; a weak, rapid pulse; pallor; jugular vein distention; anxiety; and absence of breath sounds over the affected lobe.

▶ *Polycythemia vera.* A ruddy complexion that can appear cyanotic is characteristic in this chronic myeloproliferative disorder. Other findings include hepatosplenomegaly, headache, dizziness, fatigue, aquagenic pruritus, blurred vision, chest pain, intermittent claudication, and coagulation defects.

▶ *Pulmonary edema.* In this disorder, acute central cyanosis occurs with dyspnea; orthopnea; frothy, blood-tinged sputum; tachycardia; tachypnea; dependent crackles; ventricular gallop; cold, clammy skin; weak, thready pulse; hypotension; and confusion.

▶ *Pulmonary embolism.* Acute central cyanosis occurs when a large embolus causes significant obstruction of the pulmonary circulation. Syncope and jugular vein distention also may occur. Other common signs and symptoms include dyspnea, chest pain, tachycardia, paradoxical pulse, a dry cough or a productive cough with blood-tinged sputum, low-grade fever, restlessness, and diaphoresis.

▶ *Raynaud's phenomenon.* In Raynaud's phenomenon, exposure to cold or stress initially causes the fingers or hands to blanch and turn cold, then to become cyanotic, and finally to redden with return of normal temperature. This condition is more common in women and those living in colder climates.[2] Numbness and tingling also may occur. Secondary Raynaud's phenomenon describes the same presentation when associated with other disorders, such as rheumatoid arthritis, scleroderma, or systemic lupus erythematosus.

▶ *Shock.* In shock, acute peripheral cyanosis develops in the hands and feet, which also may be cold, clammy, and pale. Other characteristic signs and symptoms include lethargy, confusion, increased capillary refill time, and a rapid, weak pulse. Tachypnea, hyperpnea, and hypotension also may be present.

▶ *Sleep apnea.* Chronic and severe sleep apnea causes pulmonary hypertension and cor pulmonale (right-sided heart failure), which can produce chronic cyanosis.

Special considerations

Provide supplemental oxygen to relieve dyspnea, improve oxygenation, and decrease cyanosis. Be sure to deliver small doses (2 L/minute) to patients with COPD, who may retain carbon dioxide. Use a low-flow oxygen rate for mild worsening of COPD. However, for acute situations, a high-flow oxygen rate may be needed initially. Remember to pay attention to the patient's respiratory drive and adjust the amount of oxygen accordingly. Position the patient comfortably to ease breathing. Give a diuretic, a bronchodilator, an antibiotic, or a cardiac drug as needed. Make sure that the patient gets sufficient rest between activities to prevent dyspnea.

Prepare the patient for such tests as arterial blood gas analysis and a complete blood count to determine the cause of cyanosis.

Pediatric pointers

Many pulmonary disorders responsible for cyanosis in adults also cause cyanosis in children. In addition, central cyanosis may result from cystic fibrosis, asthma, airway obstruction by a foreign body, acute laryngotracheobronchitis, or epiglottiditis. It also may result from congenital heart defects that cause deoxygenated venous blood returning to the heart to enter arterial circulation without first passing through the lungs, such as Tetrology of Fallot (most common), tricuspid atresia, and transposition of the great arteries.[3]

In children, circumoral cyanosis may precede generalized cyanosis. Acrocyanosis (also called *glove and bootie cyanosis*) may occur in infants from excessive crying or exposure to cold. Exercise and agitation enhance cyanosis, so provide regular rest periods and make the child comfortable. Also, administer supplemental oxygen during cyanotic episodes.

Geriatric pointers

Because elderly patients have reduced tissue perfusion, peripheral cyanosis can occur even with a slight decrease in cardiac output or systemic blood pressure.

Patient counseling

Teach patients with chronic cardiopulmonary diseases, such as heart failure, asthma, or COPD, to recognize cyanosis as a sign of severe disease and to get immediate medical attention when it occurs.

REFERENCES

1. Giuliano, K.K. and Liu, L.M. "Knowledge of Pulse Oximetry Among Critical Care Nurses." *Dimensions of Critical Care Nursing* 25(1):44-49, January/February 2006.
2. Reilly, A. and Snyder, B. "Raynaud Phenomenon: Whether It's Primary or Secondary, There Is No Cure But Treatment Can Alleviate Symptoms." *AJN* 105(8):56-65, August 2005.
3. Hockenberry, M.J. and Wilson, D. (Eds.) *Wong's Nursing Care of Infants and Children,* 8th ed. St. Louis: Mosby, 2007.

D

DECEREBRATE POSTURE

Decerebrate posture, also known as *decerebrate rigidity, abnormal extensor reflex,* and *extensor posture,* is characterized by adduction (internal rotation) and extension of the arms, with the wrists pronated and the fingers flexed. The legs are stiffly extended, with forced plantar flexion of the feet. In severe cases, the back is acutely arched (opisthotonos). This sign indicates upper brain stem damage, which may result from primary lesions, such as infarction, hemorrhage, or tumor; metabolic encephalopathy; head injury; or brain stem compression associated with increased intracranial pressure (ICP).

Decerebrate posture may be elicited by noxious stimuli or may occur spontaneously. It may be unilateral or bilateral. With concurrent brain stem and cerebral damage, decerebrate posture may affect only the arms, with the legs remaining flaccid. Or, decerebrate posture may affect one side of the body and decorticate posture the other. The two postures also may alternate as the patient's neurologic status fluctuates. Generally, the duration of each posturing episode correlates with the severity of brain stem damage Posturing may be reversed if adequate oxygenation and perfusion are restored.[1] However, if posturing occurs when there is adequate oxygenation and perfusion, there is a greater chance that the patient is in a persistent vegetative state.[1] (See *Comparing decerebrate and decorticate postures.*)

Your first priority is to ensure a patent airway. Insert an artificial airway and institute measures to prevent aspiration. (Don't disrupt spinal alignment if you suspect spinal cord injury.) Suction the patient as needed.

Next, examine spontaneous respirations. Give supplemental oxygen, and ventilate the patient with a handheld resuscitation bag if needed. Intubation and mechanical ventilation may be indicated. Keep emergency resuscitation equipment handy, but be sure to check the patient's chart for a do-not-resuscitate order.

History and physical examination

After taking vital signs, determine the patient's level of consciousness (LOC). Use the Glasgow Coma Scale (GCS) as a reference. Decerebrate posturing indicates the second-lowest measure of motor response, according to the GCS. Patients exhibiting this abnormal posturing have a decreased LOC and may be in a comatose state. Evaluate the pupils for size, equality, and response to light. Test deep tendon reflexes (DTRs) and cranial nerve reflexes, and check for doll's eye sign.

Next, explore the history of the patient's coma. If you're unable to obtain this information, look for clues to the causative disorder, such as hepatomegaly, cyanosis, diabetic skin changes, needle tracks, or obvious trauma. If a family member is available, find out when the patient's LOC began deteriorating. Did it occur abruptly? What did the patient complain of before he lost consciousness? Does he have a history of diabetes, liver disease, can-

Comparing decerebrate and decorticate postures

Decerebrate posture results from damage to the upper brain stem. In this posture, the arms are adducted and extended, with the wrists pronated and the fingers flexed. The legs are extended stiffly, with plantar flexion of the feet.

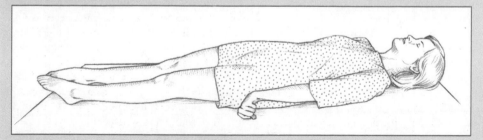

Decorticate posture results from damage to one or both corticospinal tracts. In this posture, the arms are adducted and the elbows are flexed, with the wrists and fingers flexed on the chest. The legs are extended stiffly and internally rotated, with plantar flexion of the feet.

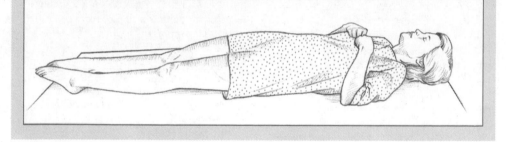

cer, blood clots, or aneurysm? Ask about any accident or traumatic injury responsible for the coma.

Medical causes

▶ *Brain stem infarction.* Decerebrate posture may occur when this primary lesion produces a coma. Other signs and symptoms vary with the severity of the infarct and may include cranial nerve palsies, bilateral cerebellar ataxia, and sensory loss. In a deep coma, all normal reflexes are usually lost, resulting in absence of doll's eye sign, a positive Babinski's reflex, and flaccidity.

▶ *Brain stem tumor.* In a brain stem tumor, decerebrate posture is a late sign that accompanies a coma. Early findings commonly include hemiparesis or quadriparesis, cranial nerve palsies, vertigo, dizziness, ataxia, and vomiting.

▶ *Cerebral lesion.* Whether the cause is trauma, tumor, abscess, or infarction, any cerebral lesion that increases ICP also may produce decerebrate posture, which typically is a sign of extensive damage.[2] Other findings vary with the lesion's site and extent but commonly include a coma, abnormal pupil size and response to light, and the classic triad of increased ICP—bradycardia, increasing systolic blood pressure, and widening pulse pressure.

▶ *Hepatic encephalopathy.* A late sign in this disorder, decerebrate posture occurs with a coma resulting from increased ICP and ammonia toxicity. Other signs include fetor hepaticus (foul-smelling breath), a positive Babinski's reflex, and hyperactive DTRs.

▶ *Hypoglycemic encephalopathy.* Characterized by extremely low blood glucose levels, this disorder may produce decerebrate posture and a coma. It also causes dilated pupils, bradypnea, and bradycardia. Muscle spasms, twitching, and seizures eventually progress to flaccidity.

▶ *Hypoxic encephalopathy.* Severe hypoxia may produce decerebrate posture—the result of brain stem compression associated with anaerobic metabolism and increased ICP. Other findings include a coma, a positive Babinski's reflex, absence of doll's eye sign, hypoactive DTRs, and possibly fixed pupils and respiratory arrest.

▶ *Meningeal tuberculosis.* In this form of extrapulmonary tuberculosis, early symptoms are vague and may include anorexia, irritability, and behavioral changes. As the disease progresses, the patient may have headache, vomiting, fever, seizures, cranial nerve palsies, and blindness. Further progression may eventually cause coma and decerebrate or decorticate posturing. Death may occur in 5 to 8 weeks if this disease is left untreated.[3]

▶ *Pontine hemorrhage.* Typically, this life-threatening disorder rapidly leads to decerebrate posture with a coma. Other signs include total paralysis, absence of doll's eye sign, a positive Babinski's reflex, and small, reactive pupils.

▶ *Posterior fossa hemorrhage.* This subtentorial lesion causes decerebrate posture. Its early signs and symptoms include vomiting, headache, vertigo, ataxia, stiff neck, drowsiness, papilledema, and cranial nerve palsies. The patient eventually slips into a coma and may have respiratory arrest.

Other causes

▶ *Diagnostic tests.* Removal of spinal fluid during a lumbar puncture to relieve high ICP may cause cerebral compression of the brain stem and cause decerebrate posture and a coma.

Special considerations

Help prepare the patient for diagnostic tests to determine the cause of his decerebrate posture. These include skull X-rays, computed tomography scan, magnetic resonance imaging, cerebral angiography, digital subtraction angiography, electroencephalogram, brain scan, and ICP monitoring.

Monitor the patient's neurologic status and vital signs every 30 minutes or as indicated.

Also, be alert for signs of increased ICP (bradycardia, increasing systolic blood pressure, and widening pulse pressure) and neurologic deterioration (altered respiratory pattern and abnormal temperature).

Pediatric pointers

Children younger than age 2 may not display decerebrate posture because the nervous system is still immature. However, if this posture occurs, it's usually the more severe opisthotonos. In fact, opisthotonos is more common in infants and young children than in adults and usually is a terminal sign. In children, the most common cause of decerebrate posture is head injury. It also occurs in Reye's syndrome—the result of increased ICP causing brain stem compression.

Patient counseling

Inform the patient's family that decerebrate posture is a reflex response—not a voluntary response to pain or a sign of recovery. Offer emotional support.

REFERENCES

1. Lower, J.S. "Fearlessly Facing Neurologic Evaluation." *LPN* 3(2):11-15, March/April 2007.
2. Frizzell, J.P. "Acute Stroke: Pathophysiology, Diagnosis, and Treatment." *AACN Clinical Issues: Advanced Practice in Acute and Critical Care* 16(4):421-440, October/December 2005.
3. Rockwood, R.R. "Extrapulmonary TB: What You Need to Know." *The Nurse Practitioner* 32(8):44-49, August 2007.

DECORTICATE POSTURE

A sign of corticospinal damage, decorticate posture (also called *decorticate rigidity* or *abnormal flexor response*) is characterized by adduction of the arms and flexion of the elbows, with wrists and fingers flexed on the chest. The legs are extended and internally rotated, with plantar flexion of the feet. This posture may occur unilaterally or bilaterally. It usually results from a stroke or head injury. It may be elicited by noxious stimuli or may occur spontaneously. The intensity of the required stimulus, the duration of the posture, and the frequency of spontaneous episodes vary with the severity and location of the cerebral injury. Posturing may be reversed if adequate oxygenation and perfusion are restored.[1] However, if posturing occurs when oxygenation and perfusion are adequate, he is more likely to be in a persistent vegetative state.[1]

Although a serious sign, decorticate posture carries a more favorable prognosis than decerebrate posture. However, decorticate posture may progress to decerebrate posture if the causative disorder extends lower in the brain stem. (See *Comparing decerebrate and decorticate postures*, page 129.)

Obtain vital signs and evaluate the patient's level of consciousness (LOC). If his consciousness is impaired, insert an oropharyngeal airway, and take measures to prevent aspiration (unless spinal cord injury is suspected). Evaluate the patient's respiratory rate, rhythm, and depth. Prepare to assist respirations with a handheld resuscitation bag or with intubation and mechanical ventilation if needed. Also, take seizure precautions.

History and physical examination

Test the patient's motor and sensory function. Evaluate pupil size, equality, and response to light. Then test cranial nerve function and deep tendon reflexes. Ask family members if the patient experienced headache, dizziness, nausea, changes in vision, numbness, or tingling. When did the patient first notice these symptoms? Is his family aware of any behavioral changes? Also, ask about a history of cerebrovascular disease, cancer, meningitis, encephalitis, upper respiratory tract infection, bleeding or clotting disorders, or recent trauma.

Medical causes

▶ *Brain abscess.* Decorticate posture may occur in a brain abscess. Related findings vary with the size and location of the abscess but may include aphasia, hemiparesis, headache, dizziness, seizures, nausea, and vomiting. The patient also may experience behavioral changes, altered vital signs, and decreased LOC.

▶ *Brain tumor.* A brain tumor may produce decorticate posture that's usually bilateral—the result of increased intracranial pressure (ICP) associated with tumor growth. Related signs and symptoms include headache, behavioral changes, memory loss, diplopia, blurred vision or vision loss, seizures, ataxia, dizziness, apraxia, aphasia, paresis, sensory loss, paresthesia, vomiting, papilledema, and signs of hormonal imbalance.

▶ *Head injury.* Decorticate posture may result from a head injury, depending on the site and severity of the injury. Other signs and symptoms include headache, nausea and vomiting, dizziness, irritability, decreased LOC, aphasia, hemiparesis, unilateral numbness, seizures, and pupillary dilation.

▶ *Meningeal tuberculosis.* In this form of extrapulmonary tuberculosis, early symptoms are vague and may include anorexia, irritability, and behavioral changes. As the disease progresses, the patient may experience headache, vomiting, fever, seizures, cranial nerve palsies, and blindness. Further progression may eventually cause coma and decerebrate or decorticate posturing. Death may occur in 5 to 8 weeks if this disease is left untreated.[2]

▶ *Stroke.* Typically, a stroke involving the cerebral cortex produces unilateral decorticate posture, also called spastic hemiplegia. Other signs and symptoms include hemiplegia (contralateral to the lesion), dysarthria, dysphagia, unilateral sensory loss, apraxia, agnosia, aphasia, memory loss, decreased LOC, urine retention, urinary incontinence, and constipation. Ocular effects include homonymous hemianopsia, diplopia, and blurred vision.

Special considerations

Monitor the patient's neurologic status and vital signs every 30 minutes to 2 hours. Be alert for signs of increased ICP, including bradycardia, increasing systolic blood pressure, and widening pulse pressure and subtle signs of neurologic deterioration.

Pediatric pointers

Decorticate posture is an unreliable sign before age 2 because of nervous system immaturity. In children, this posture usually results from head injury, but it also may occur in Reye's syndrome.

Patient counseling

Inform the patient's family that decerebrate posture is a reflex response—not a voluntary response to pain or a sign of recovery. Offer emotional support.

REFERENCES

1. Lower, J.S. "Fearlessly Facing Neurologic Evaluation." *LPN* 3(2):11-15, March/April 2007.
2. Rockwood, R.R. "Extrapulmonary TB: What You Need to Know." *The Nurse Practitioner* 32(8):44-49, August 2007.

DEEP TENDON REFLEXES, HYPERACTIVE

Deep tendon reflexes are used to assess central and peripheral nervous system function. A hyperactive deep tendon reflex (DTR) is an abnormally brisk muscle contraction that occurs in response to a sudden stretch induced by sharply tapping the muscle's tendon of insertion. This elicited sign may be graded as brisk or pathologically hyperactive. Hyperactive DTRs are commonly accompanied by clonus.

The corticospinal tract and other descending tracts govern the reflex arc—the relay cycle that produces any reflex response. A corticospinal lesion above the level of the reflex arc being tested may result in hyperactive DTRs. Abnormal neuromuscular transmission at the end of the reflex arc also may cause hyperactive DTRs. For example, a deficiency of calcium or magnesium may cause hyperactive DTRs because these electrolytes regulate neuromuscular excitability. (See *Tracing the reflex arc*, pages 134 and 135.)

Although hyperactive DTRs typically accompany other neurologic findings, they usually lack specific diagnostic value.

History and physical examination

After eliciting hyperactive DTRs, take the patient's history. Ask about spinal cord injury or other trauma and about prolonged exposure to cold, wind, or water. Could the patient be pregnant? A positive response to any of these questions requires prompt evaluation to rule out life-threatening autonomic hyperreflexia, tetanus, preeclampsia, or hypothermia. Ask about the onset and progression of related signs and symptoms. Next, perform a neurologic examination. Evaluate level of consciousness, and test motor and sensory function in the limbs. Ask about paresthesia. Check for ataxia or tremors and for speech and visual deficits. Test for Chvostek's sign (an abnormal spasm of the facial muscles elicited by light taps on the facial nerve in patients who have hypocalcemia) and Trousseau's sign (a carpal spasm induced by inflating a sphygmomanometer cuff on the upper arm to a pressure exceeding systolic blood pressure for 3 minutes in patients who have hypocalcemia or hypomagnesemia) and for carpopedal spasm. Ask about vomiting or altered urination habits. Be sure to take vital signs.

Medical causes

▶ *Amyotrophic lateral sclerosis.* This disorder produces generalized hyperactive DTRs accompanied by weakness of the hands and forearms and spasticity of the legs. Eventually, the patient develops atrophy of the neck and tongue muscles, fasciculations, weakness of the legs and, possibly, bulbar signs (dysphagia, dysphonia, facial weakness, and dyspnea).

▶ *Brain tumor.* A cerebral tumor causes hyperactive DTRs on the side opposite the lesion. Other signs and symptoms develop slowly and may include unilateral paresis or paralysis, anesthesia, visual field deficits, spasticity, and a positive Babinski's reflex.

▶ *Hepatic encephalopathy.* Generalized hyperactive DTRs occur late and are accompanied by a positive Babinski's reflex, fetor hepaticus, and a coma.

▶ *Hypocalcemia.* This disorder may produce sudden or gradual onset of generalized hyperactive DTRs with paresthesia, muscle twitching and cramping, positive Chvostek's and Trousseau's signs, carpopedal spasm, and tetany.

▶ *Hypomagnesemia.* This disorder results in gradual onset of generalized hyperactive DTRs accompanied by muscle cramps, hypotension, tachycardia, paresthesia, ataxia, tetany and, possibly, seizures.[1]

▶ *Hypothermia.* Mild hypothermia (90° to 94° F [32.2° to 34.4° C]) produces generalized hyperactive DTRs. Other signs and symptoms include shivering, fatigue, weakness, lethargy, slurred speech, ataxia, muscle stiffness, tachycardia, diuresis, bradypnea, hypotension, and cold, pale skin.

▶ *Multiple sclerosis.* Typically, hyperactive DTRs are preceded by weakness and paresthesia in one or both arms or legs. Other signs include clonus and a positive Babinski's reflex. Passive flexion of the patient's neck may cause a tingling sensation down his back. Later, ataxia, diplopia, vertigo, vomiting, urine retention, or urinary incontinence may occur.

▶ *Preeclampsia.* Occurring in pregnancy of at least 20 weeks' duration, preeclampsia may cause gradual onset of generalized hyperactive DTRs. Accompanying signs and symptoms include increased blood pressure; abnormal weight gain; edema of the face, fingers, and abdomen after bed rest; albuminuria; oliguria; severe headache; blurred or double vision; epigastric pain; nausea and vomiting; irritability; cyanosis; dyspnea; and crackles. If preeclampsia progresses to eclampsia, the patient develops seizures.

▶ *Spinal cord lesion.* Incomplete spinal cord lesions cause hyperactive DTRs below the level of the lesion. In a traumatic lesion, hyperactive DTRs follow resolution of spinal shock. In a neoplastic lesion, hyperactive DTRs gradually replace normal DTRs. Other signs and symptoms are paralysis and sensory loss below the level of the lesion, urine retention and overflow incontinence, and alternating constipation and diarrhea. A lesion above T6 also may produce autonomic hyperreflexia with diaphoresis and flushing above the level of the lesion, headache, nasal congestion, nausea, increased blood pressure, and bradycardia.

▶ *Stroke.* A stroke that affects the origin of the corticospinal tracts causes sudden onset of hyperactive DTRs on the side opposite the lesion. The patient also may have unilateral paresis or paralysis, anesthesia, visual field deficits, spasticity, and a positive Babinski's reflex.

▶ *Tetanus.* In this disorder, sudden onset of generalized hyperactive DTRs accompanies tachycardia, diaphoresis, low-grade fever, painful and involuntary muscle contractions,

trismus (lockjaw), and risus sardonicus (a masklike grin).

Special considerations

Prepare the patient for diagnostic tests to evaluate hyperactive DTRs. These may include laboratory tests for serum calcium magnesium and ammonia levels, magnetic resonance imaging, computed tomography scan, lumbar puncture, spinal X-rays, and myelography.

If motor weakness accompanies hyperactive DTRs, perform or encourage range-of-motion exercises to preserve muscle integrity and prevent deep vein thrombosis. Also, reposition the patient frequently, provide a special mattress, and massage his back and ensure adequate nutrition to prevent skin breakdown. Give a muscle relaxant and a sedative to relieve severe muscle contractions. Keep emergency resuscitation equipment on hand. Provide a quiet, calm atmosphere to decrease neuromuscular excitability. Assist with activities of daily living, and provide emotional support.

Pediatric pointers

Hyperreflexia may be a normal sign in neonates. After age 6, reflex responses are similar to those of adults. When testing DTRs in small children, use distraction techniques to promote reliable results.

Cerebral palsy commonly causes hyperactive DTRs in children. Reye's syndrome causes generalized hyperactive DTRs in stage II and absent DTRs in stage V. Adult causes of hyperactive DTRs also may appear in children.

Patient counseling

Teach the patient or family member to perform passive range-of-motion exercises. Also teach ways to help prevent or relieve muscle contractions.

REFERENCES
1   Bartlett, D. "Hydrofluoric Acid Exposure." *Nursing* 37(1):80, January 2007.

Tracing the reflex arc

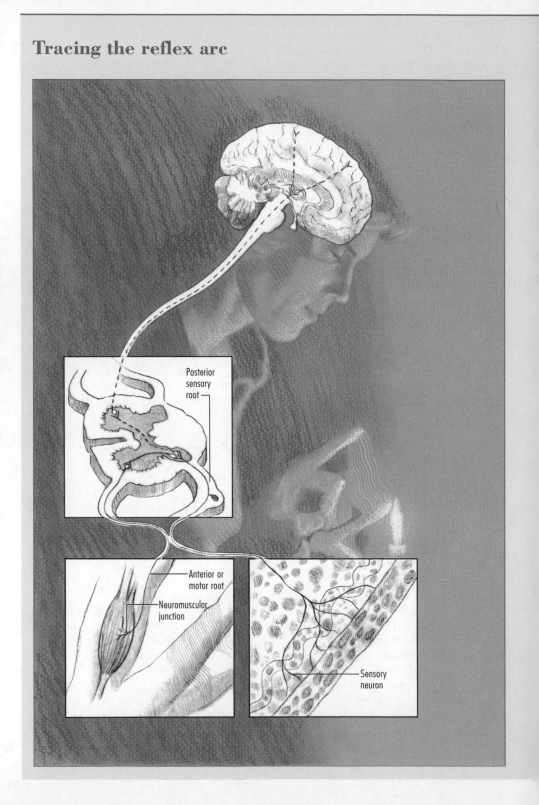

Sharply tapping a tendon starts a sensory (afferent) impulse that travels along a peripheral nerve to a spinal nerve and then to the spinal cord. The impulse enters the spinal cord through the posterior root, communicates with a motor (efferent) neuron in the anterior horn on the same side of the spinal cord, and then is transmitted through a motor nerve fiber back to the muscle. When the impulse crosses the neuromuscular junction, the muscle contracts, completing the reflex arc.

BICEPS REFLEX (C 5–6 INNERVATION)

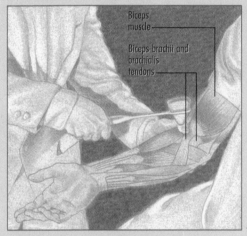

Biceps muscle

Biceps brachii and brachialis tendons

TRICEPS REFLEX (C 7–8 INNERVATION)

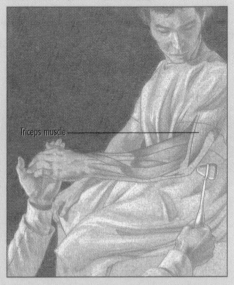

Triceps muscle

BRACHIORADIALIS REFLEX (C 5–6 INNERVATION)

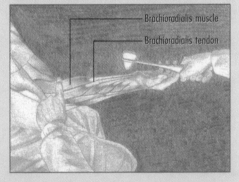

Brachioradialis muscle

Brachioradialis tendon

PATELLAR REFLEXES (L 2–4 INNERVATION)

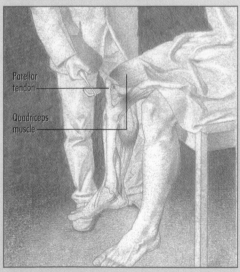

Patellar tendon

Quadriceps muscle

ACHILLES TENDON REFLEX (S 1–2 INNERVATION)

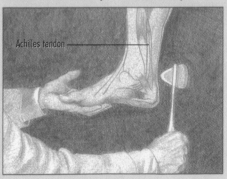

Achilles tendon

DEPRESSION

Depression is a mood disturbance characterized by feelings of sadness, despair, and loss of interest or pleasure in activities. These feelings may be accompanied by somatic complaints, such as changes in appetite, sleep disturbances, restlessness or lethargy, and decreased concentration. The patient also may have thoughts of death, suicide, or injuring herself.

Clinical depression must be distinguished from "the blues," periodic bouts of dysphoria that are less persistent and severe than the clinical disorder. The criterion for major depression is one or more episodes of depressed mood, or decreased interest or ability to take pleasure in all or most activities, lasting at least 2 weeks.

Major depression strikes up to 10% of men and 25% of women.[1] It affects all racial, ethnic, age, and socioeconomic groups, and is especially prevalent among adolescents. Depression has numerous causes, including genetic and family history, medical and psychiatric disorders, and the use of certain drugs. It can also occur in the postpartum period. A complete psychiatric and physical examination should be conducted to exclude possible medical causes.

History and physical examination

During the examination, determine how the patient feels about herself, her family, and her environment. Your goal is to explore the nature of her depression, the extent to which other factors affect it, and her coping mechanisms and their effectiveness. Begin by asking what's bothering her. How does her current mood differ from her usual mood? Then ask her to describe the way she feels about herself. What are her plans and dreams? How realistic are they? Is she generally satisfied with what she has accomplished in her work, relationships, and other interests? (See *PWB in married women.*) Ask about changes in her social interactions, sleep patterns, appetite, normal activities, or ability to make decisions and concentrate. Determine patterns of drug and alcohol use. Listen for clues that she may be suicidal. (See *Suicide: Caring for the high-risk patient,* page 138.)

Ask the patient about her family—its patterns of interaction and characteristic responses to success and failure. What part does she feel she plays in her family's life? Find out if other family members have been depressed and whether anyone important to her has been sick or has died in the past year. Finally, ask the patient about her environment. Has her lifestyle changed in the past months? Six months? Year? When she's feeling depressed, where does she go and what does she do to feel better? Find out how she feels about her role in the community and the resources that are available to her. Try to determine if she has an adequate support network to help her cope with her depression.

Medical causes

▶ *Childbirth.* Although its cause hasn't been determined, postpartum depression occurs in about 5% to 25% of women who have given birth.[2] Symptoms range from mild postpartum blues to an intense, suicidal, depressive psychosis.

▶ *Organic disorders.* Various organic disorders and chronic illnesses produce mild, moderate, or severe depression. Among these are metabolic and endocrine disorders, such as hypothyroidism, hyperthyroidism, and diabetes; infectious diseases, such as influenza, hepatitis, and encephalitis; degenerative diseases, such as Alzheimer's disease, multiple sclerosis, and multi-infarct dementia; and neoplastic disorders such as cancer.

▶ *Psychiatric disorders.* Affective disorders typically are characterized by abrupt mood swings from depression to elation (mania) or by prolonged episodes of either mood. In fact, severe depression may last for weeks. More moderate depression occurs in cyclothymic disorders and usually alternates with moderate mania. Moderate depression that's more or less constant over a 2-year period typically results from dysthymic disorders. Also, chronic anxiety disorders, such as panic and obsessive-compulsive disorder, may be accompanied by depression.

EVIDENCE-BASED PRACTICE

PWB in married women

Question: *Using a family systems framework, what factors explain married women's psychological well-being (PWB)?*

Research: Adult women experience psychological distress at greater rates than men and it has been shown that the quality of a marital relationship is linked to the experience of well-being in women. A convenience sample of 136 adult married women was used in this cross-sectional correlational-predictive study. Women were recruited during routine office visits for gynecologic care from three women's healthcare practices in the New York City area. The participants were between the ages of 21 and 75 and all were married for at least 1 year (range 1 to 47 years). Each potential participant was mailed a survey packet with a questionnaire booklet. Instruments used to analyze the responses included the PWB scale of the Mental Health Inventory, the Level of Differentiation of Self (DOS) Scale, and the interactional-emotional need fulfillment (I-ENF) and the sexual need fulfillment (SNF) subscales of the Partner Relationship Inventory.

Conclusion: Both I-ENF and SNF showed a strong, statistically significant association with PWB. The relationship between DOS and PWB was also statistically significant, but not as strong. When women's interactional, emotional, and sexual needs were being met by their husbands, their level of well-being increased. These findings suggest that DOS and need fulfillment may have a protective effect against mental health problems in married women.

Application: Assess women's relationship issues, especially if you work in a primary care or women's health setting. Ask about marital quality, and whether and how needs are being met. Identify women who report an unhappy marriage as being at risk for depression, anxiety, or other symptoms of psychological distress. Teach effective communication and refer to marriage or individual counseling as indicated and provide emotional support as needed.

Source: Steelman, J. R. "Relationship Dynamics: Understanding Married Women's Mental Health." *Advances in Nursing Science* 30(2): 151-158, 2007.

Other causes

▶ *Alcohol abuse.* Long-term alcohol use, intoxication, or withdrawal commonly produces depression.

DRUG WATCH *Various drugs cause depression as an adverse effect. Among the more common are barbiturates, chemotherapy drugs such as asparaginase, anticonvulsants such as diazepam, and antiarrhythmics such as disopyramide. Other depression-inducing drugs include centrally acting antihypertensives, such as reserpine (common with high doses), methyldopa, and clonidine; beta blockers such as propranolol; levodopa; indomethacin; cycloserine; corticosteroids; and hormonal contraceptives.*

Special considerations

Caring for a depressed patient takes time, tact, and energy. It also requires an awareness of your own vulnerability to feelings of despair that can stem from interacting with a depressed patient. Help the patient set realistic goals; encourage her to promote feelings of self-worth by expressing her opinions and making decisions. Keep in mind that one in every 7 patients with recurrent depression commits suicide.[3] Try to determine her suicide potential, and take steps to help ensure her safety. The patient may require close surveillance to prevent a suicide attempt.

Make sure the patient receives adequate nourishment and rest, and keep her environment free from stress and excessive stimulation. Arrange for ordered diagnostic tests to determine if her depression has an organic cause, and give prescribed drugs. Also arrange for follow-up counseling, or contact a mental health professional for a referral.

Suicide: Caring for the high-risk patient

One of the most common factors in suicide is hopelessness, an emotion felt by many depressed patients. Regularly assess a depressed patient for suicidal tendencies.

The patient may provide specific clues about her intentions. For example, you may notice her talking often about death or the futility of life, concealing potentially harmful items (such as knives and belts), hoarding medications, giving away personal belongings, or getting her legal and financial affairs in order. If you suspect that a patient is suicidal, follow these guidelines:

- Try to determine the patient's suicide potential. Does she have a simple, straightforward suicide plan that's likely to succeed? Does she have a strong support system (family, friends, a therapist)? A patient with low to moderate suicide potential is noticeably depressed but has a support system. She may have thoughts of suicide, but no specific plan. A patient with high suicide potential feels profoundly hopeless and has a minimal support system. She thinks about suicide often and has a plan that's likely to succeed.
- Observe precautions. Ensure the patient's safety by removing objects she could use to harm herself, such as knives, scissors, razors, belts, electrical cords, shoelaces, and drugs. Know where she is and what she's doing at all times; this may require surveillance and placing the patient in a room that's close to your station. Have someone accompany her when she leaves the unit.
- Be alert for in-hospital suicide attempts, which typically occur when there's a low staff-to-patient ratio—for example, between shifts, during evening and night shifts, or when a critical event such as a code draws attention away from the patient.
- Finally, arrange for follow-up counseling. Recognize suicidal ideation and behavior as a cry for help. Contact a mental health professional for a referral.

Pediatric pointers

Depression occurs in 2% to 6% of children and adolescents, with a sharp increase in incidence during adolescence.[1] Because emotional lability is normal in adolescence, depression can be difficult to assess and diagnose in teenagers. Clues to underlying depression may include somatic complaints, sexual promiscuity, poor grades, and abuse of alcohol or drugs.

Use of a family systems model usually helps determine the cause of depression in adolescents. Once family roles are determined, family therapy or group therapy with peers may help the patient overcome her depression. In severe cases, an antidepressant may be required.

Geriatric pointers

Signs and symptoms of depression occur in about 30% to 50% of older adults.[4] Many elderly patients have physical complaints, somatic complaints, agitation, or changes in intellectual functioning (memory impairment), making the diagnosis of depression difficult in these patients.[5] Depressed older adults who are age 85 and older have the highest risk of suicide.[5] Even a frail nursing home resident with these characteristics may have the strength to kill herself.

Patient counseling

Educate the patient about available treatment options and possible outcomes. Explain the symptoms of depression and adverse reactions to medications, and urge the patient to report them to a health care provider. Urge the patient to include nondrug strategies in depression treatment, such as relaxation techniques, daily exercise, eating a well-balanced diet, participating in support groups, and maintaining relationships with family and friends.[1]

REFERENCES

1. Thayer, K.M. and Bruce, M.L. "Recognition and Management of Major Depression." *The Nurse Practitioner* 31(5):12-23, May 2006.
2. Mitchell, A.M., Mittelstaedt, M.E., and Schott-Baer, D. "Postpartum Depression: The Reliability of Telephone Screening." *MCN The American Journal of Maternal/Child Nursing* 31(6):382-387, November/December 2006.

3. Mynatt, S. and Cunningham, P. "Unraveling Anxiety and Depression." *The Nurse Practitioner* 32(8):28-36, August 2007.
4. Walker, J.T., Lofton, S.P., Haynie, L., and Martin, T. "The Home Health Nurses' Role in Geriatric Assessment of Three Dimensions: Depression, Delirium, and Dementia." *Home Healthcare Nurse* 24(9):572-578, October 2006.
5. Butcher, H.K. and McGonigal-Kenney, M. "Depression & Dispiritedness in Later Life: A 'Gray Drizzle of Horror' Isn't Inevitable." *AJN* 105(12):52-61, December 2005.

DIAPHORESIS

Diaphoresis is profuse sweating, sometimes producing more than 1 L of sweat per hour. This sign represents an autonomic nervous system response to physical or psychogenic stress, fever, or high environmental temperature. When caused by stress, diaphoresis may be generalized or limited to the palms, soles, and forehead. When caused by fever or high environmental temperature, it's usually generalized.

Diaphoresis usually begins abruptly and may be accompanied by other autonomic system signs, such as tachycardia and increased blood pressure. However, this sign also varies with age because sweat glands function immaturely in infants and are less active in elderly people. As a result, patients in these age-groups may fail to display diaphoresis associated with its common causes. Intermittent diaphoresis may accompany chronic disorders characterized by recurrent fever; isolated diaphoresis may mark an episode of acute pain or fever. Night sweats may characterize intermittent fever because body temperature tends to return to normal between 2 A.M. and 4 A.M. before rising again. (Temperature is usually lowest around 6 A.M.)

Diaphoresis is a normal response to high external temperature. Acclimatization usually requires several days of exposure to high temperatures; during this process, diaphoresis helps maintain normal body temperature. Diaphoresis also commonly occurs during menopause, preceded by a sensation of intense heat (a hot flash). Other causes include exercise or exertion that accelerates metabolism, creating internal heat, and mild to moderate anxiety that helps initiate the fight-or-flight response. (See *Understanding diaphoresis,* pages 140 and 141.)

History and physical examination

If the patient is diaphoretic, quickly rule out the possibility of a life-threatening cause. (See *When diaphoresis signifies crisis,* page 142.) Begin the history by having the patient describe his chief complaint. Then explore related signs and symptoms. Note general fatigue and weakness. Does the patient have insomnia, headache, and changes in vision or hearing? Is he often dizzy? Does he have palpitations? Ask about pleuritic pain, cough, sputum, difficulty breathing, nausea, vomiting, abdominal pain, and altered elimination habits. Ask the female patient about amenorrhea and any changes in her menstrual cycle. Is she menopausal? Ask about paresthesia, muscle cramps or stiffness, and joint pain. Has she noticed any changes in elimination habits? Note weight loss or gain. Has she had to change her glove or shoe size lately?

Complete the history by asking about travel to tropical countries. Note recent exposure to high environmental temperatures or to pesticides. Did the patient recently get an insect bite? Check for a history of partial gastrectomy or of drug or alcohol abuse. Finally, obtain a thorough drug history.

Next, perform a physical examination. First, determine the extent of diaphoresis by inspecting the trunk and extremities as well as the palms, soles, and forehead. Also, check the patient's clothing and bedding for dampness. Note whether diaphoresis occurs during the day or at night. Observe the patient for flushing, abnormal skin texture or lesions, and an increased amount of coarse body hair. Note poor skin turgor and dry mucous membranes. Check for splinter hemorrhages and Plummer's nails (separation of the fingernail ends from the nail beds).

Then evaluate the patient's mental status and take his vital signs. Observe the patient for fasciculations and flaccid paralysis. Be alert for seizures. Note the patient's facial expression, and examine the eyes for pupillary

Understanding diaphoresis

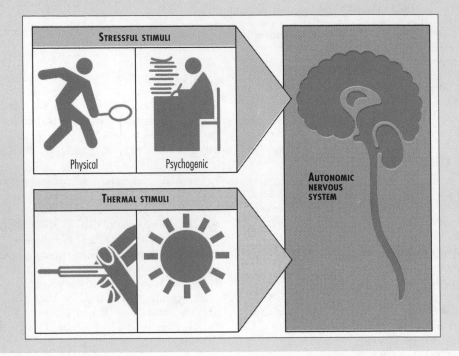

dilation or constriction, exophthalmos, and excessive tearing. Test visual fields. Also, check for hearing loss and for tooth or gum disease. Percuss the lungs for dullness, and auscultate for crackles, diminished or bronchial breath sounds, and increased vocal fremitus. Look for decreased respiratory excursion. Palpate for lymphadenopathy and hepatosplenomegaly.

Medical causes

▶ *Acquired immunodeficiency syndrome.* Night sweats may be an early feature, occurring either as a result of the disease itself or secondary to an opportunistic infection. The patient also has fever, fatigue, lymphadenopathy, anorexia, dramatic and unexplained weight loss, diarrhea, and a persistent cough.
▶ *Acromegaly.* In this slowly progressive disorder, diaphoresis is a sensitive gauge of disease activity, which involves hypersecretion of growth hormone and increased metabolic rate. The patient has a hulking appearance

with an enlarged supraorbital ridge and thickened ears and nose. Other signs and symptoms include warm, oily, thickened skin; enlarged hands, feet, and jaw; joint pain; weight gain; hoarseness; and increased coarse body hair. Increased blood pressure, severe headache, and visual field deficits or blindness also may occur.
▶ *Anxiety disorders.* Acute anxiety characterizes panic, whereas chronic anxiety characterizes phobias, conversion disorders, obsessions, and compulsions. Whether acute or chronic, anxiety may cause sympathetic stimulation, resulting in diaphoresis. The diaphoresis is most dramatic on the palms, soles, and forehead and is accompanied by palpitations, tachycardia, tachypnea, tremors, and GI distress. Psychological signs and symptoms—fear, difficulty concentrating, and behavior changes—also occur.
▶ *Autonomic hyperreflexia.* Occurring after resolution of spinal shock in a spinal cord injury above T6, hyperreflexia causes profuse

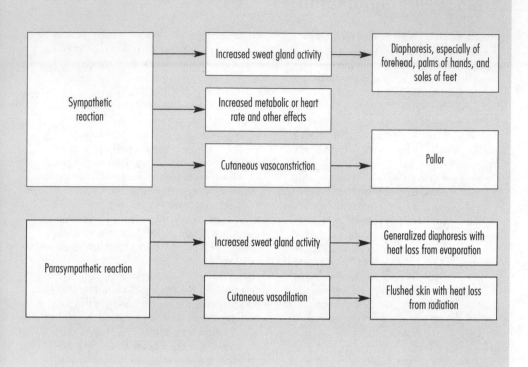

diaphoresis, pounding headache, blurred vision, and dramatically elevated blood pressure. Diaphoresis occurs above the level of the injury, especially on the forehead, and is accompanied by flushing. Other findings include restlessness, nausea, nasal congestion, and bradycardia.

▶ *Drug and alcohol withdrawal syndromes.* Withdrawal from alcohol or an opioid analgesic may cause generalized diaphoresis, dilated pupils, tachycardia, tremors, and altered mental status (confusion, delusions, hallucinations, agitation). The effects of alcohol withdrawal may appear 6 to 24 hours after the patient's last drink.[1] Those from opioid withdrawal will depend on the half-life and dose of the drug used as well as the duration of treatment.[2] Other signs and symptoms include severe muscle cramps, generalized paresthesia, tachypnea, increased or decreased blood pressure and, possibly, seizures. Nausea and vomiting are common.

▶ *Empyema.* Pus accumulation in the pleural space leads to drenching night sweats and fever. The patient also complains of chest pain, cough, and weight loss. Examination reveals decreased respiratory excursion on the affected side and absent or distant breath sounds.

▶ *Heart failure.* Typically, diaphoresis follows fatigue, dyspnea, orthopnea, and tachycardia in patients with left-sided heart failure, and jugular vein distention and dry cough in patients with right-sided heart failure. Other features include tachypnea, cyanosis, dependent edema, crackles, ventricular gallop, and anxiety.

▶ *Heat exhaustion.* Although this condition is marked by failure of heat to dissipate, it initially may cause profuse diaphoresis, fatigue, weakness, and anxiety. These signs and symptoms may progress to circulatory collapse and shock (marked by confusion, thready pulse, hypotension, tachycardia, and cold, clammy skin). Other features include an ashen gray

When diaphoresis signifies crisis

Diaphoresis is an early sign of certain life-threatening disorders. These guidelines will help you promptly detect such disorders and intervene to minimize harm to the patient.

HYPOGLYCEMIA

If you observe diaphoresis in a patient who complains of blurred vision, ask him about increased irritability and anxiety. Has the patient been unusually hungry lately? Does he have tremors? Take the patient's vital signs, noting hypotension and tachycardia. Then ask about a history of type 2 diabetes or antidiabetic therapy. If you suspect hypoglycemia, evaluate the patient's blood glucose level using a glucose reagent strip, or send a serum sample to the laboratory. Give I.V. glucose 50% as ordered to return the patient's glucose level to normal. Monitor his vital signs and cardiac rhythm. Ensure a patent airway, and be prepared to assist with breathing and circulation, if needed.

HEATSTROKE

If you observe profuse diaphoresis in a weak, tired, and apprehensive patient, suspect heatstroke, which can progress to circulatory collapse. Take vital signs, noting a normal or subnormal temperature. Check for ashen gray skin and dilated pupils. Was the patient recently exposed to high temperatures and humidity? Was he wearing heavy clothing or performing strenuous activity? Also, ask if he takes a diuretic, which interferes with normal sweating.

Then take the patient to a cool room, remove his clothing, and use a fan to direct cool air over his body. Insert an I.V. line, and prepare for electrolyte and fluid replacement. Monitor

the patient for signs of shock. Check his urine output carefully along with other sources of output (such as tubes, drains, and ostomies).

AUTONOMIC HYPERREFLEXIA

If you observe diaphoresis in a patient with a spinal cord injury above T6 or T7, ask if he has a pounding headache, restlessness, blurred vision, or nasal congestion. Take the patient's vital signs, noting bradycardia or extremely elevated blood pressure. If you suspect autonomic hyperreflexia, quickly rule out its common complications. Examine the patient for eye pain associated with intraocular hemorrhage and for facial paralysis, slurred speech, or limb weakness associated with intracerebral hemorrhage.

Quickly reposition the patient to remove any pressure stimuli. Also, check for a distended bladder or fecal impaction. Remove any kinks from the urinary catheter if needed, and administer a suppository or manually remove impacted feces. If you can't locate and relieve the causative stimulus, start an I.V. line. Prepare to give hydralazine for hypertension.

MYOCARDIAL INFARCTION OR HEART FAILURE

If the diaphoretic patient complains of chest pain and dyspnea, or has arrhythmias or ECG changes, suspect a myocardial infarction or heart failure. Connect the patient to a cardiac monitor, ensure a patent airway, and give supplemental oxygen. Start an I.V. line, and give an analgesic. Prepare for emergency resuscitation if cardiac or respiratory arrest occurs.

appearance, dilated pupils, and normal or subnormal temperature.

▶ *Hodgkin's disease.* Especially in elderly patients, early features of Hodgkin's disease may include night sweats, fever, fatigue, pruritus, and weight loss. Usually, however, this disease initially causes painless swelling of a cervical lymph node. Occasionally, a Pel-Ebstein fever pattern is present—several days or weeks of fever and chills alternating with afebrile periods with no chills. Systemic signs and symp-

toms—such as weight loss, fever, and night sweats—indicate a poor prognosis. Progressive lymphadenopathy eventually causes widespread effects, such as hepatomegaly and dyspnea.

▶ *Hypoglycemia.* Rapidly induced hypoglycemia may cause diaphoresis accompanied by irritability, tremors, hypotension, blurred vision, tachycardia, hunger, and loss of consciousness.

▶ *Immunoblastic lymphadenopathy.* Resembling Hodgkin's disease but more rare, this disorder causes episodic diaphoresis along with fever, weight loss, weakness, generalized lymphadenopathy, rash, and hepatosplenomegaly.

▶ *Infective endocarditis (subacute).* Generalized night sweats occur early in this disorder and are accompanied by intermittent low-grade fever, weakness, fatigue, anorexia, weight loss, and arthralgia. A sudden change in a murmur or the discovery of a new murmur is a classic sign. Petechiae and splinter hemorrhages are also common.

▶ *Liver abscess.* Signs and symptoms vary, depending on the extent of the abscess, but commonly include diaphoresis, right-upper-quadrant pain, weight loss, fever, chills, nausea, vomiting, and signs of anemia.

▶ *Lung abscess.* Drenching night sweats are common in this disorder. Its chief sign, however, is a cough that produces copious amounts of purulent, foul-smelling, and typically blood-tinged sputum. Other findings include fever with chills, pleuritic chest pain, dyspnea, weakness, anorexia, weight loss, headache, malaise, clubbing, tubular or amphoric breath sounds, and dullness on percussion.

▶ *Malaria.* Profuse diaphoresis marks the third stage of paroxysmal malaria, preceded by chills (first stage) and high fever (second stage). Headache, arthralgia, and hepatosplenomegaly also may occur. In the benign form of malaria, these paroxysms alternate with periods of well-being. The severe form may progress to delirium, seizures, and coma.

▶ *Ménière's disease.* Characterized by severe vertigo, tinnitus, and hearing loss, this disorder also may cause diaphoresis, nausea, vomiting, and nystagmus. Hearing loss may be progressive, and tinnitus may persist between attacks.

▶ *Myocardial infarction.* Diaphoresis usually accompanies acute, substernal, radiating chest pain in this life-threatening disorder. However, men are more likely to have diaphoresis than women.[3] Other signs and symptoms include anxiety, dyspnea, nausea, vomiting, tachycardia, irregular pulse, blood pressure change, fine crackles, pallor, and clammy skin.

▶ *Pheochromocytoma.* This disorder commonly produces diaphoresis, but its cardinal sign is persistent or paroxysmal hypertension. Other effects include headache, palpitations, tachycardia, anxiety, tremors, pallor, flushing, paresthesia, abdominal pain, tachypnea, nausea, vomiting, and orthostatic hypotension.

▶ *Pneumonia.* In patients with pneumonia, intermittent, generalized diaphoresis accompanies fever, chills, and pleuritic chest pain that increases with deep inspiration. Other features are tachypnea, dyspnea, a productive cough (with scant and mucoid or copious and purulent sputum), headache, fatigue, myalgia, abdominal pain, anorexia, and cyanosis. Auscultation reveals bronchial breath sounds.

▶ *Relapsing fever.* Profuse diaphoresis marks resolution of the crisis stage of this disorder, which typically produces attacks of high fever accompanied by severe myalgia, headache, arthralgia, diarrhea, vomiting, coughing, and eye or chest pain. Splenomegaly is common, but hepatomegaly and lymphadenopathy also may occur. The patient may develop a transient macular rash. At 3 to 10 days after onset, the febrile attack abruptly terminates in chills with increased pulse and respiratory rates. Diaphoresis, flushing, and hypotension may then lead to circulatory collapse and death. Relapse invariably occurs if the patient survives the initial attack.

▶ *Tetanus.* This disorder commonly causes profuse sweating and low-grade fever, tachycardia, and hyperactive deep tendon reflexes. Early restlessness and pain and stiffness in the jaw, abdomen, and back progress to spasms associated with lockjaw, risus sardonicus, dysphagia, and opisthotonos. Laryngospasm may result in cyanosis or sudden death by asphyxiation.

▶ *Thyrotoxicosis.* This disorder commonly produces diaphoresis accompanied by heat intolerance, weight loss despite increased appetite, tachycardia, palpitations, an enlarged thyroid, dyspnea, nervousness, diarrhea, tremors, Plummer's nails and, possibly, exophthalmos. Gallops also may occur.

▶ *Tuberculosis (TB).* Although many patients with primary infection are asymptomatic, TB may cause night sweats, low-grade fever, fatigue, weakness, anorexia, and weight loss. In reactivation, a productive cough with mucopurulent sputum, occasional hemoptysis, and chest pain may be present.

Other causes

DRUG WATCH *Sympathomimetics, some antipsychotics, thyroid hormone, corticosteroids, and antipyretics may cause diaphoresis. Aspirin and acetaminophen poisoning also cause this sign. Diaphoresis occurs early in acetaminophen toxicity, within the first 24 hours after ingestion; nausea, vomiting, pallor, lethargy, and anorexia also may occur before the patient progresses to more severe stages of toxicity.*[4]

▶ *Dumping syndrome.* The result of rapid emptying of gastric contents into the small intestine after partial gastrectomy, dumping syndrome causes diaphoresis, palpitations, profound weakness, epigastric distress, nausea, and explosive diarrhea soon after eating.

▶ *Envenomation.* Depending on the type of bite, neurotoxic effects may include diaphoresis, chills (with or without fever), weakness, dizziness, blurred vision, increased salivation, nausea and vomiting and, possibly, paresthesia and muscle fasciculations. Local features may include ecchymosis and progressively severe pain and edema. Palpation reveals tender regional lymph nodes.

▶ *Pesticide poisoning.* Among the toxic effects of pesticides are diaphoresis, nausea, vomiting, diarrhea, blurred vision, miosis, and excessive lacrimation and salivation. The patient also may display fasciculations, muscle weakness, and flaccid paralysis. Signs of respiratory depression and coma also may occur.

Special considerations

After an episode of diaphoresis, sponge the patient's face and body and change wet clothes and bed linens. To prevent skin irritation, dust skin folds in the groin and axillae and under pendulous breasts with cornstarch, or tuck gauze or cloth into the folds. Encourage regular bathing.

Replace fluids and electrolytes. Regulate infusions of I.V. saline or Ringer's lactate solution, and monitor urine output. Encourage intake of oral fluids high in electrolytes (such as Gatorade). Enforce bed rest, and maintain a quiet environment. Keep the patient's room temperature moderate to prevent additional diaphoresis.

Prepare the patient for diagnostic tests, such as blood tests, cultures, chest X-rays, immunologic studies, biopsy, computed tomography scan, and audiometry. Monitor the patient's vital signs, including temperature.

Pediatric pointers

Diaphoresis in children commonly results from environmental heat or overdressing the child; it's usually most apparent around the head. Other causes include drug withdrawal (from maternal addiction), heart failure, thyrotoxicosis, and the effects of such drugs as antihistamines, ephedrine, haloperidol, and thyroid hormone.

Assess fluid status carefully. Some fluid loss through diaphoresis may cause hypovolemia more rapidly in a child than an adult. Monitor input and output, weigh the child daily, and note the duration of each episode of diaphoresis.

Geriatric pointers

Elderly patients with acute myocardial infarction are less likely to have chest or arm pain, diaphoresis, nausea, and vomiting, but are more likely to have dyspnea, confusion, and syncope.[3]

The autonomic responses typically associated with severe acute pain, such as diaphoresis, tachycardia, tachypnea, and elevated blood pressure, may be reduced or diminished in the older adult.[5]

Elderly patients with TB may exhibit a change in activity or weight rather than the hallmark symptoms of fever and night sweats. Also, keep in mind that older patients may not exhibit diaphoresis because of a decreased sweating mechanism. For this reason, they're at increased risk for developing heatstroke in high temperatures.

REFERENCES

1. Lussier-Cushing, M., Repper-DeLisi, J., Mitchell, M.T., Lakatos, B.E., Mahmaid, F., and Lipkis-Orlando, R. "Is Your Medical/Surgical Patient Withdrawing From Alcohol?" *Nursing* 37(10):50-55, October 2007.
2. Miller, N.S., Swiney, T., and Barkin, R.L. "Effects of Opioid Prescription Medication Dependence and Detoxification on Pain Perceptions

and Self-Reports." *American Journal of Therapeutics* 13(5):436-444, September/October 2006.

3. Ryan, C.J., DeVon, H.A., Horne, R., King, K.B., Milner, K., Moser, D.K., Quinn, J.R., Rosenfeld, A., Hwang, S.Y., and Zerwic, J.J. "Symptom Clusters in Acute Myocardial Infarction: A Secondary Data Analysis." *Nursing Research* 56(2):72-81, March/April 2007.

4. Saccomano, S. and DeLuca, D. "Too Toxic." *Men in Nursing* 2(5):42-48, October 2007.

5. Hadjistavropoulos, T., et al. "An Interdisciplinary Expert Consensus Statement on Assessment of Pain in Older Persons." *The Clinical Journal of Pain* 23(Supplement 1):S1-S43, January 2007.

DIARRHEA

Usually a chief sign of an intestinal disturbance, diarrhea is an increase in the volume of stools compared with the patient's normal bowel elimination habits. It is one of the most common illnesses in the U.S.[1] It varies in severity and may be acute (lasting 7 to 14 days) or chronic (lasting more than 2 to 3 weeks).[2] Infection is the leading cause of acute diarrhea, and acute infectious diarrhea is one of the leading causes of illness and death worldwide.[2,3] Acute diarrhea also may result from stress, fecal impaction, or the effect of a drug. Irritable bowel syndrome is the leading cause of chronic diarrhea.[2] Chronic diarrhea also may result from chronic infection, obstructive bowel disease, malabsorption syndrome, an endocrine disorder, or GI surgery. Periodic diarrhea may result from food intolerance or from ingestion of spicy or high-fiber foods or caffeine.

One or more pathophysiologic mechanisms may contribute to diarrhea. (See *What causes diarrhea,* page 146.) The fluid and electrolyte imbalances it produces may cause life-threatening arrhythmias or hypovolemic shock.

If the patient's diarrhea is profuse, check for signs of shock—tachycardia, hypotension, and cool, pale, clammy skin. If you detect these signs, place the patient in the supine position and elevate his legs 20 degrees. Insert an I.V. line for fluid replacement. Monitor the patient for electrolyte imbalances, and look for an irregular pulse, muscle weakness, anorexia, and nausea and vomiting. Keep emergency resuscitation equipment handy.

History and physical examination

If the patient isn't in shock, explore signs and symptoms related to the diarrhea. Does the patient have abdominal pain and cramps? Difficulty breathing? Is he weak or fatigued? Is the stool mixed with pus or blood?[2] Has he noticed a pattern? Find out his drug history. Has he had GI surgery or radiation therapy recently? Ask the patient to briefly describe his diet. Does he have any known food allergies? Ask about sources of drinking water, and find out if the patient has had recent recreational water exposure, such as in a swimming pool or hot tub.[4] Lastly, find out if he's under unusual stress or has traveled recently.

Proceed with a brief physical examination. Evaluate hydration, check skin turgor and mucous membranes, and take blood pressure with the patient lying, sitting, and standing. Inspect the abdomen for distention, and palpate for tenderness. Auscultate bowel sounds. Check for tympany over the abdomen. Take the patient's temperature, and note any chills. Also, look for a rash. Conduct a rectal examination and a pelvic examination if indicated.

Medical causes

▶ *Anthrax, GI.* This disease follows ingestion of contaminated meat from an animal infected with *Bacillus anthracis*. Early signs and symptoms include decreased appetite, nausea, vomiting, and fever. Later signs and symptoms include severe bloody diarrhea, abdominal pain, and hematemesis.

▶ *Carcinoid syndrome.* In this disorder, severe diarrhea occurs with flushing—usually of the head and neck—that's commonly caused by emotional stimuli or the ingestion of food, hot water, or alcohol. Other signs and symptoms include abdominal cramps, dyspnea, anorexia, weight loss, weakness, palpitations, valvular heart disease, and depression.

▶ *Celiac disease.* In celiac disease, caused by a sensitivity to gluten, diarrhea is due to malabsorption that occurs secondary to villous atrophy of the small intestine. Other signs and symptoms may include bloating, iron-

What causes diarrhea

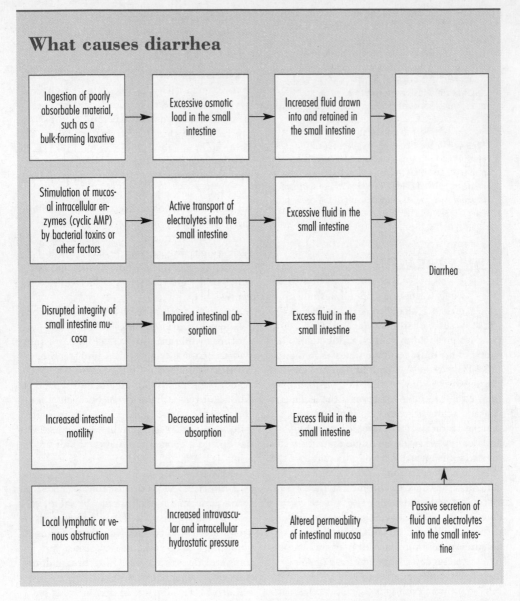

deficiency anemia, weight loss, and vague abdominal pain.

▶ *Cholera*. After ingesting water or food contaminated by the bacterium *Vibrio cholerae,* the patient experiences massive, abrupt watery diarrhea and vomiting. Other signs and symptoms include thirst (due to severe water and electrolyte loss), weakness, muscle cramps, decreased skin turgor, oliguria, tachycardia, and hypotension. Without treatment, death can occur within hours from volume depletion and vascular collapse.

▶ Clostridium difficile *infection*. The patient may be asymptomatic or may have soft, unformed stools or watery diarrhea that may be foul smelling or grossly bloody; abdominal pain, cramping, and tenderness; fever; and a white blood cell count as high as 20,000/µl. In severe cases, the patient may develop toxic megacolon, colonic perforation, or peritonitis. (See Clostridium difficile: *Emergence of a new strain.*)

▶ *Crohn's disease*. This recurring inflammatory disorder produces diarrhea, abdominal

Clostridium difficile: Emergence of a new strain

According to some sources, 15% to 20% of hospitalized patients may be colonized with *Clostridium difficile*.[5] Although many of these patients don't become ill, they do function as a reservoir of bacteria in the hospital, which raises the risk of contaminating the hospital environment, health care workers, and other patients. In those who do become ill, *C. difficile* infection can cause serious complications, such as pseudomembranous colitis, toxic megacolon, and even death.[1,5]

Recent reports of increased frequency and severity of *C. difficile* infection have led researchers to suspect the emergence of a previously uncommon, more virulent strain.[5] It produces more *C. difficile* toxins, thus producing a more severe infection. Besides being resistant to clindamycin and cephalosporins, like the previous strain, the new strain also is resistant to fluoroquinolone antibiotics. And unlike the previous strain, it can occur without the patient having recently taken antibiotics.[5]

To prevent the spread of infection by all strains of *C. difficile*, follow these guidelines:
• Be aware that any patient with acute diarrhea could have *C. difficile* infection.
• Implement contact precautions for any patient with possible or confirmed *C. difficile* infection. Provide a private room, if possible.
• Prevent cross-contamination between patients by dedicating equipment for each patient's use. Electronic rectal thermometers that use probe covers have been a source of transmission in the past.
• Wash your hands often with soap and water. Alcohol doesn't kill *C. difficile* spores, so cleaning your hands with alcohol-based hand gel won't remove the organisms.[1,5]
• Make sure that bleach-based cleaning products are used by environmental services to clean rooms and equipment.

---

pain with guarding and tenderness, and nausea. The patient also may display fever, chills, weakness, anorexia, and weight loss.

▶ *Escherichia coli O157:H7.* Watery or bloody diarrhea, nausea, vomiting, fever, and abdominal cramps occur after the patient eats undercooked beef or other foods contaminated with this particular strain of bacteria. Hemolytic uremic syndrome (HUS), which causes red blood cell destruction and eventually acute renal failure, is a complication of *E. coli* O157:H7 that occurs in 3% to 5% of patients with confirmed infection.[6] Children age 5 and younger and elderly people are at increased risk of HUS.

▶ *Infections.* Acute viral, bacterial, and protozoal infections (such as cryptosporidiosis) cause the sudden onset of watery diarrhea as well as abdominal pain or cramps, nausea, vomiting, and fever. Significant fluid and electrolyte loss may cause signs of dehydration and shock. Chronic tuberculosis and fungal and parasitic infections may produce a less severe but more persistent diarrhea, accompanied by epigastric distress, vomiting, weight loss and, possibly, passage of blood and mucus.

▶ *Intestinal obstruction.* Partial intestinal obstruction increases intestinal motility, resulting in diarrhea, abdominal pain with tenderness and guarding, nausea and, possibly, distention.

▶ *Irritable bowel syndrome.* Diarrhea may be prominent or may alternate with constipation or normal bowel function. Related findings include abdominal pain, tenderness, and distention; dyspepsia; and nausea.

▶ *Ischemic bowel disease.* This life-threatening disorder causes sudden onset of bloody diarrhea with abdominal pain. If severe, shock may occur, requiring surgery.

▶ *Lactose intolerance.* Diarrhea occurs within several hours of ingesting milk or milk products in patients with this disorder. It's accompanied by cramps, abdominal pain, borborygmi, bloating, nausea, and flatus.

▶ *Large-bowel cancer.* In this disorder, bloody diarrhea is seen with a partial obstruction. Other signs and symptoms include abdominal pain, anorexia, weight loss, weakness, fatigue, exertional dyspnea, and depression.

▶ *Listeriosis.* This infection, caused by ingestion of food contaminated with the bacterium *Listeria monocytogenes,* primarily affects pregnant women, neonates, and those with weakened immune systems. Findings include diarrhea, fever, myalgia, abdominal pain, nausea, and vomiting. Fever, headache, nuchal rigidity, and altered level of consciousness may occur if the infection spreads to the nervous system and causes meningitis. Listeriosis during pregnancy may lead to premature delivery, infection of the neonate, or stillbirth.

▶ *Malabsorption syndrome.* Occurring after meals, diarrhea is accompanied by steatorrhea, abdominal distention, and muscle cramps. The patient also displays anorexia, weight loss, bone pain, anemia, weakness, and fatigue. He may bruise easily and have night blindness.

▶ *Pseudomembranous enterocolitis.* This potentially life-threatening disorder commonly follows antibiotic administration. It produces copious watery, green, foul-smelling, bloody diarrhea that rapidly causes signs of shock. Other signs and symptoms include colicky abdominal pain, distention, fever, and dehydration.

▶ *Q fever.* This infection is caused by the bacterium *Coxiella burnetii* and causes diarrhea along with fever, chills, severe headache, malaise, chest pain, and vomiting. In severe cases, hepatitis or pneumonia may follow.

▶ *Rotavirus gastroenteritis.* This disorder commonly starts with a fever, nausea, and vomiting, followed by diarrhea. The illness can be mild to severe and last from 3 to 9 days. Diarrhea and vomiting may result in dehydration.

▶ *Thyrotoxicosis.* In this disorder, diarrhea is accompanied by nervousness, tremors, diaphoresis, weight loss despite increased appetite, dyspnea, palpitations, tachycardia, enlarged thyroid, heat intolerance and, possibly, exophthalmos.

▶ *Ulcerative colitis.* The hallmark of this disorder is recurrent bloody diarrhea with pus or mucus. Other signs and symptoms include tenesmus, hyperactive bowel sounds, cramp-

ing lower abdominal pain, low-grade fever, anorexia and, possibly, nausea and vomiting. Weight loss, anemia, and weakness are late findings.

▶ *Waterborne illnesses.* Waterborne illnesses cause infection when a person consumes contaminated water, and can cause diarrhea as well as such signs and symptoms as fever, nausea, vomiting, abdominal pain or cramping, bloating, and dehydration. Infectious agents may include parasites such as *Cryptosporidium* and *Giardia intestinalis,* bacteria such as *Campylobacter jejuni* and *Salmonella enterica typhimurium,* and viruses such as noroviruses, rotaviruses, adenoviruses, astroviruses, and hepatitis A.[4]

Other causes

DRUG WATCH *Many antibiotics— such as ampicillin, cephalosporins, tetracyclines, and clindamycin—cause diarrhea. Other drugs that may cause diarrhea include magnesium-containing antacids, lactulose, dantrolene, ethacrynic acid, mefenamic acid, methotrexate, metyrosine and, with high doses, cardiac glycosides and quinidine. Laxative abuse can cause acute or chronic diarrhea.*

▶ *Foods.* Foods that contain certain oils may inhibit the food's absorption, causing acute uncontrollable diarrhea and rectal leakage. High consumption of caffeine or sorbitol-containing foods may cause diarrhea. Herbal remedies, such as ginkgo biloba, ginseng, and licorice, may cause diarrhea.

▶ *Lead poisoning.* Alternating diarrhea and constipation may be accompanied by abdominal pain, anorexia, nausea, and vomiting. The patient complains of a metallic taste, headache, and dizziness and displays a bluish gingival lead line.

▶ *Treatments.* Gastrectomy, gastroenterostomy, and pyloroplasty may produce diarrhea. High-dose radiation therapy may produce enteritis associated with diarrhea.

Special considerations

Give oral or I.V. fluid replacements to help the patient maintain adequate hydration.[2] Monitor electrolyte levels and hematocrit. When appropriate, give an analgesic for pain and an opioid as ordered to decrease intestinal motility, unless the patient may have a stool infection. Ensure the patient's privacy during defecation, and empty bedpans promptly. Clean the perineum thoroughly, and apply ointment to prevent skin breakdown. Measure liquid stools and carefully observe intake and output; weigh the patient daily. A stool specimen may be ordered for diagnostic evaluation.[2]

To prevent diarrhea, dilute drugs that are hyperosmotic or that contain sorbitol before giving them, and flush enteral tubes with water before and after drug administration.[2]

Food- or water-borne illnesses should be reported to the local public health agency or to the hospital infection control practitioner.[4]

Pediatric pointers
Diarrhea in children commonly results from infection, although chronic diarrhea may result from malabsorption syndrome, an anatomic defect, or allergies. Because dehydration and electrolyte imbalance occur rapidly in children, diarrhea can be life-threatening. Diligently monitor all episodes of diarrhea, and replace lost fluids immediately.

Geriatric pointers
In the elderly patient with new-onset segmental colitis, always consider ischemia before labeling the patient as having Crohn's disease.

Patient counseling
Explain the purpose of diagnostic tests to the patient. These tests may include blood studies, stool cultures, X-rays, and endoscopy.

Advise the patient to avoid spicy or high-fiber foods (such as fruits), caffeine, high-fat foods, and milk. The patient with watery diarrhea may benefit from eating foods that are easily digested, such as bananas, rice, applesauce, and toast (the BRAT diet).[1] Suggest smaller, more frequent meals if he has had GI surgery or disease. If appropriate, teach the patient stress-reducing measures, such as guided imagery and deep-breathing techniques, or recommend counseling.

Stress the need for medical follow-up to patients with inflammatory bowel disease (particularly ulcerative colitis), who have an increased risk of developing colon cancer.

REFERENCES
1. Amerine, E. and Keirsey, M. "Managing Acute Diarrhea." *Nursing* 36(9):64hn1, 64hn2, 64hn4, September 2006.
2. Sabol, V. and Carlson, K. "Diarrhea: Applying Research to Bedside Practice." *AACN Advanced Critical Care* 18(1):32-44, January/March 2007.
3. Cheng, A., McDonald, J., and Thielman, N. "Infectious Diarrhea in Developed and Developing Countries." *Journal of Clinical Gastroenterology* 39(9):757-773, October 2005.
4. Chalupka, S. "Tainted Water on Tap: What to Tell Patients About Preventing Illness from Drinking Water." *AJN* 105(11):40-52, November 2005.
5. Todd, B. "Clostridium Difficile: Familiar Pathogen, Changing Epidemiology." *AJN* 106(5):33-36, May 2006.
6. Raffaelli, R.M., et al. "Child-Care Associated Outbreak of Escherichia coli O157:H7 and Hemolytic Uremic Syndrome." *The Pediatric Infectious Disease Journal* 26(10):951-953, October 2007.

DIZZINESS

A common symptom, dizziness is a sensation of imbalance or faintness, sometimes associated with giddiness, weakness, confusion, and blurred or double vision. Episodes of dizziness are usually brief; they may be mild or severe with an abrupt or gradual onset. Dizziness may be aggravated by standing up quickly and eased by lying down and by resting.

Dizziness typically results from inadequate blood flow and oxygen supply to the cerebrum and spinal cord. It's a key symptom in certain serious disorders, such as hypertension and vertebrobasilar artery insufficiency, and it also may occur in anxiety, respiratory and cardiovascular disorders, and postconcussion syndrome. In many cases, medical and psychological factors interact to cause dizziness.[1]

Dizziness is commonly confused with vertigo—a sensation of revolving in space or of surroundings revolving around oneself. However, unlike dizziness, vertigo is commonly accompanied by nausea, vomiting, nystagmus, staggering gait, and tinnitus or hearing loss and may be caused by inner ear diseases, brainstem ischemia, or Ménière disease.[2] Dizziness and vertigo may occur together, as in postconcussion syndrome.

If the patient complains of dizziness, first ensure his safety by preventing falls, and then determine the severity and onset of the dizziness. Ask the patient to describe it. Is it associated with headache or blurred vision? Next, take the patient's blood pressure while he's lying, sitting, and standing to check for orthostatic hypotension. Ask about a history of high blood pressure. Determine if the patient is at risk for hypoglycemia. Tell the patient to lie down, and recheck his vital signs every 15 minutes. Start an I.V. line, and prepare to administer drugs as ordered.

History and physical examination

Ask about a history of diabetes and cardiovascular disease. Is the patient taking drugs prescribed for high blood pressure? If so, when did he take his last dose?

If the patient's blood pressure is normal, obtain a more complete history. Ask if he's had a myocardial infarction, heart failure, kidney disease, or atherosclerosis, which may predispose him to cardiac arrhythmias, hypertension, and a transient ischemic attack. Does he have a history of anemia, chronic obstructive pulmonary disease, anxiety disorders, or head injury? Obtain a complete drug history.

Next, explore the patient's dizziness. How often does it occur? How long does each episode last? Does the dizziness abate spontaneously? Does it lead to loss of consciousness? Find out if dizziness is triggered by sitting or standing up suddenly or by stooping over. Does being in a crowd make the patient feel dizzy? Ask about emotional stress. Has the patient been irritable or anxious lately? Does he have insomnia or difficulty concentrating? Look for fidgeting and eyelid twitching. Does the patient startle easily? Also, ask about palpitations, chest pain, diaphoresis, shortness of breath, and chronic cough.

Next, perform a physical examination. Begin with a quick neurocheck, assessing the patient's level of consciousness (LOC), motor and sensory function, and reflexes. Then inspect for poor skin turgor and dry mucous membranes, signs of dehydration. Auscultate

heart rate and rhythm. Inspect for barrel chest, clubbing, cyanosis, and use of accessory muscles. Also auscultate breath sounds. Take the patient's blood pressure while he's lying, sitting, and standing to check for orthostatic hypotension. Test capillary refill time in the extremities, and palpate for edema.

Medical causes

▶ *Anemia.* Anemia typically causes dizziness that's aggravated by postural changes or exertion. Other signs and symptoms include pallor, dyspnea, fatigue, tachycardia, bounding pulse, and increased capillary refill time.
▶ *Cardiac arrhythmias.* Dizziness lasts for several seconds or longer and may precede fainting in arrhythmias. The patient may experience palpitations; irregular, rapid, or thready pulse and, possibly, hypotension. He also may experience weakness, blurred vision, paresthesia, and confusion.
▶ *Carotid sinus hypersensitivity.* This disorder is characterized by brief episodes of dizziness that usually terminate in fainting. These episodes are caused by stimulation of one or both carotid arteries by seemingly minor sensations or actions, such as wearing a tight collar or moving the head. Other signs and symptoms include sweating, nausea, and pallor.
▶ *Emphysema.* Dizziness may follow exertion or the chronic productive cough that's characteristic of this disorder. Other signs and symptoms include dyspnea, anorexia, weight loss, malaise, use of accessory muscles, pursed-lip breathing, tachypnea, peripheral cyanosis, and diminished breath sounds. Barrel chest and clubbing may occur.
▶ *Generalized anxiety disorder.* This disorder produces persistent anxiety (for at least 1 month), insomnia, difficulty concentrating, irritability and, possibly, continuous dizziness that may intensify as the anxiety worsens. The patient may show signs of motor tension—for example, twitching or fidgeting, muscle aches, a furrowed brow, and a tendency to be startled. He also may display signs of autonomic hyperactivity, such as diaphoresis, palpitations, cold and clammy hands, dry mouth, paresthesia, indigestion, hot or cold flashes, frequent urination, diarrhea, a lump in the

throat, pallor, and increased pulse and respiratory rates.

▶ *Hypertension.* In patients with hypertension, dizziness may precede fainting, but it also may be relieved by rest. Other common signs and symptoms include headache and blurred vision. Retinal changes include hemorrhage, sclerosis of retinal blood vessels, exudate, and papilledema.

▶ *Hyperventilation syndrome.* Episodes of hyperventilation cause dizziness that usually lasts a few minutes; however, if these episodes occur often, dizziness may persist between them. Other effects include apprehension, diaphoresis, pallor, dyspnea, chest tightness, palpitations, trembling, fatigue, and peripheral and circumoral paresthesia.

▶ *Hypoglycemia.* Dizziness is a central nervous system (CNS) disturbance that can result from fasting hypoglycemia. It's typically accompanied by headache, clouding of vision, restlessness, and mental status changes.

▶ *Hypovolemia.* Dizziness may be accompanied by other signs of fluid volume deficit, such as dry mucous membranes, decreased blood pressure, and increased heart rate.

▶ *Orthostatic hypotension.* This condition produces dizziness that may terminate in fainting or disappear with rest. Related findings include dim vision, spots before the eyes, pallor, diaphoresis, hypotension, tachycardia and, possibly, signs of dehydration.

▶ *Panic disorder.* Dizziness may accompany acute attacks of panic in patients with this disorder. Other findings include anxiety, dyspnea, palpitations, chest pain, a choking or smothering sensation, vertigo, paresthesia, hot and cold flashes, diaphoresis, and trembling or shaking. The patient may feel like he's dying or losing his mind.

▶ *Postconcussion syndrome.* Occurring 1 to 3 weeks after a head injury, this syndrome is marked by dizziness, headache (throbbing, aching, bandlike, or stabbing), emotional lability, alcohol intolerance, fatigue, anxiety and, possibly, vertigo. Dizziness and other symptoms are intensified by mental or physical stress. The syndrome may persist for years, but symptoms eventually abate.

▶ *Rift Valley fever.* Typical signs and symptoms of this disorder include dizziness, fever, myalgia, weakness, and back pain. A small percentage of patients may develop encephalitis or may progress to hemorrhagic fever, which can lead to shock and hemorrhage. Inflammation of the retina may result in some permanent vision loss.

▶ *Transient ischemic attack (TIA).* Lasting from a few seconds to 24 hours, a TIA commonly signals an impending stroke and may be triggered by turning the head to the side. Besides dizziness of varying severity, TIAs are marked by unilateral or bilateral diplopia, blindness or visual field deficits, ptosis, tinnitus, hearing loss, paresis, and numbness. Other findings may include dysarthria, dysphagia, vomiting, hiccups, confusion, decreased LOC, and pallor.

Other causes

DRUG WATCH *Anxiolytics, CNS depressants, opioids, decongestants, antihistamines, antihypertensives, neuroleptics, and vasodilators commonly cause dizziness.*

▶ *Herbal supplements.* Remedies such as St. John's wort can produce dizziness.

Special considerations

Prepare the patient for diagnostic tests, such as blood studies, arteriography, computed tomography scan, EEG, magnetic resonance imaging, and tilt-table studies.

Pediatric pointers

Dizziness is less common in children than in adults. Many children have trouble describing this symptom and instead complain of tiredness, stomachache, or feeling sick. If you suspect dizziness, also assess the patient for vertigo, a more common symptom in children that may result from a vision disorder, an ear infection, or antibiotic therapy.

Geriatric pointers

Older adults are at increased risk for heatstroke, a condition marked by a core body temperature of at least 104° F (40° C) with signs and symptoms of central nervous system impairment such as dizziness, confusion, and delirium that may progress to seizures and coma.[3] Vitamin B_{12} deficiency, which occurs in 15% 25% of older adults, can cause dizziness as well as paresthesia, weakness, tremors, mood disorders, impaired balance, dementia, and visual disturbances.[4]

Patient counseling

Teach the patient ways to control dizziness. If he's hyperventilating, have him breathe and rebreathe into his cupped hands or a paper bag. If he feels dizzy in an upright position, tell him to lie down and rest and then to rise slowly. Advise a patient with carotid sinus hypersensitivity to avoid wearing garments that constrict the neck. Instruct the patient who risks a TIA from vertebrobasilar insufficiency to turn his body instead of sharply turning his head to one side.

Explain that vestibular rehabilitation, provided by a physical therapist, can help to decrease dizziness and improve the sense of balance by promoting central nervous system compensation for inner ear disorders.[5]

REFERENCES

1. Staab, J.P. "Assessment and Management of Psychological Problems in the Dizzy Patient." *CONTINUUM: Lifelong Learning in Neurology* 12(4):189-213, August 2006.
2. Pendrak, T. "Orthostatic Hypotension: Catching the Fall in Blood Pressure." *LPN* 1(5):4-7, September/October 2005.
3. Lewis, A.M. "Heatstroke in Older Adults: In This Population It's A Short Step from Heat Exhaustion." *AJN* 107(6):52-56, June 2007.
4. Pacholok, S. "Simple Steps to Stamp Out Vitamin B12 Deficiency." *Nursing* 37(1):67-69, January 2007.
5. Pullen, R.L. "Spin Control: Caring for A Patient With Inner Ear Disease." *Nursing* 36(5):48-51, May 2006.

DYSARTHRIA

Dysarthria, which refers to poorly articulated speech, is characterized by slurring and a labored, irregular speech rhythm. It may be accompanied by a nasal voice tone caused by palate weakness. Whether it occurs abruptly or gradually, dysarthria is usually evident in ordinary conversation. It's confirmed by asking the patient to produce a few simple sounds and words, such as "ba," "sh," and "cat." However, dysarthria is occasionally confused with aphasia, which is loss of the ability to produce or comprehend speech.

Dysarthria results from brain stem damage that affects cranial nerves IX, X, or XII. Degenerative neurologic disorders and cerebellar disorders commonly cause dysarthria. In fact, dysarthria is a cardinal sign of olivopontocerebellar degeneration. It also may result from ill-fitting dentures.

If the patient has dysarthria, ask if he has trouble swallowing. Then determine respiratory rate and depth. Measure vital capacity with a Wright respirometer if available. Assess blood pressure and heart rate. Tachycardia, slightly increased blood pressure, and shortness of breath are usually early signs of respiratory muscle weakness.

Ensure a patent airway. Place the patient in Fowler's position and suction him if necessary. Administer oxygen and keep emergency resuscitation equipment nearby. Anticipate intubation and mechanical ventilation in progressive respiratory muscle weakness. Withhold oral fluids in the patient with associated dysphagia.

If dysarthria isn't accompanied by respiratory muscle weakness and dysphagia, continue to assess for other neurologic deficits. Compare muscle strength and tone in the limbs, and evaluate tactile sensation. Ask the patient about numbness or tingling. Test deep tendon reflexes (DTRs), and note gait ataxia. Assess cerebellar function by observing rapid alternating movement, which should be smooth and coordinated. Next, test visual fields and ask about double vision. Check for signs of facial weakness such as ptosis. Finally, determine level of consciousness (LOC) and mental status.

History and physical examination

Explore the dysarthria completely. When did it begin? Has it gotten better? Speech improves with resolution of a transient ischemic attack, but not in a completed stroke. Ask if dysarthria worsens during the day. Then obtain a drug and alcohol history. Also, ask about a history of seizures. Observe dentures for a proper fit.

Medical causes

▶ *Alcoholic cerebellar degeneration.* This disorder commonly causes chronic, progressive dysarthria along with ataxia, diplopia, ophthalmoplegia, hypotension, and altered mental status.

▶ *Amyotrophic lateral sclerosis.* Dysarthria occurs when this disorder affects the bulbar nuclei; it may worsen as the disease progresses. Other signs and symptoms include dysphagia; difficulty breathing; muscle atrophy and weakness, especially of the hands and feet; fasciculations; spasticity; hyperactive DTRs in the legs; and occasionally excessive drooling. Progressive bulbar palsy may cause crying spells or inappropriate laughter.

▶ *Basilar artery insufficiency.* This disorder causes random, brief episodes of bilateral brain stem dysfunction, resulting in dysarthria. Accompanying it are diplopia, vertigo, facial numbness, ataxia, paresis, and visual field loss, all of which can last from minutes to hours.

▶ *Botulism.* The hallmark of this disorder is acute cranial nerve dysfunction that causes dysarthria, dysphagia, diplopia, and ptosis. Early findings include dry mouth, sore throat, weakness, vomiting, and diarrhea. Later, descending weakness or paralysis of muscles in the extremities and trunk causes hyporeflexia and dyspnea.

▶ *Multiple sclerosis.* When demyelination affects the brain stem and cerebellum, the patient displays dysarthria accompanied by nystagmus, blurred or double vision, dysphagia, ataxia, and intention tremor. Exacerbations and remissions of these signs and symptoms are common. Other findings include paresthesia, spasticity, intention tremor, hyperreflexia, muscle weakness or paralysis, constipation, emotional lability, and urinary frequency, urgency, and incontinence.

▶ *Myasthenia gravis.* This neuromuscular disorder causes dysarthria associated with a nasal voice tone. Typically, the dysarthria worsens during the day and may temporarily improve with short rest periods. Other findings include dysphagia, drooling, facial weakness, diplopia, ptosis, dyspnea, and muscle weakness.

▶ *Olivopontocerebellar degeneration.* Dysarthria, a cardinal sign of this disorder, accompanies cerebellar ataxia and spasticity.

▶ *Parkinson's disease.* This disorder produces dysarthria and a monotone voice. It also produces muscle rigidity, bradykinesia, an involuntary tremor that usually begins in the fingers, difficulty walking, muscle weakness, and stooped posture. Other findings include masklike facies, dysphagia and, occasionally, drooling.

▶ *Shy-Drager syndrome.* Marked by chronic orthostatic hypotension, this syndrome eventually causes dysarthria as well as cerebellar ataxia, bradykinesia, masklike facies, dementia, impotence and, possibly, stooped posture and incontinence.

▶ *Stroke.* Some 8% to 30% of stroke patients develop dysarthria.[1] A brain stem stroke is characterized by bulbar palsy, resulting in the triad of dysarthria, dysphonia, and dysphagia. The dysarthria is most severe at the onset of the stroke; it may lessen or disappear with rehabilitation and training. Other findings include facial weakness, diplopia, hemiparesis, spasticity, drooling, dyspnea, and decreased LOC.

A massive bilateral cerebral stroke causes pseudobulbar palsy. Bilateral weakness produces dysarthria that's most severe at the stroke's onset. This sign is accompanied by dysphagia, drooling, dysphonia, bilateral hemianopsia, and aphasia. Sensory loss, spasticity, and hyperreflexia also may occur.

Other causes

▶ *Drugs.* Dysarthria can occur when anticonvulsant dosage is too high. Ingestion of large doses of barbiturates also may cause dysarthria.

▶ *Manganese poisoning.* Chronic manganese poisoning causes progressive dysarthria accompanied by weakness, fatigue, confusion, hallucinations, drooling, hand tremors, limb stiffness, spasticity, gross rhythmic movements of the trunk and head, and a propulsive gait.

▶ *Mercury poisoning.* Chronic mercury poisoning causes progressive dysarthria accompanied by weakness, fatigue, depression, lethargy, irritability, confusion, ataxia, and tremors.

Special considerations

Encourage the patient with dysarthria to speak slowly so he can be understood. Give him time to express himself, and encourage him to use gestures. Dysarthria usually requires consultation with a speech pathologist.

If the patient has trouble swallowing, monitor him closely to prevent aspiration.[2]

Pediatric pointers

Dysarthria in children usually results from brain stem glioma, a slow-growing tumor that mainly affects children. It also may result from cerebral palsy.

Dysarthria may be difficult to detect, especially in an infant or a young child who hasn't perfected speech. Be sure to look for other neurologic deficits, too. Encourage a child with dysarthria to speak; a child's potential for rehabilitation is typically greater than an adult's.

Geriatric pointers

Dysarthria is the second most common speech and language disorder in the elderly.[1]

Patient counseling

Instruct the patient and his family about communication techniques. Encourage the patient to express his feelings. Provide guidelines on foods or liquids that should be avoided due to risk for aspiration. Refer the patient to a speech therapist.

REFERENCES

1. Jordan, L.C. and Hillis, A.E. "Disorders of Speech and Language: Aphasia, Apraxia, and Dysarthria." *Current Opinion in Neurology* 19(6):580-585, December 2006.
2. Palmieri, R.L. "Take Aim at Amyotrophic Lateral Sclerosis." *Nursing* 35(11):32hn1-32hn2, November 2005.

DYSPHAGIA

Dysphagia—difficulty swallowing—is a common symptom that's usually easy to localize. It may be constant or intermittent and is classified by the phase of swallowing it affects. (See *Classifying dysphagia*.) Among the factors that interfere with swallowing are severe pain, obstruction, abnormal peristalsis, impaired gag reflex, and excessive, scanty, or thick oral secretions.

Dysphagia is the most common—and sometimes the only—symptom of an esophageal disorder. However, it also may result from oropharyngeal, respiratory, neurologic, and collagen disorders or from the effects of toxins and treatments. Dysphagia increases the risk of choking and aspiration and may lead to malnutrition and dehydration.

If the patient suddenly complains of dysphagia and has signs of respiratory distress, such as dyspnea and stridor, suspect an airway obstruction and quickly perform abdominal thrusts. Prepare to give oxygen by mask or nasal cannula or to assist with endotracheal intubation.

History and physical examination

If the patient's dysphagia doesn't suggest an airway obstruction, begin a health history. Ask the patient if swallowing is painful. If so, is the pain constant or intermittent? Have the patient point to where dysphagia feels most intense. Does eating alleviate or aggravate the symptom? Are solids or liquids more difficult to swallow? If the answer is liquids, ask if hot, cold, and lukewarm fluids affect him differently. Does the symptom disappear after he tries to swallow a few times? Is swallowing easier if he changes position? Ask if he has recently experienced vomiting, regurgitation, weight loss, anorexia, hoarseness, dyspnea, or a cough.

To evaluate the patient's swallowing reflex, place your finger along his thyroid notch and instruct him to swallow. If you feel his larynx rise, the reflex is intact. Next, have him cough to assess his cough reflex. Check his gag reflex if you're sure he has a good swallow or cough reflex. Listen closely to his speech for signs of muscle weakness. Does he have aphasia or dysarthria? Is his voice nasal, hoarse, or breathy? Assess the patient's mouth carefully. Check for dry mucous membranes and thick, sticky secretions. Observe for tongue and facial weakness and obvious obstructions (for example, enlarged tonsils). Assess the patient for disorientation, which may make him neglect to swallow.

Classifying dysphagia

Because swallowing occurs in three distinct phases, dysphagia can be classified by the phase it affects. Each phase suggests a specific pathology.

PHASE 1

Swallowing begins in the *transfer phase* with chewing and moistening of food with saliva. The tongue presses against the hard palate to transfer chewed food to the back of the throat; cranial nerve V then stimulates the swallowing reflex. Phase 1 dysphagia typically results from a neuromuscular disorder.

PHASE 2

In the *transport phase,* the soft palate closes against the pharyngeal wall to prevent nasal regurgitation. At the same time, the larynx rises and the vocal cords close to keep food out of the lungs; breathing stops momentarily as the throat muscles constrict to move food into the esophagus. Phase 2 dysphagia usually indicates spasm or cancer.

PHASE 3

Peristalsis and gravity work together in the *entrance phase* to move food through the esophageal sphincter and into the stomach. Phase 3 dysphagia results from lower esophageal narrowing by diverticula, esophagitis, and other disorders.

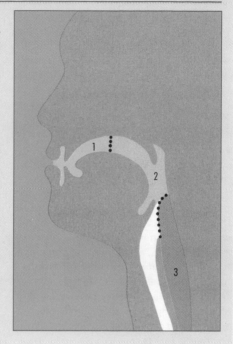

Medical causes

▶ *Achalasia.* Most common in patients ages 20 to 40 (although it also occurs in older people), this disorder produces phase 3 dysphagia for solids and liquids. The dysphagia develops gradually and may be caused or worsened by stress. Occasionally, it's preceded by esophageal colic. Regurgitation of undigested food, especially at night, may cause wheezing, coughing, or choking as well as halitosis. Weight loss, cachexia, hematemesis and, possibly, heartburn are late findings.

▶ *Airway obstruction.* Life-threatening upper airway obstruction is marked by signs of respiratory distress, such as crowing and stridor. Phase 2 dysphagia occurs with gagging and dysphonia. When hemorrhage obstructs the trachea, dysphagia is usually painless and rapid in onset. When inflammation causes the obstruction, dysphagia may be painful and develop slowly.

▶ *Amyotrophic lateral sclerosis.* Besides dysphagia, this disorder causes muscle weakness and atrophy, fasciculations, dysarthria, dyspnea, shallow respirations, tachypnea, slurred speech, hyperactive deep tendon reflexes, and emotional lability.

▶ *Botulism.* This type of food poisoning causes phase 1 dysphagia and dysuria, usually within 36 hours of toxin ingestion. Other early findings include blurred or double vision, dry mouth, sore throat, nausea, vomiting, and diarrhea. Symmetrical descending weakness or paralysis occurs gradually.

▶ *Bulbar paralysis.* Phase 1 dysphagia occurs along with drooling, difficulty chewing, dysarthria, and nasal regurgitation in this disorder. Dysphagia for both solids and liquids is painful and progressive. Accompanying features may include arm and leg spasticity, hyperreflexia, and emotional lability.

▶ *Dysphagia lusoria.* This disorder is caused by compression of the esophagus by a congenital vascular abnormality (usually an aberrant right subclavian artery arising from the left side of the aortic arch). Phase 3 dysphagia symptoms may start in childhood or may develop later from changes in the aberrant vessel such as arteriosclerosis.

▶ *Esophageal cancer.* Phase 2 or 3 dysphagia is the earliest and most common symptom of esophageal cancer. Typically, this painless, progressive symptom is accompanied by rapid weight loss.[1] As the cancer advances, dysphagia becomes painful and constant. In addition, the patient complains of steady chest pain, cough with hemoptysis, hoarseness, and sore throat. He also may develop nausea and vomiting, fever, hiccups, hematemesis, melena, and halitosis.

▶ *Esophageal compression (external).* Usually caused by a dilated carotid or aortic aneurysm, this rare condition causes phase 3 dysphagia as the primary symptom. Other features depend on the cause of the compression.

▶ *Esophageal diverticulum.* This disorder causes phase 3 dysphagia when the enlarged diverticulum obstructs the esophagus. Other signs and symptoms include food regurgitation, chronic cough, hoarseness, chest pain, and halitosis.

▶ *Esophageal leiomyoma.* A relatively rare benign tumor, esophageal leiomyoma may cause phase 3 dysphagia along with retrosternal pain or discomfort. In addition, the patient experiences weight loss and a feeling of fullness.

▶ *Esophageal obstruction by foreign body.* Sudden onset of phase 2 or 3 dysphagia, gagging, coughing, and esophageal pain characterize this potentially life-threatening condition. Dyspnea may occur if the obstruction compresses the trachea.

▶ *Esophageal spasm.* The most striking symptoms of this disorder are phase 2 dysphagia for solids and liquids and dull or squeezing substernal chest pain. The pain may last up to an hour and may radiate to the neck, arm, back, or jaw; however, it may be relieved by drinking a glass of water. Bradycardia also may occur.

▶ *Esophageal stricture.* Usually caused by scar tissue or ingestion of a chemical, this condition causes phase 3 dysphagia. Drooling, tachypnea, and gagging also may be evident.

▶ *Esophagitis.* Corrosive esophagitis, resulting from ingestion of alkalies or acids, causes severe phase 3 dysphagia. Accompanying it are marked salivation, hematemesis, tachypnea, fever, and intense pain in the mouth and anterior chest that's aggravated by swallowing. Signs of shock, such as hypotension and tachycardia, also may occur.

Candidal esophagitis causes phase 2 dysphagia, sore throat and, possibly, retrosternal pain on swallowing. In reflux esophagitis, phase 3 dysphagia is a late symptom that usually accompanies stricture development. The patient complains of heartburn, which is aggravated by strenuous exercise, bending over, or lying down and is relieved by sitting up or taking an antacid.

Other features include regurgitation; frequent, effortless vomiting; a dry, nocturnal cough; and substernal chest pain that may mimic angina pectoris. If the esophagus ulcerates, signs of bleeding, such as melena and hematemesis, may occur along with weakness and fatigue.

▶ *Gastric carcinoma.* Infiltration of the cardia or esophagus by gastric carcinoma causes phase 3 dysphagia along with nausea, vomiting, and pain that may radiate to the neck, back, or retrosternum. In addition, perforation causes massive bleeding with coffee-ground vomitus or melena.

▶ *Hypocalcemia.* Although tetany is its main sign, severe hypocalcemia may cause neuromuscular irritability, producing phase 1 dysphagia with numbness and tingling in the nose, ears, fingertips, and toes and around the mouth. Carpopedal spasms, muscle twitching, and laryngeal spasms also may occur.

▶ *Laryngeal cancer (extrinsic).* Phase 2 dysphagia and dyspnea develop late in this disorder. Accompanying features include muffled voice, stridor, pain, halitosis, weight loss, ipsilateral otalgia, chronic cough, and cachexia. Palpation reveals enlarged cervical nodes.

▶ *Laryngeal nerve damage.* Commonly the result of radical neck surgery, superior laryngeal nerve damage may produce painless phase 2 dysphagia.

▶ *Lower esophageal ring.* Narrowing of the lower esophagus can cause an attack of phase 3 dysphagia that may recur several weeks or months later. During the attack, the patient complains of a foreign body sensation in the lower esophagus, which may be relieved by drinking water or vomiting. Esophageal rupture produces severe lower chest pain followed by a feeling of something giving way.

▶ *Mediastinitis.* Varying with the extent of esophageal perforation, mediastinitis can cause insidious or rapid onset of phase 3 dysphagia. The patient displays chills, fever, and severe retrosternal chest pain that may radiate to the epigastrium, back, or shoulder. The pain may be aggravated by breathing, coughing, or sneezing. Other findings include tachycardia, subcutaneous crepitation in the suprasternal notch, and falling blood pressure.

▶ *Myasthenia gravis.* Fatigue and progressive muscle weakness characterize this disorder and account for painless phase 1 dysphagia and possibly choking. Typically, dysphagia follows ptosis and diplopia. Other features include masklike facies, nasal voice, frequent nasal regurgitation, and head bobbing. Shallow respirations and dyspnea may occur with respiratory muscle weakness. Signs and symptoms worsen during menses and with exposure to stress, cold, or infection.

▶ *Oral cavity tumor.* Painful phase 1 dysphagia is accompanied by hoarseness and ulcerating lesions in patients with this type of tumor.

▶ *Parkinson's disease.* Dysphagia occurs in about half of people with Parkinson's disease.[1] Phase 1 dysphagia is painless but progressive and may cause choking. Other signs and symptoms include bradykinesia, tremors, muscle rigidity, dysarthria, masklike facies, muffled voice, increased salivation and lacrimation, constipation, stooped posture, a propulsive gait, incontinence, and sexual dysfunction.

▶ *Pharyngitis (chronic).* This condition causes painful phase 2 dysphagia for solids and liquids. Rarely serious, it's accompanied by a dry, sore throat; a cough; and thick mucus in the throat.

▶ *Plummer-Vinson syndrome.* This syndrome causes phase 3 dysphagia for solids in some women with severe iron deficiency anemia.

Related features include upper esophageal pain; atrophy of the oral or pharyngeal mucous membranes; tooth loss; a smooth, red, sore tongue; dry mouth; chills; inflamed lips; spoon-shaped nails; pallor; and splenomegaly.

▶ *Rabies.* Severe phase 2 dysphagia for liquids results from painful pharyngeal muscle spasms occurring late in this rare, life-threatening disorder. In fact, the patient may become dehydrated and possibly apneic. Dysphagia also causes drooling and, in 50% of patients, hydrophobia. Eventually, rabies causes progressive flaccid paralysis that leads to peripheral vascular collapse, coma, and death.

▶ *Scleroderma (progressive systemic sclerosis).* The esophagus is affected in about 80% of people with scleroderma.[1] Typically, dysphagia is preceded by Raynaud's phenomenon in patients with this disorder. The dysphagia may be mild at first and described as a feeling of food sticking behind the breastbone. The patient also complains of heartburn after meals that's aggravated by lying down. As the disease progresses, dysphagia worsens until only liquids can be swallowed. It may be accompanied by other GI effects, including weight loss, abdominal distention, diarrhea, and malodorous, floating stools. Other characteristic late features include joint pain and stiffness, masklike face, and thick, taut, shiny skin.

▶ *Stroke.* About half of stroke survivors have dysphagia.[1] They also may have complications such as aspiration pneumonia, dehydration, and malnutrition. Because these conditions may be life-threatening, early and aggressive dysphagia management is called for to reduce morbidity and mortality.[1,2] Other signs and symptoms of stroke may include unilateral limb weakness or numbness, speech difficulties, headache, vision disturbances, dizziness, anxiety, and altered level of consciousness.

▶ *Syphilis.* Rarely, tertiary-stage syphilis causes ulceration and stricture of the upper esophagus, resulting in phase 3 dysphagia. The dysphagia may be accompanied by regurgitation after meals and heartburn that's aggravated by lying down or bending over.

▶ *Systemic lupus erythematosus.* This disorder may cause progressive phase 2 dysphagia.

However, its primary signs and symptoms include nondeforming arthritis, a characteristic butterfly rash, and photosensitivity.

▶ *Tetanus.* Phase 1 dysphagia usually develops about 1 week after the patient receives a puncture wound. Other characteristics include marked muscle hypertonicity, hyperactive deep tendon reflexes, tachycardia, diaphoresis, drooling, and low-grade fever. Painful, involuntary muscle spasms account for lockjaw (trismus), risus sardonicus, opisthotonos, boardlike abdominal rigidity, and intermittent tonic seizures.

Other causes

DRUG WATCH *Dysphagia may occur as an adverse effect from nitrates, calcium channel blockers, calcium tablets, iron supplements, vitamin C supplements, aspirin, tetracycline, and some anticholinergics and antipsychotics.[3]*

▶ *Lead poisoning.* Painless, progressive dysphagia may result from lead poisoning. Related findings include a lead line on the gums, metallic taste, papilledema, ocular palsy, footdrop or wristdrop, and signs of hemolytic anemia, such as abdominal pain and fever. The patient may be depressed and display severe mental impairment and seizures.

▶ *Procedures.* A recent tracheostomy or repeated or prolonged intubation may cause temporary dysphagia.

▶ *Radiation therapy.* When used to treat oral cancer, radiation therapy may cause scant salivation and temporary dysphagia.

Special considerations

Stimulate salivation by talking with the patient about food, adding a lemon slice or dill pickle to his tray, and providing mouth care before and after meals. Moisten his food with a little liquid if he has decreased salivation. Administer an anticholinergic or antiemetic to control excess salivation. If he has a weak or absent cough reflex, begin tube feedings or esophageal drips of special formulas.

Patients with dysphagia may be unable to swallow tablets or capsules, and many drugs (such as those in extended-release form or those that are enteric coated) are not appropriate to be crushed or chewed. To ease drug administration for these patients, find out if the drug is available in liquid or suspension form for use orally or by feeding tube. Or, a different drug with similar effects that's available in liquid form may need to be considered. Or, different routes of the same drug (I.V., rectal, patch) may be needed, if available.[4]

Consult with the dietitian to select foods with distinct temperatures and textures. The patient should avoid sticky foods, such as bananas and peanut butter. If he produces mucus, avoid uncooked milk products. Arrange for a therapist to assess the patient for his aspiration risk and to teach him swallowing exercises that may help decrease his risk. At mealtimes, take measures to minimize the patient's risk of choking and aspiration. Place him in an upright position, and have him flex his neck forward slightly and keep his chin at midline. Instruct the patient to swallow multiple times before taking the next bite or sip. Separate solids from liquids; it depends on the individual whether solids or liquids are harder to swallow.

Prepare the patient for diagnostic tests, including endoscopy, esophageal manometry, esophagography, and the esophageal acidity test, to pinpoint the cause of dysphagia.

Pediatric pointers

In looking for dysphagia in an infant or a small child, pay close attention to his sucking and swallowing ability. Coughing, choking, or regurgitation during feeding suggests dysphagia.

Corrosive esophagitis and esophageal obstruction by a foreign body are more common causes of dysphagia in children than in adults. However, dysphagia also may result from congenital anomalies, such as annular stenosis, dysphagia lusoria, and esophageal atresia.

Geriatric pointers

Dysphagia is commonly the presenting complaint of patients older than age 50 with head or neck cancer. The incidence of these cancers increases markedly in this age-group.

Patient counseling

Advise the patient to prepare foods that are easy to swallow. The National Dysphagia Diet (NDD) consists of guidelines for patients with dysphagia developed by a multidisciplinary panel for the American Dietetic Association. The NDD recommends dietary modifications based on the severity of dysphagia, and includes sample diets, food preparation methods, and resource lists for patients and health care professionals.[5] Explain measures he can take to reduce the risk of choking and aspiration, such as positioning during eating and after the meal has been consumed. Encourage the patient's family or caregiver to take a first aid or cardiopulmonary course that provides techniques for managing choking.

REFERENCES

1. Achem, S.R. and DeVault, K.R. "Dysphagia in Aging." *Journal of Clinical Gastroenterology* 39(5):357-371, May/June 2005.
2. Alverzo, J.P., Brigante, M.A., and McNish, M.D. "Improving Stroke Outcomes." *AJN* 107(11):72A-72G, November 2007.
3. Peters, V.L. "Feeding Patients with Swallowing Disorders." *LPN* 2(2):13-17, March/April 2006.
4. Rex, T. "Pharmaceutical Considerations for Patients with Dysphagia." *Gastroenterology Nursing* 28(2):143-144, March/April 2005.
5. National Dysphagia Diet Task Force. "National Dysphagia Diet: Standardization for Optimal Care." Chicago, IL: American Dietetic Association, 2002.

DYSPNEA

Typically a symptom of cardiopulmonary dysfunction, dyspnea is the sensation of difficult or uncomfortable breathing. It's usually described as breathlessness or shortness of breath. It's a common symptom in patients with acute or chronic illness, as well as those with terminal disease.[1] Moderate dyspnea has been reported in up to 55% of patients with cancer at the end of life.[2] Its severity varies greatly and usually is unrelated to the severity of the underlying cause. Dyspnea may arise suddenly or slowly and may subside rapidly or persist for years.

Most people normally develop dyspnea when they exert themselves, and its severity depends on their physical condition. In a healthy person, dyspnea is quickly relieved by rest. Pathologic causes of dyspnea include pulmonary, cardiac, neuromuscular, and allergic disorders. It also may be caused by anxiety.

If a patient complains of shortness of breath, quickly look for signs of respiratory distress, such as tachypnea, cyanosis, restlessness, and accessory muscle use. Prepare to give oxygen by nasal cannula or endotracheal tube. Avoid using a mask to deliver oxygen because it may be uncomfortable and worsen feelings of breathlessness.[1] Ensure patent I.V. access, and begin cardiac monitoring and oxygen saturation monitoring to detect arrhythmias and low oxygen saturation, respectively. Expect to insert a chest tube for severe pneumothorax and to start continuous positive airway pressure (CPAP).

History and physical examination

Because dyspnea is a subjective symptom, the patient's description of it is crucial.[1] If the patient can answer questions without increasing his distress, take a complete history. (See *Differential diagnosis: Dyspnea*, pages 160 to 163.) Ask if the shortness of breath began suddenly or gradually. Is it constant or intermittent? Does it occur during activity or while at rest? If the patient has had dyspneic attacks before, ask if they're increasing in severity. Can he identify what aggravates or alleviates these attacks? Does he have a productive or nonproductive cough or chest pain? Ask about recent trauma, and note a history of upper respiratory tract infection, deep vein phlebitis, or other disorders. Ask the patient if he smokes or is exposed to toxic fumes or irritants on the job. Find out if he also has orthopnea, paroxysmal nocturnal dyspnea, or progressive fatigue. Include a psychological assessment, noting signs and symptoms of anxiety or depression.[1]

During the physical examination, look for signs of chronic dyspnea, such as accessory muscle hypertrophy (especially in the shoulders and neck). Also look for pursed-lip exhalation, clubbing, peripheral edema, barrel chest, diaphoresis, and jugular vein distention. (See *Improving dyspnea in patients with COPD,* page 164.)

Differential diagnosis: Dyspnea

Differential diagnosis for dyspnea is based on the history of the present illness and a physical examination focused on the abdomen and the respiratory, cardiovascular, and neurologic systems.

SIGNS AND SYMPTOMS	POSSIBLE DIAGNOSIS	CONFIRMING TESTS
• Acute dyspneic attacks • Audible or auscultated wheezing • Dry cough • Hyperpnea • Chest tightness • Accessory muscle use • Nasal flaring • Intercostal and supraclavicular retractions • Tachypnea • Tachycardia • Diaphoresis • Prolonged expiration • Flushing or cyanosis • Apprehension	• Acute asthma	• Laboratory tests (complete blood count [CBC], arterial blood gas [ABG] analysis, allergy skin testing) • Pulmonary function tests • Chest X-ray • Peak flow meter
• Acute dyspnea • Sudden pleuritic chest pain • Tachycardia • Low-grade fever • Tachypnea • Nonproductive or productive cough with blood-tinged sputum • Pleural friction rub • Crackles • Possible hemoptysis • Diffuse wheezing • Dullness on percussion • Decreased breath sounds • Diaphoresis • Restlessness • Acute anxiety • Signs of shock (possibly)	• Pulmonary embolism	• Imaging studies (chest X-ray, pulmonary $\dot{V}/\dot{Q}$ or pulmonary angiography, spiral chest computed tomography scan) • Electrocardiography (ECG)
• Gradually developing dyspnea • Chronic paroxysmal nocturnal dyspnea • Orthopnea • Tachypnea • Tachycardia • Palpitations • S$_3$ • Fatigue • Dependent peripheral edema • Hepatomegaly	• Heart failure • Acute onset heart failure if patient also has jugular vein distention (JVD), bibasilar crackles, oliguria, hypotension	• Physical examination • Laboratory tests (CBC, cardiac enzymes) • Imaging studies (chest X-ray, echocardiogram) • ECG

TREATMENT AND FOLLOW-UP

- Avoidance of allergens and tobacco
- Medication (beta blockers, inhaled beta$_2$-agonists, inhaled corticosteroid [nedocromil or cromolyn if younger than age 12], leukotriene receptor agonist, systemic corticosteroids during infections and exacerbations, mast cell stabilizer)
- Peak expiratory flow monitoring

Follow-up: For acute exacerbation, return visit within 24 hours, then every 3 to 5 days, then every 1 to 3 months; referral to pulmonologist, if the treatment is ineffective

- Oxygen therapy
- Medication (anticoagulants, thrombolytic therapy)

Follow-up: Reevaluation within the first week after hospitalization

- Medication (angiotensin-converting enzyme inhibitor, diuretics, carvedilol [possibly], digoxin [possibly]), inotropic agents

Follow-up: Return visit within 1 week after discharge, at 4 weeks, and then every 3 months; referral to cardiologist if chronic

(continued)

Check blood pressure, and auscultate the lungs for crackles, abnormal heart sounds or rhythms, egophony, bronchophony, and whispered pectoriloquy. Note any signs of heart failure, such as third heart sounds or jugular vein distention. Finally, palpate the abdomen for hepatomegaly, and assess the patient for edema.

Medical causes

▶ *Acute respiratory distress syndrome (ARDS).* This life-threatening form of noncardiogenic pulmonary edema usually produces acute dyspnea as the first complaint. As respiratory distress progresses, the patient develops restlessness, anxiety, decreased mental acuity, tachycardia, and crackles and rhonchi in both lung fields. Other findings include cyanosis, tachypnea, motor dysfunction, and intercostal and suprasternal retractions. Severe ARDS can produce signs of shock, such as hypotension and cool, clammy skin.

▶ *Amyotrophic lateral sclerosis.* Also known as Lou Gehrig's disease, this disorder causes slow onset of dyspnea that worsens with time. Other features include dysphagia, dysarthria, muscle weakness and atrophy, fasciculations, shallow respirations, tachypnea, and emotional lability.

▶ *Anemia.* Dyspnea usually develops gradually in anemia, which commonly causes fatigue, weakness, and syncope; severe anemia also may cause tachycardia, tachypnea, restlessness, anxiety, and thirst.

▶ *Anthrax, inhalation.* Anthrax is an acute infectious disease that's caused by the gram-positive, spore-forming bacterium *Bacillus anthracis.* Although the disease most commonly occurs in wild and domestic grazing animals, such as cattle, sheep, and goats, spores can live in the soil for many years. The disease can occur in humans exposed to infected animals, tissue from infected animals, or biological agents. Most natural cases occur in agricultural regions worldwide. Anthrax may occur in cutaneous, inhalation, or GI forms.

Inhalation anthrax is caused by inhalation of aerosolized spores. The disease typically occurs in two stages with a period of recovery after the initial signs and symptoms. Dyspnea is a symptom of the second stage of this disorder along with fever, stridor and hypotension;

Differential diagnosis: Dyspnea *(continued)*

SIGNS AND SYMPTOMS	POSSIBLE DIAGNOSIS	CONFIRMING TESTS
• Dry cough • Anorexia • Weight gain • Loss of mental acuity • Hemoptysis		
• Acute dyspnea • Sudden, stabbing chest pain that may radiate to the arms, face, back, or abdomen • Anxiety • Restlessness • Dry cough • Cyanosis • Decreased vocal fremitus • Tachypnea • Tympany • Decreased or absent breath sounds on the affected side • Asymmetrical chest expansion • Splinting • Accessory muscle use	• Pneumothorax • Tension pneumothorax if patient also has tracheal deviation, decreased blood pressure, tachycardia, JVD	• ABG • Chest X-ray

Other differential diagnoses include acute respiratory distress syndrome, anemia, aspiration of a foreign body, cardiac arrhythmias, chronic obstructive pulmonary disease, cor pulmonale, emphysema, flail chest, inhalation injury, interstitial fibrosis, lung cancer, myocardial infarction, pleural effusion, pneumonia, and pulmonary edema.

the patient usually dies within 24 hours. Initial signs and symptoms are flulike and include fever, chills, weakness, cough, and chest pain.

▶ *Aspiration of a foreign body.* Acute dyspnea marks this life-threatening condition, along with paroxysmal intercostal, suprasternal, and substernal retractions. The patient also may display accessory muscle use, inspiratory stridor, tachypnea, decreased or absent breath sounds, asymmetrical chest expansion, anxiety, cyanosis, diaphoresis, and hypotension.

▶ *Asthma.* Acute dyspneic attacks occur in this chronic disorder along with audible wheezing, a dry cough, accessory muscle use, nasal flaring, intercostal and supraclavicular retractions, tachypnea, tachycardia, diaphoresis, prolonged expiration, flushing or cyanosis, and apprehension. Drugs that block beta receptors can worsen asthma attacks.

▶ *Avian influenza.* These potentially life-threatening viruses are spread to humans through contact with infected poultry or surfaces contaminated with infected bird excretions. Within 1 to 5 days of exposure to avian influenza, the patient typically develops flulike symptoms, such as fever, sore throat, cough, and muscle aches. Those with severe forms of the virus may develop dyspnea caused by acute respiratory distress or pneumonia. To date, the most virulent strain of this virus has not yet surfaced in humans in the United States, but a recent outbreak in Asian countries has had a mortality rate of about 50% among infected humans.

▶ *Blast lung injury.* The result of a forceful percussive wave following an explosive deto-

TREATMENT AND FOLLOW-UP

Pneumothorax:
- Chest tube insertion
- Oxygen therapy

Follow-up: Return visit in 1 to 2 weeks after hospitalization

Tension pneumothorax:
- Immediate needle decompression followed by chest tube insertion
- Oxygen therapy

Follow-up: Return visit in 1 to 2 weeks after hospitalization

nation, blast lung injury is commonly characterized by dyspnea and hypoxia. Worldwide terrorist activity has recently increased the incidence of this condition, which also may cause cyanosis, chest pain, wheezing, and hemoptysis. Chest X-ray, the primary diagnostic tool, reveals a characteristic "butterfly" pattern. Many of these patients suffer concomitant injuries and require complex management, usually in an intensive care setting.

▶ *Cardiac arrhythmias.* Acute or gradual dyspnea can result from decreased cardiac output in a patient with arrhythmias. The pulse rate may be rapid, slow, or irregular, with frequent premature or escape beats. Alternating pulse may be present. Other symptoms include palpitations, chest pain, diaphoresis, light-headedness, weakness, and vertigo.

▶ *Cor pulmonale.* Chronic dyspnea begins gradually with exertion and progressively worsens until it occurs even at rest. Most patients with cor pulmonale have an underlying cardiac or pulmonary disease. Other findings may include a chronic productive cough, wheezing, tachypnea, jugular vein distention, dependent edema, hepatomegaly, increasing fatigue, weakness, and light-headedness.

▶ *Emphysema.* This chronic disorder gradually causes progressive exertional dyspnea as well as barrel chest, accessory muscle hypertrophy, diminished breath sounds, anorexia, weight loss, malaise, peripheral cyanosis, tachypnea, pursed-lip breathing, prolonged expiration and, possibly, a chronic productive cough. Clubbing is a late sign. The patient may have a history of smoking, an alpha$_1$-antitrypsin deficiency, or exposure to an occupational irritant.

▶ *Flail chest.* In this condition, dyspnea results suddenly from multiple rib fractures and is accompanied by paradoxical chest movement, severe chest pain, hypotension, tachypnea, tachycardia, and cyanosis. Bruising and decreased or absent breath sounds occur over the affected side.

▶ *Guillain-Barré syndrome.* This syndrome, which usually follows a fever and upper respiratory tract infection, causes slowly worsening dyspnea along with fatigue, ascending muscle weakness and, eventually, paralysis.

▶ *Heart failure.* Dyspnea usually develops gradually in patients with heart failure. Chronic paroxysmal nocturnal dyspnea, orthopnea, tachypnea, tachycardia, palpitations, ventricular gallop, fatigue, dependent peripheral edema, hepatomegaly, dry cough, weight gain, and loss of mental acuity may occur. With acute onset, heart failure may produce jugular vein distention, bibasilar crackles, oliguria, and hypotension.

▶ *Interstitial fibrosis.* Besides dyspnea, this disorder causes chest pain, a dry cough, crackles, weight loss and, possibly, cyanosis and pleural friction rub.

▶ *Lung cancer.* Dyspnea develops slowly and worsens progressively in late-stage lung cancer. Other findings include fever, hemoptysis, a productive cough, wheezing, clubbing, chest pain, and pleural friction rub.

Improving dyspnea in patients with COPD

Question: *Is pursed-lips breathing or expiratory muscle training more effective in improving dyspnea and functional performance in patients with chronic obstructive pulmonary disease (COPD)?*

Research: Exertional dyspnea associated with COPD is typically managed with drugs and self-care strategies, such as breathing pattern retraining. In this study, 40 patients from an outpatient pulmonary clinic were randomized to one of three groups: pursed-lips breathing (PLB), expiratory muscle training, or the control group. Criteria for inclusion were a clinical diagnosis of COPD, expiratory airflow limitation evidenced by pulmonary function testing, and self-report of shortness of breath while walking.

During the baseline visit, subjects completed a 6-minute walk then sat while their breathing frequency and duty cycle were monitored using respiratory inductive plethysmography for 25 minutes. They also completed questionnaires and received breathing pattern retraining according to their assigned group. Each participant made four weekly visits to the research laboratory to reinforce the teaching and assure adherence to the assigned protocol.

Subjects in the expiratory muscle training group used a special device to increase expiratory resistance. PLB was taught by demonstra-

tion. Practice sessions for both groups were 10 minutes/day for the first week, 15 minutes/day for the second week, 20 minutes/day by the third week, and 25 minutes/day by the fourth week.

Conclusion: After 12 weeks, only the PLB group had significant improvement in exertional dyspnea and functional status.

Application: Educate patients how to perform PLB using verbal instruction and demonstration. Encourage patients to practice this strategy and increase the amount of time they perform PLB as tolerated. Provide support and tell patients that they may not notice improvement immediately. Recommend sustained practice.

Source: Nield, M. A., Soo Hoo, G. W., Roper, J. M., and Santiago, S. "Efficacy of Pursed-Lips Breathing: A Breathing Pattern Retraining Strategy for Dyspnea Reduction." *Journal of Cardiopulmonary Rehabilitation & Prevention,* 27(4):237-244, 2007.

▶ *Monkeypox.* Dyspnea is one of the less common symptoms of this rare viral disease. Infected people also may have fever, muscle aches, sore throat, chills, and lymphadenopathy. A papular rash appears 1 to 3 days after the fever starts. The virus is similar to smallpox, but symptoms are milder and the disease is rarely fatal in developed countries.

▶ *Myasthenia gravis.* This neuromuscular disorder causes bouts of dyspnea as the respiratory muscles weaken. In myasthenic crisis, acute respiratory distress may occur, with shallow respirations and tachypnea.

▶ *Myocardial infarction.* Sudden dyspnea occurs with crushing substernal chest pain that may radiate to the back, neck, jaw, and arms. Other signs and symptoms include nausea, vomiting, diaphoresis, vertigo, hypertension

or hypotension, tachycardia, anxiety, and pale, cool, clammy skin.

▶ *Plague.* Caused by *Yersinia pestis,* plague is one of the most virulent and, if untreated, most lethal bacterial infections known. Clinical forms include bubonic (the most common), septicemic, and pneumonic plagues. The pneumonic form can be contracted by inhaling respiratory droplets from an infected person or inhaling the organism that has been dispersed in the air through biological warfare. Among the symptoms of the pneumonic form are dyspnea, a productive cough, chest pain, tachypnea, hemoptysis, increasing respiratory distress, and cardiopulmonary insufficiency.

▶ *Pleural effusion.* Dyspnea develops slowly and worsens progressively in this disorder. Initial findings include a pleural friction rub accompanied by pleuritic pain that worsens with coughing or deep breathing. Other findings include a dry cough; dullness on percussion; egophony, bronchophony, and whispered pectoriloquy; tachycardia; tachypnea; weight loss; and decreased breath sounds, chest motion, and tactile fremitus. Fever may occur if infection is present.

▶ *Pneumonia.* Dyspnea occurs suddenly in pneumonia and is usually accompanied by fever, shaking chills, pleuritic chest pain that worsens with deep inspiration, and a productive cough. Fatigue, headache, myalgia, anorexia, abdominal pain, crackles, rhonchi, tachycardia, tachypnea, cyanosis, decreased breath sounds, and diaphoresis also may occur.

▶ *Pneumothorax.* This life-threatening disorder causes acute dyspnea unrelated to the severity of pain. Sudden, stabbing chest pain may radiate to the arms, face, back, or abdomen. Other signs and symptoms include anxiety, restlessness, dry cough, cyanosis, decreased vocal fremitus, tachypnea, tympany, decreased or absent breath sounds on the affected side, asymmetrical chest expansion, splinting, and accessory muscle use. In patients with tension pneumothorax, tracheal deviation occurs in addition to these typical findings. Decreased blood pressure and tachycardia also may occur.

▶ *Poliomyelitis (bulbar).* Dyspnea develops gradually in this disorder and worsens progressively. Additional signs and symptoms include fever, facial weakness, dysphasia, hypoactive deep tendon reflexes, decreased mental acuity, dysphagia, nasal regurgitation, and hypopnea.

▶ *Pulmonary edema.* Commonly preceded by signs of heart failure, such as jugular vein distention and orthopnea, this life-threatening disorder causes acute dyspnea. Other features include tachycardia, tachypnea, crackles in both lung fields, a ventricular gallop (third heart sound [S_3]), oliguria, thready pulse, hypotension, diaphoresis, cyanosis, and marked anxiety. The patient's cough may be dry or may produce copious amounts of pink, frothy sputum.

▶ *Pulmonary embolism.* This life-threatening disorder is characterized by acute dyspnea that's usually accompanied by sudden pleuritic chest pain. Related findings include tachycardia, low-grade fever, tachypnea, a nonproductive cough or a productive cough with blood-tinged sputum, pleural friction rub, crackles, diffuse wheezing, dullness on percussion, decreased breath sounds, diaphoresis, restlessness, and acute anxiety. A massive embolism may cause signs of shock, such as hypotension and cool, clammy skin.

▶ *Sepsis.* This potentially fatal disorder gradually causes dyspnea along with chills and sudden fever. As dyspnea worsens, it may be accompanied by tachycardia, tachypnea, restlessness, anxiety, decreased mental acuity, and warm, flushed, dry skin. Late findings include hypotension; oliguria; cool, clammy skin; and rapid, thready pulse.

▶ *Severe acute respiratory syndrome (SARS).* SARS is an acute infectious disease of unknown etiology; however, a novel coronavirus has been implicated as a possible cause. Although most cases have been reported in Asia (China, Vietnam, Singapore, Thailand), cases have cropped up in Europe and North America. After an incubation period of 2 to 7 days, the illness generally begins with a fever (usually greater than 100.4° F [38° C]). Other symptoms include headache, malaise, a nonproductive cough, and dyspnea. The severity of the illness is highly variable, ranging from mild illness to pneumonia and, in some cases, progressing to respiratory failure and death.

▶ *Shock.* Dyspnea arises suddenly and worsens progressively in this life-threatening disorder. Related findings include severe hypotension, tachypnea, tachycardia, decreased peripheral pulses, decreased mental acuity, restlessness, anxiety, and cool, clammy skin.

▶ *Tuberculosis.* Dyspnea commonly occurs with chest pain, crackles, and a productive cough. Other findings are night sweats, fever, anorexia and weight loss, vague dyspepsia, palpitations on mild exertion, and dullness on percussion.

▶ *Tularemia.* Also known as *rabbit fever,* this infectious disease causes dyspnea along with fever, chills, headache, generalized myalgia, a nonproductive cough, pleuritic chest pain, and empyema.

Other causes

▶ *Inhalation injury.* Dyspnea may develop suddenly or over several hours after inhalation of chemicals or hot gases. Increasing hoarseness, a persistent cough, sooty or bloody sputum, and oropharyngeal edema also may be present. The patient also may exhibit thermal burns, singed nasal hairs, and orofacial burns as well as crackles, rhonchi, wheezing, and signs of respiratory distress.

Special considerations

Monitor the dyspneic patient closely. Be as calm and reassuring as possible to reduce his anxiety, and help him into a comfortable position—usually high Fowler's or a forward-leaning position.[1] Support him with pillows, loosen his clothing, and give oxygen if appropriate. Oxygen is helpful for patients who are hypoxic; to improve the patient's ability to exercise or otherwise function; to ease discomfort at the end of life; and for patients requiring mechanical ventilation.[1]

Prepare the patient for diagnostic studies, such as arterial blood gas analysis, chest X-rays, and pulmonary function tests. Give a bronchodilator, an antiarrhythmic, a diuretic, and an analgesic, as needed, to dilate bronchioles, correct cardiac arrhythmias, promote fluid excretion, and relieve pain, respectively. Opioid analgesics, particularly morphine, are used to decrease the patient's central respiratory drive and reduce the sensation of breathlessness, and are recommended for patients in the terminal stage of disease.[1,3]

Pediatric pointers

Normally, a child's respirations are abdominal in infancy and gradually change to costal by age 7. Suspect dyspnea in an infant who breathes costally, in an older child who breathes abdominally, or in any child who uses his neck or shoulder muscles to help him breathe.

Both acute epiglottiditis and laryngotracheobronchitis (croup) can cause severe dyspnea in a child and may even lead to respiratory or cardiovascular collapse. Expect to administer oxygen, using a hood or cool mist tent.

Geriatric pointers

About one-third of adults older than age 70 who live at home have dyspnea.[1] Older patients often have atypical symptoms with illness, and dyspnea may be the only symptom an elderly patient has during myocardial infarction. Older patients with dyspnea related to chronic illness may not be aware initially of a significant change in their breathing pattern.

Patient counseling

Encourage pursed-lip breathing and diaphragmatic breathing if these strategies have been found to provide the patient with relief.[1] Cool air blowing across the face has been useful in relieving early dyspnea.[1] Using a fan or opening a window can be used for this. Complementary therapies, such as acupuncture, acupressure, relaxation therapy, massage therapy, or aromatherapy, also may help to relieve dyspnea and the resulting anxiety.[1] Gentle, low-intensity arm exercises using light weights, cans of food, or bottles of water can help support respiratory muscles and ease dyspnea.[4]

Tell the patient that oxygen therapy isn't always indicated for dyspnea. Urge a patient with chronic dyspnea to pace his daily activities. A patient with chronic dyspnea may benefit from a pulmonary rehabilitation program. After rehabilitation, encourage the patient to maintain an exercise program to relieve dyspnea.[2,5]

REFERENCES

1. Spector, N., Connolly, M.A., and Carlson, K.K. "Dyspnea: Applying Research to Bedside Practice." *AACN Advanced Critical Care* 18(1):45-58, January/March 2007.
2. Williams, C. "Dyspnea." *The Cancer Journal* 12(5):365-373, September/October 2006.
3. Tice, M. "Managing Breathlessness: Providing Comfort at the End of Life." *Home Healthcare Nurse* 24(4):207-210, April 2006.
4. Dahlin, C. "It Takes My Breath Away END STAGE COPD: Part 2: Pharmacologic and Nonpharmacologic Management of Dyspnea and Other Symptoms." *Home Healthcare Nurse* 24(4):218-224, April 2006.
5. Heppner, P.S., Morgan, C., Kaplan, R.M., and Ries, A.L. "Regular Walking and Long-Term Maintenance of Outcomes After Pulmonary Rehabilitation." *Journal of Cardiopulmonary Rehabilitation* 26(1):44-53, January/February 2006.

DYSURIA

Dysuria—painful or difficult urination—is commonly accompanied by urinary frequency, urgency, or hesitancy. This symptom usually reflects lower urinary tract infection (UTI)—the most common bacterial infection in women.[1]

Dysuria results from lower urinary tract irritation or inflammation, which stimulates nerve endings in the bladder and urethra. The onset of pain provides clues to its cause. For example, pain just before voiding usually indicates bladder irritation or distention, whereas pain at the start of urination typically results from bladder outlet irritation. Pain at the end of voiding may signal bladder spasms; in women, it may indicate vaginal candidiasis.

History and physical examination

If the patient complains of dysuria, have him describe its severity and location. When did he first notice it? Did anything cause it? Does anything aggravate or alleviate it?

Next, ask about previous urinary or genital tract infections. Has the patient recently undergone an invasive procedure, such as cystoscopy or urethral dilatation, or had a urinary catheter inserted? Also, ask if he has a history of intestinal disease. Ask a female patient about menstrual disorders and use of products that irritate the urinary tract, such as bubble bath, bath salts, feminine deodorants, contraceptive gels, or perineal lotions. Also ask her about vaginal discharge or pruritus.

During the physical examination, inspect the urethral meatus for discharge, irritation, or other abnormalities. A pelvic or rectal examination may be needed.

Medical causes

▶ *Appendicitis.* Occasionally, appendicitis causes dysuria that persists throughout voiding and is accompanied by bladder tenderness. Appendicitis is characterized by periumbilical abdominal pain that shifts to McBurney's point, anorexia, nausea, vomiting, constipation, slight fever, abdominal rigidity and rebound tenderness, and tachycardia.

▶ *Bladder cancer.* In this mainly male disorder, dysuria throughout voiding is a late symptom associated with urinary frequency and urgency, nocturia, hematuria, and perineal, back, or flank pain.

▶ *Cystitis.* Dysuria throughout voiding is common in all types of cystitis, as are urinary frequency, nocturia, straining to void, and hematuria. Bacterial cystitis, the most common cause of dysuria in women, also may produce urinary urgency, perineal and lower back pain, suprapubic discomfort, fatigue and, possibly, a low-grade fever. In chronic interstitial cystitis, dysuria is accentuated at the end of voiding. In tubercular cystitis, symptoms also may include urinary urgency, flank pain, fatigue, and anorexia. In viral cystitis, severe dysuria occurs with gross hematuria, urinary urgency, and fever. Women are more prone to cystitis than men because they have a shorter urethra. For men, age is a factor: Older men have a 15% higher risk of developing cystitis.

▶ *Diverticulitis.* Inflammation near the bladder may cause dysuria throughout voiding. Other effects include urinary frequency and urgency, nocturia, hematuria, fever, abdominal pain and tenderness, perineal pain, constipation or diarrhea and, possibly, an abdominal mass.

▶ *Paraurethral gland inflammation.* Dysuria throughout voiding is accompanied by urinary frequency and urgency, diminished urine stream, mild perineal pain and, occasionally, hematuria in this disorder.

▶ *Prostatitis.* Acute prostatitis commonly causes dysuria throughout or toward the end of voiding as well as a reduced urine stream, urinary frequency and urgency, hematuria, suprapubic fullness, fever, chills, fatigue, myalgia, nausea, vomiting, and constipation. In chronic prostatitis, urethral narrowing causes dysuria throughout voiding. Related effects are urinary frequency and urgency; diminished urine stream; perineal, back, and buttocks pain; urethral discharge; nocturia; and, at times, hematospermia and ejaculatory pain.

▶ *Pyelonephritis (acute).* More common in women than men, this disorder causes dysuria throughout voiding. Other features include persistent high fever with chills, costovertebral angle tenderness, unilateral or bilateral flank pain, weakness, urinary urgency and frequency, nocturia, straining on urination, and hematuria. Nausea, vomiting, and anorexia also may occur.

▶ *Reiter's syndrome.* In this mainly male disorder, dysuria occurs 1 to 2 weeks after sexual contact. Initially, the patient has a mucopurulent discharge, urinary urgency and frequency, meatal swelling and redness, suprapubic pain, anorexia, weight loss, and low-grade fever. Hematuria, conjunctivitis, arthritic symptoms, a papular rash, and oral and penile lesions may follow.

▶ *Urethral syndrome.* Occurring in sexually active women, this syndrome mimics urethritis. Dysuria throughout voiding may occur with urinary frequency, diminished urine stream, suprapubic aching and cramping, tenesmus, and low back and unilateral flank pain. In the absence of pyuria, symptoms will usually resolve without intervention.

▶ *Urethritis.* Mainly found in sexually active men, this infection causes dysuria throughout voiding. It's accompanied by a reddened meatus and a copious, yellow, purulent discharge (gonorrheal infection) or a white or clear mucoid discharge (chlamydial infection).[2,3]

▶ *Urinary obstruction.* Outflow obstruction by urethral strictures or calculi produces dysuria throughout voiding. (In a complete obstruction, bladder distention develops and dysuria precedes voiding.) Other features are diminished urine stream, urinary frequency and urgency, and a sensation of fullness or bloating in the lower abdomen or groin.

▶ *Vaginitis.* Characteristically, dysuria occurs throughout voiding as urine touches inflamed or ulcerated labia. Other findings include urinary frequency and urgency, nocturia, hematuria, perineal pain, and vaginal discharge and odor.

Other causes

▶ *Chemical irritants.* Dysuria may result from irritating substances, such as bubble bath salts and feminine deodorants; it's usually most intense at the end of voiding. Spermicides may cause dysuria in both sexes as well as urinary frequency and urgency, a diminished urine stream and, possibly, hematuria.

🔷 **DRUG WATCH** *Monoamine oxidase inhibitors and metyrosine can cause dysuria.*

Special considerations

Monitor vital signs and intake and output. Give prescribed drugs, and prepare the patient for such tests as urinalysis and cystoscopy.

Pediatric pointers

Dysuria as a symptom of UTI typically is seen in children over age 2.[4] It also may signal acute glomerulonephritis and is a physical symptom of sexual abuse.[4]

Geriatric pointers

Be aware that elderly patients tend to under-report their symptoms, and that the pain or fever that typically occurs in UTI may be replaced with feelings of confusion or general malaise in this population.[5] Older men have an increased incidence of nonsexually related UTIs and postmenopausal women have an increased incidence of noninfectious dysuria.

Patient counseling

Teach patients to recognize the signs and symptoms of UTI, such as cloudy urine, burning or pain on urination, urgency, frequency, flank pain, and a low-grade fever, to facilitate early treatment. Teach the patient how to prevent UTIs. Cranberry juice has been found to prevent recurrent UTIs.[1] Instruct female patients to prevent bacterial contamination by wiping the perineum from front to back after defecation.

REFERENCES

1. Sheffield, J. and Cunningham, F.G. "Urinary Tract Infection in Women." *Obstetrics and Gynecology* 106(5, Part 1):1085-1092, November 2005.
2. Miller, K.E. "Diagnosis and Treatment of Neisseria gonorrhoeae Infections." *American Family Physician* 73(10):1779-1784, 1786, May 2006.
3. Miller, K.E. "Diagnosis and Treatment of Chlamydial Trachomatis Infections." *American Family Physician* 73(8):1411-1416, April 2006.
4. Hockenberry, M.J. and Wilson, D. (Eds.) *Wong's Nursing Care of Infants and Children,* 8th ed. St. Louis: Mosby, 2007.
5. Neal-Boylan, L. "Health Assessment of the Very Old Person at Home." *Home Healthcare Nurse* 25(6):388-98, June 2007.

EDEMA, GENERALIZED

A common sign in severely ill patients, generalized edema is the excessive accumulation of interstitial fluid throughout the body. Its severity varies widely; slight edema may be difficult to detect, especially if the patient is obese, whereas massive edema is immediately apparent.

Generalized edema typically is chronic and progressive. It may result from cardiac, renal, endocrine, or hepatic disorders as well as from severe burns, malnutrition, or the effects of certain drugs and treatments.

Common factors responsible for edema are hypoalbuminemia and excess sodium ingestion or retention, both of which influence plasma osmotic pressure. (See *Understanding fluid balance,* page 170.) Cyclic edema from increased aldosterone secretion may occur in premenopausal women.

Quickly determine the location and severity of edema, including the degree of pitting. (See *Edema: Pitting or nonpitting?* page 172.) If the patient has severe edema, promptly take his vital signs, and check for jugular vein distention and cyanotic lips. Auscultate the lungs and heart. Be alert for signs of heart failure or pulmonary congestion, such as crackles, muffled heart sounds, or ventricular gallop. Unless the patient is hypotensive, place him in Fowler's position to promote lung expansion. Insert an I.V. device and prepare to give I.V. isotonic maintenance fluids; intermittent infusion of a colloid such as albumin also may be ordered.[1] Prepare to give oxygen and an I.V. diuretic. Have emergency resuscitation equipment nearby.

History and physical examination

When the patient's condition permits, obtain a complete medical history. First, note when the edema began. Does it move throughout the course of the day—for example, from the arms to the legs, the orbits, or the sacral area? Is edema worse in the morning or at the end of the day? Is it affected by position changes? Is it accompanied by shortness of breath or pain in the arms or legs? Find out how much weight the patient has gained. Has his urine output changed in quantity or quality?

Next, ask about previous burns or cardiac, renal, hepatic, endocrine, or GI disorders. Have the patient describe his diet so you can determine whether he has from protein malnutrition. Explore his drug history, and note recent I.V. therapy.

Begin the physical examination by comparing the patient's arms and legs for symmetrical edema. Also, note ecchymoses and cyanosis. Assess the back, sacrum, and hips of a bedridden patient for dependent edema. Palpate peripheral pulses, noting whether hands and feet feel cold. Finally, perform a complete cardiac and respiratory assessment.

Medical causes

▶ *Angioneurotic edema or angioedema.* Recurrent attacks of acute, painless, nonpitting edema involving the skin and mucous membranes—especially those of the respiratory tract, face, neck, lips, larynx, hands, feet, gen-

Understanding fluid balance

Normally, fluid moves freely between the interstitial and intravascular spaces to maintain homeostasis. Four basic pressure mechanisms control the shift of fluid across the capillary membrane that separates these spaces:
• capillary hydrostatic pressure (internal fluid pressure on the capillary membrane)
• interstitial fluid pressure (external fluid pressure on the capillary membrane)
• osmotic pressure (fluid-attracting pressure from protein concentration in the capillary)
• interstitial osmotic pressure (fluid-attracting pressure from protein concentration outside the capillary).

Here's how these pressures maintain homeostasis. At the capillary's arterial end, capillary hydrostatic pressure normally exceeds plasma osmotic pressure, forcing fluid out of the capillary. At the capillary's venous end, the reverse is true: Plasma osmotic pressure exceeds capillary hydrostatic pressure, drawing fluid into the capillary. Normally, the lymphatic system transports excess interstitial fluid back to the intravascular space.

Edema results when this balance is upset by increased capillary permeability, lymphatic obstruction, persistently increased capillary hydrostatic pressure, decreased plasma osmotic or interstitial fluid pressure, or dilation of precapillary sphincters.

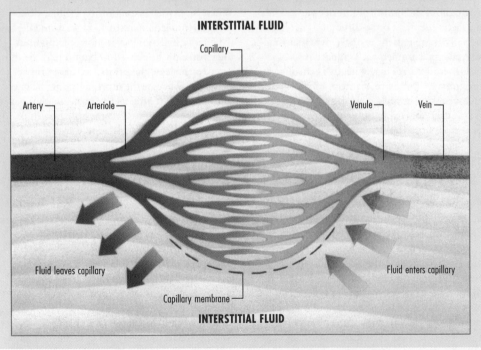

itals, or viscera—may result from a food or drug allergy or emotional stress, or they may be hereditary. Abdominal pain, nausea, vomiting, and diarrhea accompany visceral edema; dyspnea and stridor accompany life-threatening laryngeal edema.
▶ *Burns*. Edema and related tissue damage vary with the severity of the burn. Severe gen-

eralized edema (4+) may occur within 2 days of a major burn; localized edema may occur with a less severe burn.
▶ *Cirrhosis*. A late sign of chronic cirrhosis, edema usually starts in the legs and thighs and may progress to anasarca (extreme generalized edema). Accompanying signs and symptoms include abdominal pain, anorexia, nau-

sea and vomiting, hepatomegaly, ascites, jaundice, pruritus, bleeding tendencies, musty breath, lethargy, mental changes, and asterixis.

▶ *Heart failure.* Severe, generalized pitting edema—occasionally anasarca—may follow leg edema late in heart failure. The edema may improve with exercise or elevation of the limbs and typically is worse at the end of the day. Among other classic late findings are hemoptysis, cyanosis, marked hepatomegaly, clubbing, crackles, and a ventricular gallop. Typically, the patient has tachypnea, palpitations, hypotension, weight gain despite anorexia, nausea, slowed mental response, diaphoresis, and pallor. Dyspnea, orthopnea, tachycardia, and fatigue typify left-sided heart failure; jugular vein distention, hepatomegaly, and peripheral edema typify right-sided heart failure.

▶ *Malnutrition.* Anasarca in this disorder may mask dramatic muscle wasting. Malnutrition also typically causes muscle weakness; lethargy; anorexia; diarrhea; apathy; dry, wrinkled skin; and signs of anemia, such as dizziness and pallor.

▶ *Myxedema.* In this severe form of hypothyroidism, generalized nonpitting edema is accompanied by dry, flaky, inelastic, waxy, pale skin; a puffy face; and an upper eyelid droop. Observation also reveals masklike facies, hair loss or coarsening, and psychomotor slowing. Other findings include hoarseness, weight gain, fatigue, cold intolerance, bradycardia, hypoventilation, constipation, abdominal distention, menorrhagia, impotence, and infertility.

▶ *Nephrotic syndrome.* Although nephrotic syndrome is characterized by generalized pitting edema, the edema is initially localized around the eyes. Anasarca develops in severe cases, increasing body weight by up to 50%. Other common signs and symptoms are ascites, anorexia, fatigue, malaise, depression, and pallor.

▶ *Pericardial effusion.* In pericardial effusion, generalized pitting edema may be most prominent in the arms and legs. It may be accompanied by chest pain, dyspnea, orthopnea, a nonproductive cough, pericardial friction rub, jugular vein distention, dysphagia, and fever.

▶ *Pericarditis (chronic constrictive).* Like right-sided heart failure, this disorder usually begins with pitting edema of the arms and legs that may progress to generalized edema. Other signs and symptoms include ascites, Kussmaul's sign, dyspnea, fatigue, weakness, abdominal distention, and hepatomegaly.

▶ *Protein-losing enteropathy.* Increased albumin levels lead to progressive generalized pitting edema in this disorder. The patient also may have a mild fever and abdominal pain with bloody diarrhea and steatorrhea.

▶ *Renal failure.* Generalized pitting edema is a late sign of acute renal failure. In chronic renal failure, edema is less likely to become generalized; its severity depends on the degree of fluid overload. Both forms of renal failure cause oliguria, anorexia, nausea and vomiting, drowsiness, confusion, hypertension, dyspnea, crackles, dizziness, and pallor.

▶ *Septic shock.* A late sign of this life-threatening disorder, generalized edema typically develops rapidly as altered capillary permeability allows fluid and protein to leak from the vascular spaces into the surrounding tissue.[2] The edema is pitting and moderately severe. Accompanying it may be cool skin, hypotension, oliguria, tachycardia, cyanosis, thirst, anxiety, and signs of respiratory failure.

Other causes

DRUG WATCH *Any drug that causes sodium retention may cause or aggravate generalized edema. Examples include antihypertensives, corticosteroids, androgenic and anabolic steroids, estrogens, and nonsteroidal anti-inflammatory drugs, such as ibuprofen and naproxen.*

▶ *Treatments.* I.V. saline solution infusions and internal feedings may cause sodium and fluid overload, resulting in generalized edema, especially in patients with cardiac or renal disease.

Special considerations

Position the patient with his limbs above heart level to promote drainage. Periodically reposition him to avoid pressure ulcers. If the patient develops dyspnea, lower his limbs, raise the head of the bed, and give oxygen. Massage reddened areas, especially where dependent edema has formed (for example, the

Edema:
Pitting or nonpitting?

To see if your patient has pitting edema, press your finger against a swollen area. Then, after 5 seconds, quickly remove your finger and watch what happens.

If an indentation remains where you compressed the tissue, the patient has pitting edema. The pressure from your finger forced fluid into the underlying tissues, and the resulting depression will fill slowly. To determine the severity of pitting edema, estimate the indentation's depth in centimeters: 1+ (1 cm), 2+ (2 cm), 3+ (3 cm), or 4+ (4 cm).

In nonpitting edema, pressure leaves no indentation because fluid has coagulated in the tissues. Typically, the skin feels unusually tight and firm.

PITTING EDEMA (4+)

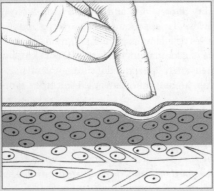

NONPITTING EDEMA

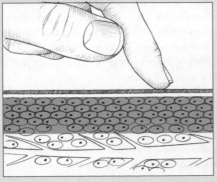

back, sacrum, hips, and buttocks). Prevent skin breakdown in these areas by placing a pressure mattress, lamb's wool pad, or flotation ring on the patient's bed. Restrict fluids and sodium, and give a diuretic or I.V. albumin.

Monitor intake and output and daily weight. Also monitor serum electrolyte levels, especially sodium and albumin. Prepare the patient for blood and urine tests, X-rays, echocardiography, or an electrocardiogram.

Pediatric pointers
Renal failure in children commonly causes generalized edema. Monitor fluid balance closely. Remember that fever or diaphoresis can lead to fluid loss, so promote fluid intake.

Kwashiorkor (protein-deficiency malnutrition) is more common in children than in adults and causes anasarca.

Geriatric pointers
Elderly patients are more likely to develop edema for several reasons, including decreased cardiac and renal function and, in some cases, poor nutritional status. Use caution when giving older patients I.V. fluids or drugs that can raise sodium levels and thereby increase fluid retention.

Patient counseling
Teach patients with known heart failure or renal failure to watch for edema; explain that it's an important sign of decompensation that indicates the need for immediate adjustment of therapy. Stress the importance of taking his weight daily, at the same time every day.

REFERENCES
1. Bixby, M. "Third-Spacing: Where Has All the Fluid Gone?" *Nursing Made Incredibly Easy!* 4(5):42-53, September-October 2006.
2. Wood, S., Lavieri, M.C., Durkin, T. "What You Need to Know About Sepsis," *Nursing* 37(3):46-51, March 2007.

EPISTAXIS

A common sign, epistaxis (nosebleed) can be spontaneous or induced and may spring from the front or back of the nose. Most nosebleeds occur in the anterior-inferior nasal septum (Little's area or Kiesselbach's plexus[1,2]), but some occur at the point where the inferior turbinates meet the nasopharynx. Bleeding points are difficult to identify in posterior epistaxis.[1,2] Usually unilateral, they seem bilateral when blood runs from the bleeding side behind the nasal septum and out the opposite side. Epistaxis ranges from mild oozing to severe—possibly life-threatening—blood loss.

A rich supply of fragile blood vessels makes the nose particularly vulnerable to bleeding. Air moving through the nose can dry and irritate the mucous membranes, forming crusts that bleed when they're removed; dry mucous membranes also are more susceptible to infections, which can produce epistaxis as well. Trauma is another common cause of epistaxis. Additional causes include septal deviations; hematologic, coagulation, renal, and GI disorders; and certain drugs and treatments.

If your patient has severe epistaxis, quickly take his vital signs. Be alert for tachypnea, hypotension, and other signs of hypovolemic shock. Insert a large-gauge I.V. line for rapid fluid and blood replacement, and attempt to control bleeding by pinching the nares closed. (However, if you suspect a nasal fracture, don't pinch the nares. Instead, place gauze under the patient's nose to absorb the blood.)

Have a hypovolemic patient lie down and turn his head to the side to prevent blood from draining down the back of his throat, which could cause aspiration or vomiting of swallowed blood. If the patient isn't hypovolemic, have him sit upright and tilt his head forward. Constantly check airway patency. If the patient's condition is unstable, begin cardiac monitoring and give supplemental oxygen by mask.

History and physical examination

If your patient isn't in distress, take a history. Does he have a history of recent trauma? How often has he had nosebleeds in the past? Have the nosebleeds been long or unusually severe? Has the patient recently had surgery in the sinus area? Ask about a history of hypertension, bleeding or liver disorders, and other recent illnesses. Ask if the patient bruis-

es easily. Find out what drugs he uses, especially anti-inflammatories such as aspirin and anticoagulants such as warfarin.

Begin the physical examination by inspecting the patient's skin for other signs of bleeding, such as ecchymoses and petechiae, and noting any jaundice, pallor, or other abnormalities. When examining a trauma patient, look for related injuries, such as eye trauma or facial fractures.

Medical causes

▶ *Angiofibroma (juvenile).* This rare disorder usually occurs in adolescent boys and is characterized by severe recurrent epistaxis and nasal obstruction.

▶ *Aplastic anemia.* This disorder develops insidiously, eventually producing nosebleeds as well as ecchymoses, retinal hemorrhages, menorrhagia, petechiae, bleeding from the mouth, and signs of GI bleeding. Fatigue, dyspnea, headache, tachycardia, and pallor also may occur.

▶ *Barotrauma.* Commonly seen in airline passengers and scuba divers, barotrauma may cause severe, painful epistaxis when the patient has an upper tract respiratory infection.

▶ *Biliary obstruction.* This disorder produces bleeding tendencies, including epistaxis. Typical features are colicky right–upper-quadrant pain after eating fatty food, nausea, vomiting, fever, flatulence and, possibly, jaundice.

▶ *Cirrhosis.* Epistaxis is a late sign that occurs with other bleeding tendencies (bleeding gums, easy bruising, hematemesis, melena) in cirrhosis. Other typical late findings include ascites, abdominal pain, shallow respirations, hepatomegaly or splenomegaly, and fever of 101° F to 103° F (38.3° C to 39.4° C). The patient also may have muscle atrophy, enlarged superficial abdominal veins, severe pruritus, extremely dry skin, poor tissue turgor, abnormal pigmentation, spider angiomas, palmar erythema and, possibly, jaundice and central nervous system disturbances.

▶ *Coagulation disorders.* Such disorders as hemophilia and thrombocytopenic purpura can cause epistaxis along with ecchymoses, petechiae, and bleeding from the gums, mouth, and I.V. puncture sites. Menorrhagia and signs of GI bleeding, such as melena and hematemesis, can also occur.

▶ *Glomerulonephritis (chronic).* This disorder produces epistaxis as well as hypertension, proteinuria, hematuria, headache, edema, oliguria, hemoptysis, nausea, vomiting, pruritus, dyspnea, malaise, and fatigue.

▶ *Hepatitis.* When hepatitis interferes with the clotting mechanism, epistaxis and other abnormal bleeding tendencies can result. Other signs and symptoms typically include jaundice, clay-colored stools, pruritus, hepatomegaly, abdominal pain, fever, fatigue, weakness, dark amber urine, anorexia, nausea, and vomiting.

▶ *Hereditary hemorrhagic telangiectasia (Rendu-Osler-Weber disease).* This disease causes frequent, sometimes daily, epistaxis as well as hemoptysis and GI bleeding. It's characterized by telangiectases—pinpoint, purplish red spots or flat, spiderlike lesions—on the mucous membranes of the lips, mouth, tongue, nose, and GI tract and occasionally on the trunk and fingertips.

▶ *Hypertension.* Severe hypertension can produce severe epistaxis, usually in the posterior nose, with pulsation above the middle turbinate. It may be accompanied by dizziness, a throbbing headache, anxiety, peripheral edema, nocturia, nausea, vomiting, drowsiness, and mental impairment.

▶ *Infectious mononucleosis.* In patients with this infectious disorder, blood may ooze from the nose. Characteristic features include sore throat, cervical lymphadenopathy, and a fluctuating fever with an evening peak of 101° F to 102° F (38.3° C to 38.9° C).

▶ *Influenza.* When influenza affects the capillaries, a slow, oozing nosebleed results. Other signs and symptoms of influenza include a dry cough, chills, fever, malaise, myalgia, sore throat, hoarseness or loss of voice, conjunctivitis, facial flushing, headache, rhinitis, and rhinorrhea.

▶ *Leukemia.* In *acute leukemia,* sudden epistaxis is accompanied by a high fever and other types of abnormal bleeding, such as bleeding gums, ecchymoses, petechiae, easy bruising, and prolonged menses. These may follow less-noticeable signs and symptoms, such as weakness, lassitude, pallor, chills, recurrent infections, and a low-grade fever. Acute leukemia also may cause dyspnea, fatigue, malaise, tachycardia, palpitations, a systolic ejection murmur, and abdominal or bone pain.

In *chronic leukemia,* epistaxis is a late sign that may be accompanied by other types of abnormal bleeding, extreme fatigue, weight loss, hepatosplenomegaly, bone tenderness, edema, macular or nodular skin lesions, pallor, weakness, dyspnea, tachycardia, palpitations, and headache.

▶ *Maxillofacial injury.* A pumping arterial bleed usually causes severe epistaxis in a maxillofacial injury. Other signs and symptoms include facial pain, numbness, swelling, and asymmetry; open-bite malocclusion or inability to open the mouth; diplopia; conjunctival hemorrhage; lip edema; and buccal, mucosal, and soft-palatal ecchymoses.

▶ *Nasal fracture.* A nasal fracture may cause unilateral or bilateral epistaxis with nasal swelling, pain, and deformity; crepitation of the nasal bones; and periorbital ecchymoses and edema.

▶ *Nasal tumor.* Blood may ooze from the nose when a tumor disrupts the nasal vasculature. Benign tumors usually bleed when touched, but malignant tumors produce spontaneous unilateral epistaxis along with a foul discharge, cheek swelling, and—in the late stage—pain.

▶ *Orbital floor fracture.* This type of trauma may damage the maxillary sinus mucosa and, on rare occasions, cause epistaxis. More typical features include periorbital edema and ecchymoses, diplopia, infraorbital numbness, enophthalmos, limited eye movement, and facial asymmetry.

▶ *Polycythemia vera.* A common sign of polycythemia vera, spontaneous epistaxis may be accompanied by bleeding gums; ecchymoses; ruddy cyanosis of the face, nose, ears, and lips; and congestion of the conjunctiva, retina, and oral mucous membranes. Other signs and symptoms vary according to the affected body system but may include headache, dizziness, tinnitus, vision disturbances, hypertension, chest pain, intermittent claudication, early satiety and fullness, marked splenomegaly, epigastric pain, pruritus, and dyspnea.

▶ *Renal failure.* Chronic renal failure is more likely than acute renal failure to cause epistaxis and a tendency to bruise easily. More common signs and symptoms are oliguria or anuria, anorexia, weight loss, abdominal pain, diarrhea, nausea, vomiting, tissue wasting, dry mucous membranes, uremic breath odor, Kussmaul's respirations, deteriorating mental status, and tachycardia.

Skin changes include pruritus, pallor, yellow-bronze pigmentation, purpura, excoriation, uremic frost, and brown arcs under the nail margins. Neurologic signs and symptoms may include muscle twitching, fasciculations, asterixis, paresthesia, and footdrop. Cardiovascular effects include hypertension, arrhythmias, signs of heart failure or pericarditis, and peripheral edema.

▶ *Sarcoidosis.* Oozing epistaxis may be accompanied by a nonproductive cough, substernal pain, malaise, and weight loss in this disorder. Related findings include tachycardia, arrhythmias, parotid gland enlargement, cervical lymphadenopathy, skin lesions, hepatosplenomegaly, and arthritis in the ankles, knees, and wrists.

▶ *Scleroma.* In this disorder, oozing epistaxis occurs with a watery nasal discharge that becomes foul-smelling and crusty. Progressive anosmia and turbinate atrophy also may occur.

▶ *Sinusitis (acute).* In this disorder, a bloody or blood-tinged nasal discharge may become purulent and copious after 24 to 48 hours. Other signs and symptoms include nasal congestion, pain, and tenderness; malaise; headache; a low-grade fever; and red, edematous nasal mucosa.

▶ *Skull fracture.* Depending on the type of fracture, epistaxis can be direct (when blood flows directly down the nares) or indirect (when blood drains through the eustachian tube and into the nose). Abrasions, contusions, lacerations, or avulsions are common. A severe skull fracture may cause severe headache, decreased level of consciousness, hemiparesis, dizziness, seizures, projectile vomiting, and decreased pulse and respiratory rates.

A basilar fracture also may cause bleeding from the pharynx, ears, and conjunctivae as well as raccoon eyes and Battle's sign. Cerebrospinal fluid or even brain tissue may leak from the nose or ears. A sphenoid fracture also may cause blindness, whereas a temporal fracture also may cause unilateral deafness or facial paralysis.

▶ *Syphilis.* Epistaxis is most common in patients with tertiary syphilis, as posterior septum ulcerations produce a foul, bloody nasal discharge. It may be accompanied by a painful nasal obstruction and nasal deformity. Occasionally, primary syphilis causes painful nasal crusting and bleeding accompanied by the characteristic chancre sores.

▶ *Systemic lupus erythematosus (SLE).* Usually affecting women younger than age 50, SLE causes oozing epistaxis. More characteristic signs and symptoms include butterfly rash, lymphadenopathy, joint pain and stiffness, nausea, vomiting, myalgia, anorexia, and weight loss.

▶ *Typhoid fever.* Oozing epistaxis and dry cough are common signs of typhoid fever, which also may cause sudden chills and high fever, vomiting, abdominal distention, constipation or diarrhea, splenomegaly, hepatomegaly, "rose-spot" rash, jaundice, anorexia, weight loss, and profound fatigue.

Other causes

▶ *Chemical irritants.* Some chemicals—including phosphorus, sulfuric acid, ammonia, printer's ink, and chromates—irritate the nasal mucosa, producing epistaxis.

DRUG WATCH *Anticoagulants, such as warfarin, and anti-inflammatories, such as aspirin, can cause epistaxis.*

▶ *Illicit drug use.* Cocaine use, especially if frequent, can cause epistaxis.

▶ *Surgery and procedures.* Epistaxis rarely results from facial or nasal surgery, including septoplasty, rhinoplasty, antrostomy, endoscopic sinus procedures, orbital decompression, and dental extraction.

▶ *Vigorous nose blowing.* This may rupture superficial blood vessels, especially in elderly people and young people, causing nosebleeds.

Special considerations

Until the bleeding is completely under control, monitor the patient for signs of hypovolemic shock, such as tachycardia and clammy skin. If external pressure doesn't control the bleeding, insert cotton that has been impregnated with a vasoconstrictor and local anesthetic into the patient's nose.

Controlling epistaxis with nasal packing

When epistaxis persists despite application of direct pressure and cautery, the patient may need nasal packing. Anterior packing may be used if the patient has severe bleeding in the anterior nose. This involves inserting horizontal layers of petroleum jelly gauze strips into the nostrils near the turbinates.

Posterior packing may be needed if the patient has severe bleeding in the posterior nose or if blood from anterior bleeding starts flowing backward. This type of packing consists of a gauze pack secured by three strong silk sutures. After the nose is anesthetized, sutures are pulled through the nostrils with a soft catheter and the pack is positioned behind the soft palate. Two of the sutures are tied to a gauze roll under the patient's nose, which keeps the pack in place. The third suture is taped to his cheek.

Instead of a gauze pack, an indwelling urinary or nasal epistaxis catheter may be inserted through the nose into the area behind the soft palate and inflated with 10 ml of water to compress the bleeding point.

PRECAUTIONS

If your patient has nasal packing, follow these guidelines:
- Watch for signs of respiratory distress such as dyspnea, which may occur if the packing slips and obstructs the airway.
- Keep emergency equipment (flashlights, scissors, and hemostat) at the patient's bedside. Expect to cut the cheek suture (or deflate the

catheter) and remove the pack at the first sign of airway obstruction.
- Avoid tension on the cheek suture, which could cause the posterior pack to slip out of place.
- Keep the call bell within easy reach.
- Monitor vital signs often. Watch for signs of hypoxia, such as tachycardia and restlessness.
- Elevate the head of the patient's bed, and remind him to breathe through his mouth.
- Administer humidified oxygen as needed.
- Instruct the patient not to blow his nose for 48 hours after the packing is removed.

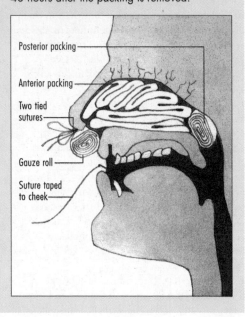

Posterior packing

Anterior packing

Two tied sutures

Gauze roll

Suture taped to cheek

If bleeding persists, expect to insert anterior or posterior nasal packing. (See *Controlling epistaxis with nasal packing.*) Give humidified oxygen by face mask to a patient with posterior packing. If nasal packing fails to control bleeding, examination under general anesthesia may be needed.[1]

A complete blood count may be ordered to evaluate blood loss and detect anemia. Clotting studies, such as prothrombin time and partial thromboplastin time, may be required to test coagulation time. Prepare the patient for X-rays if he has had a recent trauma. Any

patient with recurrent epistaxis should be evaluated for hereditary hemorrhagic telangiectasia.[3]

Pediatric pointers

Children are more likely to have anterior nosebleeds, usually the result of nose-picking or allergic rhinitis. Biliary atresia, cystic fibrosis, hereditary afibrinogenemia, and nasal trauma due to a foreign body can also cause epistaxis. Rubeola may cause an oozing nosebleed along with the characteristic maculopapular rash. Two rare childhood diseases—pertussis and diphtheria—can also cause oozing epistaxis.

Children with epistaxis should be evaluated for anemia and an underlying coagulation disorder.[4] Suspect a bleeding disorder if you see excess umbilical cord bleeding at birth or profuse bleeding during circumcision. Epistaxis occurs in 90% of patients with hereditary hemorrhagic telangiectasia, and commonly starts at adolescence or even childhood.[3] This bleeding tends to increase with age.[3]

Geriatric pointers
Elderly patients are more likely to have posterior nosebleeds.[1]

Patient counseling
Teach the patient proper pinching techniques for applying pressure to the nose. For prevention, tell him to apply liberal amounts of petroleum jelly to nostrils to prevent drying, cracking, and picking. Also recommend using of a humidifier at night and trimming fingernails.

REFERENCES
1. Thornton, M.A., et al. "Posterior Epistaxis: Identification of Common Bleeding Sites," *The Laryngoscope* 115(4):588-590, April 2005.
2. Douglas, R., and Wormald, P.J. "Update on Epstaxis," *Current Opinion in Otolaryngology & Head and Neck Surgery* 15(3):180-183, June 2007.
3. Ragsdale, J.A. "Hereditary Hemorrhagic Telangiectasia: From Epistaxis to Life-Threatening GI Bleeding," *Gastroenterology Nursing* 30(4):293-299, July-August 2007.
4. Damrose, J.F., and Maddalozzo, J. "Pediatric Epistaxis," *The Laryngoscope* 116(3):387-393, March 2006.

ERYTHEMA

Dilated or congested blood vessels produce red skin, a condition called *erythema* or *erythroderma*, the most common sign of skin inflammation or irritation. Erythema may be localized or generalized and may occur suddenly or gradually. Skin color can range from bright red in patients with acute conditions to pale violet or brown in those whose conditions are chronic. Erythema

Rare causes of erythema

In exceptional cases, your patient's erythema may be caused by one of these rare disorders:
- *acute febrile neutrophilic dermatosis*, which produces erythematous lesions on the face, neck, and limbs after a high fever
- *erythema abigne*, which produces lacy erythema and telangiectases after exposure to radiant heat
- *erythema chronicum migrans*, which produces erythematous macules and papules on the trunk, upper arms, or thighs after a tick bite
- *erythema gyratum repens*, which produces wavy bands of erythema and is commonly related to internal malignancy
- *toxic epidermal necrolysis*, which causes severe, widespread erythema, tenderness, bullae formation, and exfoliation; this disorder usually is caused by medications and may be fatal because of epidermal destruction and its consequences.

must be differentiated from purpura, which causes redness from bleeding into the skin. When pressure is applied directly to the skin, erythema blanches momentarily, but purpura doesn't.

Erythema usually results from changes in the arteries, veins, and small vessels that lead to increased small-vessel perfusion. Drugs and neurogenic mechanisms can allow extra blood to enter the small vessels. Erythema also may result from trauma and tissue damage; changes in supporting tissues, which increase vessel visibility; and a number of rare disorders. (See *Rare causes of erythema*.)

If your patient suddenly develops progressive erythema with a rapid pulse, dyspnea, hoarseness, and agitation, he may be experiencing anaphylactic shock. Quickly take his vital signs. Provide emergency respiratory support and give epinephrine.

Differential diagnosis: Erythema

POSSIBLE CAUSES	SIGNS AND SYMPTOMS	DIAGNOSIS
Burns	*First degree* • Pressure that causes skin blanching • Tenderness at the site • Involvement of superficial epidermal layers *Second degree* • Deep or superficial blisters • Increased tenderness at the site • Variable involvement of epidermis and part of dermis *Third degree* • Tough and leathery affected area • Nontender • Destruction of all skin elements	• History of exposure to heat, chemicals, or electricity • Physical examination • Chest X-ray for smoke inhalation
Erythema multiforme	• Hivelike erythema with blisters • Pathognomonic petechial or "iris" lesions • Symmetrical lesions (less than 3 cm) on the face, hands, and feet • Involvement of less than 20% of body surface area	• Physical examination • Skin biopsy
Seborrheic dermatitis	• Dull red or yellow lesions on the scalp, eyebrows, ears, and nasolabial folds • Butterfly rash on the face, chest, or trunk	• Physical examination • Skin biopsy • Allergy patch test
Atopic dermatitis	• Intense pruritus • Small papules that redden, weep, scale, and lichenify, commonly occurring in skin folds of the extremities, neck, and eyelids	• Physical examination • Skin biopsy • Allergy patch test
Contact dermatitis	• History of exposure to irritant • Vesicles, blisters, ulcerations that appear on exposed skin	• Physical examination • Skin biopsy • Allergy patch test

History and physical examination

If the patient isn't in anaphylaxis, obtain a detailed health history. (See *Differential diagnosis: Erythema*.) Find out how long the patient has had the erythema and where it first began. Dark-skinned patients may have trouble seeing erythema; as a result, they may present with related diseases in a more advanced state. Has he had any related pain or itching? Has he recently had a fever, an upper respiratory tract infection, or joint pain? Does he have a history of skin disease or other illness? Does he or anyone in his family have allergies, asthma, or eczema? Find out if he has been exposed to someone who has had a similar rash or who is now ill. Did he have a recent fall or injury in the erythematous area?

Obtain a complete drug history, including recent immunizations. Ask about food intake and exposure to chemicals.

TREATMENT AND FOLLOW-UP

- Removal of cause of injury
- Rule of nines to estimate extent of injury and guide treatment
- I.V. hydration
- Medication (analgesics, nonsteroidal anti-inflammatory drugs, topical antibacterial)

Follow-up: As needed (depending on severity of burn), referral to burn center if injury is severe

- Treatment of underlying cause
- Medication (analgesics, antipruritics)

Follow-up: None unless complications develop

- Medication (antiseborrheic shampoo, selenium or zinc lotion, steroid cream)

Follow-up: Reevaluation every 2 to 12 weeks as needed

- Topical corticosteroids

Follow-up: Reevaluation every 2 to 12 weeks as needed

- Cool compresses with astringent
- Soaks with oatmeal
- Medication (topical and systemic corticosteroids, antihistamines, antibiotics)

Follow-up: Reevaluation every 2 to 12 weeks as needed

Begin the physical examination by assessing the extent, distribution, and intensity of erythema. Look for edema and other skin lesions, such as urticaria, scales, papules, and purpura. Examine the affected area for warmth, and gently palpate it to check for tenderness or crepitus.

Medical causes

▶ *Allergic reactions.* Foods, drugs, chemicals, and other allergens can cause an allergic reaction and erythema. A localized allergic reaction also produces hivelike eruptions and edema.

Anaphylaxis, a life-threatening reaction, produces relatively sudden erythema in the form of urticaria. It also produces flushing; facial edema; diaphoresis; weakness; sneezing; bronchospasm with dyspnea and tachypnea; shock with hypotension and cool, clammy skin; and possibly airway edema with hoarseness and stridor.

▶ *Burns.* In thermal burns, erythema and swelling appear first, possibly followed by deep or superficial blisters and other signs of damage that vary with the severity of the burn. Burns from ultraviolet rays, such as sunburn, cause delayed erythema and tenderness on exposed areas of the skin.

▶ *Candidiasis.* When this fungal infection affects the skin, it produces erythema and a scaly, papular rash under the breasts and at the axillae, neck, umbilicus, and groin (intertrigo). Small pustules commonly occur at the periphery of the rash (satellite pustulosis).

▶ *Cellulitis.* This bacterial infection of the skin and subcutaneous tissue causes erythema, tenderness, and edema.

▶ *Dermatitis.* Erythema commonly occurs in this family of inflammatory disorders. In *atopic dermatitis*, erythema and intense pruritus precede the development of small papules that may redden, weep, scale, and lichenify. These usually occur at skin folds of the limbs, neck, and eyelids.

Contact dermatitis occurs after exposure to an irritant. It quickly produces erythema and vesicles, blisters, or ulcerations on exposed skin.

In *seborrheic dermatitis*, erythema appears with dull red or yellow lesions. Sharply marginated, these lesions are sometimes ring shaped and covered with greasy scales. They usually occur on the scalp, eyebrows, ears, and nasolabial folds, but they may form a butterfly rash on the face or move to the chest or to skin folds on the trunk. This disorder is common in patients infected with the human immunodeficiency virus and in infants (cradle cap).

▶ *Dermatomyositis.* This disorder, most common in women older than age 50, produces a dusky lilac rash on the face, neck, upper torso, and nail beds. Gottron's papules (violet, flat-topped lesions) may appear on finger joints.

▶ *Erysipelas.* This skin infection caused by group A beta-hemolytic streptococci is characterized by an abrupt onset of reddish, well-demarcated, tender, warm, sometimes elevated lesions, mainly on the face and neck but sometimes also on the limbs. Flaccid, pus-filled bullae may develop after 2 to 3 days. Extension into deeper tissues is rare. Other signs and symptoms include fever, chills, cervical lymphadenopathy, vomiting, headache, sore throat, warmth and tenderness in the affected area and, possibly, alopecia.

▶ *Erythema annulare centrifugum.* Small, pink infiltrated papules appear on the trunk, buttocks, and inner thighs, slowly spreading at the margins and clearing in the center. Itching, scaling, and tissue hardening may occur.

▶ *Erythema marginatum rheumaticum.* Related to rheumatic fever, this disorder causes erythematous lesions that are superficial, flat, and slightly hardened. They shift, spread rapidly, and may last for hours or days, recurring after a time.

▶ *Erythema multiforme.* This acute inflammatory skin disease develops as a result of drug sensitivity after an infection (most commonly herpes simplex or a mycoplasmal infection), allergies, or pregnancy. One-half of the cases are of idiopathic origin.

Erythema multiforme minor produces reddish pink iris-shaped, urticarial, localized lesions with little or no mucous membrane involvement. Most lesions occur on flexor surfaces of the limbs. Burning or itching may occur before or with lesion development. Lesions appear in crops and last 2 to 3 weeks. After 1 week, they become flat or hyperpigmented. Early signs and symptoms may include a mild fever, cough, and sore throat.

Erythema multiforme major usually occurs as a cutaneous adverse drug reaction; causes widespread symmetrical, bullous lesions that may become confluent; and includes erosions of the mucous membranes. Erythema usually is preceded by blisters on the lips, tongue, and buccal mucosa and a sore throat. Other early signs and symptoms include cough, vomiting, diarrhea, coryza, and epistaxis. Later signs and symptoms include fever, prostration,

trouble with oral intake because of mouth and lip lesions, conjunctivitis from ulceration, vulvitis, and balanitis. The most severe form of this disorder is known as Stevens-Johnson syndrome, a multisystem disorder that occasionally is fatal. In addition to all signs and symptoms mentioned above, patients develop exfoliation of the skin from disruptions of bullae, although less than 10% of the body surface area is affected. These areas resemble second-degree thermal burns and should be cared for as such. Fever may rise to 102° F to 104° F (38.9° C to 40° C). The patient also may have tachypnea; a weak, rapid pulse; chest pain; malaise; and muscle or joint pain.

▶ *Erythema nodosum.* Sudden bilateral eruption of tender erythematous nodules characterizes this disorder. These firm, round, protruding lesions usually appear in crops on the shins, knees, and ankles but may occur on the buttocks, arms, calves, and trunk as well. Other effects include mild fever, chills, malaise, muscle and joint pain and, possibly, swollen feet and ankles. Erythema nodosum occurs with various diseases, most notably inflammatory bowel disease, sarcoidosis, tuberculosis, and streptococcal and fungal infections.

▶ *Frostbite.* First-degree frostbite turns the affected body part a lifeless gray color, followed by an intense bluish red flush on rewarming. Blisters, lack of feeling, and tissue necrosis may follow.

▶ *Gout.* This disease, which typically affects men ages 40 to 60, is characterized by tight and erythematous skin over an inflamed, edematous joint.

▶ *Intertrigo.* In this superficial fungal infection, skin friction usually causes symmetrical erythema and possibly soreness and itching. Typically, erythema occurs in skin folds, such as in the groin; in severe cases, the skin may become bright red with erosion and maceration.

▶ *Kawasaki syndrome.* This acute illness of unknown cause, which affects mainly children younger than age 5, commonly produces a rash or erythema. The rash may desquamate in the subacute phase or after treatment.[1] No test is available for Kawasaki syndrome, which can cause serious heart damage and death if not detected and treated immediately.

Additional characteristic signs include fever, conjunctival injection, extreme irritability, enlarged papillae on the tongue, and lymphadenopathy. Patients are treated with I.V. immune globulin and aspirin therapy.[1,2]

▶ *Liver disease (chronic).* Any chronic liver disease, such as cirrhosis, can cause local vasodilation and palmar erythema along with jaundice, pruritus, spider angiomas, xanthomas, and characteristic systemic signs.

▶ *Lupus erythematosus.* Both discoid and systemic lupus erythematosus (SLE) can produce a characteristic butterfly rash. This erythematous eruption may range from a blush with swelling to a scaly, sharply demarcated, macular rash with plaques that may spread to the forehead, chin, ears, chest, and other sun-exposed parts of the body.

In *discoid lupus erythematosus,* other signs and symptoms may include telangiectasia, hyperpigmentation, ear and nose deformity, and mouth, tongue, and eyelid lesions.

In *SLE,* acute onset of erythema may be accompanied by photosensitivity and mucous membrane ulcers, especially in the nose and mouth. Mottled erythema may occur on the hands, with edema around the nails and macular reddish purple lesions on the fingers. Telangiectasia occurs at the base of the nails or eyelids along with purpura, petechiae, ecchymoses, and urticaria. Other findings vary according to the body systems affected but typically include low-grade fever, malaise, weakness, headache, arthralgia, arthritis, depression, lymphadenopathy, fatigue, anorexia, weight loss, nausea, vomiting, diarrhea, and constipation.

▶ *Necrotizing fasciitis.* This streptococcal infection usually begins with an area of mild erythema at the site of insult, which soon changes from red to purple and then blue. The appearance of fluid-filled blisters and bullae indicates the rapid progression of the necrotizing process. By days 7 to 10, dead skin begins to separate at the margins of the erythema, revealing extensive necrosis of the underlying tissue layers. Other findings include fever, hypovolemia and, in later stages, hypotension and respiratory insufficiency—signs of overwhelming sepsis that require supportive care.

▶ *Polymorphous light eruption.* This condition produces erythema, vesicles, plaques, and multiple small papules on sun-exposed areas, which may later eczematize, lichenify, and excoriate. Pruritus also may occur.

▶ *Psoriasis.* Silvery white scales over a thickened erythematous base usually affect the elbows, knees, chest, scalp, and intergluteal folds. The fingernails may become thick and pitted.

▶ *Raynaud's disease.* In this disorder, the skin on the hands and feet typically blanches and cools after exposure to cold and stress and later becomes warm and purplish red.

▶ *Rheumatoid arthritis.* In a flare-up of this disorder, erythema occurs over the affected joints along with heat, swelling, pain, and stiffness. Earlier symptoms include malaise, fatigue, myalgia, prolonged morning stiffness, and clumsiness. As the disease progresses, muscle atrophy, palmar erythema, generalized edema, mottled skin, and structural deformities occur.

▶ *Rosacea.* Scattered erythema initially develops across the center of the face, followed by superficial telangiectases, papules, pustules, and nodules. Rhinophyma may occur on the lower half of the nose.

▶ *Rubella.* Typically, flat solitary lesions join to form a blotchy pink erythematous rash that spreads rapidly to the trunk and limbs in this disorder. Occasionally, small red lesions (Forschheimer spots) occur on the soft palate. Lesions clear in 4 to 5 days. The rash usually follows a fever (up to 102° F [38.9° C]), headache, malaise, sore throat, a gritty eye sensation, lymphadenopathy, pain in the joints, and coryza.

▶ *Staphylococcal scalded skin syndrome.* This endotoxin-mediated epidermolytic disease is caused by a clinically unapparent *Staphylococcus aureus* infection and mainly affects infants (Ritter's disease) and small children. It's characterized by erythema and widespread exfoliation of superficial epidermal layers, resembling scalded skin. Other signs and symptoms include low-grade fever and irritability. Care must be taken to maintain hydration and prevent secondary infections of denuded areas; hospitalization commonly is required. Death may occur, especially in infants with extensive disease.

Drugs that may cause erythema

Suspect drug-induced erythema in any patient who develops this sign within 1 week of starting a drug. Erythematous lesions can vary in size, shape, type, and amount, but they almost always appear suddenly and symmetrically on the trunk and inner arms. The following drugs can produce erythematous lesions:

allopurinol	co-trimoxazole	indomethacin	quinidine
anticoagulants	diazepam	iodide bromides	salicylates
antimetabolites	erythromycin	isoniazid	sulfonamides
barbiturates	gentamicin	lithium	sulfonylureas
cephalosporins	gold	nitrofurantoin	tetracyclines
chlordiazepoxide	griseofulvin	penicillin	thiazides
codeine	hormonal contra-	phenothiazines	
corticosteroids	ceptives	phenytoin	

REMINDERS

• Topical drugs cause more adverse cutaneous reactions than parenteral drugs do, and parenteral drugs cause more cutaneous reactions than oral drugs do.[3]

• Some drugs—particularly barbiturates, hormonal contraceptives, salicylates, sulfonamides, and tetracycline—can cause a "fixed" drug eruption, in which lesions appear anywhere on the body and then flake off after a few days, leaving a brownish purple pigmentation. Repeated use of that drug causes the original lesions to recur and new ones to develop.

• Applying topical steroids to the face for longer than 2 weeks can cause a rosacea-like rash on the face and neck called *steroid rosacea.*[4] After stopping topical steroid therapy that lasts 2 weeks or more, the patient may develop severe erythema and burning on the face, neck, and genitals. This is known as *steroid addiction syndrome.*[4]

▶ *Thrombophlebitis.* Although this disorder sometimes is asymptomatic, it can produce erythema over the inflamed vein. Fever, chills, and malaise may accompany severe localized pain, warmth, and induration; distal edema; and a positive Homans' sign.

▶ *Toxic shock syndrome.* This infectious disorder, which is caused by a toxin-producing *S. aureus* infection, causes sudden, diffuse erythema in the form of a macular rash. It's accompanied by a sudden high fever, myalgia, vomiting, severe diarrhea, and sudden hypotension that may lead to shock. Desquamation occurs after 1 to 2 weeks, especially on the palms and soles. This syndrome usually affects young women and may be related to the use of tampons during menses.

Other causes

▶ *Drugs.* Many drugs commonly cause erythema. (See *Drugs that may cause erythema.*)

▶ *Herbs.* Ingestion of the fruit pulp of ginkgo biloba can cause severe erythema and edema of the mouth and rapid vesicles. St. John's wort can cause heightened photosensitivity, resulting in erythema or "sunburn."

▶ *Radiation and other treatments.* Radiation therapy may produce dull erythema and edema within 24 hours. As the erythema fades, the skin becomes light brown and mildly scaly. Any treatment that causes an allergic reaction can also cause erythema.

Special considerations

Because erythema can cause fluid loss, closely monitor and replace fluids and electrolytes, especially in patients with burns or widespread erythema. Be sure to withhold all medications until the cause of the erythema has been identified. Then expect to administer an antibiotic and a topical or systemic corticosteroid.

For a patient with itching skin, expect to give soothing baths or apply open wet dressings containing starch, bran, or sodium bicarbonate; also administer an antihistamine and an analgesic as needed. Advise a patient with leg erythema to keep his legs elevated above heart level. For a burn patient with erythema, immerse the affected area in cold water, or apply a sheet soaked in cold water to reduce pain, edema, and erythema.

Prepare the patient for diagnostic tests, such as skin biopsy to detect cancerous lesions, cultures to identify infectious organisms, and sensitivity studies to confirm allergies.

Pediatric pointers

Many newborns develop a pink papular rash (erythema toxicum neonatorum) that starts within the first 4 days after birth and spontaneously disappears by the tenth day. Neonates and infants can also develop erythema from infections and other disorders. For instance, candidiasis can produce thick white lesions over an erythematous base on the oral mucosa as well as diaper rash with beefy red erythema.

Roseola, rubeola, scarlet fever, granuloma annulare, and cutis marmorata also cause erythema in children.

Geriatric pointers

Many elderly patients have well-demarcated purple macules or patches, usually on the back of the hands and on the forearms. Known as *actinic purpura,* this condition results from blood leaking through fragile capillaries. The lesions disappear on their own.

Patient counseling

Teach patients with a chronic disease, such as SLE or psoriasis, about the character of their typical rashes so they can be alert to any flare-ups of their disease. Also, advise such patients to avoid sun exposure by using of protective clothing and wide-brimmed hats, and to use sunscreen with UVA and UVB protection when appropriate.[5] To avoid steroid rosacea and steroid addiction syndrome, tell the patient to avoid using steroids on the face for greater than 2 weeks.[4]

REFERENCES
1. Satou, G.M., et al. "Kawasaki Disease: Diagnosis, Management, and Long-Term Implications," *Cardiology in Review* 15(4):163-169, July-August 2007.
2. Hockenberry, M.J., and Wilson, D. (Eds.) *Wong's Nursing Care of Infants and Children,* 8th ed. St. Louis: Mosby, 2007.
3. Hayden, M.L. "Did That Medication Cause This Rash?" *Nursing* 35(9):62-64, September 2005.
4. Smith, M.C., et al. "Facing Up to Withdrawal from Topical Steroids," *Nursing* 37(9):60-61, September 2007.
5. Rooney, J. "Systemic Lupus Erythematosus: Unmasking a Great Imitator," *Nursing* 35(11):54-60, November 2005.

FATIGUE

Fatigue is a feeling of excessive tiredness, lack of energy, or exhaustion accompanied by a strong desire to rest or sleep. This common symptom is distinct from weakness, which involves the muscles, but may accompany it.

Fatigue is a normal and important response to physical overexertion, prolonged emotional stress, and sleep deprivation. However, it can also be a nonspecific symptom of a psychological or physiologic disorder, especially viral or bacterial infection and endocrine, cardiovascular, or neurologic disease.

Fatigue reflects both hypermetabolic and hypometabolic states in which nutrients needed for cellular energy and growth are lacking because of overly rapid depletion, impaired replacement mechanisms, insufficient hormone production, or inadequate nutrient intake or metabolism.

History and physical examination

Obtain a careful history to identify the patient's fatigue pattern. Fatigue that worsens with activity and improves with rest generally indicates a physical disorder; the opposite pattern, a psychological disorder. Fatigue lasting longer than 4 months, constant fatigue that's unrelieved by rest, and transient exhaustion that quickly gives way to bursts of energy are findings associated with psychological disorders.

Ask about related symptoms and any recent viral or bacterial illness or stressful changes in lifestyle. Explore nutritional habits and any appetite or weight changes. Carefully review the patient's medical and psychiatric history for any chronic disorders that commonly produce fatigue, and ask about a family history of such disorders.

Obtain a thorough drug history, noting use of any opioid or drug with fatigue as an adverse effect. Ask about alcohol and drug use patterns. Determine the patient's risk of carbon monoxide poisoning, and ask whether the patient has a carbon monoxide detector.

Observe the patient's general appearance for overt signs of depression or organic illness. Is he unkempt or expressionless? Does he appear tired or sickly, or have a slumped posture? If warranted, evaluate his mental status, noting especially mental clouding, attention deficits, agitation, or psychomotor retardation.

Medical causes

▶ *Acquired immunodeficiency syndrome.* Besides fatigue, this syndrome may cause fever, night sweats, weight loss, diarrhea, and a cough, followed by several concurrent opportunistic infections.

▶ *Adrenocortical insufficiency.* Mild fatigue, the hallmark of this disorder, initially appears after exertion and stress but later becomes more severe and persistent. Weakness and weight loss typically accompany GI disturbances, such as nausea, vomiting, anorexia, abdominal pain, and chronic diarrhea; hyperpigmentation; orthostatic hypotension; and a weak, irregular pulse.

▶ *Anemia.* Fatigue after mild activity is commonly the first symptom of anemia. Associated findings vary but generally include pallor, tachycardia, and dyspnea.

▶ *Anxiety.* Chronic, unremitting anxiety invariably produces fatigue, often characterized as nervous exhaustion. Other persistent findings include apprehension, indecisiveness, restlessness, insomnia, trembling, and increased muscle tension.

▶ *Cancer.* Unexplained fatigue is commonly the earliest sign of cancer. Fatigue occurs in 70% to 100% of patients with cancer, and cancer treatment may make it worse.[1] Related findings reflect the type, location, and stage of the tumor and typically include pain, nausea, vomiting, anorexia, weight loss, abnormal bleeding, and a palpable mass.

▶ *Chronic fatigue syndrome.* This syndrome, whose cause is unknown, is characterized by incapacitating fatigue. Other findings are sore throat, myalgia, and cognitive dysfunction.

▶ *Chronic obstructive pulmonary disease (COPD).* The earliest and most persistent symptoms of this disease are progressive fatigue and dyspnea.[2] Fatigue occurs most commonly in the afternoon, and it may be caused by physical activity. The patient also may have a chronic and usually productive cough, weight loss, barrel chest, cyanosis, slight dependent edema, and poor exercise tolerance.

▶ *Cirrhosis.* Severe fatigue typically occurs late in this disorder, accompanied by weight loss, bleeding tendencies, jaundice, hepatomegaly, ascites, dependent edema, severe pruritus, and decreased level of consciousness.

▶ *Cushing's syndrome (hypercortisolism).* This disorder typically causes fatigue, related in part to accompanying sleep disturbances. Cardinal signs include truncal obesity with slender limbs, buffalo hump, moon face, purple striae, acne, and hirsutism; increased blood pressure and muscle weakness may also occur.

▶ *Depression.* Persistent fatigue unrelated to exertion nearly always accompanies chronic depression. Associated somatic complaints include headache, anorexia (occasionally, increased appetite), constipation, and sexual dysfunction. The patient may also experience insomnia, slowed speech, agitation or bradykinesia, irritability, loss of concentration, feelings of worthlessness, and persistent thoughts of death.

▶ *Diabetes mellitus.* Fatigue, the most common symptom of this disorder, may begin insidiously or abruptly. Related findings include weight loss, blurred vision, polyuria, polydipsia, and polyphagia.

▶ *Heart failure.* Persistent fatigue and lethargy characterize this disorder. Left-sided heart failure produces exertional and paroxysmal nocturnal dyspnea, orthopnea, and tachycardia. Right-sided heart failure produces jugular vein distention and possibly a slight but persistent nonproductive cough. In both types, later signs and symptoms include mental status changes, nausea, anorexia, weight gain and, possibly, oliguria. Cardiopulmonary findings include tachypnea, inspiratory crackles, palpitations and chest tightness, hypotension, narrowed pulse pressure, ventricular gallop, pallor, diaphoresis, clubbing, and dependent edema.

▶ *Hypopituitarism.* Fatigue, lethargy, and weakness usually develop slowly. Other insidious effects may include irritability, anorexia, amenorrhea or impotence, decreased libido, hypotension, dizziness, headache, visual disturbances, and cold intolerance.

▶ *Hypothyroidism.* Fatigue occurs early in this disorder, along with forgetfulness, cold intolerance, weight gain, metrorrhagia, and constipation.

▶ *Infection.* Fatigue is often the most prominent symptom—and sometimes the only one—in a *chronic infection.* Low-grade fever and weight loss may accompany signs and symptoms that reflect the type and location of the infection, such as burning on urination or swollen, painful gums. Subacute bacterial endocarditis is an example of a chronic infection that causes fatigue and acute hemodynamic decompensation.

In an *acute infection,* brief fatigue typically accompanies headache, anorexia, arthralgia, chills, high fever, and such infection-specific signs as a cough, vomiting, or diarrhea.

▶ *Lyme disease.* Besides fatigue and malaise, signs and symptoms of this tick-borne disease include intermittent headache, fever, chills, an expanding red rash, and muscle and joint aches. Later, patients may develop arthritis, fluctuating meningoencephalitis, and cardiac abnormalities, such as a brief, fluctuating atrioventricular heart block.

▶ *Malnutrition.* Easy fatigability, lethargy, and apathy are common findings in patients with protein-calorie malnutrition. Patients may also exhibit weight loss, muscle wasting, sensations of coldness, pallor, edema, and dry, flaky skin.

▶ *Myasthenia gravis.* The cardinal symptoms of this disorder are easy fatigability and muscle weakness, which worsen as the day progresses. They also worsen with exertion and abate with rest. Related findings depend on the specific muscles affected.

▶ *Myocardial infarction.* Fatigue can be severe but is typically overshadowed by chest pain. Related findings include dyspnea, anxiety, pallor, cold sweats, increased or decreased blood pressure, and abnormal heart sounds. Fatigue commonly lingers as a problem after acute myocardial infarction.[3]

▶ *Narcolepsy.* One or more of the following characterizes this disorder: hypersomnia, hypnagogic hallucinations, cataplexy, sleep paralysis, and insomnia. Fatigue is a common symptom as well.

▶ *Renal failure. Acute renal failure* commonly causes sudden fatigue, drowsiness, and lethargy. Oliguria, an early sign, is followed by severe systemic effects: ammonia breath odor, nausea, vomiting, diarrhea or constipation, and dry skin and mucous membranes. Neurologic findings include muscle twitching, personality changes, and altered level of consciousness, which may progress to seizures and coma.

Chronic renal failure produces insidious fatigue and lethargy along with marked changes in all body systems, including GI disturbances, ammonia breath odor, Kussmaul's respirations, bleeding tendencies, poor skin turgor, severe pruritus, paresthesia, visual disturbances, confusion, seizures, and coma.

▶ *Restrictive lung disease.* Chronic fatigue may accompany the characteristic signs and symptoms: dyspnea, cough, and rapid, shallow respirations. Cyanosis first appears with exertion; later, even at rest.

▶ *Rheumatoid arthritis.* Fatigue, weakness, and anorexia precede localized articular findings: joint pain, tenderness, warmth, and swelling along with morning stiffness.

▶ *Systemic lupus erythematosus.* Fatigue usually occurs along with generalized aching, malaise, low-grade fever, headache, and irritability. Primary signs and symptoms include joint pain and stiffness, butterfly rash, and photosensitivity. Also common are Raynaud's phenomenon, patchy alopecia, and mucous membrane ulcers.

▶ *Thyrotoxicosis.* In this disorder, fatigue may accompany characteristic signs and symptoms, including an enlarged thyroid, tachycardia and palpitations, tremors, weight loss despite increased appetite, diarrhea, dyspnea, nervousness, diaphoresis, heat intolerance, amenorrhea and, possibly, exophthalmos.

▶ *Valvular heart disease.* All types of valvular heart disease commonly produce progressive fatigue and a cardiac murmur. Other signs and symptoms vary but typically include exertional dyspnea, cough, and hemoptysis.

Other causes

▶ *Carbon monoxide poisoning.* Fatigue occurs along with headache, dyspnea, and confusion; apnea and unconsciousness may occur eventually.

DRUG WATCH *Fatigue may result from various drugs, notably antihypertensives and sedatives. In those receiving cardiac glycoside therapy, fatigue may indicate toxicity.*

▶ *Surgery.* Most types of surgery cause temporary fatigue, probably from the combined effects of hunger, anesthesia, and sleep deprivation.

Special considerations

If fatigue results from organic illness, help the patient determine which daily activities he may need help with and how he should pace himself to ensure sufficient rest. You can help him reduce chronic fatigue by alleviating pain, which may interfere with rest, or nausea, which may lead to malnutrition. He may benefit from referral to a community health nurse or housekeeping service. If fatigue results from a psychogenic cause, refer him for psychological counseling.

Assess the patient for signs and symptoms of anemia, especially those at high risk, including patients with cancer and pregnant or postpartum women. Reaching a hemoglobin of 11 to 12 g/dl produces the greatest effect in reducing fatigue.[4,5]

Pediatric pointers

When evaluating a child for fatigue, ask his parents if they've noticed any change in his activity level. Fatigue without an organic cause occurs normally during accelerated growth phases in preschool-age and prepubescent children. However, psychological causes of fatigue must be considered; for example, a depressed child may try to escape problems at home or school by taking refuge in sleep. In the pubescent child, consider the possibility of drug abuse, particularly of hypnotics and tranquilizers.

Geriatric pointers

Always ask older patients about fatigue because this symptom may be insidious and mask more serious underlying conditions in this age-group. Temporal arthritis, which is much more common in people older than age 60, is usually characterized by fatigue, weight loss, jaw claudication, proximal muscle weakness, headache, visual disturbances, and anemia.

Patient counseling

Regardless of the cause of fatigue, you may need to help the patient alter his lifestyle to achieve a balanced diet, a program of regular exercise, and adequate rest. Counsel him about setting priorities, keeping a reasonable schedule, and developing good sleep habits. Teach stress management techniques as appropriate.

REFERENCES

1. Olson, K., Krawchuk, A., and Quddusi, T. "Fatigue in Individuals with Advanced Cancer in Active Treatment and Palliative Settings." *Cancer Nursing* 30(4):E1-E10, July/August 2007.
2. Kapella, M.C., Larson, J.L., Munu, K., Covey, M.K., and Berry, J.K. "Subjective Fatigue, Influencing Variables, and Consequences in Chronic Obstructive Pulmonary Disease." *Nursing Research* 55(1):10-17, January/February 2006.
3. Brink, E. and Grankvist, G. "Associations Between Depression, Fatigue, and Life Orientation in Myocardial Infarction Patients." *The Journal of Cardiovascular Nursing* 21(5):407-411, September/October 2006.
4. Mitchell, S.A. and Berger, A.M. "Cancer-Related Fatigue: The Evidence Base for Assessment and Management." *The Cancer Journal* 12(5):374-387, September/October 2006.
5. Corwin, E.J. and Arbour, M. "Postpartum Fatigue and Evidence-Based Interventions." *MCN The American Journal of Maternal/Child Nursing* 32(4):215-220, July/August 2007.

FEVER

Fever, or *pyrexia*, occurs in about 29% to 36% of all hospitalized patients. It refers to a regulated rise in core body temperature or an elevation in temperature set-point.[1] Fever can arise from numerous disorders. Because these disorders can affect virtually any body system, fever in the absence of other signs usually has little diagnostic significance. A persistent high fever, though, represents an emergency. (See *How fever develops,* page 188.)

Fever can be classified as low (oral reading of 99° to 100.4° F [37.2° to 38° C]), moderate (100.5° to 104° F [38.1° to 40° C]), or high (above 104° F). Fever over 106° F (41.1° C) causes unconsciousness and, if sustained, leads to permanent brain damage. Don't confuse fever with hyperthermia, which is related to heat illness or malignant hyperthermia and results from the body's inability to effectively release or eliminate heat.

Fever also may be classified as remittent, intermittent, sustained, relapsing, or undulant. *Remittent fever,* the most common type, is characterized by daily temperature fluctuations above the normal range. *Intermittent fever* is marked by a daily temperature drop into the normal range and then a rise back to above normal. An intermittent fever that fluctuates widely, typically producing chills and sweating, is called *hectic* (or *septic*) *fever.* *Sustained fever* involves persistent temperature elevation with little fluctuation. *Relapsing fever* consists of alternating feverish and afebrile periods. *Undulant fever* refers to a gradual increase in temperature that stays high for a few days and then decreases gradually.

How fever develops

Body temperature is regulated by the hypothalamic thermostat, which has a specific set point under normal conditions. Fever can result from a resetting of this set point or from an abnormality in the thermoregulatory system itself, as shown in this flowchart.

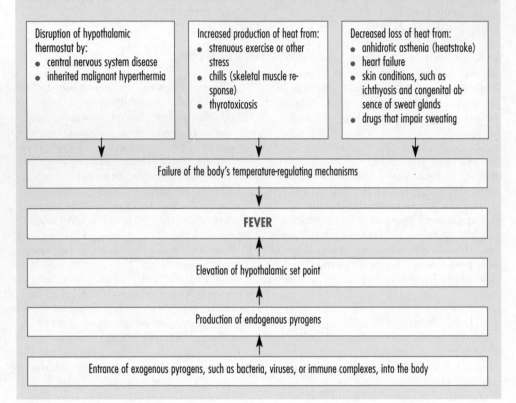

Disruption of hypothalamic thermostat by:
- central nervous system disease
- inherited malignant hyperthermia

Increased production of heat from:
- strenuous exercise or other stress
- chills (skeletal muscle response)
- thyrotoxicosis

Decreased loss of heat from:
- anhidrotic asthenia (heatstroke)
- heart failure
- skin conditions, such as ichthyosis and congenital absence of sweat glands
- drugs that impair sweating

Failure of the body's temperature-regulating mechanisms

FEVER

Elevation of hypothalamic set point

Production of endogenous pyrogens

Entrance of exogenous pyrogens, such as bacteria, viruses, or immune complexes, into the body

---

Fever can be either brief (less than 3 weeks) or prolonged. Prolonged fevers include fever of unknown origin, a classification used when careful examination fails to detect an underlying cause.

If you detect a fever higher than 103.1° F (39.5° C), take the patient's other vital signs and determine his level of consciousness (LOC). Give an antipyretic, and consider starting rapid cooling measures: Apply a cooling blanket, or use a convective cooling device such as a fan. To prevent shivering (which can increase metabolic demand) during cooling measures, use warmer temperatures that still provide a cooling effect.[1] These methods may evoke a cooling response; to prevent this, con-

stantly monitor the patient's rectal temperature.

History and physical examination

If the patient's fever is only mild to moderate, ask him when it began and how high his temperature reached. Did the fever disappear, only to reappear later? Did he experience any other symptoms, such as chills, fatigue, or pain?

Obtain a complete medical history, noting especially immunosuppressive treatments or disorders, infection, trauma, surgery, diagnostic testing, and use of anesthesia or other drugs. Ask about recent travel because certain diseases are endemic.

Let the history findings direct your physical examination. (See *Differential diagnosis: Fever,* pages 190 and 191.) Because fever can accompany diverse disorders, the examination may range from a brief evaluation of one body system to a comprehensive review of all systems.

Medical causes

▶ *Anthrax, cutaneous.* In this disorder, the patient may experience a fever along with lymphadenopathy, malaise, and headache. After the bacterium *Bacillus anthracis* enters a cut or abrasion on the skin, the infection begins as a small, painless or pruritic macular or papular lesion resembling an insect bite. Within 1 to 2 days, the lesion develops into a vesicle and then into a painless ulcer with a characteristic black necrotic center.

▶ *Anthrax, GI.* After ingesting contaminated meat from an animal infected with the bacterium *Bacillus anthracis,* the patient experiences fever, anorexia, nausea, vomiting and, possibly, abdominal pain, severe bloody diarrhea, and hematemesis.

▶ *Anthrax, inhalation.* This acute infectious disease initially produces flulike signs and symptoms, including fever, chills, weakness, cough, and chest pain. The disease generally occurs in two stages with a period of recovery after the initial symptoms. The second stage develops abruptly and causes rapid deterioration marked by fever, dyspnea, stridor, and hypotension; death generally results within 24 hours.

▶ *Avian influenza.* Avian influenza, also known as bird flu, is an infection caused by viruses that originate in the intestines of wild birds but are highly contagious to domesticated birds, such as chickens, turkeys, and geese. Infected poultry and surfaces contaminated with infected bird excretions have recently led to human infections and deaths in several Asian countries. Fever is commonly an initial symptom of these viruses along with other conventional influenza symptoms, such as muscle aches, sore throat, and cough. Individuals infected with the most virulent avian virus, influenza A (H5N1), may develop pneumonia, acute respiratory distress, and other life-threatening complications.

▶ *Escherichia coli O157:H7.* Fever, bloody diarrhea, nausea, vomiting, and abdominal cramps occur after eating undercooked beef or other foods contaminated with this strain of bacteria. Children younger than age 5 and elderly patients may develop hemolytic uremic syndrome, which can ultimately lead to acute renal failure.

▶ *Immune complex dysfunction.* When present, fever usually remains low, although moderate elevations may accompany erythema multiforme. Fever may be remittent or intermittent, as in acquired immunodeficiency syndrome (AIDS) or systemic lupus erythematosus, or sustained, as in polyarteritis. As one of several vague, prodromal complaints (such as fatigue, anorexia, and weight loss), fever produces nocturnal diaphoresis and accompanies such associated signs and symptoms as diarrhea and a persistent cough (in AIDS) or morning stiffness (in rheumatoid arthritis). Other disease-specific findings include headache and vision loss (in temporal arteritis); pain and stiffness in the neck, shoulders, back, or pelvis (in ankylosing spondylitis and polymyalgia rheumatica); skin and mucous membrane lesions (in erythema multiforme); and urethritis with urethral discharge and conjunctivitis (in Reiter's syndrome).

▶ *Infectious and inflammatory disorders.* Fever ranges from low (in Crohn's disease or ulcerative colitis) to extremely high (in those with bacterial pneumonia, necrotizing fasciitis, Ebola virus or *Hantavirus* pulmonary syndrome). It may be remittent, as in infectious mononucleosis or otitis media; hectic (recurring daily with sweating, chills, and flushing), as in a lung abscess, influenza, or endocarditis; sustained, as in meningitis; or relapsing, as in malaria. Fever may arise abruptly, as in toxic shock syndrome or Rocky Mountain spotted fever, or insidiously, as in mycoplasmal pneumonia. In patients with hepatitis, fever may represent a disease prodrome; in those with appendicitis, it follows the acute stage. Its sudden late appearance with tachycardia, tachypnea, and confusion heralds life-threatening septic shock in patients with peritonitis or gram-negative bacteremia.

Differential diagnosis: Fever

Patients with fever commonly experience fatigue, malaise, and anorexia. Additional symptoms can help you differentiate between these common causes of fever.

POSSIBLE CAUSES	ADDITIONAL SIGNS AND SYMPTOMS	DIAGNOSIS
Thermoregulatory dysfunction	• Sudden onset of fever that rises rapidly and remains high • Temperature that may rise to 107° F (41.7° C) • Vomiting • Anhidrosis • Decreased level of consciousness (LOC) • Hot, flushed skin • Tachycardia • Tachypnea • Hypotension	Patient history with additional signs or symptoms that would indicate source of thermoregulatory dysfunction (such as heatstroke, thyroid storm, neuroleptic malignant syndrome, malignant hyperthermia, lesions of the central nervous system)
Neoplasms	• Prolonged fever of varying elevations • Nocturnal diaphoresis • Weight loss • Lymphadenopathy • Palpable mass	Varies based on other signs and symptoms but usually includes imaging studies (computed tomography scan, magnetic resonance imaging)
Infection and inflammatory disorders	• Low or extremely high temperature that may be intermittent or sustained and may rise abruptly or insidiously • Chills • Diaphoresis • Weakness • Additional signs that may involve every system	Varies based on other signs and symptoms
Immune complex dysfunction	• Low-grade fever that may be remittent, intermittent, or sustained • Nocturnal diaphoresis	Varies based on other signs and symptoms
West Nile encephalitis	• Mild to moderate fever • Headache • Myalgia • Rash • Swollen lymph glands • Neck stiffness • Decreased LOC • Seizures	History of recent mosquito bite, West Nile activity reported in locality, blood culture

Other signs and symptoms involve every system. The cyclic variations of hectic fever typically produce alternating chills and diaphoresis. General systemic complaints include weakness, anorexia, and malaise.

▶ *Kawasaki syndrome.* Fever, typically high and spiking, is the primary characteristic of

TREATMENT AND FOLLOW-UP

- Cooling techniques to decrease temperature
- Treatment of cause
- Antipyretics

Follow-up: As needed (depending on cause of dysfunction)

- Varies with type and location of neoplasm but may include medication (antipyretics, chemotherapy), radiation therapy, and surgery

Follow-up: Referral to oncologist

- Varies with source of fever but usually includes antipyretics

Follow-up: As needed (depending on source of infection)

- Varies with specific cause of fever but usually includes antipyretics

Follow-up: As needed (depending on cause of fever)

- Supportive treatment
- Treatment of symptoms
- Medication (antipyretics, analgesics)

Follow-up: As needed (depending on severity of infection)

this acute illness. The diagnosis of Kawasaki syndrome is confirmed when fever persists for 5 or more days (or until administration of I.V. gamma globulin if given before the fifth day)

and is accompanied by other signs, including conjunctival injection, erythema, lymphadenopathy, and peripheral limb swelling. This syndrome occurs worldwide, with the highest incidence in Japan. It primarily affects children under age 5, is more prevalent in boys, and can cause serious heart damage and death without prompt treatment with I.V. gamma globulin.

▶ *Listeriosis.* Signs and symptoms of this infection include fever, myalgia, abdominal pain, nausea, vomiting, and diarrhea. If the infection spreads to the nervous system, it may cause meningitis, whose symptoms include fever, headache, nuchal rigidity, and change in LOC. Listeriosis during pregnancy may lead to premature delivery, infection of the neonate, or stillbirth.

▶ *Monkeypox.* Fever is one of the initial symptoms that occurs in almost all patients infected with this rare viral disease. A papular rash that may be localized or generalized appears within 1 to 3 days after the fever begins. Other symptoms commonly include sore throat, chills, and lymphadenopathy. There is no treatment for monkeypox, but the disease is rarely fatal in developed countries and usually lasts 2 to 4 weeks.

▶ *Neoplasms.* Primary neoplasms and metastases can produce prolonged fever of varying elevations. For instance, acute leukemia may manifest insidiously with a low fever, pallor, and bleeding tendencies, or more abruptly with a high fever, frank bleeding, and prostration. Occasionally, Hodgkin's disease produces undulant fever or Pel-Ebstein fever, an irregularly relapsing fever.

Besides fever and nocturnal diaphoresis, neoplastic disease commonly causes anorexia, fatigue, malaise, and weight loss. Examination may reveal lesions, lymphadenopathy, palpable masses, and hepatosplenomegaly.

▶ *Plague.* Caused by *Yersinia pestis,* plague is one of the most virulent bacterial infections known. The bubonic form of plague is transmitted to man from the bite of infected fleas and causes fever, chills, and swollen, inflamed, and tender lymph nodes near the site of the bite. Septicemic plague may develop as a complication of untreated bubonic or pneumonic plague, and occurs when bacteria enter the bloodstream and multiply. Pneumonic plague manifests as a sudden onset of chills, fever, headache, and myalgia after person-to-person transmission by respiratory droplets. Other signs and symptoms of the pneumonic form include a productive cough, chest pain, tachypnea, dyspnea, hemoptysis, increasing respiratory distress, and cardiopulmonary insufficiency.

▶ *Q fever.* This rickettsial disease caused by *Coxiella burnetii* causes fever (which may last up to 2 weeks), chills, severe headache, malaise, chest pain, nausea, vomiting, and diarrhea. In severe cases, the patient may develop hepatitis or pneumonia.

▶ *Respiratory syncytial virus (RSV).* Fever is one of the initial symptoms of this common illness that affects most children by age 2. Healthy adults and children older than age 3 usually develop a low-grade fever along with other common coldlike symptoms of runny nose, cough, and wheezing. Many children younger than age 3 have a high-grade fever and possibly a severe cough, rapid breathing, and high-pitched expiratory wheezing. Infants with RSV typically have lethargy, poor eating, irritability, and trouble breathing; severe cases may require hospitalization. To avoid repeated RSV infection, parents and caregivers should practice infection-control techniques, such as proper hand-washing and avoiding contact with contaminated surfaces.

▶ *Rhabdomyolysis.* This disorder results in muscle breakdown and release of the muscle cell contents (myoglobin) into the bloodstream. Signs and symptoms include fever, muscle weakness or pain, nausea, vomiting, malaise, and dark urine. Acute renal failure, the most common complication rhabdomyolysis, results from renal structure obstruction and injury during the kidneys' attempt to filter the myoglobin from the bloodstream.

▶ *Rift Valley fever.* Typical signs and symptoms of this infection include fever, myalgia, weakness, dizziness, and back pain. A small percentage of patients may develop encephalitis or may progress to hemorrhagic fever that can lead to shock and hemorrhage. Inflammation of the retina may result in some permanent vision loss.

▶ *Severe acute respiratory syndrome (SARS).* SARS is an acute infectious disease of unknown etiology; however, a novel coronavirus has been implicated as a possible cause. Although most cases have been reported in Asia (China, Vietnam, Singapore, Thailand), cases have cropped up in Europe and North America. After an incubation period of 2 to 7 days, the illness generally begins with a fever (usually greater than 100.4° F [38° C]). Other symptoms include headache, malaise, a nonproductive cough, and dyspnea. SARS may produce only mild symptoms, or it may progress to pneumonia and, in some cases, even respiratory failure and death.

▶ *Smallpox (variola major).* Initial signs and symptoms of this virus include high fever, malaise, prostration, severe headache, backache, and abdominal pain. A maculopapular rash develops on the mucosa of the mouth, pharynx, face, and forearms and then spreads to the trunk and legs. Within 2 days, the rash becomes vesicular and later pustular. The lesions develop at the same time, appear identical, and are more prominent on the face and limbs. The pustules are round, firm, and deeply embedded in the skin. After 8 or 9 days, they form a crust, which later separates from the skin, leaving a pitted scar. Death may result from encephalitis, extensive bleeding, or secondary infection.

▶ *Thermoregulatory dysfunction.* Sudden onset of fever that rises rapidly and remains as high as 107° F (41.7° C) occurs in life-threatening disorders, such as heatstroke, thyroid storm, neuroleptic malignant syndrome, and malignant hyperthermia, and in lesions of the central nervous system (CNS). A low or moderate fever occurs in dehydrated patients.

Prolonged high fever commonly produces vomiting, anhidrosis, decreased level of consciousness (LOC), and hot, flushed skin. Related cardiovascular effects may include tachycardia, tachypnea, and hypotension. Other disease-specific findings include skin changes (dry skin and mucous membranes, poor skin turgor) and oliguria in dehydration; mottled cyanosis in malignant hyperthermia; diarrhea in thyroid storm; and ominous signs of increased intracranial pressure (decreased LOC with bradycardia, widened pulse pressure, and increased systolic pressure) in CNS tumor, trauma, or hemorrhage.

▶ *Tularemia.* This infectious disease, also known as "rabbit fever," causes abrupt onset of fever, chills, headache, generalized myalgia, nonproductive cough, dyspnea, pleuritic chest pain, and empyema.

▶ *Typhus.* In this rickettsial disease, the patient initially experiences headache, myalgia, arthralgia, and malaise. These symptoms are followed by an abrupt onset of fever, chills, nausea, vomiting, and—in some cases—a maculopapular rash.

▶ *West Nile encephalitis.* This brain infection is caused by West Nile virus, a mosquito-borne flavivirus commonly found in Africa, West Asia, and the Middle East and rarely in North America. Most patients have mild signs and symptoms, including fever, headache, body aches, rash, and swollen lymph glands. More severe infection is marked by high fever, headache, neck stiffness, stupor, disorientation, coma, tremors and, occasionally, paralysis or seizures. Death rarely occurs.

Other causes

▶ *Diagnostic tests.* Immediate or delayed fever occasionally follows radiographic tests that use a contrast medium.

DRUG WATCH *Fever and rash commonly result from hypersensitivity to antifungals, sulfonamides, penicillins, cephalosporins, tetracyclines, barbiturates, phenytoin, quinidine, iodides, methyldopa, procainamide, and some antitoxins. Fever can accompany chemotherapy, especially with bleomycin, vincristine, and asparaginase. It can result from drugs that impair sweating, such as anticholinergics, phenothiazines, and monoamine oxidase inhibitors. A drug-induced fever typically disappears after the drug is discontinued. Fever can also stem from toxic doses of salicylates, amphetamines, and tricyclic antidepressants.*

Inhaled anesthetics and muscle relaxants can trigger malignant hyperthermia in patients with this inherited trait.

▶ *Treatments.* A remittent or intermittent low fever may occur for several days after surgery. Transfusion reactions characteristically produce an abrupt onset of fever and chills.

Special considerations

Regularly monitor the patient's temperature, and record it on a chart for easy follow-up of the temperature curve. Temperature can be most accurately measured orally, rectally, or via external auditory canal; axillary temperatures should be avoided because they are not as accurate as other methods.[1] (See *Effectiveness of body temperature monitoring methods,* page 194.) In critically ill patients, the most accurate sites for temperature measurement are the pulmonary artery and the bladder through the use of a thermistor.[1] Provide increased fluid and nutritional intake. Give antipyretics (acetaminophen, NSAIDs) for a fever greater than 102.2° F (39° C). When giving a prescribed antipyretic, minimize chills and diaphoresis by following a regular dosage schedule. Promote patient comfort by maintaining a stable room temperature and providing frequent changes of bedding and clothing. Prepare the patient for laboratory tests, such as complete blood count and cultures of blood, urine, sputum, and wound drainage.

Pediatric pointers

Infants and young children experience higher and more prolonged fevers, more rapid temperature increases, and greater temperature fluctuations than older children and adults.

Keep in mind that seizures commonly accompany extremely high fever, so take appropriate precautions. Also, instruct parents not to give aspirin to a child with varicella or flu-like symptoms because of the risk of precipitating Reye's syndrome.

Common pediatric causes of fever include varicella, croup syndrome, dehydration, meningitis, mumps, otitis media, pertussis, roseola infantum, rubella, rubeola, and tonsillitis. Fever can also occur as a reaction to immunizations and antibiotics.

Alternating antipyretic drugs, such as acetaminophen and ibuprofen, may be more effective in reducing fever in children than using a single drug.[2]

Geriatric pointers

Elderly people may have an altered sweating mechanism that predisposes them to heatstroke when exposed to high temperatures; they may also have an impaired thermoregulatory mechanism, making temperature change a much less reliable measure of disease severity.

EVIDENCE-BASED PRACTICE

Effectiveness of body temperature monitoring methods

Question: *Are there significant differences between left tympanic temperature, right tympanic temperature, and oral temperature?*

Research: Accurate body temperature monitoring provides valuable information that impacts patient care. Inaccurate measurements can lead to diagnostic and treatment errors. In this study, the convenience sample consisted of 66 patients at an urban hospital in the central United States. Subjects were ages 19 to 96.

Both tympanic temperatures were measured 2 minutes apart. Oral temperature was measured using an electronic device placed in the posterior sublingual pocket. All measurements were documented on a data collection sheet designed to gather pertinent data, such as the presence of a hearing aid, oxygen, or a fan; if the patient's ear was down against a pillow or up; and the room temperature.

Conclusion: Analysis of the data revealed a significant difference between the left tympanic

temperature and the oral temperature. Of note, there was no consistency regarding one ear always having the lowest temperature and the other being higher when the ear was against the pillow.

Application: To effectively track changes in temperature, choose the optimal site for each patient and use that site consistently. Ensure that all staff members using tympanic thermometers are properly trained to use the device and that the thermometers are calibrated as recommended by the manufacturer.

Source: Spitzer, O. P. "Comparing Tympanic Temperatures in Both Ears to Oral Temperature in the Critically Ill Adult." *Dimensions of Critical Care Nursing,* 27(1):24-29, 2008.

Patient counseling

If the patient has not been admitted to the hospital, ask him to measure his oral temperature at home and record the time and value. Explain to him that fever is a response to an underlying condition and that it plays an important role in fighting infection. For this reason, advise him not to take an antipyretic until his body temperature reaches 101° F (38.3° C).

REFERENCES

1. Henker, R. and Carlson, K.K. "Fever: Applying Research to Bedside Practice." *AACN Advanced Critical Care* 18(1):76-87, January/March 2007.
2. Sarrell, E.M., Wieliensky, E., and Cohen, H.A. "Antipyretic Treatment in Young Children with Fever: Acetaminophen, Ibuprofen, or Both Alternating in a Randomized Double-Blind Study." *Archives of Pediatrics and Adolescent Medicine* 160(2):197-202, February 2006.

● FLANK PAIN

Pain in the flank, the area extending from the ribs to the ilium, is a leading indicator of renal and upper urinary tract disease or trauma. Depending on the cause, this symptom may vary from a dull ache to severe stabbing or throbbing pain, and may be unilateral or bilateral and constant or intermittent. It's aggravated by costovertebral angle (CVA) percussion and, in patients with renal or urinary tract obstruction, by increased fluid intake and ingestion of alcohol, caffeine, or diuretics. Unaffected by position changes, flank pain typically responds only to analgesics or, of course, to treatment of the underlying disorder.

If the patient sustained trauma, quickly look for a visible or palpable flank mass, related injuries, CVA pain, hematuria, Turner's sign, and signs of shock (such as tachycardia and cool, clammy skin). If one or more of these signs is present, insert an I.V. line to allow fluid or drug infusion. Insert an indwelling urinary catheter to monitor urine output and evaluate hematuria. Obtain blood samples for typing and crossmatching, complete blood count, and electrolyte levels.

History and physical examination

If the patient's condition isn't critical, take a thorough history. Ask about the pain's onset and apparent precipitating events. Have him describe the pain's location, intensity, pattern, and duration. Find out if anything aggravates or alleviates it.

Ask the patient about any changes in his normal pattern of fluid intake and urine output. Explore his history for urinary tract infection (UTI) or obstruction, renal disease, or recent streptococcal infection.

During the physical examination, palpate the patient's flank area and percuss the CVA to determine the extent of pain.

Medical causes

▶ *Abdominal aortic aneurysm, ruptured or dissected.* Severe flank pain may occur. Other signs and symptoms include severe abdominal or back pain, hematuria, a pulsating abdominal mass, and hypertension.[1] Shock is a late sign.

▶ *Bladder cancer.* Dull, constant flank pain may be unilateral or bilateral and may radiate to the leg, back, and perineum. Commonly, the first sign of bladder cancer is gross, painless, intermittent hematuria, often with clots. Related effects may include urinary frequency and urgency, nocturia, dysuria, or pyuria; bladder distention; pain in the bladder, rectum, pelvis, back, or legs; diarrhea; vomiting; and sleep disturbances.

▶ *Calculi.* Renal and ureteral calculi produce intense unilateral, colicky flank pain. Typically, initial CVA pain radiates to the flank, suprapubic region, and perhaps the genitalia; abdominal and low back pain are also possible. Nausea and vomiting commonly accompany severe pain. Associated findings include CVA tenderness, hematuria, hypoactive bowel sounds and, possibly, signs and symptoms of UTI (urinary frequency and urgency, dysuria,

nocturia, fatigue, low-grade fever, and tenesmus).

▶ *Cortical necrosis (acute).* Unilateral flank pain is usually severe in this disorder. Accompanying findings include gross hematuria, anuria, leukocytosis, and fever.

▶ *Cystitis (bacterial).* Unilateral or bilateral flank pain occurs secondarily to an ascending UTI in bacterial cystitis. The patient may also report perineal, low back, and suprapubic pain. Other effects include dysuria, nocturia, hematuria, urinary frequency and urgency, tenesmus, fatigue, and low-grade fever.

▶ *Glomerulonephritis (acute).* Flank pain in patients with this disorder is bilateral, constant, and of moderate intensity. The most common findings are moderate facial and generalized edema, hematuria, oliguria or anuria, and fatigue. Additional effects include slightly increased blood pressure, low-grade fever, malaise, headache, nausea, and vomiting. Other signs of pulmonary congestion include dyspnea, tachypnea, and crackles.

▶ *Obstructive uropathy.* In an acute obstruction, flank pain may be excruciating; in a gradual obstruction, it's typically a dull ache. In both types, the pain may also localize in the upper abdomen and radiate to the groin. Nausea and vomiting, abdominal distention, anuria alternating with periods of oliguria and polyuria, and hypoactive bowel sounds may also occur. Additional findings—a palpable abdominal mass, CVA tenderness, and bladder distention—vary with the site and cause of the obstruction.

▶ *Pancreatitis (acute).* Bilateral flank pain may develop as severe epigastric or left-upper-quadrant pain radiates to the back. A severe attack causes extreme pain, nausea and persistent vomiting, abdominal tenderness and rigidity, hypoactive bowel sounds and, possibly, restlessness, low-grade fever, tachycardia, hypotension, and positive Turner's and Cullen's signs.

▶ *Papillary necrosis (acute).* In this disorder, intense bilateral flank pain occurs with renal colic, CVA tenderness, and abdominal pain and rigidity. Urinary signs and symptoms— oliguria or anuria, hematuria, and pyuria— are associated with high fever, chills, vomiting, and hypoactive bowel sounds.

▶ *Perirenal abscess.* Intense unilateral flank pain and CVA tenderness accompany dysuria, persistent high fever, chills and, in some patients, a palpable abdominal mass.

▶ *Polycystic kidney disease.* Dull, aching, bilateral flank pain is commonly the earliest symptom of this renal disorder. The pain can become severe and colicky if cysts rupture and clots migrate or cause an obstruction. Nonspecific early findings include polyuria, increased blood pressure, and signs and symptoms of UTI. Later findings include hematuria and perineal, low back, and suprapubic pain.

▶ *Pyelonephritis (acute).* Intense, constant, unilateral or bilateral flank pain develops over a few hours or days along with typical urinary features: dysuria, nocturia, hematuria, urgency, frequency, and tenesmus. Other common findings include persistent high fever, chills, anorexia, weakness, fatigue, generalized myalgia, abdominal pain, and marked CVA tenderness.

▶ *Renal cancer.* Unilateral flank pain, gross hematuria, and a palpable flank mass form the classic clinical triad in renal cancer. Flank pain is usually dull and vague, although severe colicky pain can occur during bleeding or passage of clots. Associated signs and symptoms include fever, increased blood pressure, and urine retention. Weight loss, leg edema, nausea, and vomiting are indications of advanced disease.

▶ *Renal infarction.* Unilateral, constant, severe flank pain and tenderness typically accompany persistent, severe upper abdominal pain in this disorder. The patient may also develop CVA tenderness, anorexia, nausea and vomiting, fever, hypoactive bowel sounds, hematuria, and oliguria or anuria.

▶ *Renal trauma.* Variable bilateral or unilateral flank pain, a visible or palpable flank mass, and CVA or abdominal pain (which may be severe and radiate to the groin) are common findings in renal trauma. Other findings include hematuria, oliguria, abdominal distention, Turner's sign, hypoactive bowel sounds, and nausea and vomiting. Severe injury may produce signs of shock, such as tachycardia and cool, clammy skin.

▶ *Renal vein thrombosis.* Severe unilateral flank and low back pain with CVA and epigastric tenderness typify the rapid onset of venous obstruction. Other features include fever, hematuria, and leg edema. Bilateral flank pain, oliguria, and other uremic signs and symptoms (nausea, vomiting, and uremic fetor) typify bilateral obstruction.

Other causes

▶ *Treatments.* Flank pain can be a sign of an acute hemolytic transfusion reaction, which occurs when a patient is administered a blood product that's incompatible with his own.[2] Other signs and symptoms include fever, chills, diaphoresis, and a sense of impending doom.

Special considerations

Give analgesics. Continue to monitor the patient's vital signs, and maintain a precise record of the patient's intake and output.

Diagnostic evaluation may involve serial urine and serum analysis, excretory urography, flank ultrasonography, computed tomography scan, voiding cystourethrography, cystoscopy, and retrograde ureteropyelography, urethrography, and cystography.

Pediatric pointers

Assessment of flank pain can be difficult if a child can't describe the pain. In such cases, transillumination of the abdomen and flanks may help to detect bladder distention and identify masses. Common causes of flank pain in children include obstructive uropathy, acute poststreptococcal glomerulonephritis, infantile polycystic kidney disease, and nephroblastoma.

Patient counseling

Provide information on the importance of increased fluid intake, unless contraindicated. Explain signs and symptoms that are imperative to report. Emphasize the importance of taking drugs as prescribed. Stress the importance of keeping follow-up appointments.

REFERENCES
1. Gendreau-Webb, R. "Is It a Kidney Stone or Abdominal Aortic Aneurysm?" *Nursing* 36(5) ED Insider: 22-24, Spring 2006.
2. Kyles, D. "Is Your Patient Having a Transfusion Reaction?" *Nursing* 37(4):64hn1-64hn4, April 2007.

G

GAG REFLEX, ABNORMAL

The gag reflex, or *pharyngeal reflex,* is a protective mechanism that prevents aspiration of food, fluid, and vomitus. It normally can be elicited by touching the posterior wall of the oropharynx with a tongue depressor or by suctioning the throat. Prompt elevation of the palate, constriction of the pharyngeal musculature, and a sensation of gagging indicate a normal gag reflex. An abnormal— decreased or absent—gag reflex interferes with the ability to swallow and, more important, increases the risk of life-threatening aspiration.

An impaired gag reflex can result from any lesion that affects its mediators: cranial nerves IX (glossopharyngeal) and X (vagus), the pons, or the medulla. It also can occur during a coma, in muscle diseases such as severe myasthenia gravis, or as a temporary result of anesthesia.

If you detect an abnormal gag reflex, immediately stop the patient's oral intake to prevent aspiration. Quickly evaluate his level of consciousness (LOC). If it's decreased, place him in a side-lying position to prevent aspiration; if not, place him in Fowler's position. Keep suction equipment at hand.

History and physical examination

Ask the patient (or a family member if the patient can't communicate) about the onset and duration of swallowing difficulties, if any. Are liquids more difficult to swallow than solids? Is swallowing more difficult at certain times of the day (as occurs in the bulbar palsy associated with myasthenia gravis)? If the patient also has trouble chewing, suspect more widespread neurologic involvement because chewing involves different cranial nerves.

Explore the patient's medical history for vascular and degenerative disorders. Then assess his respiratory status for evidence of aspiration, and perform a neurologic examination. Assess the patient's gag reflex by lightly stimulating each side of the back of the throat and noting the response.[1]

Medical causes

▶ *Basilar artery occlusion.* This disorder may suddenly diminish or obliterate the gag reflex. It also causes diffuse sensory loss, dysarthria, facial weakness, extraocular muscle palsies, quadriplegia, and decreased LOC.

▶ *Brain stem glioma.* This lesion causes gradual loss of the gag reflex. Related symptoms reflect bilateral brain stem involvement and include diplopia and facial weakness. Involvement of the corticospinal pathways causes spasticity and paresis of the arms and legs as well as gait disturbances.

▶ *Bulbar palsy.* Loss of the gag reflex reflects temporary or permanent paralysis of muscles supplied by cranial nerves IX and X. Other indicators of this paralysis include jaw and facial muscle weakness, dysphagia, loss of sensation at the base of the tongue, increased salivation, fasciculations and, possibly, trouble articulating and breathing.

▶ *Myasthenia gravis.* In severe myasthenia, the motor limb of the gag reflex is reduced.

Weakness worsens with repetitive use and also may involve other muscles.

▶ *Wallenberg's syndrome.* Paresis of the palate and an impaired gag reflex usually develop within hours to days of thrombosis. The patient may have analgesia and thermanesthesia, occurring ipsilaterally on the face and contralaterally on the body, as well as vertigo. He also may have nystagmus, ipsilateral ataxia of the arm and leg, and signs of Horner's syndrome (unilateral ptosis and miosis, hemifacial anhidrosis).

Other causes

▶ *Anesthesia.* General and local (throat) anesthesia can produce temporary loss of the gag reflex.

Special considerations

Continually assess the patient's ability to swallow. If his gag reflex is absent, provide tube feedings; if it's merely diminished, try pureed foods. Advise the patient to take small amounts and eat slowly while sitting or in high Fowler's position. Stay with him while he eats, and watch for choking. Remember to keep suction equipment handy in case of aspiration. Keep accurate intake and output records, and assess the patient's nutritional status daily.

Refer the patient to a therapist to determine his aspiration risk and develop an exercise program to strengthen specific muscles.

Prepare the patient for diagnostic studies, such as swallow studies, computed tomography scan, magnetic resonance imaging, EEG, lumbar puncture, and arteriography.

Pediatric pointers

Brain stem glioma is an important cause of abnormal gag reflex in children. Children with neurodevelopmental disabilities may have an absent, weakened, or hyperactive gag reflex.[2] A weak or absent gag reflex also may occur in infant botulism, along with hypotonia, lethargy, and poor feeding.[3]

Patient counseling

Discuss diet and fluid restrictions and positioning requirements related to food and liquid consumption. Encourage the family to consider taking a course that will teach techniques to relieve an airway obstruction. If speech therapy is indicated, encourage the patient to begin as soon as possible and follow through with the suggestions and ongoing therapy. Teach the family about aspiration pneumonia and how to prevent it.

REFERENCES

1. "Assessing the Cranial Nerves." *Nursing* 36(11):47-49, Novemeber 2006.
2. Crisp, C.L. "Nasogastric Tube Insertion in a Child With Neurodevelopmental Disabilities: Size Does Matter: A Case Study." *Gastroenterology Nursing* 29(2):108-110, March/April 2006.
3. Clemmens, M.R. and Bell, L. "Infant Botulism Presenting with Poor Feeding and Lethargy: A Review of 4 Cases." *Pediatric Emergency Care* 23(7):492-494, July 2007.

GALLOP, ATRIAL

An atrial (or presystolic) gallop is an extra heart sound (known as S_4) that's heard or commonly palpated immediately before the first heart sound, late in diastole. This low-pitched sound is heard best with the bell of the stethoscope pressed lightly against the cardiac apex. Some clinicians say that an S_4 has the cadence of the "Ten" in Tennessee (Ten = S_4; nes = S_1; see = S_2).[1,2]

An atrial gallop typically results from hypertension, conduction defects, valvular disorders, heart failure, or other problems such as ischemia. Occasionally, it helps differentiate angina from other causes of chest pain. It results from abnormal forceful atrial contraction caused by resistance to ventricular filling or by decreased left ventricular compliance. An atrial gallop usually originates from left atrial contraction, is heard at the apex, and doesn't vary with inspiration. A left-sided S_4 can occur in hypertensive heart disease, coronary artery disease, aortic stenosis, and cardiomyopathy. It also may originate from right atrial contraction. A right-sided S_4 indicates pulmonary hypertension and pulmonary stenosis. It's heard best at the lower left sternal border and intensifies with inspiration.[3]

Locating heart sounds

When auscultating heart sounds, remember that certain sounds are heard best in specific areas. Use the auscultatory points shown here to locate heart sounds quickly and accurately. Then expand your auscultation to nearby areas. Note that the numbers indicate pertinent intercostal spaces.

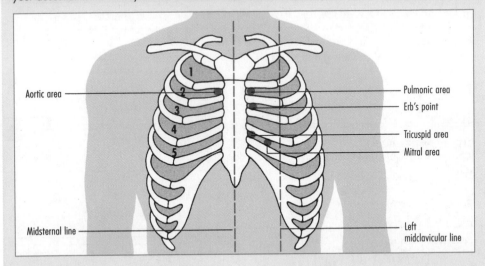

Aortic area

Pulmonic area

Erb's point

Tricuspid area

Mitral area

Midsternal line

Left midclavicular line

An atrial gallop seldom occurs in normal hearts; however, it may occur in elderly people and in athletes with physiologic hypertrophy of the left ventricle.

Suspect myocardial ischemia if you auscultate an atrial gallop in a patient with chest pain. (See *Locating heart sounds*, and *Interpreting heart sounds*, pages 200 and 201.) Take the patient's vital signs and quickly assess for signs of heart failure, such as dyspnea, crackles, and distended jugular veins. If you detect these signs, connect the patient to a cardiac monitor and obtain an electrocardiogram. Give an antianginal and oxygen. If the patient has dyspnea, elevate the head of the bed. Then auscultate for abnormal breath sounds. If you detect coarse crackles, ensure patent I.V. access and give oxygen and diuretics as needed. If the patient has bradycardia, he may require atropine and a pacemaker.

History and physical examination

When the patient's condition permits, ask about a history of hypertension, angina,

valvular stenosis, or cardiomyopathy. If appropriate, have him describe the frequency and severity of anginal attacks.

Medical causes

▶ *Anemia.* In this disorder, an atrial gallop may accompany increased cardiac output. Other findings may include fatigue, pallor, dyspnea, tachycardia, bounding pulse, crackles, and a systolic bruit over the carotid arteries.

▶ *Angina.* An intermittent atrial gallop characteristically occurs during an anginal attack and disappears when angina subsides. This gallop may be accompanied by a paradoxical second heart sound (S_2) or a new murmur. Typically, the patient complains of anginal chest pain—a feeling of tightness, pressure, achiness, or burning that usually radiates from the retrosternal area to the neck, jaws, left shoulder, and arm. He also may exhibit dyspnea, tachycardia, palpitations, increased blood pressure, dizziness, diaphoresis, belching, nausea, and vomiting.

Interpreting heart sounds

Detecting subtle variations in heart sounds requires both concentration and practice. Once you recognize normal heart sounds, the abnormal sounds become more obvious.

HEART SOUND AND CAUSE	TIMING AND CADENCE
First heart sound (S_1) Vibrations associated with mitral and tricuspid valve closure	systole diastole systole diastole S_1 S_2 S_1 S_2 S_1 LUB dub LUB dub
Second heart sound (S_2) Vibrations associated with aortic and pulmonic valve closure	systole diastole systole diastole S_1 S_2 S_1 S_2 S_1 lub DUB lub DUB
Ventricular gallop (S_3) Vibrations produced by rapid blood flow into the ventricles	systole diastole systole diastole S_1 $S_2 S_3$ S_1 $S_2 S_3$ S_1 lub dubDEE lub dubDEE ken tucKY ken tucKY
Atrial gallop (S_4) Vibrations produced by an increased resistance to sudden, forceful ejection of atrial blood	systole diastole systole diastole S_1 S_2 $S_4 S_1$ S_2 $S_4 S_1$ DEElub dub DEElub TENnes see TENnes
Summation gallop Vibrations produced in middiastole by simultaneous ventricular and atrial gallops, usually caused by tachycardia	systole diastole systole diastole systole S_1 $S_2 S_3 S_4 S_1$ $S_2 S_3 S_4 S_1$ $S_2 S_3 S_4$

▶ *Aortic insufficiency (acute).* This disorder causes an atrial gallop accompanied by a soft, short diastolic murmur along the left sternal border. S_2 may be soft or absent. Sometimes a soft, short midsystolic murmur may be heard over the second right intercostal space. Related cardiopulmonary findings may include tachycardia, a ventricular gallop (S_3), dyspnea, jugular vein distention, crackles and, possibly, angina. The patient also may be fatigued and have cool extremities.
▶ *Aortic stenosis.* This disorder usually causes an atrial gallop, especially if valvular obstruction is severe. Auscultation reveals a

AUSCULTATION TIPS

Best heard with the diaphragm of the stethoscope at the apex (mitral area).

Best heard with the diaphragm of the stethoscope in the second or third right and left parasternal intercostal spaces with the patient sitting or in a supine position.

Best heard through the bell of the stethoscope at the apex with the patient in the left lateral position. May be visible and palpable during early diastole at the midclavicular line between the fourth and fifth intercostal spaces.

Best heard through the bell of the stethoscope at the apex with the patient in the left semilateral position. May be visible in late diastole at the midclavicular line between the fourth and fifth intercostal spaces. May also be palpable in the midclavicular area with the patient in the left lateral decubitus position.

Best heard through the bell of the stethoscope at the apex with the patient in the left lateral position. May be louder than S_1 or S_2. May be visible and palpable during diastole.

harsh, crescendo-decrescendo, systolic ejection murmur that's loudest at the right sternal border near the second intercostal space. Dyspnea, angina, and syncope are other cardinal findings. The patient also may have crackles, palpitations, fatigue, and diminished carotid pulses.

▶ *Atrioventricular (AV) block.* First-degree AV block may cause an atrial gallop accompanied by a faint first heart sound (S_1). Although the patient may have bradycardia, he's usually asymptomatic. In second-degree AV block, an atrial gallop is easily heard. If bradycardia develops, the patient also may have hypotension, light-headedness, dizziness, and fatigue. An atrial gallop is also common in third-degree AV block. It varies in intensity with S_1 and is loudest when atrial systole coincides with early, rapid ventricular filling during diastole. The patient with third-degree AV block may be asymptomatic or have hypotension, light-headedness, dizziness, or syncope, depending on the ventricular rate. Bradycardia also may aggravate or provoke angina or symptoms of heart failure such as dyspnea.

▶ *Cardiomyopathy.* An atrial gallop may reflect all types of cardiomyopathy—dilated (most common), hypertrophic, or restrictive (least common).[4] Other findings may include dyspnea, orthopnea, crackles, fatigue, syncope, chest pain, palpitations, edema, jugular vein distention, a ventricular gallop, and transient or sustained bradycardia that's usually associated with tachycardia.

▶ *Hypertension.* One of the earliest findings in systemic arterial hypertension is an atrial gallop. The patient may be asymptomatic, or he may have headache, weakness, epistaxis, tinnitus, dizziness, and fatigue.

▶ *Mitral insufficiency.* In acute mitral insufficiency, auscultation may reveal an atrial gallop accompanied by an S_3, a ventricular gallop that's heard best at the apex or over the precordium. This murmur radiates to the axilla and back and along the left sternal border. Other features may include fatigue, dyspnea, tachypnea, orthopnea, tachycardia, crackles, and jugular vein distention.

▶ *Myocardial infarction (MI).* An atrial gallop is a classic sign of life-threatening MI; in fact, it may persist even after the infarction heals. Typically, the patient reports crushing substernal chest pain that may radiate to the back, neck, jaw, shoulder, and left arm. Other signs and symptoms include dyspnea, restlessness, anxiety, a feeling of impending doom, diaphoresis, pallor, clammy skin, nausea, vomiting, and increased or decreased blood pressure.

▶ *Pulmonary embolism.* This life-threatening disorder causes a right-sided atrial gallop that's usually heard along the lower left sternal border with a loud pulmonic closure sound. Other features include tachycardia, tachypnea, fever, chest pain, dyspnea, decreased breath sounds, crackles, a pleural friction rub, apprehension, diaphoresis, syncope, and cyanosis. The patient may have a productive cough with blood-tinged sputum or a nonproductive cough.

▶ *Thyrotoxicosis.* This disorder may produce atrial and ventricular gallops. Its cardinal features include an enlarged thyroid gland, tachycardia, bounding pulse, widened pulse pressure, palpitations, weight loss despite increased appetite, diarrhea, tremors, dyspnea, nervousness, difficulty concentrating, diaphoresis, heat intolerance, exophthalmos, weakness, fatigue, and muscle atrophy.

Special considerations
Prepare the patient for diagnostic tests, such as electrocardiography, echocardiography, cardiac catheterization, CT angiogram, laboratory tests such as creatine kinase-MB and, possibly, a lung scan.

Pediatric pointers
An atrial gallop may occur normally in children, especially after exercise. However, it also may result from congenital heart defects, such as atrial septal defect, ventricular septal defect, patent ductus arteriosus, and severe pulmonary valvular stenosis.

Geriatric pointers
Because the absolute intensity of an atrial gallop doesn't decrease with age, as it does with an S_1, the relative intensity of S_4 increases compared with S_1. This explains the increased frequency of an audible S_4 in elderly patients and why this sound may be considered a normal finding in older patients.

Patient counseling
Inform the patient about ways to reduce his cardiac risks. Teach him the correct way to measure his pulse rate. Emphasize conditions that require medical attention. Stress the importance of follow-up appointments.

REFERENCES
1. Quigley, P. "Valve Jobs Aren't Just for '57 Chevys: Expertly Sorting through the Various Types of Valvular Disorders." *Nursing Made Incredibly Easy!* 3(3):20-35, May/June 2005.
2. "Now Hear This: How to Identify Heart Sounds." *LPN* 3(1):5-7, January/February 2007.
3. Jacobs, M. and Meyer, T. "The Push Is On in Pulmonary Hypertension." *Nursing Made Incredibly Easy!* 4(3):42-52, May/June 2006.
4. Bruce, J. "Getting to the Heart of Cardiomyopathies." *Nursing* 36(Cardiac Insider):16-20, Spring 2006.

GENITAL LESIONS IN MALE PATIENTS

Among the diverse lesions that may affect the male genitals are warts, papules, ulcers, scales, and pustules. These common lesions may be painful or painless, singular or multiple. They may be limited to the genitals, or they also may occur elsewhere on the body. (See *Recognizing common male genital lesions.*)

Genital lesions may result from infection, neoplasms, parasites, allergy, or the effects of drugs. They can profoundly affect the patient's self-image and relationships. In fact, the patient may hesitate to seek medical attention because he fears cancer or a sexually transmitted infection (STI).

Genital lesions that arise from an STI could mean that the patient is at risk for human immunodeficiency virus (HIV) infection. Genital ulcers make HIV transmission between sexual partners more likely. Unfortunately, if the patient is treating himself, he may alter the lesions, making differential diagnosis especially difficult.

It is important to note that denial, embarrassment, fear, and other factors cause many men to delay seeking treatment for genital lesions. Therefore, the lesions may become quite extensive by the time the patient seeks care.[1]

Recognizing common male genital lesions

A wide variety of lesions may affect the male genitalia. Some of the more common ones and their causes appear below.

Penile cancer causes a painless ulcerative lesion on the glans or foreskin, possibly with a foul-smelling discharge.

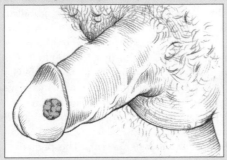

A **fixed drug eruption** causes a bright red to purplish lesion on the glans penis.

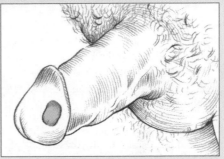

Genital warts are marked by clusters of flesh-colored papillary growths that may be barely visible or several inches in diameter.

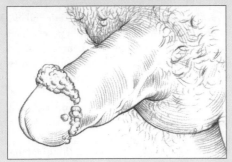

Genital herpes begins as a swollen, slightly pruritic wheal and later becomes a group of small vesicles or blisters on the foreskin, glans, or penile shaft.

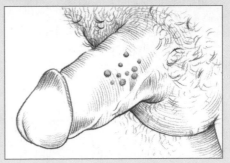

Tinea cruris (commonly known as *jock itch*) produces itchy patches of well-defined, slightly raised, scaly lesions that usually affect the inner thighs and groin.

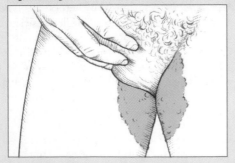

Chancroid causes a painful ulcer that's usually less than 2 cm in diameter and bleeds easily. The lesion may be deep and covered by a gray or yellow exudate at its base.

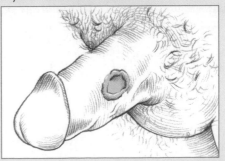

History and physical examination

Begin by asking the patient when he first noticed the lesion. Did it erupt after he began taking a new drug or after a trip out of the country? Has he had similar lesions before? If so, did he get medical treatment for them? Find out if he has been treating the lesion himself. If so, how? Does the lesion itch? If so, is the itching constant or does it bother him only at night? Note whether the lesion is painful. Ask for a description of any drainage from the lesion. Next, take a complete sexual history, noting the frequency of relations, the number of sexual partners, and the pattern of condom use.

Before you examine the patient, observe his clothing. Do his pants fit properly? Tight pants or underwear, especially those made of nonabsorbent fabrics, can promote the growth of bacteria and fungi. Examine the entire skin surface, noting the location, size, color, and pattern of the lesions. Do genital lesions resemble lesions on other parts of the body? Palpate for nodules, masses, and tenderness. Also, look for bleeding, edema, or signs of infection, such as purulent drainage or erythema. Finally, take the patient's vital signs.

Medical causes

▶ *Balanitis and balanoposthitis.* Typically, balanitis (glans infection) and posthitis (prepuce infection) occur together (balanoposthitis), causing painful ulceration on the glans, foreskin, or penile shaft. Ulceration usually is preceded by 2 to 3 days of prepuce irritation and soreness, followed by a foul discharge and edema. The patient may then develop features of acute infection, such as fever with chills, malaise, and dysuria. Without treatment, the ulcers may deepen and multiply. Eventually, the entire penis and scrotum may become gangrenous, resulting in life-threatening sepsis.

▶ *Bowen's disease.* This painless, premalignant lesion usually occurs on the penis or scrotum but may appear elsewhere. It appears as a brownish red, raised, scaly, indurated, well-defined plaque that may have an ulcerated center.

▶ *Candidiasis.* When this infection involves the anogenital area, it produces erythematous, weepy, circumscribed lesions, usually under the prepuce. Vesicles and pustules also may develop.

▶ *Chancroid.* This STI is characterized by the eruption of one or more lesions, usually on the groin, inner thigh, or penis. Within 24 hours, the lesion changes from a reddened area to a small papule. (A similar papule may erupt on the tongue, lip, breast, or umbilicus.) It then becomes an inflamed pustule that rapidly ulcerates. This painful—and usually deep—ulcer bleeds easily and commonly has a purulent gray or yellow exudate covering its base. Rarely more than 2 cm in diameter, it's typically irregular in shape. The inguinal lymph nodes also enlarge, become very tender, and may drain pus.

▶ *Erythroplasia of Queyrat.* This premalignant lesion is a form of Bowen's disease that appears exclusively under the foreskin of an uncircumcised penis. It typically appears as a red, raised, well-defined, velvety, indurated plaque that may have an ulcerated center.

▶ *Folliculitis and furunculosis.* Hair follicle infection may cause red, sharply pointed, tender and swollen lesions with central pustules. If folliculitis progresses to furunculosis, these lesions become hard, painful nodules that may gradually enlarge and rupture, discharging pus and necrotic material. Rupture relieves the pain, but erythema and edema may persist for days or weeks.

▶ *Fournier's gangrene.* In this life-threatening form of cellulitis, the scrotum suddenly becomes tense, swollen, painful, red, warm, and glossy. As gangrene develops, the scrotum also becomes moist. Fever and malaise may accompany these scrotal changes.

▶ *Genital herpes.* Caused by herpesvirus type I or II, this STI produces fluid-filled vesicles on the glans penis, foreskin, or penile shaft and, occasionally, on the mouth or anus. Usually painless at first, these vesicles may rupture and become extensive, shallow, painful ulcers accompanied by redness, marked edema, and tender, inguinal lymph nodes. Other findings may include fever, malaise, and dysuria. If the vesicles recur in the same area, the patient usually feels localized numbness and tingling before they erupt. Associated inflammation is typically less marked.

▶ *Genital warts.* Genital warts, an STI caused by the human papillomavirus, initially develops on the subpreputial sac, urethral meatus or, less commonly, the penile shaft and then spreads to the perineum and the perianal area. These painless warts start as tiny red or pink swellings that may grow to 8 cm to 12 cm and become pedunculated.[2] Multiple swellings are common, giving the warts a cauliflower-like appearance. Infected warts are malodorous.

▶ *Granuloma inguinale.* Initially, this rare, chronic STI causes a single painless macule or papule on the external genitalia that ulcerates and becomes a raised, beefy red lesion with a granulated, friable border. Later, other painless lesions may erupt and blend together on the glans penis, foreskin, or penile shaft. Lesions also may develop on the nose, mouth, or pharynx. Eventually, these lesions become infected, malodorous, and painful and may be accompanied by fever, weight loss, malaise, and signs of anemia such as weakness. Later, they're marked by fibrosis, keloidal scarring, and depigmentation.

▶ *Leukoplakia.* This precancerous disorder is characterized by white, scaly patches on the glans and prepuce accompanied by skin thickening and occasionally fissures.

▶ *Lichen planus.* Small, shiny, polygonal, violet papules develop on the glans penis in this disorder. These papules are less than 3 cm in diameter and have white, lacy, milky striations. They may be linear or coalesce into plaques. Occasionally, oral lesions precede genital lesions; lesions also may appear on the lower back, ankles, and lower legs. Accompanying findings may include pruritus, distorted nails, and alopecia.

▶ *Lymphogranuloma venereum.* One to three weeks after sexual exposure, this STI may produce a penile erosion or papule that heals rapidly and spontaneously; in fact, it often goes unnoticed. A few days or weeks later, the inguinal and subinguinal nodes enlarge, becoming painful, fluctuant masses. If these nodes become infected, they rupture and form sinus tracts, discharging a thick, yellow, granular secretion. Eventually, a scar or chronic indurated mass forms in the inguinal area.

Systemic signs and symptoms include a rash, fever with chills, headache, migratory joint and muscle pain, malaise, and weight loss.

▶ *Pediculosis pubis.* This parasitic infestation is characterized by erythematous, pruritic papules in the pubic area and around the anus, abdomen, and thigh. Inspection may detect grayish white specks (lice eggs) attached to hair shafts. Skin irritation from scratching in these areas is common.

▶ *Penile cancer.* This rare cancer occurs in only 1% of American men every year, and it occurs least commonly in those who are circumcised at birth.[1] Early signs and symptoms include a painless, enlarging wartlike lesion on the glans or foreskin and itching or burning under the forskin. The patient may have localized pain, however, if the foreskin becomes unretractable. As the cancer progresses, examination may reveal a foul-smelling discharge from the prepuce, a firm lump in the glans, and enlarged lymph nodes. Late signs and symptoms may include dysuria, pain, bleeding from the lesion, and urine retention and bladder distention from obstruction of the urinary tract.

▶ *Psoriasis.* Red, raised, scaly plaques typically affect the scalp, chest, knees, elbows, and lower back. When they occur on the groin or on the shaft and glans of the penis, the plaques are usually redder; on an uncircumcised penis, the characteristic silver scales are absent. The patient commonly reports itching and, possibly, pain from dry, cracked, encrusted lesions. Nail pitting and joint stiffness also may occur.

▶ *Scabies.* In this disorder, mites that burrow under the skin may cause crusted lesions or large papules on the glans and shaft of the penis and on the scrotum. Lesions also may occur on the wrists, elbows, axillae, and waist. They're usually raised, threadlike, and 1 to 10 cm long and have a swollen nodule or red papule that contains the mite. Nocturnal pruritus is typical and commonly leads to excoriation.

▶ *Seborrheic dermatitis.* Initially, this disorder causes erythematous, dry or moist, greasy, scaling papules with yellow crusts that enlarge to form annular plaques. These pruritic plaques may affect the glans and shaft of the penis, scrotum, and groin as well as the scalp, chest, eyebrows, back, axillae, and umbilicus.

▶ *Syphilis.* Two to four weeks after exposure to the spirochete *Treponema pallidum,* one or more primary lesions, or chancres, may erupt on the genitals; occasionally, they also erupt elsewhere on the body, typically on the mouth or perianal area. In men, the glans, coronal sulcus, and foreskin are the most common sites.[3] The chancre usually starts as a small, red, fluid-filled papule and then erodes to form a painless, firm, indurated, shallow ulcer with a clear base and a scant yellow serous discharge or, less commonly, a hard papule. This lesion gradually involutes and disappears. Painless, unilateral regional lymphadenopathy is also typical.

▶ *Tinea cruris.* Also called *jock itch,* this superficial fungal infection usually causes sharply defined, slightly raised, scaling patches on the inner thigh or groin (often bilaterally) and, less commonly, on the scrotum and penis. Pruritus may be severe.

▶ *Urticaria.* This common allergic reaction is characterized by intensely pruritic hives, which may appear on the genitalia, especially on the foreskin or shaft of the penis. These distinct, raised, evanescent wheals are surrounded by an erythematous flare.

Other causes

DRUG WATCH *Barbiturates and broad-spectrum antibiotics, such as tetracycline and sulfonamides, may cause a fixed drug eruption and genital lesions.*

Special considerations

Many disorders produce penile lesions that resemble those of syphilis. Expect to screen every patient with penile lesions for STIs, using the dark-field examination and the Venereal Disease Research Laboratory test. You may need to prepare the patient for a biopsy to confirm or rule out penile cancer. Provide emotional support if cancer is suspected.

To prevent cross-contamination, wash your hands before and after every patient contact. Wear gloves when handling urine or performing catheter care. Dispose of all needles carefully, and double-bag all material contaminated by secretions.

Pediatric pointers

In infants, contact dermatitis (diaper rash) may produce minor irritation or bright red, weepy, excoriated lesions. Use of disposable diapers and careful cleaning of the penis and scrotum can help reduce diaper rash.

In children, impetigo may cause pustules with thick, yellow, weepy crusts. Like adults, children may develop genital warts, but they'll need more reassurance that the treatment (excision) won't hurt or castrate them. Any child with an STI must be evaluated for signs of sexual abuse.

Adolescents ages 15 to 19 have a high incidence of STIs and related genital lesions. The spirochete that causes syphilis can pass through the human placenta, producing congenital syphilis.

Geriatric pointers

Elderly adults who are sexually active with multiple partners have as high a risk of developing STIs as do younger adults. However, because of decreased immunity, poor hygiene, poor symptom reporting and, possibly, concurrent conditions, they may present with different symptoms. Seborrheic dermatitis lasts longer and is more extensive in bedridden patients and those with Parkinson's disease.

Patient counseling

Explain to the patient how to use prescribed ointments or creams. Advise him to use a heat lamp to dry moist lesions or to take sitz baths to relieve crusting and itching. Also, instruct him to report any changes in the lesions.

Explain to male patients that condoms effectively prevent many STIs when used correctly. Advise them to use a new condom for each coitus; to avoid damaging the condom with a sharp object, such as fingernails or teeth; to put the condom on the erect penis before any genital contact; to use only water-based lubricants; to hold the condom firmly while withdrawing the penis; to always withdraw the penis while it's still erect to avoid premature condom loss; and to check the expiration date on the individual condom packet. Teach the patient that hormonal contraceptives, diaphragms, foams, and jellies don't protect against STIs.

REFERENCES

1. Rundio, A. "Spindle Cell Variation, Squamous Cell Carcinoma of the Glans Penis." *Nurse Practitioner* 32(2):11-17, February 2007.
2. Gustavo, E., et al. "Human-Papillomavirus–Related Lesions of the Penis." *Pathology Case Reviews* 10(1):14-20, January/February 2005.
3. Lautenschlager, S. "Cutaneous Manifestations of Syphilis: Recognition and Management." *American Journal of Clinical Dermatology* 7(5):291-304, 2006.

GYNECOMASTIA

Gynecomastia refers to increased breast size in boys and men from excessive development of the mammary glands. This change may be barely palpable or immediately obvious. Usually bilateral, gynecomastia may include breast tenderness and milk secretion. This common condition occurs in about 30% to 65% of adult men.[1]

Normally, several hormones regulate breast development. Estrogens, growth hormone, and corticosteroids stimulate ductal growth, while progesterone and prolactin stimulate growth of the alveolar lobules. Although the pathophysiology of gynecomastia isn't fully understood, a hormonal imbalance—particularly a change in the estrogen-androgen ratio and an increase in prolactin—is a likely contributing factor. This explains why gynecomastia commonly results from the effects of estrogens and other drugs. It also may result from hormone-secreting tumors and from endocrine, genetic, hepatic, or adrenal disorders. Physiologic gynecomastia may occur in neonatal, pubertal, and geriatric males because of normal fluctuations in hormone levels.

History and physical examination

Begin the history by asking the patient when he first noticed his breast enlargement. How old was he at the time? Since then, have his breasts gotten progressively larger, smaller, or stayed the same? Does he also have breast tenderness or discharge? Have him describe the discharge, if any. Ask him if he ever had his nipples pierced and, if so, if he developed complications. Take a thorough drug history, including prescription, over-the-counter, herbal, and street drugs. Then explore related signs and symptoms, such as testicular mass or pain, loss of libido, decreased potency, and loss of chest, axillary, or facial hair.

Focus the physical examination on the breasts, testicles, and penis. As you examine the breasts, note any asymmetry, dimpling, abnormal pigmentation, or ulceration. Observe the testicles' size and symmetry; palpate them to detect nodules, tenderness, or unusual consistency. Look for normal penile development after puberty, and note hypospadias.

Medical causes

▶ *Adrenal carcinoma.* Estrogen production by an adrenal tumor may produce a feminizing syndrome in males characterized by bilateral gynecomastia, loss of libido, impotence, testicular atrophy, and reduced facial hair growth. Cushingoid signs, such as moon face and purple striae, also may occur.

▶ *Breast cancer.* Painful unilateral gynecomastia develops rapidly in men with breast cancer, which accounts for only 0.7% of all breast cancer diagnoses.[2] Palpation may reveal a hard or stony lump suggesting a malignant tumor. Examination also may detect changes in breast symmetry; skin changes, such as thickening, dimpling, peau d'orange, or ulceration; a warm, reddened area; and nipple changes, such as itching, burning, erosion, deviation, flattening, retraction, or watery, bloody, or purulent discharge.

▶ *Cirrhosis.* A late sign of cirrhosis, bilateral gynecomastia results from failure of the liver to inactivate circulating estrogens. It's often accompanied by testicular atrophy, decreased libido, impotence, and loss of facial, chest, and axillary hair. Other late signs and symptoms include mental changes, bleeding tendencies, spider angiomas, palmar erythema, severe pruritus and dry skin, fetor hepaticus, enlarged superficial abdominal veins and, possibly, jaundice and hepatomegaly.

▶ *Hermaphroditism.* In true hermaphroditism, ovarian and testicular tissues coexist, resulting in external genitalia with both feminine and masculine characteristics. At puberty, the patient typically develops marked bilateral gynecomastia. About 50% of hermaphrodites also have male menstruation in the form of cyclic hematuria.

▶ *Hypothyroidism.* Typically, this disorder produces bilateral gynecomastia along with bradycardia, cold intolerance, weight gain despite anorexia, and mental dullness. The patient may display periorbital edema and puffiness in the face, hands, and feet. His hair appears brittle and sparse and his skin is dry, pale, cool, and doughy.

▶ *Klinefelter's syndrome.* Painless bilateral gynecomastia first appears during adolescence in this genetic disorder. Before puberty, symptoms also include abnormally small testicles and slight mental deficiency; after puberty, sparse facial hair, a small penis, decreased libido, and impotence.

▶ *Liver cancer.* This type of cancer may produce bilateral gynecomastia and other characteristics of feminization, such as testicular atrophy, impotence, and reduced facial hair growth. The patient may complain of severe epigastric or right-upper-quadrant pain associated with a right-upper-quadrant mass. A large tumor also may produce a bruit on auscultation. Related findings may include anorexia, weight loss, dependent edema, fever, cachexia and, possibly, jaundice or ascites.

▶ *Lung cancer.* Bronchogenic carcinoma or metastasis to the lung from testicular choriocarcinoma may result in bilateral gynecomastia. Other effects vary according to the tumor's primary site but usually include anorexia, weight loss, fatigue, chronic cough, hemoptysis, clubbing, dyspnea, and diffuse chest pain. Fever and wheezing may occur.

▶ *Malnutrition.* Painful unilateral gynecomastia (known as refeeding gynecomastia) may occur when the malnourished patient begins to take nourishment again. Other effects of malnutrition include apathy, muscle wasting, weakness, limb paresthesia, anorexia, nausea, vomiting, and diarrhea. Inspection may reveal dull, sparse, dry hair; brittle nails; dark, swollen cheeks and lips; dry, flaky skin; and, occasionally, edema and hepatomegaly.

▶ *Pituitary tumor.* This hormone-secreting tumor causes bilateral gynecomastia accompanied by galactorrhea, impotence, and decreased libido. Other hormonal effects may include enlarged hands and feet, coarse facial features with prognathism, voice deepening, weight gain, increased blood pressure, diaphoresis, heat intolerance, hyperpigmentation, and thickened, oily skin. Paresthesia or sensory loss and muscle weakness commonly affect the limbs. If the tumor expands, it may cause blurred vision, diplopia, headache, or partial bitemporal hemianopia that may progress to blindness.

▶ *Reifenstein's syndrome.* This genetic disorder produces painless bilateral gynecomastia at puberty. Other signs may include hypospadias, testicular atrophy, and an underdeveloped penis.

▶ *Renal failure (chronic).* This disorder may produce bilateral gynecomastia accompanied by decreased libido and impotence. Among its more characteristic features, however, are ammonia breath odor, oliguria, fatigue, decreased mental acuity, seizures, muscle cramps, and peripheral neuropathy. Common GI effects include anorexia, nausea, vomiting, and constipation or diarrhea. The patient also typically has bleeding tendencies, pruritus, yellow-brown or bronze skin and, occasionally, uremic frost and increased blood pressure.

▶ *Testicular failure (secondary).* Commonly associated with mumps and other infectious disorders, secondary testicular failure produces bilateral gynecomastia that appears after normal puberty. This disorder also may cause sparse facial hair, decreased libido, impotence, and testicular atrophy.

▶ *Testicular tumor.* Choriocarcinomas, Leydig's cell tumors, and other testicular tumors typically cause bilateral gynecomastia, nipple tenderness, and decreased libido. Because these tumors are usually painless, testicular swelling may be the patient's initial complaint. A firm mass and a heavy sensation in the scrotum may occur.

▶ *Thyrotoxicosis.* Bilateral gynecomastia may occur in 10% to 40% of patients.[1] Cardinal findings include an enlarged thyroid gland, tachycardia, palpitations, weight loss despite increased appetite, diarrhea, tremors, dyspnea, nervousness, diaphoresis, heat intolerance, loss of libido, impotence, and possibly exophthalmos. An atrial or ventricular gallop also may occur.

Other causes

DRUG WATCH *When gynecomastia is an effect of drugs, it's typically painful and unilateral. Estrogens used to* treat prostate cancer, including estramustine, directly affect the estrogen-androgen ratio. Drugs that have an estrogen-like effect, such as cardiac glycosides and human chorionic gonadotropin, may do the same. Regular use of alcohol, marijuana, or heroin reduces plasma testosterone levels, causing gyneco-mastia. Other drugs—such as flutamide, spironolactone, cimetidine, and ketocona-zole—produce this sign by interfering with androgen production or action. Some com-mon drugs, including phenothiazines, tri-cyclic antidepressants, and antihypertensives, may produce gynecomastia, but the mecha-nism of action is unknown.

▶ Treatments. Gynecomastia may develop within weeks of starting hemodialysis for chronic renal failure. It also may follow major surgery or testicular irradiation.

Special considerations

To make the patient as comfortable as possi-ble, apply cold compresses to his breasts and administer analgesics. Prepare him for diag-nostic tests, including chest and skull X-rays and blood hormone levels.

Pediatric pointers

In neonates, gynecomastia may be associated with galactorrhea ("witch's milk"). It occurs as a result of maternal hormones remaining in the neonate.[3] This sign usually disappears within a few weeks but may persist until age 2.

Physiologic gynecomastia that occurs dur-ing puberty happens in 50% to 70% of boys, usually around age 14.[1] This gynecomastia usually is asymmetrical and tender; it com-monly resolves within 2 years and rarely per-sists beyond age 20.

Patient counseling

Because gynecomastia may alter the patient's body image, provide emotional support. Reas-sure the patient that treatment can reduce gy-necomastia. Some patients are helped by ta-moxifen, an antiestrogen that can reduce gy-necomastia in 60% to 90% of patients,[1] or by testolactone, an inhibitor of testosterone-to-estrogen conversion. Surgical removal of breast tissue may be an option if drug treat-ment fails.

REFERENCES

1. Pearlman, G. and Carlson, H.E. "Gynecomastia: An Update." *The Endocrinologist* 16(2):109-115, March/April 2006.
2. Donovan, T.M. and Flynn, M. "What Makes a Man a Man?: The Lived Experience of Male Breast Cancer." *Cancer Nursing* 30(6):464-470, November/December 2007.
3. Hockenberry, M.J. and Wilson, D. (Eds.) *Wong's Nursing Care of Infants and Children*, 8th ed. St. Louis: Mosby, 2007.

HEADACHE

The most common neurologic symptom, headaches may be localized or generalized, producing mild to severe pain. About 90% of all headaches are benign and can be described as vascular, muscle-contraction, or a combination of both. (See *Comparing benign headaches*.) Occasionally, though, headaches indicate a severe neurologic disorder associated with intracranial inflammation, increased intracranial pressure (ICP), or meningeal irritation. They may also result from an ocular or sinus disorder, tests, drugs, or other treatments.

Other causes of headache include fever, eyestrain, dehydration, and systemic febrile illnesses. Headaches may occur in certain metabolic disturbances—such as hypoxemia, hypercapnia, hyperglycemia, and hypoglycemia—but they aren't a diagnostic or prominent symptom in these disorders. Some individuals get headaches after seizures or from coughing, sneezing, heavy lifting, or stooping.

History and physical examination

If the patient reports a headache, ask him to describe its characteristics and location. How often does he get a headache? How long does a typical headache last? Try to identify precipitating factors, such as eating certain foods or exposure to bright lights. Ask what helps to relieve the headache. Is the patient under stress? Has he had trouble sleeping?

Take a drug and alcohol history, and ask about head trauma within the last 4 weeks. Has the patient recently experienced nausea, vomiting, photophobia, or visual changes? Does he feel drowsy, confused, or dizzy? Has he recently developed seizures, or does he have a history of seizures?

Begin the physical examination by evaluating the patient's level of consciousness (LOC). Then check his vital signs. Perform a focused neurological examination.[1] Be alert for signs of increased ICP: widened pulse pressure, bradycardia, altered respiratory pattern, and increased blood pressure. Check pupil size and response to light, and note any neck stiffness. (See *Differential diagnosis: Headache*, pages 212 and 213.)

Medical causes

▶ *Anthrax, cutaneous.* Along with a macular or papular lesion that develops into a vesicle and finally a painless ulcer, this disorder may produce a headache, lymphadenopathy, fever, and malaise.

▶ *Brain abscess.* In this disorder, the headache is localized to the abscess site; it usually intensifies over a few days and is aggravated by straining. Accompanying the headache may be nausea, vomiting, and focal or generalized seizures. The patient's LOC varies from drowsiness to deep stupor. Depending on the abscess site, associated signs and symptoms may include aphasia, impaired visual acuity, hemiparesis, ataxia, tremors, and personality changes. Signs of infection, such as fever and pallor, usually develop late;

Comparing benign headaches

Of the many patients who report headaches, only about 10% have an underlying medical disorder. The other 90% have benign headaches, which may be classified as muscle-contraction (tension), vascular (migraine and cluster), or a combination of both.

As you review this table, you'll see that the two major types—muscle-contraction and vascular headaches—are quite different. In a combined headache, features of both appear; this type of headache may affect the patient with a severe muscle-contraction headache or a late-stage migraine. Treatment of a combined headache includes analgesics and sedatives.

CHARACTERISTICS	MUSCLE-CONTRACTION HEADACHES	VASCULAR HEADACHES
Incidence	• Most common type, accounting for 80% of all headaches	• More common in women and those with a family history of migraines • Onset after puberty
Precipitating factors	• Stress, anxiety, tension, improper posture, and body alignment • Prolonged muscle contraction without structural damage • Eye, ear, and paranasal sinus disorders that produce reflex muscle contractions	• Hormone fluctuations • Alcohol • Emotional upset • Too little or too much sleep • Foods, such as chocolate, cheese, monosodium glutamate, and cured meats; caffeine withdrawal • Weather changes, such as shifts in barometric pressure
Intensity and duration	• Produce an aching tightness or a band of pain around the head, especially in the neck and in occipital and temporal areas • Occur frequently and usually last for several hours	• May begin with an awareness of an impending migraine or a 5- to 15-minute prodrome of neurologic deficits, such as visual disturbances, dizziness, unsteady gait, or tingling of the face, lips, or hands • Produce severe, constant, throbbing pain that is typically unilateral and may be incapacitating • Last for 4 to 6 hours
Related signs and symptoms	• Tense neck and facial muscles	• Anorexia, nausea, and vomiting • Occasionally photophobia, sensitivity to loud noises, weakness, and fatigue • Depending on the type (cluster headache or classic, common, or hemiplegic migraine), possibly chills, depression, eye pain, ptosis, tearing, rhinorrhea, diaphoresis, and facial flushing • Triptans, such as sumatriptan, rizatriptan, and zolmitriptan, to relieve acute migraine headaches.
Alleviating factors	• Mild analgesics, muscle relaxants, or other drugs during an attack • Measures to reduce stress, such as biofeedback, relaxation techniques, and counseling; posture correction to prevent attacks	• Amitriptyline, methysergide, and propranolol to prevent vascular headache • Ergot alkaloids or serotonin-receptor drugs at the first sign of a migraine • Rest in a quiet, darkened room • Elimination of irritating foods from diet

Differential diagnosis: Headache

HISTORY OF PRESENT ILLNESS
Focused physical examination includes: Neurologic and musculoskeletal systems; head, eyes, ears, nose, and throat; mental health; and lymph nodes.

POSSIBLE CAUSES	SIGNS AND SYMPTOMS	DIAGNOSIS	TREATMENT AND FOLLOW-UP
Sinusitis	• Dull periorbital headache • Unilateral or bilateral frontal or maxillary sinus pain that's increased by palpation or bending over • Fever • Malaise • Nasal turbinate edema • Sore throat • Nasal discharge	• Physical examination • Transillumination • Sinus X-ray	• Medication (decongestants, analgesics, antibiotics) *Follow-up:* None unless signs and symptoms worsen or recur
Brain abscess	• Localized headache that increases over a few days • Possible nausea and vomiting • Focal or generalized seizures • Drowsiness		
Subdural hematoma	• Decreased level of consciousness (LOC) • Acute drowsiness, confusion, or agitation • Pounding headache • Giddiness • Personality changes • Dizziness • Confusion	• Possible history of head trauma • Lumbar puncture • Imaging studies (computed tomography scan, magnetic resonance imaging, arteriography)	• Medication (antibiotics, if indicated; analgesics; anticonvulsants; osmotic diuretics) • Surgery if appropriate • Chemotherapy or radiation therapy if malignancy is present *Follow-up:* Referral to neurologist or neurosurgeon
Encephalitis	• Severe, generalized headache • Deteriorating LOC within 48 hours of initial headache • Fever • Nuchal rigidity • Irritability • Seizures • Nausea and vomiting • Photophobia		
Epidural hemorrhage	• Progressively severe headache • Unilateral seizures • Decreased LOC • Hemiparesis or hemiplegia • High-grade fever		

Differential diagnosis: Headache *(continued)*

POSSIBLE CAUSES	SIGNS AND SYMPTOMS	DIAGNOSIS	TREATMENT AND FOLLOW-UP
Cerebral aneurysm (ruptured)	• Sudden severe, possibly unilateral headache • Possible nausea and vomiting • Change in LOC • Vision changes		
Intracranial hemorrhage	• Severe generalized headache • Rapid, steady decrease in LOC • Hemiparesis or hemiplegia • Aphasia • Dizziness • Nausea and vomiting • Irregular respirations • Positive Babinski's reflex	• Possible history of head trauma • Lumbar puncture • Imaging studies (computed tomography scan, magnetic resonance imaging, arteriography)	• Medication (antibiotics, if indicated; analgesics; anticonvulsants; osmotic diuretics) • Surgery if appropriate • Chemotherapy or radiation therapy if malignancy is present *Follow-up:* Referral to neurologist or neurosurgeon
Brain tumor	• Localized or generalized headache • Intermittent deep pain that's more intense in the morning and increases with Valsalva's maneuver • Personality changes • Changes in LOC		

however, if the abscess remains encapsulated, these signs may not appear.

▶ *Brain tumor.* Headache, an ealy symptom of brain tumor, is often described as localized and occuring near the tumor site.[2] The pain is usually persistent and is most intense at night, and may even waken the patient from sleep.[2] It's aggravated by activities that increase ICP, such as coughing, stooping, Valsalva's maneuver, and changes in head position, and it's relieved by sitting and rest. Associated signs and symptoms include personality changes, altered LOC, motor and sensory dysfunction, and eventually signs of increased ICP, such as vomiting, increased systolic blood pressure, and widened pulse pressure.

▶ *Cerebral aneurysm (ruptured).* Cerebral aneurysm is a life-threatening disorder that's characterized by a sudden excruciating headache, which may be unilateral and usually peaks within minutes of the rupture. The patient's description of this headache as the worst of his life is a classic presentation of a ruptured aneurysm.[3] The patient may lose consciousness immediately or display a variably altered LOC. Depending on the severity and location of the bleeding, he may also exhibit nausea and vomiting; signs and symptoms of meningeal irritation, such as nuchal rigidity and blurred vision; hemiparesis; and other features.

▶ *Ebola virus.* A sudden headache commonly occurs on the 5th day of this deadly illness. Additionally, the patient has a history of malaise, myalgia, high fever, diarrhea, abdominal pain, dehydration, and lethargy. A maculopapular rash develops between the 5th and 7th days of the illness. Other possible findings include pleuritic chest pain; a dry, hacking cough; pronounced pharyngitis; hematemesis; melena; and bleeding from the nose, gums, and vagina. Death usually occurs in the second week of the illness, preceded by massive blood loss and shock.

▶ *Encephalitis.* A severe, generalized headache is characteristic with this disorder. Within 48 hours, the patient's LOC typically deteriorates, perhaps from lethargy to coma. Other signs and symptoms include fever, nuchal rigidity, irritability, seizures, nausea and vomiting, photophobia, cranial nerve palsies such as ptosis, and focal neurologic deficits, such as hemiparesis and hemiplegia.

▶ *Epidural hemorrhage (acute).* Head trauma and a sudden, brief loss of consciousness usually precede this hemorrhage, which causes a progressively severe headache that's accompanied by nausea and vomiting, bladder distention, confusion, and then a rapid decrease in LOC. Other signs and symptoms include unilateral seizures, hemiparesis, hemiplegia, high fever, decreased pulse rate and bounding pulse, widened pulse pressure, increased blood pressure, a positive Babinski's reflex, and decerebrate posture.

If the patient slips into a coma, his respirations deepen and become stertorous, then shallow and irregular, and eventually cease. Pupil dilation may occur on the same side as the hemorrhage.

▶ *Glaucoma, acute angle-closure.* This type of glaucoma is an ophthalmic emergency that may cause an excruciating headache as well as acute eye pain, blurred vision, halo vision, nausea, and vomiting. Assessment reveals conjunctival injection, a cloudy cornea, and a moderately dilated, fixed pupil.

▶ Hantavirus *pulmonary syndrome.* Noncardiogenic pulmonary edema distinguishes this viral disease, which was first reported in the United States in 1993. Common reasons for seeking treatment include flulike signs and symptoms—headache, myalgia, fever, nausea, vomiting, and a cough—followed by respiratory distress. Fever, hypoxia, and (in some patients) serious hypotension typify the hospital course. Other signs and symptoms include a rising respiratory rate (28 breaths/minute or more) and an increased heart rate (120 beats/minute or more).

▶ *Hypertension.* This disorder may cause a slightly throbbing occipital headache on awakening that decreases in severity during the day. However, if the patient's diastolic blood pressure exceeds 120 mm Hg, the headache remains constant. Other signs and symptoms include an atrial gallop, restlessness, confusion, nausea and vomiting, blurred vision, seizures, and altered LOC.

▶ *Influenza.* A severe generalized or frontal headache usually begins suddenly with the flu. Accompanying signs and symptoms may last for 3 to 5 days and include stabbing retro-orbital pain, weakness, diffuse myalgia, fever, chills, coughing, rhinorrhea and, occasionally, hoarseness.

▶ *Intracerebral hemorrhage.* In some patients, this hemorrhage produces a severe generalized headache. Other signs and symptoms vary with the size and location of the hemorrhage. A large hemorrhage may produce a rapid, steady decrease in LOC, perhaps resulting in a coma. Other common findings include hemiplegia, hemiparesis, abnormal pupil size and response, aphasia, dizziness, nausea, vomiting, seizures, decreased sensation, irregular respirations, positive Babinski's reflex, decorticate or decerebrate posture, and increased blood pressure.

▶ *Listeriosis.* If this infection spreads to the nervous system, it may cause meningitis, whose signs and symptoms include headache, nuchal rigidity, fever, and change in LOC. Earlier signs and symptoms of listeriosis include fever, myalgia, abdominal pain, nausea, vomiting, and diarrhea. Listeriosis during pregnancy may lead to premature delivery, infection of the neonate, or stillbirth.

▶ *Meningitis.* This disorder is marked by the sudden onset of a severe, constant, generalized headache that worsens with movement. Fever and chills are other early signs. As meningitis progresses, it also causes nuchal rigidity, positive Kernig's and Brudzinski's signs, hyperreflexia, altered LOC, seizures, ocular palsies, facial weakness, hearing loss, vomiting and, possibly, opisthotonos and papilledema.

▶ *Plague.* The pneumonic form of this lethal bacterial infection causes a sudden onset of headache, chills, fever, and myalgia. Pulmonary findings include a productive cough, chest pain, tachypnea, dyspnea, hemoptysis, respiratory distress, and cardiopulmonary insufficiency.

▶ *Postconcussion syndrome.* A generalized or localized headache may develop 1 to 30 days after head trauma and last for 2 to 3 weeks.

This characteristic symptom may be described as an aching, pounding, pressing, stabbing, or throbbing pain. The patient's neurologic examination is normal, but he may experience giddiness or dizziness, blurred vision, fatigue, insomnia, inability to concentrate, and noise and alcohol intolerance.

▶ *Q fever.* Signs and symptoms of this disease include severe headaches, fever, chills, malaise, chest pain, nausea, vomiting, and diarrhea. The fever may last up to 2 weeks and, in severe cases, the patient may develop hepatitis or pneumonia.

▶ *Severe acute respiratory syndrome (SARS).* SARS is an acute infectious disease of unknown etiology; however, a novel coronavirus has been implicated as a possible cause. Although most cases have been reported in Asia (China, Vietnam, Singapore, Thailand), cases have cropped up in Europe and North America. After an incubation period of 2 to 7 days, the illness typically starts with a fever (usually greater than 100.4° F [38° C]). Other symptoms include headache, malaise, a nonproductive cough, and dyspnea. SARS may produce only mild symptoms, or it may progress to pneumonia and, in some cases, even respiratory failure and death.

▶ *Sinusitis (acute).* This disorder is usually marked by a dull periorbital headache that's usually aggravated by bending over or touching the face and is relieved by sinus drainage. Fever, sinus tenderness, nasal turbinate edema, sore throat, malaise, cough, and nasal discharge may accompany the headache.

▶ *Smallpox (variola major).* Initial signs and symptoms of this virus include a severe headache, backache, abdominal pain, high fever, malaise, prostration, and a maculopapular rash on the mucosa of the mouth, pharynx, face, and forearms and then on the trunk and legs. The rash becomes vesicular, then pustular. After 8 or 9 days, the pustules form a crust, which later separates from the skin, leaving a pitted scar. Death may result from encephalitis, extensive bleeding, or secondary infection.

▶ *Subarachnoid hemorrhage.* This hemorrhage commonly produces a sudden, violent headache along with nuchal rigidity, nausea and vomiting, seizures, dizziness, ipsilateral pupil dilation, and altered LOC that may rapidly progress to coma. The patient also exhibits positive Kernig's and Brudzinski's signs, photophobia, blurred vision and, possibly, a fever. Focal signs and symptoms (such as hemiparesis, hemiplegia, sensory or vision disturbances, and aphasia) and signs of elevated ICP (such as bradycardia and increased blood pressure) may also occur.

▶ *Subdural hematoma.* Typically associated with head trauma, both acute and chronic subdural hematomas may cause headache and decreased LOC. An *acute subdural hematoma* also produces drowsiness, confusion, and agitation that may progress to coma. Later findings include signs of increased ICP and focal neurologic deficits such as hemiparesis.

A *chronic subdural hematoma* produces a dull, pounding headache that fluctuates in severity and is located over the hematoma. Weeks or months after the initial head trauma, the patient may experience giddiness, personality changes, confusion, seizures, and progressively worsening LOC. Late signs may include unilateral pupil dilation, sluggish pupil reaction to light, and ptosis.

▶ *Temporal arteritis.* A throbbing unilateral headache in the temporal or frontotemporal region may be accompanied by vision loss, hearing loss, confusion, and fever. The temporal arteries are tender, swollen, nodular, and sometimes erythematous.

▶ *Tularemia.* Signs and symptoms following inhalation of the bacterium *Francisella tularensis* include abrupt onset of headache, fever, chills, generalized myalgia, a nonproductive cough, dyspnea, pleuritic chest pain, and empyema.

▶ *Typhus.* In typhus, initial symptoms of headache, myalgia, arthralgia, and malaise are followed by an abrupt onset of chills, fever, nausea, and vomiting. A maculopapular rash may also occur.

▶ *West Nile encephalitis.* This brain infection is caused by West Nile virus, a mosquito-borne flavivirus commonly found in Africa, West Asia, the Middle East and, rarely, in North America. Most patients have mild signs and symptoms, including fever, headache, body aches, rash, and swollen lymph glands. More severe infection is marked by high fever, headache, neck stiffness, stupor, disorientation, coma, tremors, and paralysis.

Other causes

▶ *Diagnostic tests.* A headache is the most common complication of lumbar puncture.[4] Myelogram may produce a throbbing frontal headache that worsens on standing.

DRUG WATCH *A wide variety of drugs can cause headaches. For example, indomethacin produces headaches in many patients, usually in the morning. Vasodilators and drugs with a vasodilating effect, such as nitrates, typically cause a throbbing headache. Headaches also may follow withdrawal from caffeine (a cerebral vasoconstrictor), opioids, estrogen, systemic serotonin-reuptake inhibitors, tricyclic antidepressants, and corticosteroids.[5]*

▶ *Food additives.* Monosodium glutamate, found in soy sauces and other foods, can cause a diffuse, throbbing headache within 30 minutes of ingestion.[5] Aspartame, found in artifical sweeteners, can also cause headaches.[5]

▶ *Herbs.* Herbal remedies, such as St. John's wort, ginseng, and ephedra (banned by the Food and Drug Administration) can cause various adverse reactions, including headaches.

▶ *Traction.* Cervical traction with pins commonly causes a headache, which may be generalized or localized to pin insertion sites.

Special considerations

Continue to monitor the patient's vital signs and LOC. If the patient always reports pain localized to one side, imaging studies should be ordered to rule out structural problems.[6] Watch for any change in the headache's severity or location. To help ease the headache, administer an analgesic, darken the patient's room, and minimize other stimuli. Explain the rationale of these interventions to the patient. Patients with migraine headaches may also have anxiety or depression; be sure to assess psychological status and provide emotional support as needed.[6]

Prepare the patient for diagnostic tests, such as skull X-rays, computed tomography scan, lumbar puncture, or cerebral arteriography.

Pediatric pointers

If a child is too young to describe his symptom, suspect a headache if you see him banging or holding his head. In an infant, a shrill cry or bulging fontanels may indicate increased ICP and headache. In a school-age child, ask the parents about the child's recent scholastic performance and about any problems at home that may produce a tension headache.

Twice as many young boys have migraine headaches as girls. In children older than age 3, headache is the most common symptom of a brain tumor.

Patient counseling

Encourage the patient to keep a headache diary including frequency, severity, and possible or known triggers, as well as what treatment he used and his response to treatment.[1] Counsel the patient to avoid triggers (environmental, hormonal, emotional, dietary, drug-related, or lifestyle-related).[1]

REFERENCES

1. Holcomb, S.S. "Guidelines for Migraine Treatment." *The Nurse Practitioner* 30(7):12-15, July 2005.
2. Franges, E.Z. "When A Headache Is Really A Brain Tumor." *The Nurse Practitioner* 31(4):47-51, April 2006.
3. Olson, D. and Halley, N. "Cerebral Aneurysm Rupture—Are You Prepared?" *Nursing* 37(3):64cc1-64cc4, March 2007.
4. Lawes, R. "Uncovering the Layers of Meningitis and Encephalitis." *Nursing Made Incredibly Easy!* 5(4):26-35, July/August 2007.
5. Butt, T.F. and Evans, B. "Drug-Induced Headache." *Adverse Drug Reaction Bulletin* (240):919-922, October 2006.
6. O'Malley, P. "Oh! My Aching Head—Safely Managing Migraine Headaches: Update for the Clinical Nurse Specialist." *Clinical Nurse Specialist* 19(4):187-189, July/August 2005.

HEARING LOSS

Affecting nearly 28 million Americans,[1] hearing loss may be temporary or permanent and partial or complete. This common symptom may involve reception of low-, middle-, or high-frequency tones. If the hearing loss doesn't affect speech frequencies, the patient may be unaware of it.

Normally, sound waves enter the external auditory canal and travel to the middle ear's tympanic membrane and ossicles (incus, malleus, and stapes) and then into the inner ear's cochlea. The cochlear division of the eighth cranial (auditory) nerve carries the sound impulse to the brain. This type of sound transmission, called air conduction, is normally better than bone conduction—sound transmission through bone to the inner ear.

Hearing loss can be classified as conductive, sensorineural, mixed, or functional. Conductive hearing loss results from external or middle ear disorders that block sound transmission. This type of hearing loss usually responds to medical or surgical intervention (or in some cases, both). Sensorineural hearing loss results from disorders of the inner ear or of the eighth cranial nerve. Mixed hearing loss combines aspects of conductive and sensorineural hearing loss. Functional hearing loss results from psychological factors rather than identifiable organic damage.

Hearing loss may also result from trauma, infection, allergy, tumors, certain systemic and hereditary disorders, and the effects of ototoxic drugs and treatments. In most cases, though, it results from presbycusis, a type of sensorineural hearing loss that usually affects people older than age 50. Other physiologic causes of hearing loss include cerumen (earwax) impaction; barotitis media (unequal pressure on the eardrum) associated with descent in an airplane or elevator, diving, or close proximity to an explosion; and chronic exposure to noise over 90 decibels, which can occur on the job, with certain hobbies, or from listening to live or recorded music.

History and physical examination

If the patient reports hearing loss, ask him to describe it fully. Is it unilateral or bilateral? Continuous or intermittent? Ask about a family history of hearing loss. Then obtain the patient's medical history, noting chronic ear infections, ear surgery, and ear or head trauma. Has the patient recently had an upper respiratory tract infection? After taking a drug history, have the patient describe his occupation and work environment.

Next, explore associated signs and symptoms. Does the patient have ear pain? If so, is it unilateral or bilateral? Continuous or intermittent? Ask the patient if he has noticed discharge from one or both ears? If so, have him describe its color and consistency, and note when it began. Does he hear ringing, buzzing, hissing, or other noises in one or both ears? If so, are the noises constant or intermittent? Does he experience any dizziness? If so, when did he first notice it?

Begin the physical examination by inspecting the external ear for inflammation, boils, foreign bodies, and discharge. Then apply pressure to the tragus and mastoid to elicit tenderness. If you detect tenderness or external ear abnormalities, ask the physician whether an otoscopic examination should be done. During the otoscopic examination, note any color change, perforation, bulging, or retraction of the tympanic membrane, which normally looks like a shiny, pearl gray cone.

Next, evaluate the patient's hearing acuity, using the ticking watch and whispered voice tests. Then perform the Weber and Rinne tests to obtain a preliminary evaluation of the type and degree of hearing loss. (See *Differentiating conductive from sensorineural hearing loss,* page 218.)

Medical causes

▶ *Acoustic neuroma.* This eighth cranial nerve tumor causes unilateral, progressive, sensorineural hearing loss. The patient may also develop tinnitus, vertigo, and—with cranial nerve compression—facial paralysis.

▶ *Adenoid hypertrophy.* Eustachian tube dysfunction gradually causes conductive hearing loss accompanied by intermittent ear discharge. The patient also tends to breathe through his mouth and may have a sensation of ear fullness.

▶ *Allergies.* Conductive hearing loss may result when an allergy produces eustachian tube and middle ear congestion. Other features include ear pain or a feeling of fullness, nasal congestion, and conjunctivitis.

▶ *Aural polyps.* If a polyp occludes the external auditory canal, partial hearing loss may

Differentiating conductive from sensorineural hearing loss

The Weber and Rinne tests can help determine whether the patient's hearing loss is conductive or sensorineural. The Weber test evaluates bone conduction; the Rinne test, bone and air conduction. Using a 512-Hz tuning fork, perform these preliminary tests as described below.

WEBER TEST

Place the base of a vibrating tuning fork firmly against the midline of the patient's skull at the forehead. Ask her if she hears the tone equally well in both ears. If she does, the Weber test is graded *midline*—a normal finding. In an abnormal Weber test (graded *right* or *left*), sound is louder either in the impaired ear, suggesting a conductive hearing loss in that ear, or in the normal ear, suggesting a sensorineural loss in the opposite ear.

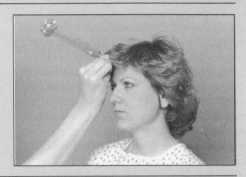

RINNE TEST

Hold the base of a vibrating tuning fork against the patient's mastoid process to test bone conduction (BC). Then quickly move the vibrating fork in front of her ear canal to test air conduction (AC). Ask her to tell you which location has the louder or longer sound. Repeat the procedure for the other ear. In a positive Rinne test, the AC sound lasts longer or is louder than the BC sound—a normal finding. In a negative test, the opposite is true: the BC sound lasts as long as or longer than AC sound. In sensorineural loss, the AC sound lasts longer than the BC sound, but the BC sound is louder.

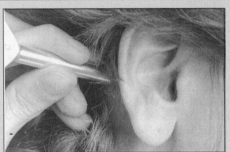

After performing both tests, correlate the results with other assessment data.

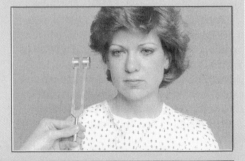

IMPLICATIONS OF RESULTS

Conductive hearing loss produces:
- abnormal Weber test result
- negative Rinne test result
- improved hearing in noisy areas
- normal ability to discriminate sounds
- difficulty hearing when chewing
- a quiet speaking voice.

Sensorineural hearing loss produces:
- positive Rinne test
- poor hearing in noisy areas
- difficulty hearing high-frequency sounds
- complaints that others mumble or shout
- tinnitus
- loud speaking voice.

occur. The polyp typically bleeds easily and is covered by a purulent discharge.

▶ *Cholesteatoma.* Gradual hearing loss is characteristic in this disorder and may be accompanied by vertigo and, at times, facial paralysis. Examination reveals eardrum perforation, pearly white balls in the ear canal and, possibly, a discharge.

▶ *Cyst.* Ear canal obstruction by a sebaceous or dermoid cyst causes progressive conductive hearing loss. On inspection, the cyst looks like a soft mass.

▶ *External ear canal tumor (malignant).* Progressive conductive hearing loss is characteristic and is accompanied by deep, boring ear pain; a purulent discharge; and eventually facial paralysis. Examination may detect the granular, bleeding tumor.

▶ *Furuncle.* Reversible conductive hearing loss may occur when one of these painful, hard nodules forms in the ear. The patient may report a sense of fullness in the ear and pain on palpation of the tragus or auricle. Rupture relieves the pain and produces a purulent, necrotic discharge.

▶ *Glomus jugulare tumor.* Initially, this benign tumor causes mild, unilateral conductive hearing loss that becomes progressively more severe. The patient may report tinnitus that sounds like his heartbeat. Associated signs and symptoms include gradual congestion in the affected ear, throbbing or pulsating discomfort, bloody otorrhea, facial nerve paralysis, and vertigo. Although the tympanic membrane is normal, a reddened mass appears behind it.

▶ *Glomus tympanum tumor.* This cancerous middle ear tumor causes slowly progressive hearing loss and throbbing or pulsating tinnitus. It usually bleeds easily when manipulated. Late features include ear pain, dizziness, and total unilateral deafness.

▶ *Granuloma.* A rare cause of conductive hearing loss, a granuloma may also produce fullness in the ear, deep-seated pain, and a bloody discharge.

▶ *Head trauma.* Sudden conductive or sensorineural hearing loss may result from ossicle disruption, ear canal fracture, tympanic membrane perforation, or cochlear fracture associated with head trauma. Typically, the patient reports a headache and has bleeding from his

ear. Neurologic features vary and may include impaired vision and altered level of consciousness.

▶ *Herpes zoster oticus (Ramsay Hunt syndrome).* This syndrome causes sudden severe, unilateral mixed hearing loss, which may be accompanied by vesicles in the external ear, tinnitus, vertigo, ear pain, malaise, and transient ipsilateral facial paralysis.

▶ *Hypothyroidism.* This disorder may produce reversible sensorineural hearing loss. Other effects include bradycardia, weight gain despite anorexia, mental dullness, cold intolerance, facial edema, brittle hair, and dry skin that's pale, cool, and doughy.

▶ *Ménière's disease.* Initially, this inner ear disorder produces intermittent, unilateral sensorineural hearing loss that involves only low tones. Later, hearing loss becomes constant and affects other tones. Other signs and symptoms include intermittent severe vertigo, nausea and vomiting, a feeling of fullness in the ear, a roaring or hollow-seashell tinnitus, diaphoresis, and nystagmus.

▶ *Multiple sclerosis.* Rarely, this disorder causes sensorineural hearing loss associated with myelin destruction of the central auditory pathways. The hearing loss may be sudden and unilateral or intermittent and bilateral. Other traits include impaired vision, paresthesia, muscle weakness, gait ataxia, intention tremor, urinary disturbances, and emotional lability.

▶ *Myringitis.* Rarely, *acute infectious myringitis* produces conductive hearing loss when fluid accumulates in the middle ear or a large bleb totally obstructs the ear canal. Small, reddened inflamed blebs may develop in the canal, on the tympanic membrane, or in the middle ear and may produce a bloody discharge if they rupture. Other findings may include severe ear pain, mastoid tenderness, and fever.

Chronic granular myringitis produces gradual hearing loss with pruritus and a purulent discharge.

▶ *Nasopharyngeal cancer.* This type of cancer causes mild unilateral conductive hearing loss when it compresses the eustachian tube. Bone conduction is normal, and inspection reveals a retracted tympanic membrane backed by fluid. When this tumor obstructs the nasal airway, the patient may exhibit nasal speech and a bloody nasal and postnasal discharge. Cranial nerve involvement produces other findings, such as diplopia and rectus muscle paralysis.

▶ *Osteoma.* Commonly affecting women and swimmers, osteoma may cause sudden or intermittent conductive hearing loss. Typically, bony projections are visible in the ear canal, but the tympanic membrane appears normal.

▶ *Otitis externa.* Conductive hearing loss resulting from debris in the ear canal characterizes both acute and malignant otitis externa. In *acute otitis externa,* ear canal inflammation produces pain, itching, and a foul-smelling, sticky yellow discharge. Severe tenderness is typically elicited by chewing, opening the mouth, and pressing on the tragus or mastoid. The patient may also develop a low-grade fever, regional lymphadenopathy, a headache on the affected side, and mild to moderate pain around the ear that may later intensify. Examination may reveal greenish white debris or edema in the canal.

In *malignant otitis externa,* debris is also visible in the canal. This life-threatening disorder, which most commonly occurs in diabetics, causes sensorineural hearing loss, pruritus, tinnitus, and severe ear pain.

▶ *Otitis media.* This middle ear inflammation typically produces unilateral conductive hearing loss. In *acute suppurative otitis media,* the hearing loss develops gradually over a few hours and usually is accompanied by an upper respiratory tract infection with sore throat, cough, nasal discharge, and headache. Related signs and symptoms include dizziness, a sensation of fullness in the ear, intermittent or constant ear pain, fever, nausea, and vomiting. Rupture of the bulging, swollen tympanic membrane relieves the pain and produces a brief bloody and purulent discharge. Hearing returns after the infection subsides.

Hearing loss also develops gradually in patients with *chronic otitis media.* Assessment may reveal a perforated tympanic membrane, purulent ear drainage, earache, nausea, and vertigo.

Commonly associated with an upper respiratory tract infection or nasopharyngeal cancer, *serous otitis media* commonly produces a stuffy feeling in the ear and pain that worsens at night. Examination reveals a retracted— and perhaps discolored—tympanic membrane and possibly air bubbles behind the membrane.

▶ *Otosclerosis.* In this hereditary disorder, unilateral conductive hearing loss usually begins when the patient is in his early twenties and may gradually progress to bilateral mixed hearing loss. The patient may report tinnitus and an ability to hear better in a noisy environment.

Otosclerosis affects twice as many women as men and may worsen during pregnancy.

▶ *Skull fracture.* Auditory nerve injury causes sudden unilateral sensorineural hearing loss. Accompanying signs and symptoms include ringing tinnitus, blood behind the tympanic membrane, scalp wounds, and other findings.

▶ *Syphilis.* In tertiary syphilis, sensorineural hearing loss may develop suddenly or gradually and usually affects one ear more than the other. It's usually accompanied by a gumma lesion—a chronic, superficial nodule or a deep, granulomatous lesion on the skin or mucous membranes. The lesion is solitary, asymmetrical, painless, and indurated. The patient also may have signs of liver, respiratory, cardiovascular, or neurologic dysfunction.

▶ *Temporal arteritis.* This disorder may produce unilateral sensorineural hearing loss accompanied by throbbing unilateral facial pain, pain behind the eye, temporal or frontotemporal headache, and occasionally vision loss. The hearing loss usually is preceded by a prodrome of malaise, anorexia, weight loss, weakness, and myalgia that lasts for several days. Examination may reveal a nodular, swollen temporal artery. Low-grade fever, confusion, and disorientation may also occur.

▶ *Temporal bone fracture.* This fracture can cause sudden unilateral sensorineural hearing loss accompanied by hissing tinnitus. The tympanic membrane may be perforated, depending on the fracture's location. Loss of consciousness, Battle's sign, and facial paralysis may also occur.

▶ *Tuberculosis.* This pulmonary infection may spread to the ear, resulting in eardrum perforation, mild conductive hearing loss, and cervical lymphadenopathy.

▶ *Tympanic membrane perforation.* Commonly caused by trauma from sharp objects or rapid pressure changes, perforation of the tympanic membrane causes abrupt hearing loss along with ear pain, tinnitus, vertigo, and a sensation of fullness in the ear.

▶ *Wegener's granulomatosis.* Conductive hearing loss develops slowly in this rare necrotizing, granulomatous vasculitis. This multisystem disorder may also cause cough, pleuritic chest pain, epistaxis, hemorrhagic skin lesions, oliguria, and nasal discharge.

Other causes

DRUG WATCH *Ototoxic drugs typically produce ringing or buzzing tinnitus and a feeling of fullness in the ear. Chloroquine, cisplatin, vancomycin, and aminoglycosides (especially neomycin, kanamycin, and amikacin) may cause irreversible hearing loss. Loop diuretics, such as furosemide, ethacrynic acid, and bumetanide, usually produce a brief, reversible hearing loss. Quinine, quinidine, and high doses of erythromycin or salicylates (such as aspirin) also may cause reversible hearing loss.*

▶ *Radiation therapy.* Irradiation of the middle ear, thyroid, face, skull, or nasopharynx may cause eustachian tube dysfunction, resulting in hearing loss.

▶ *Surgery.* Myringotomy, myringoplasty, simple or radical mastoidectomy, or fenestrations may cause scarring that interferes with hearing.

Special considerations

When talking with the patient, remember to face him and speak slowly.[2] Don't shout at the patient or cover your mouth when speaking.[2] Also avoid smoking, eating, or chewing gum when talking.

Prepare the patient for audiometry and auditory evoked-response testing. After testing, the patient may require a hearing aid or cochlear implant to improve his hearing.

Pediatric pointers

About 2 in 1,000 infants are born profoundly deaf in the United States each year.[3] In about half these infants, hereditary disorders (such as Paget's disease and Alport's, Hurler's, and Klippel-Feil syndromes) cause the typically sensorineural hearing loss. Nonhereditary dis-

orders associated with congenital sensorineural hearing loss include albinism, onychodystrophy, cochlear dysplasia, and Pendred's, Usher's, Waardenburg's, and Jervell and Lange-Nielsen syndromes. Sensorineural hearing loss may also result from maternal use of ototoxic drugs, birth trauma, and anoxia during or after birth.

Mumps is the most common cause of unilateral sensorineural hearing loss in children. Other causes are meningitis, measles, influenza, and acute febrile illness.

Congenital conductive hearing loss may be caused by atresia, ossicle malformation, and other abnormalities. Otitis media with effusion can cause hearing loss in children, which may be mild to moderate and intermittent or constant.[4] Putting foreign objects in the ears can also cause conductive hearing loss.

Hearing disorders in children may lead to speech, language, and learning problems. Early identification and treatment of hearing loss is thus crucial for the development of speech and language, and has prompted universal hearing screens for all infants before discharge from the newborn nursery.[5] Indeed, recent research shows that hearing impaired infants who receive treatment for hearing loss before the age of 6 months are likely to develop language that's equal to infants with normal hearing.[5]

When assessing an infant or a young child for hearing loss, remember that you can't use a tuning fork. Instead, test the startle reflex in infants younger than age 6 months, or have an audiologist test brain stem evoked response in neonates, infants, and young children. Also, obtain a gestational, perinatal, and family history from the parents.

Geriatric pointers

Hearing loss increases with age and affects about 25% to 40% of adults older than age 65, more than 80% of those older than age 85.[3] Changes with aging that predispose older patients to hearing loss include a thickened and less flexible tympanic membrane that impairs vibration transmission; a stiffened stapes that can limit the conduction of sound waves to the cochlea; and an accumulation of dry cerumen that can impact the external ear canal.[2] In older patients, presbycusis may be aggravated by exposure to noise as well as other factors.

Patient counseling

Instruct the patient to avoid exposure to loud noise and to use ear protection to arrest hearing loss. If the patient has an upper respiratory tract infection, tell him to avoid flying and driving. Encourage the patient to use hearing aids as appropriate; they have been improved in recent years and are beneficial with most types of hearing loss.[3] Remind patients to keep the batteries charged.[2] Provide the patient with strategies to maximize the function of hearing aids in noisy settings (like a restaurant), such as sitting with his back against the wall to limit the direction of sound, trying to sit in the center of the conversation, and to select a seat with enough light to allow for good face visualization.[2]

REFERENCES

1. Munson, B.L. "Now, Listen Up! Understanding Hearing Loss and Deafness." *Nursing Made Incredibly Easy!* 4(2):38-47, March/April 2006.
2. Wallhagen, M.I., Pettengill, E., and Whiteside, M. "Sensory Impairment in Older Adults: Part 1: Hearing Loss." *AJN* 106(10):40-48, October 2006.
3. Mattox, D.E. "Assessment and Management of Tinnitus and Hearing Loss." *CONTINUUM: Lifelong Learning in Neurology* 12(4):135-150, August 2006.
4. Carlson, L.H. "Otitis Media: New Information On An Old Disease." *The Nurse Practitioner* 30(3):31-41, March 2005.
5. Spivak, L. and Sokol, H. "Beyond Newborn Screening: Early Diagnosis and Management of Hearing Loss in Infants." *Advances in Neonatal Care* 5(2):104-112, April 2005.

● HEMATEMESIS

Hematemesis, the vomiting of blood, usually indicates GI bleeding above the ligament of Treitz, which suspends the duodenum at its junction with the jejunum. Bright red or blood-streaked vomitus indicates fresh or recent bleeding. Dark red, brown, or black vomitus (the color and consistency of coffee grounds) indicates that

Rare causes of hematemesis

Two rare disorders commonly cause hematemesis. *Malaria* produces this and other GI signs, but its most characteristic effects are chills, fever, headache, muscle pain, and splenomegaly. *Yellow fever* also causes hematemesis as well as sudden fever, bradycardia, jaundice, and severe prostration.

In rare cases, two relatively common disorders may cause hematemesis. When acute diverticulitis affects the duodenum, GI bleeding and resultant hematemesis occur with abdominal pain and fever. With GI involvement, secondary syphilis can cause hematemesis; more characteristic signs and symptoms include a primary chancre, rash, fever, malaise, anorexia, weight loss, and headache.

blood has been retained in the stomach and partially digested.

Although hematemesis usually results from a GI disorder, it may stem from a coagulation disorder or from a treatment that irritates the GI tract. Swallowed blood from epistaxis or oropharyngeal erosion may also cause bloody vomitus. Hematemesis may be precipitated by straining, emotional stress, and the use of anti-inflammatory drugs or alcohol. In a patient with esophageal varices, hematemesis may be caused by trauma from swallowing hard or partially chewed food. (See *Rare causes of hematemesis*.)

Hematemesis is always an important sign, but its severity depends on the amount, source, and intensity of the bleeding. Massive hematemesis (vomiting of 500 to 1,000 ml of blood) may be life-threatening.

If the patient has massive hematemesis, check his vital signs. If you detect signs of shock—such as tachypnea, hypotension, and tachycardia—place the patient in a supine position. Don't raise his feet into a modified Trendelenburg position because it offers no benefit for hypovolemic patients.[1] Start a large-bore I.V. line for emergency fluid replacement. Also, obtain a blood sample for

Managing hematemesis with intubation

A patient with hematemesis will need to have a GI tube inserted to allow blood drainage, to aspirate gastric contents, or to facilitate gastric lavage if necessary. Here are the most common tubes and their uses.

NASOGASTRIC TUBES	WIDE-BORE GASTRIC TUBES	ESOPHAGEAL TUBES

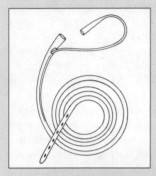 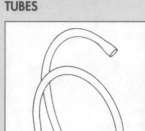 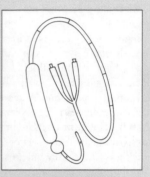

The *Salem-Sump tube* (above), a double-lumen nasogastric (NG) tube, is used to remove stomach fluid and gas or to aspirate gastric contents. It may also be used for gastric lavage, drug administration, or feeding. Its main advantage over the *Levin tube*—a single-lumen NG tube—is that it allows atmospheric air to enter the patient's stomach so the tube can float freely instead of risking adhesion and damage to the gastric mucosa.

The *Edlich tube* (above) has one wide-bore lumen with four openings near the closed distal tip. A funnel or syringe can be connected at the proximal end. Like the other tubes, the Edlich can aspirate a large volume of gastric contents quickly.

The *Ewald tube,* a wide-bore tube that allows quick passage of a large amount of fluid and clots, is especially useful for gastric lavage in patients with profuse GI bleeding and in those who have ingested poison. Another wide-bore tube, the *double-lumen Levacuator,* has a large lumen for evacuation of gastric contents and a small one for lavage.

The *Sengstaken-Blakemore tube* (above), a triple-lumen double-balloon esophageal tube, provides a gastric aspiration port that allows drainage from below the gastric balloon. It can also be used to instill medication. A similar tube, the *Linton shunt,* can aspirate esophageal and gastric contents without risking necrosis because it has no esophageal balloon. The *Minnesota esophagogastric tamponade tube,* which has four lumina and two balloons, provides pressure-monitoring ports for both balloons without the need for Y-connectors.

typing and crossmatching, hemoglobin level, and hematocrit, and give oxygen. Emergency endoscopy may be needed to locate the source of bleeding. Prepare to insert a nasogastric (NG) tube for suction or iced lavage. A Sengstaken-Blakemore tube may be used to compress esophageal varices. (See *Managing hematemesis with intubation.*)

History and physical examination

If hematemesis isn't immediately life-threatening, begin with a thorough history. First, have the patient describe the amount, color, and consistency of the vomitus. When did he first notice this sign? Has he ever had hematemesis before? Find out if he also has bloody or black tarry stools. Note whether hematemesis is usually preceded by nausea, flatulence, diarrhea, or weakness. Has he recently had bouts of retching with or without vomiting?

Next, ask about a history of ulcers or of liver or coagulation disorders. Find out how much alcohol the patient drinks, if any. Does he regularly take aspirin or another nonsteroidal anti-inflammatory drug (NSAID), such as phenylbutazone or indomethacin? These drugs may cause erosive gastritis or ulcers.

Begin the physical examination by checking for orthostatic hypotension, an early warning sign of hypovolemia. Take blood pressure and pulse with the patient in the supine, sitting, and standing positions. A decrease of 10 mm Hg or more in systolic pressure or an increase of 10 beats/minute or more in pulse rate indicates volume depletion. After obtaining other vital signs, inspect the mucous membranes, nasopharynx, and skin for any signs of bleeding or other abnormalities. Finally, palpate the abdomen for tenderness, pain, or masses. Note lymphadenopathy.

Medical causes

▶ *Achalasia.* Hematemesis is a rare effect of this disorder, which usually causes passive regurgitation and painless, progressive dysphagia. Regurgitation of undigested food may cause hoarseness, coughing, aspiration, and recurrent pulmonary infections.

▶ *Anthrax, GI.* GI anthrax is caused by eating meat contaminated with the gram-positive, spore-forming bacterium *Bacillus anthracis.* Initial signs and symptoms of anorexia, nausea, vomiting, and fever may progress to hematemesis, abdominal pain, and severe bloody diarrhea.

▶ *Coagulation disorders.* Any disorder that disrupts normal clotting, such as thrombocytopenia or hemophilia, may result in GI bleeding and moderate to severe hematemesis. Bleeding may occur in other body systems as well, resulting in such signs as epistaxis and ecchymosis. Additional effects depend on the specific coagulation disorder.

▶ *Esophageal cancer.* A late sign of this cancer, hematemesis may be accompanied by steady chest pain that radiates to the back. Other features include substernal fullness, se-

vere dysphagia, nausea, vomiting with nocturnal regurgitation and aspiration, hemoptysis, fever, hiccups, sore throat, melena, and halitosis.

▶ *Esophageal injury by caustic substances.* Ingestion of corrosive acids or alkalies produces esophageal injury associated with grossly bloody or coffee-ground vomitus. Hematemesis is accompanied by epigastric and anterior or retrosternal chest pain that's intensified by swallowing. With ingestion of alkaline agents, the oral and pharyngeal mucosa may produce a soapy white film. The mucosa becomes brown and edematous with time. Dysphagia, marked salivation, and fever may develop in 3 to 4 weeks and worsen as strictures form.

▶ *Esophageal rupture.* The severity of hematemesis depends on the cause of the rupture. When an instrument damages the esophagus, hematemesis is usually slight. However, rupture due to Boerhaave's syndrome (increased esophageal pressure from vomiting or retching) or other esophageal disorders typically causes more severe hematemesis. This life-threatening disorder may also produce severe retrosternal, epigastric, neck, or scapular pain accompanied by chest and neck edema. Examination reveals subcutaneous crepitation in the chest wall, supraclavicular fossa, and neck. The patient may also show signs of respiratory distress, such as dyspnea and cyanosis.

▶ *Esophageal varices (ruptured).* Life-threatening rupture of esophageal varices may produce coffee-ground or massive bright red vomitus. Signs of shock, such as hypotension and tachycardia, may follow or even precede hematemesis if the stomach fills with blood before vomiting occurs. Other symptoms may include abdominal distention and melena or painless hematochezia (ranging from slight oozing to massive rectal hemorrhage).

▶ *Gastric cancer.* Painless bright red or dark brown vomitus is a late sign of this uncommon cancer, which usually begins insidiously with upper abdominal discomfort. The patient then develops anorexia, mild nausea, and chronic dyspepsia that's unrelieved by antacids and worsened by food. Later symptoms may include fatigue, weakness, weight loss, feelings of fullness, melena, altered bowel habits, and signs of malnutrition, such as muscle wasting and dry skin.

▶ *Gastritis (acute).* Hematemesis and melena are the most common signs of acute gastritis. They may even be the only signs, although mild epigastric discomfort, nausea, fever, and malaise may also occur. Massive blood loss precipitates signs of shock. Typically, the patient has a history of alcohol abuse or has used aspirin or another NSAID. Gastritis may also occur secondary to *Helicobacter pylori* infection.

▶ *Gastroesophageal reflux disease.* Although rare in this disorder, hematemesis may produce significant blood loss. It's accompanied by pyrosis, flatulence, dyspepsia, and postural regurgitation that can be aggravated by lying down or stooping over. Related effects include dysphagia, retrosternal angina-like chest pain, weight loss, halitosis, and signs of aspiration, such as dyspnea and recurrent pulmonary infections.

▶ *Leiomyoma.* This benign tumor occasionally involves the GI tract, eroding the mucosa or vascular supply to produce hematemesis. Other features vary with the tumor's size and location. For example, esophageal involvement may cause dysphagia and weight loss.

▶ *Mallory-Weiss syndrome.* Characterized by a mucosal tear of the mucous membrane at the junction of the esophagus and the stomach, this syndrome may produce hematemesis and melena. It's commonly triggered by severe vomiting, retching, or straining (as from coughing), usually in alcoholics or in people whose pylorus is obstructed. Severe bleeding may precipitate signs of shock, such as tachycardia, hypotension, dyspnea, and cool, clammy skin.

▶ *Peptic ulcer.* Hematemesis may occur when a peptic ulcer penetrates an artery, vein, or highly vascular tissue. Massive—and possibly life-threatening—hematemesis is typical when an artery is penetrated. Other features include melena or hematochezia, chills, fever, and signs and symptoms of shock and dehydration, such as tachycardia, hypotension, poor skin turgor, and thirst. Most patients have a history of nausea, vomiting, epigastric tenderness, and epigastric pain that's relieved by foods or antacids. Some may also have a his-

tory of habitual use of tobacco, alcohol, or NSAIDs.

Other causes

▶ *Treatments.* Traumatic NG or endotracheal intubation may cause hematemesis from swallowed blood. Nose or throat surgery also may cause this sign in the same way.

Special considerations

Closely monitor the patient's vital signs, and watch for signs of shock. Check the patient's stools regularly for occult blood, and keep accurate intake and output records. Place the patient on bed rest in a low or semi-Fowler's position to prevent aspiration of vomitus. Keep suctioning equipment nearby, and use it as needed. Provide frequent oral hygiene and emotional support—the sight of bloody vomitus can be very frightening. Administer a histamine$_2$ blocker I.V.; vasopressin may be needed for ruptured esophageal varices. As the bleeding declines, monitor the pH of gastric contents, and give hourly doses of antacids by NG tube as needed.

Pediatric pointers

Hematemesis is much less common in children than in adults and may be related to foreign-body ingestion. In cases of iron poisoning (most common in children under 6 years of age), iron corrodes the GI mucosa and causes hematemesis, as well as nausea, vomiting, diarrhea, and melena.[2] Occasionally, neonates develop hematemesis after swallowing maternal blood during delivery or breastfeeding from a cracked nipple. Hemorrhagic disease of the neonate and esophageal erosion may also cause hematemesis in infants; such cases require immediate fluid replacement.

Geriatric pointers

In elderly patients, hematemesis may be caused by a vascular anomaly, an aortoenteric fistula, or upper GI cancer. In addition, chronic obstructive pulmonary disease, chronic hepatic or renal failure, and chronic NSAID use all predispose elderly people to hemorrhage secondary to coexisting ulcerative disorders.

Patient counseling

Explain diagnostic tests, such as endoscopy, barium swallow, and variceal banding. Explain laboratory tests, such as serum electrolyte levels, complete blood count, prothrombin time, partial thromboplastin time, and international normalized ratio. Provide information on drugs that the patient should avoid, such as aspirin or anticoagulants, and instruct the patient on non-drug measures, such as relaxation and stress management, which help minimize symptoms. Stress the importance of avoiding alcohol.

REFERENCES

1. Bridges, N. and Jarquin-Valdivia, A.A. "Use of the Trendelenburg Position as The Resuscitation Position: To T or Not to T?" *American Journal of Critical Care* 14(5):364-368, September 2005.
2. Aldridge, M.D. "Acute Iron Poisoning: What Every Pediatric Intensive Care Unit Nurse Should Know." *Dimensions of Critical Care Nursing* 26(2):43-48, March/April 2007.

● HEMATOCHEZIA

The passage of bloody stools, known as *hematochezia* or *rectal bleeding,* usually indicates—and may be the first sign of—GI bleeding below the ligament of Treitz. However, this sign—usually preceded by hematemesis—also may accompany rapid hemorrhage of 1 L or more from the upper GI tract.

Hematochezia ranges from formed, blood-streaked stools to liquid, bloody stools that may be bright red, dark mahogany, or maroon. This sign usually develops abruptly and with abdominal pain.

Although hematochezia commonly accompanies a GI disorder, it also may result from a coagulation disorder, exposure to toxins, or certain diagnostic tests. Always a significant sign, hematochezia may precipitate life-threatening hypovolemia.

If the patient has severe hematochezia, check his vital signs. If you detect signs of shock, such as hypotension and tachycardia, place the patient in a supine position. Don't raise his feet into a modified Trendelenberg position because it offers no benefit for hypovolemic patients.[1] Prepare to give oxygen, and start a large-bore I.V. line for emergency fluid replacement. Next, obtain a blood sample for typing and crossmatching, hemoglobin level, and hematocrit. Insert a nasogastric tube. Iced lavage may be indicated to control bleeding. Endoscopy may be needed to detect the source of the bleeding.

History and physical examination

If the hematochezia isn't immediately life-threatening, ask the patient to fully describe the amount, color, and consistency of his bloody stools. (If possible, also inspect and characterize the stools yourself.) How long have the stools been bloody? Do they always look the same, or does the amount of blood seem to vary? Ask about other signs and symptoms.

Next, explore the patient's medical history, focusing on GI and coagulation disorders. Ask about the use of GI irritants, such as alcohol, aspirin, and other nonsteroidal anti-inflammatory drugs.

Begin the physical examination by checking for orthostatic hypotension, an early sign of shock. Take the patient's blood pressure and pulse while he's lying down and standing.

Examine the skin for petechiae or spider angiomas. Palpate the abdomen for tenderness, pain, or masses. Also, note lymphadenopathy. Finally, a digital rectal examination must be done to rule out rectal masses or hemorrhoids.

Medical causes

▶ *Amyloidosis.* Hematochezia occasionally occurs when this disorder affects the GI tract. Massive, rapid hematochezia may precipitate signs of shock, such as hypotension and tachycardia. Other signs and symptoms include hypoactive or absent bowel sounds, abdominal pain, malabsorption, diarrhea, and renal disease. The patient also may have a stiff, enlarged tongue, resulting in dysarthria.

▶ *Anal fissure.* Slight hematochezia characterizes this disorder; blood may streak the stools or appear on toilet tissue. Accompanying hematochezia is severe rectal pain that may make the patient reluctant to defecate, thereby causing constipation.

▶ *Angiodysplastic lesions.* Most common in elderly patients, these arteriovenous lesions of the ascending colon typically cause chronic, bright red rectal bleeding. Occasionally, they may result in life-threatening blood loss and signs of shock, such as tachycardia and hypotension.

▶ *Anorectal fistula.* Blood, pus, mucus, and occasionally stool may drain from this type of fistula. Other effects include rectal pain and pruritus.

▶ *Coagulation disorders.* Patients with a coagulation disorder (such as thrombocytopenia or disseminated intravascular coagulation) may have GI bleeding marked by moderate to severe hematochezia. Bleeding may also occur in other body systems, producing such signs as epistaxis and purpura. Other findings vary with the specific coagulation disorder.

▶ *Colitis. Ischemic colitis* commonly causes bloody diarrhea, especially in elderly patients. Rectal bleeding may be slight or massive and usually is accompanied by severe, cramping lower abdominal pain and hypotension. Other effects include abdominal tenderness, distention, and absent bowel sounds. Severe colitis may cause life-threatening hypovolemic shock and peritonitis.

Ulcerative colitis typically causes bloody diarrhea that may also contain mucus. Blood loss may be slight or massive and is preceded by mild to severe abdominal cramps. Associated signs and symptoms include fever, tenesmus, anorexia, nausea, vomiting, hyperactive bowel sounds and, occasionally, tachycardia. Weight loss and weakness occur late.

▶ *Colon cancer.* Bright red rectal bleeding with or without pain is a telling sign, especially in cancer of the left colon. This type of tumor usually causes early signs of obstruction, such as rectal pressure, bleeding, and intermittent fullness or cramping. As the disease progresses, the patient also develops obstipation, diarrhea or ribbon-shaped stools, and pain that's typically relieved by passage of stools or flatus. Stools are grossly bloody.

Cancer of the right colon may initially cause melena and abdominal aching, pressure, and dull cramps. As the disease progresses, the patient also may have diarrhea, anorexia,

weight loss, anemia, weakness and fatigue, vomiting, an abdominal mass, and signs of obstruction, such as abdominal distention and abnormal bowel sounds.

▶ *Colorectal polyps.* A classic sign of colorectal polyps in patients of any age is bright red rectal bleeding that is painless and is associated with normal stool frequency and consistency.[2] These polyps are the most common cause of intermittent hematochezia in adults younger than age 60, but they don't always produce symptoms. When located high in the colon, polyps may cause blood-streaked stools that yield a positive response when tested with guaiac. If the polyps are located closer to the rectum, they may bleed freely.

▶ *Crohn's disease.* Hematochezia isn't a common sign of this disorder unless the perineum is involved. If rectal bleeding does occur, it's likely to be massive. The chief clinical features of Crohn's disease include fever, abdominal distention and pain with guarding, diarrhea, hyperactive bowel sounds, anorexia, nausea, and fatigue. Palpation may reveal a mass in the colon.

▶ *Diverticulitis.* Most common in elderly patients, this disorder can suddenly cause mild to moderate rectal bleeding after the patient feels the urge to defecate. The bleeding may end abruptly or may progress to life-threatening blood loss with signs of shock. Other signs and symptoms may include left-lower-quadrant pain that's relieved by defecation, alternating episodes of constipation and diarrhea, anorexia, nausea and vomiting, rebound tenderness, and a distended tympanic abdomen.

▶ *Dysentery.* Bloody diarrhea is common in infection with *Shigella, Amoeba,* and *Campylobacter,* but rare with *Salmonella.* Abdominal pain or cramps, tenesmus, fever, and nausea may also occur.

▶ *Esophageal varices (ruptured).* In this life-threatening disorder, hematochezia may range from slight rectal oozing to grossly bloody stools and may be accompanied by mild to severe hematemesis or melena. Signs of shock, such as tachycardia and hypotension, may follow or occasionally precede overt signs of bleeding. Typically, the patient has a history of chronic liver disease.

▶ *Food poisoning (staphylococcal)*. The patient may have bloody diarrhea 1 to 6 hours after ingesting food toxins. Accompanying signs and symptoms, which last a few hours, include severe, cramping abdominal pain, nausea and vomiting, and prostration.

▶ *Hemorrhoids*. Hematochezia may accompany external hemorrhoids, which typically cause painful defecation, resulting in constipation. Less painful internal hemorrhoids usually produce more chronic bleeding with bowel movements, which may eventually lead to signs of anemia, such as weakness and fatigue.

▶ *Leptospirosis*. The severe form of this infection—Weil's syndrome—produces hematochezia or melena with other signs of bleeding, such as epistaxis and hemoptysis. Bleeding typically is preceded by a sudden frontal headache, severe thigh and lumbar myalgia, cutaneous hyperesthesia, and conjunctival suffusion. Bleeding is followed by chills, a rapidly rising fever, and perhaps nausea and vomiting. Fever, headache, and myalgia usually intensify and persist for weeks. Other findings may include right-upper-quadrant tenderness, hepatomegaly, and jaundice.

▶ *Peptic ulcer*. Upper GI bleeding is a common complication in this disorder. The patient may display hematochezia, hematemesis, or melena, depending on the intensity and amount of bleeding. If the peptic ulcer penetrates an artery or vein, massive bleeding may precipitate signs of shock, such as hypotension and tachycardia. Other findings may include chills, fever, nausea and vomiting, and signs of dehydration, such as dry mucous membranes, poor skin turgor, and thirst. Most patients have a history of epigastric pain that's relieved by foods or antacids; some also have a history of habitual use of tobacco, alcohol, or nonsteroidal anti-inflammatory drugs.

▶ *Rectal melanoma (malignant)*. This rare form of rectal cancer typically causes recurrent rectal bleeding that arises from a painless, asymptomatic mass.

▶ *Small-intestine cancer*. This disorder occasionally produces slight hematochezia or blood-streaked stools. Its characteristic features include colicky pain and postprandial vomiting. Other common signs and symptoms include anorexia, weight loss, and fever. Palpation may reveal abdominal masses.

▶ *Typhoid fever*. About 10% of patients with typhoid fever develop hematochezia, which is occasionally massive. However, melena is more common. Both signs of bleeding occur late and may be accompanied by marked abdominal distention, diarrhea, significant weight loss, mental dullness, and profound fatigue. Earlier signs and symptoms are pathognomonic rose spots, headache, chills, fever, constipation, dry cough, conjunctivitis, and epistaxis.

▶ *Ulcerative proctitis*. In this disorder, the patient typically has an intense urge to defecate but passes only bright red blood, pus, or mucus. Other common findings include acute constipation and tenesmus.

Other causes

▶ *Heavy metal poisoning*. Bloody diarrhea is accompanied by cramping abdominal pain, nausea, and vomiting. Other signs may include tachycardia, hypotension, seizures, paresthesia, depressed or absent deep tendon reflexes, and an altered level of consciousness.

▶ *Tests*. Certain procedures, especially colonoscopy, polypectomy, and proctosigmoidoscopy, may cause rectal bleeding. Bowel perforation is rare.

Special considerations

Place the patient on bed rest and check his vital signs often, watching for signs of shock, such as hypotension, tachycardia, weak pulse, and tachypnea. Monitor the patient's intake and output hourly. Remember to provide emotional support because hematochezia may frighten the patient.

Prepare the patient for blood tests and GI procedures, such as endoscopy and GI X-rays. Visually examine the patient's stools and test them for occult blood. If necessary, send a stool specimen to the laboratory to check for parasites.

Pediatric pointers

In neonates, hematochezia may be a result of swallowed maternal blood during delivery, or it may be an initial symptom of necrotizing enterocolitis.[3]

Hematochezia is much less common in children than in adults. It may result from structural disorders, such as intussusception and Meckel's diverticulum, and from inflammatory disorders, such as peptic ulcer disease and ulcerative colitis.

In children, ulcerative colitis typically produces chronic, rather than acute, signs and symptoms and may also cause slow growth and maturation related to malnutrition. Suspect sexual abuse in all cases of rectal bleeding in children.

Geriatric pointers

Because older people have an increased risk of colon cancer, hematochezia should be evaluated with colonoscopy after perirectal lesions have been ruled out as the cause of bleeding.

Patient counseling

Provide information to the patient on signs and symptoms to report immediately. Discuss proper bowel elimination habits. Explain dietary recommendations and restrictions. Teach the patient about self-care after discharge, and consult a home health care nurse to provide support, as appropriate.

REFERENCES

1. Bridges, N. and Jarquin-Valdivia, A.A. "Use of the Trendelenburg Position as the Resuscitation Position: To T or Not to T?" *American Journal of Critical Care* 14(5):364-368, September 2005.
2. Attard, T.M. and Young, R.J. "Diagnosis and Management of Gastrointestinal Polyps: Pediatric Considerations." *Gastroenterology Nursing* 29(1):16-22, January/February 2006.
3. Lambert, D.K., et al. "Necrotizing Enterocolitis in Term Neonates: Data from a Multihospital Health-Care System." *Journal of Perinatology* 27(7):437-43, July 2007.

● HEMATURIA

A cardinal sign of renal and urinary tract disorders, hematuria is the abnormal presence of blood in urine. Strictly defined, it means three or more red blood cells (RBCs) per high-power microscopic field in the urine. Microscopic hematuria is confirmed

Confirming hematuria

If the patient's urine appears blood tinged, be sure to rule out pseudohematuria, in which red or pink urine is caused by urinary pigments. First, carefully observe the urine specimen. If it contains a red sediment, it's probably true hematuria.

Then check the patient's history for use of drugs associated with pseudohematuria, including rifampin, chlorzoxazone, phenazopyridine, phenothiazines, doxorubicin, phenytoin, and laxatives containing phenolphthalein.

Ask about the patient's intake of beets, berries, or foods with red dyes that may color the urine red. Be aware that porphyrinuria and excess urate excretion can also cause pseudohematuria.

Finally, test the urine using a chemical reagent strip. This test can confirm even microscopic hematuria and can also estimate the amount of blood present.

by an occult blood test, whereas macroscopic hematuria is immediately visible. However, macroscopic hematuria must be distinguished from pseudohematuria. (See *Confirming hematuria.*) Macroscopic hematuria may be continuous or intermittent, is often accompanied by pain, and may be aggravated by prolonged standing or walking.

Hematuria may be classified by the stage of urination it mainly affects. Bleeding at the start of urination—*initial hematuria*—usually indicates urethral pathology. Bleeding at the end of urination—*terminal hematuria*—usually indicates pathology of the bladder neck, posterior urethra, or prostate. Bleeding throughout urination—*total hematuria*—usually indicates pathology above the bladder neck.

Hematuria may result from one of two mechanisms: rupture or perforation of vessels in the renal system or urinary tract, or impaired glomerular filtration, which allows RBCs to seep into the urine. The color of the bloody urine provides a clue to the source of the bleeding. Usually, dark or brownish blood indicates renal or upper urinary tract bleeding, whereas bright red blood indicates lower urinary tract bleeding.

Although hematuria usually results from renal and urinary tract disorders, it may also result from certain GI, prostate, vaginal, or coagulation disorders or from the effects of certain drugs. Invasive therapy and diagnostic tests that involve instrumentation of the renal and urologic systems also may cause hematuria. Nonpathologic hematuria may result from fever and hypercatabolic states. Transient hematuria may follow strenuous exercise.

History and physical examination

After detecting hematuria, take a pertinent health history. If hematuria is macroscopic, ask the patient when he first noticed blood in his urine. Does it vary in severity between voidings? Is it worse at the beginning, middle, or end of urination? Has it occurred before? Is the patient passing any clots? To rule out artifactual hematuria, ask about bleeding hemorrhoids or the onset of menses, if appropriate. Ask if pain or burning accompanies the episodes of hematuria.

Ask about recent abdominal or flank trauma. Has the patient been exercising strenuously? Note a history of renal, urinary, prostatic, or coagulation disorders. Then obtain a drug history, noting the use of anticoagulants or aspirin.

Begin the physical examination by palpating and percussing the abdomen and flanks. Next, percuss the costovertebral angle (CVA) to elicit tenderness. Check the urinary meatus for bleeding or other abnormalities. Using a chemical reagent strip, test a urine specimen for protein. A vaginal or digital rectal examination may be needed.

Medical causes

▶ *Appendicitis.* About 15% of patients with appendicitis have either microscopic or macroscopic hematuria accompanied by bladder tenderness, dysuria, and urinary urgency. More typical findings include constant right-lower-quadrant pain (especially over McBurney's point), nausea and vomiting, anorexia, abdominal rigidity, rebound tenderness, constipation, tachycardia, and low-grade fever.

▶ *Bladder cancer.* Chronic or intermittent gross hematuria is the presenting sign of bladder cancer in most patients.[1] Bladder cancer may also produce pain in the bladder, rectum, pelvis, flank, back, or leg. Other common features are nocturia, dysuria, urinary frequency and urgency, vomiting, diarrhea, and insomnia.

▶ *Bladder trauma.* A characteristic finding in traumatic rupture or perforation of the bladder, gross hematuria is typically accompanied by lower abdominal pain. The patient also may develop anuria despite a strong urge to void; swelling of the scrotum, buttocks, or perineum; and signs of shock, such as tachycardia and hypotension.

▶ *Calculi.* Both bladder and renal calculi produce hematuria, which may be associated with signs of urinary tract infection, such as dysuria and urinary frequency and urgency. *Bladder calculi* also may cause gross hematuria, referred pain to the lower back or penile or vulvar area and, occasionally, bladder distention.

Renal calculi may produce microscopic or gross hematuria. The cardinal symptom, though, is colicky pain that travels from the CVA to the flank, suprapubic region, and external genitals when a calculus is passed. The pain may be excruciating at its peak. Other signs and symptoms may include nausea and vomiting, restlessness, fever, chills, abdominal distention and, possibly, decreased bowel sounds.

▶ *Coagulation disorders.* Macroscopic hematuria commonly is the first sign of hemorrhage in coagulation disorders, such as thrombocytopenia or disseminated intravascular coagulation. Among other features are epistaxis, purpura (petechiae and ecchymosis), and signs of GI bleeding.

▶ *Cortical necrosis (acute).* Accompanying gross hematuria in this renal disorder are intense flank pain, anuria, leukocytosis, and fever.

▶ *Cystitis.* Hematuria is a telling sign in all types of cystitis. *Bacterial cystitis* usually produces macroscopic hematuria with urinary urgency and frequency, dysuria, nocturia, and tenesmus. The patient complains of perineal and lumbar pain, suprapubic discomfort, and fatigue and occasionally has a low-grade fever.

More common in women, *chronic interstitial cystitis* occasionally causes gross hematuria. Other features include urinary frequency, dysuria, nocturia, and tenesmus. Both microscopic and macroscopic hematuria may occur in *tubercular cystitis,* which may also cause urinary urgency and frequency, dysuria, tenesmus, flank pain, fatigue, and anorexia. *Viral cystitis* usually produces hematuria, urinary urgency and frequency, dysuria, nocturia, tenesmus, and fever.

▶ *Diverticulitis.* When this disorder involves the bladder, it usually causes microscopic hematuria, urinary frequency and urgency, dysuria, and nocturia. Characteristic findings include left-lower-quadrant pain, abdominal tenderness, constipation or diarrhea and, occasionally, a palpable, firm, fixed, and tender abdominal mass. The patient also may develop mild nausea, flatulence, and a low-grade fever.

▶ *Endocarditis (subacute infective).* Occasionally, this disorder produces embolization, resulting in renal infarction and microscopic or gross hematuria. Common related findings are constant fever, chills, night sweats, fatigue, pallor, anorexia, weight loss, polyarthralgia, petechiae, flank pain, severe back pain, stiff neck, cardiac murmurs, tachycardia, and splenomegaly.

▶ *Glomerulonephritis. Acute glomerulonephritis* usually begins with gross hematuria that tapers off to microscopic hematuria and RBC casts, which may persist for months. It may also produce oliguria or anuria, proteinuria, mild fever, fatigue, flank and abdominal pain, generalized edema, increased blood pressure, nausea, vomiting, and signs of lung congestion, such as crackles and a productive cough.

Chronic glomerulonephritis usually causes microscopic hematuria accompanied by proteinuria, generalized edema, and increased blood pressure. Signs and symptoms of uremia may also occur in advanced disease.

▶ *Nephritis (interstitial).* Typically, this infection causes microscopic hematuria. However, some patients with acute interstitial nephritis may develop gross hematuria. Other findings are fever, maculopapular rash, and oliguria or

anuria. In chronic interstitial nephritis, the patient has dilute—almost colorless—urine that may be accompanied by polyuria and increased blood pressure.

▶ *Nephropathy (obstructive).* This disorder may cause microscopic or macroscopic hematuria, but urine is rarely grossly bloody. The patient may report colicky flank and abdominal pain, CVA tenderness, and anuria or oliguria that alternates with polyuria.

▶ *Polycystic kidney disease.* This hereditary disorder may cause recurrent microscopic or gross hematuria. It commonly produces no symptoms before age 40 but may cause increased blood pressure, polyuria, dull flank pain, and signs of urinary tract infection, such as dysuria and urinary frequency and urgency. Later, the patient develops a swollen, tender abdomen and lumbar pain that's aggravated by exertion and relieved by lying down. He may also have proteinuria and colicky abdominal pain from the ureteral passage of clots or calculi.

▶ *Prostatic hyperplasia (benign).* About 20% of patients with an enlarged prostate have macroscopic hematuria, usually when a significant obstruction is present. The hematuria is usually preceded by diminished urinary stream, tenesmus, and a feeling of incomplete voiding. It may be accompanied by urinary hesitancy, frequency, and incontinence; nocturia; perineal pain; and constipation. Inspection reveals a midline mass representing the distended bladder; rectal palpation reveals an enlarged prostate.

▶ *Prostatitis.* Whether acute or chronic, prostatitis may cause macroscopic hematuria, usually at the end of urination. It may also produce urinary frequency and urgency and dysuria followed by visible bladder distention.

Acute prostatitis also produces fatigue, malaise, myalgia, polyarthralgia, fever with chills, nausea, vomiting, perineal and low back pain, and decreased libido. Rectal palpation reveals a tender, swollen, boggy, firm prostate.

Chronic prostatitis commonly follows an acute attack. It may cause persistent urethral discharge, dull perineal pain, ejaculatory pain, and decreased libido.

▶ *Pyelonephritis (acute).* This infection typically produces microscopic or macroscopic hematuria that progresses to gross hematuria. After the infection resolves, microscopic hematuria may persist for a few months. Related signs and symptoms include persistent high fever, unilateral or bilateral flank pain, CVA tenderness, shaking chills, weakness, fatigue, dysuria, urinary frequency and urgency, nocturia, and tenesmus. The patient also may have nausea, vomiting, anorexia, and signs of paralytic ileus, such as hypoactive or absent bowel sounds and abdominal distention.

▶ *Renal cancer.* The classic triad of signs and symptoms includes gross hematuria; dull, aching flank pain; and a smooth, firm, palpable flank mass. Colicky pain may accompany the passage of clots. Other findings include fever, CVA tenderness, and increased blood pressure. In advanced disease, the patient may develop weight loss, nausea and vomiting, and leg edema with varicoceles.

▶ *Renal infarction.* Typically, this disorder produces gross hematuria. The patient may complain of constant, severe flank and upper abdominal pain accompanied by CVA tenderness, anorexia, and nausea and vomiting. Other findings include oliguria or anuria, proteinuria, hypoactive bowel sounds and, a day or two after the infarction, fever and increased blood pressure.

▶ *Renal papillary necrosis (acute).* This disorder usually produces gross hematuria, which may be accompanied by intense flank pain, CVA tenderness, abdominal rigidity and colicky pain, oliguria or anuria, pyuria, fever, chills, vomiting, and hypoactive bowel sounds. Arthralgia and hypertension are common.

▶ *Renal trauma.* About 90% of patients with renal trauma have microscopic or gross hematuria.[2] Other signs and symptoms may include flank pain, a palpable flank mass, oliguria, hematoma or ecchymosis over the upper abdomen or flank, nausea and vomiting, and hypoactive bowel sounds. Severe trauma may cause signs of shock, such as tachycardia and hypotension.

▶ *Renal tuberculosis.* Gross hematuria often is the first sign of this disorder. It may be accompanied by urinary frequency, dysuria, pyuria, and flank pain.[3]

▶ *Renal vein thrombosis.* Gross hematuria usually occurs in this type of thrombosis. In an abrupt venous obstruction, the patient has severe flank and lumbar pain as well as epigastric and CVA tenderness. Other features include fever, pallor, proteinuria, peripheral edema and, when the obstruction is bilateral, oliguria or anuria and other uremic signs. The kidneys are easily palpable. Gradual venous obstruction causes signs of nephrotic syndrome, proteinuria and, occasionally, peripheral edema.

▶ *Schistosomiasis.* This infection usually causes intermittent hematuria at the end of urination. It may be accompanied by dysuria, colicky renal and bladder pain, and palpable lower abdominal masses.

▶ *Sickle cell anemia.* In this hereditary disorder, gross hematuria may result from congestion of the renal papillae. Other signs and symptoms may include pallor, dehydration, chronic fatigue, polyarthralgia, leg ulcers, dyspnea, chest pain, impaired growth and development, hepatomegaly and, possibly, jaundice. Auscultation reveals tachycardia and systolic and diastolic murmurs.

▶ *Systemic lupus erythematosus.* Gross hematuria and proteinuria may occur when this disorder involves the kidneys. Cardinal features include nondeforming joint pain and stiffness, a butterfly rash, photosensitivity, Raynaud's phenomenon, seizures or psychoses, recurrent fever, lymphadenopathy, oral or nasopharyngeal ulcers, anorexia, and weight loss.

▶ *Urethral trauma.* Hematuria may occur initially, possibly with blood at the urinary meatus, local pain, and penile or vulvar ecchymosis.

▶ *Vaginitis.* When this infection spreads to the urinary tract, it may produce macroscopic hematuria. Related signs and symptoms may include urinary frequency and urgency, dysuria, nocturia, perineal pain, pruritus, and a malodorous vaginal discharge.

▶ *Vasculitis.* Hematuria is usually microscopic in this disorder. Other signs and symptoms include malaise, myalgia, polyarthralgia, fever, increased blood pressure, pallor and, occasionally, anuria. Other features, such as urticaria and purpura, may reflect the etiology of vasculitis.

Other causes

▶ *Diagnostic tests.* Renal biopsy is the diagnostic test most often associated with hematuria. This sign may also result from biopsy or manipulative instrumentation of the urinary tract, as in cystoscopy.

DRUG WATCH *Drugs that commonly cause hematuria include analgesics, anticoagulants, aspirin (toxicity), cyclophosphamide, metyrosine, penicillin, rifampin, and thiabendazole.*

▶ *Herbs.* When taken with an anticoagulant, herbal remedies such as garlic and ginkgo biloba can cause excessive bleeding and hematuria.

▶ *Treatments.* Any therapy that involves manipulative instrumentation of the urinary tract, such as transurethral prostatectomy, may cause microscopic or macroscopic hematuria. Hematuria may also result from radiation cystitis, a complication of external beam radiation therapy for prostate and cervical cancers.[4] After a kidney transplant, a patient may have hematuria with or without clots, which may require indwelling urinary catheter irrigation.

Special considerations

Because hematuria may frighten and upset the patient, be sure to provide emotional support. Check his vital signs at least every 4 hours and monitor intake and output, including the amount and pattern of hematuria. If the patient has an indwelling urinary catheter in place, ensure its patency and irrigate it if needed to remove clots and tissue that may impede urine drainage. Administer prescribed analgesics, and enforce bed rest as indicated. Prepare the patient for diagnostic tests, such as blood and urine studies, cystoscopy, and renal X-rays or biopsy.

Pediatric pointers

In critically ill neonates, hematuria may be a complication of umbilical artery catheterization, possibly related to renal thrombi formation.[5] Many of the causes described above also produce hematuria in children. However, cyclophosphamide is more likely to cause hematuria in children than in adults.

Common causes of hematuria that chiefly affect children include congenital anomalies, such as obstructive uropathy and renal dysplasia; birth trauma; hematologic disorders, such as vitamin K deficiency, hemophilia, and hemolytic-uremic syndrome; certain neoplasms, such as Wilms' tumor, bladder cancer, and rhabdomyosarcoma; allergies; and foreign bodies in the urinary tract. Artifactual hematuria may result from recent circumcision.

Geriatric pointers

Evaluation of hematuria in elderly patients should include a urine culture, excretory urography or sonography, and consultation with a urologist.

Patient counseling

Teach the patient how to collect serial urine specimens using the three-glass technique. This technique helps determine whether hematuria marks the beginning, end, or entire course of urination.

REFERENCES

1. Campbell, B.D. "Bladder Cancer: Revealing News about a Hidden Threat." *Nursing* 36(4):54-57, April 2006.
2. Davis, K.A., et al. "Predictors of the Need for Nephrectomy After Renal Trauma." *Journal of Trauma: Injury, Infection, and Critical Care* 60(1):164-170, January 2006.
3. Rockwood, R.R. "Extrapulmonary TB: What You Need to Know." *The Nurse Practitioner* 32(8):44-49, August 2007.
4. Gray, M. and Sims, T. "Prostate Cancer: Prevention and Management of Localized Disease." *The Nurse Practitioner* 31(9):14-29, September 2006.
5. Furdon, S.A., Horgan, M.J., Bradshaw, W.T., and Clark, D.A. "Nurses' Guide to Early Detection of Umbilical Arterial Catheter Complications in Infants." *Advances in Neonatal Care* 6(5):242-256, October 2006.

HEMOPTYSIS

Frightening to the patient and often ominous, hemoptysis is the expectoration of blood or bloody sputum from the lungs or tracheobronchial tree. It's sometimes confused with bleeding from the mouth, throat, nasopharynx, or GI tract. (See *Identifying he-*

Identifying hemoptysis

These guidelines will help you distinguish hemoptysis from epistaxis, hematemesis, and brown, red, or pink sputum.

HEMOPTYSIS

Often frothy because it's mixed with air, hemoptysis typically produces bright red sputum with an alkaline pH (tested with nitrazine paper). It's strongly suggested by respiratory signs and symptoms, including a cough, a tickling sensation in the throat, and blood produced from repeated coughing episodes. (You can rule out epistaxis because the patient's nasal passages and posterior pharynx are usually clear.)

HEMATEMESIS

Hematemesis usually originates in the GI tract; the patient vomits or regurgitates coffee-ground material that contains food particles, tests positive for occult blood, and has an acid pH. However, he may vomit bright red blood or swallowed blood from the oral cavity and nasopharynx. After an episode of hematemesis, the patient's stools may have traces of blood. Many patients with hematemesis also complain of dyspepsia.

BROWN, RED, OR PINK SPUTUM

Brown, red, or pink sputum can result from oxidation of inhaled bronchodilators. Sputum that looks like old blood may result from rupture of an amebic abscess into the bronchus. Red or brown sputum may occur in a patient with pneumonia caused by the enterobacterium *Serratia marcescens*. Currant-jelly sputum occurs with *Klebsiella* infections.

vascular, or coagulation disorders and, rarely, from a ruptured aortic aneurysm. In up to 15% of patients, the cause is unknown. The most common causes of massive hemoptysis are lung cancer, bronchiectasis, active tuberculosis, and cavitary pulmonary disease from necrotic infections or tuberculosis.

A number of pathophysiologic processes can cause hemoptysis. (See *What happens in hemoptysis.*)

If the patient coughs up copious amounts of blood, endotracheal intubation may be needed. Suction often to remove blood. Lavage may be needed to loosen tenacious secretions or clots. Massive hemoptysis can cause airway obstruction and asphyxiation. Insert an I.V. line to allow fluid replacement, drug administration, and blood transfusions if needed. An emergency bronchoscopy should be performed to identify the bleeding site. Monitor blood pressure and pulse to detect hypotension and tachycardia, and draw an arterial blood sample for laboratory analysis to monitor respiratory status.

History and physical examination

If the hemoptysis is mild, ask the patient when it began. Has he ever coughed up blood before? How much blood is he coughing up now and how often? Ask about a history of cardiac, pulmonary, or bleeding disorders. If he's receiving anticoagulant therapy, find out which drug, its dosage and schedule, and the duration of therapy. Is he taking other prescription drugs? Does he smoke? Ask the patient if he has recently had any infections or been exposed to tuberculosis. When was his last tine test and what were the results?

Take the patient's vital signs and examine his nose, mouth, and pharynx for sources of bleeding. Inspect the configuration of his chest and look for abnormal movement during breathing, use of accessory muscles, and retractions. Observe his respiratory rate, depth, and rhythm. Finally, examine his skin for lesions.

Next, palpate the patient's chest for diaphragm level and for tenderness, respiratory excursion, fremitus, and abnormal pulsations; then percuss for flatness, dullness, resonance, hyperresonance, and tympany. Finally, auscul-

moptysis.) Expectoration of 200 ml of blood in a single episode suggests severe bleeding; expectoration of 400 ml in 3 hours or more than 600 ml in 16 hours signals a life-threatening crisis.

In the United States, hemoptysis usually results from inflammatory lung disease or lung cancer.[1] Worldwide, however, tuberculosis is the leading cause of hemoptysis.[1] It also may result from inflammatory, infectious, cardio-

What happens in hemoptysis

Hemoptysis results when bronchial or pulmonary vessels bleed into the respiratory tract. Bleeding reflects alterations in the vascular walls and in blood-clotting mechanisms. It can result from any of the following pathophysiologic processes:
• hemorrhage and diapedesis of red blood cells from the pulmonary microvasculature into the alveoli
• necrosis of lung tissue that causes inflammation and rupture of blood vessels or hemorrhage into the alveolar spaces
• rupture of an aortic aneurysm into the tracheobronchial tree
• rupture of distended endobronchial blood vessels from pulmonary hypertension caused by mitral stenosis
• rupture of a pulmonary arteriovenous fistula, of bronchial or pulmonary artery collateral channels, or of pulmonary venous collateral channels
• sloughing of a caseous lesion into the tracheobronchial tree
• ulceration and erosion of the bronchial epithelium.

tate the lungs, noting especially the quality and intensity of breath sounds. Also auscultate for heart murmurs, bruits, and pleural friction rubs.

Obtain a sputum specimen and examine it for overall quantity, for the amount of blood it contains, and for its color, odor, and consistency.

Medical causes

▶ *Aortic aneurysm (ruptured)*. Rarely, an aortic aneurysm ruptures into the tracheobronchial tree, causing hemoptysis and sudden death.
▶ *Blast lung injury*. Although people with this type of injury may not have obvious external chest trauma, they sometimes show other indications of internal damage, such as hemoptysis. Health care providers should evaluate survivors of explosive detonations for other classic signs and symptoms of a blast lung injury, such as chest pain, cyanosis, dyspnea, and wheezing. Treatment includes careful administration of fluids and oxygen to ensure tissue perfusion.
▶ *Bronchial adenoma*. This insidious disorder causes recurring hemoptysis in up to 30% of patients along with a chronic cough and local wheezing.
▶ *Bronchiectasis*. Inflamed bronchial surfaces and eroded bronchial blood vessels cause hemoptysis, which can vary from blood-tinged sputum to blood (in about 20% of patients). The patient typically has a chronic cough producing copious amounts of foul-smelling, purulent sputum. He also may have coarse crackles, clubbing (a late sign), fever, weight loss, fatigue, weakness, malaise, and dyspnea on exertion.
▶ *Bronchitis (chronic)*. The first sign of this disorder is typically a productive cough that lasts at least 3 months. Eventually this leads to production of blood-streaked sputum; massive hemorrhage is unusual. Other respiratory effects include dyspnea, prolonged expirations, wheezing, scattered rhonchi, accessory muscle use, barrel chest, tachypnea, and clubbing (a late sign).
▶ *Coagulation disorders*. Such disorders as thrombocytopenia and disseminated intravascular coagulation can cause hemoptysis, multisystem hemorrhaging (for example, GI bleeding or epistaxis), and purpuric lesions.
▶ *Laryngeal cancer*. Hemoptysis occurs in this cancer, but hoarseness is usually the initial sign. Other findings may include dysphagia, dyspnea, stridor, cervical lymphadenopathy, and neck pain.
▶ *Lung abscess*. In about 50% of patients, this disorder produces blood-streaked sputum resulting from bronchial ulceration, necrosis, and granulation tissue. Common related findings include a cough producing large amounts of purulent, foul-smelling sputum; fever with chills; diaphoresis; anorexia; weight loss; headache; weakness; dyspnea; pleuritic or dull chest pain; and clubbing. Auscultation reveals tubular or cavernous breath sounds and crackles. Percussion reveals dullness on the affected side.
▶ *Lung cancer*. Ulceration of the bronchus commonly causes recurring hemoptysis (an

early sign), which can vary from blood-streaked sputum to blood. Related findings include a productive cough, dyspnea, fever, anorexia, weight loss, wheezing, and chest pain (a late symptom).

▶ *Plague.* The pneumonic form of this acute bacterial infection, caused by *Yersinia pestis,* can produce hemoptysis, a productive cough, chest pain, tachypnea, dyspnea, increasing respiratory distress, and cardiopulmonary insufficiency. Pneumonic plague begins abruptly with chills, fever, headache, and myalgia.

▶ *Pneumonia.* In up to 50% of patients, *Klebsiella* pneumonia produces dark brown or red (currant-jelly) sputum, which is so tenacious that the patient has trouble expelling it from his mouth. This type of pneumonia begins abruptly with chills, fever, dyspnea, a productive cough, and severe pleuritic chest pain. Other findings may include cyanosis, prostration, tachycardia, decreased breath sounds, and crackles.

Pneumococcal pneumonia causes pinkish or rusty mucoid sputum. It begins with sudden shaking chills; a rapidly rising temperature; and, in over 80% of patients, tachycardia and tachypnea. Within a few hours, the patient typically develops a productive cough along with severe, stabbing, pleuritic pain that leads to rapid, shallow, grunting respirations with splinting. Examination reveals respiratory distress with dyspnea and accessory muscle use, crackles, and dullness on percussion over the affected lung. Malaise, weakness, myalgia, and prostration accompany a high fever.

▶ *Pulmonary arteriovenous fistula.* Occurring in young adults, this genetic disorder causes intermittent hemoptysis along with cyanosis, clubbing, mild dyspnea, fatigue, vertigo, syncope, confusion, and speech and visual impairments. The patient may bleed from the nose, mouth, or lips. Ruby red patches appear on the face, tongue, skin, mucous membranes, or nail beds.

▶ *Pulmonary contusion.* Blunt chest trauma commonly causes a cough with hemoptysis. Other signs and symptoms that appear over several hours include dyspnea, tachypnea, chest pain, tachycardia, hypotension, crackles, and decreased or absent breath sounds over the affected area. Severe respiratory distress—with oppressive dyspnea, nasal flaring, use of accessory muscles, extreme anxiety, cyanosis, and diaphoresis—may develop at any time.

▶ *Pulmonary edema.* Severe cardiogenic or noncardiogenic pulmonary edema commonly causes frothy, blood-tinged pink sputum, which accompanies severe dyspnea, orthopnea, gasping, anxiety, cyanosis, diffuse crackles, a ventricular gallop, and cold, clammy skin. This life-threatening condition may also cause tachycardia, lethargy, cardiac arrhythmias, tachypnea, hypotension, and a thready pulse.

▶ *Pulmonary embolism with infarction.* Hemoptysis is a common finding in this life-threatening disorder, although massive hemoptysis is rare. Typical initial symptoms are dyspnea and anginal or pleuritic chest pain. Other common clinical features include tachycardia, tachypnea, low-grade fever, and diaphoresis. Less common features include splinting of the chest, leg edema, and—with a large embolus—cyanosis, syncope, and jugular vein distention. Examination reveals decreased breath sounds, pleural friction rub, crackles, diffuse wheezing, dullness on percussion, and signs of circulatory collapse (weak, rapid pulse and hypotension), cerebral ischemia (transient loss of consciousness and seizures), and hypoxemia (restlessness and, particularly in elderly patients, hemiplegia and other focal neurologic deficits).

▶ *Pulmonary hypertension (primary).* Hemoptysis, exertional dyspnea, and fatigue typically develop late in this disorder. Angina-like pain usually occurs with exertion and may radiate to the neck but not to the arms. Other findings include arrhythmias, syncope, cough, and hoarseness.

▶ *Pulmonary tuberculosis.* Blood-streaked or blood-tinged sputum commonly occurs in this disorder; massive hemoptysis may occur in advanced cavitary tuberculosis. Accompanying respiratory findings include a chronic productive cough, fine crackles after coughing, dyspnea, dullness on percussion, increased tactile fremitus and, possibly, amphoric breath sounds. The patient may also develop night sweats, malaise, fatigue, fever, anorexia, weight loss, and pleuritic chest pain.

▶ *Silicosis.* This chronic disorder causes a productive cough with mucopurulent sputum that later becomes blood streaked. Occasionally, massive hemoptysis may occur. Other findings include fine end-inspiratory crackles at lung bases, exertional dyspnea, tachypnea, weight loss, fatigue, and weakness.

▶ *Systemic lupus erythematosus.* In 50% of patients with this disorder, pleuritis and pneumonitis cause hemoptysis, a cough, dyspnea, pleuritic chest pain, and crackles. Related findings are a butterfly rash in the acute phase, nondeforming joint pain and stiffness, photosensitivity, Raynaud's phenomenon, seizures or psychoses, anorexia with weight loss, and lymphadenopathy.

▶ *Tracheal trauma.* Torn tracheal mucosa may cause hemoptysis, hoarseness, dysphagia, neck pain, airway occlusion, and respiratory distress.

▶ *Wegener's granulomatosis.* Necrotizing, granulomatous vasculitis characterizes this multisystem disorder. Findings include hemoptysis, chest pain, cough, wheezing, dyspnea, epistaxis, severe sinusitis, and hemorrhagic skin lesions.

Other causes
▶ *Diagnostic tests.* Lung or airway injury from bronchoscopy, laryngoscopy, mediastinoscopy, or lung biopsy can cause bleeding and hemoptysis.

Special considerations
Comfort and reassure the patient, who may react to this alarming sign with anxiety and apprehension. If necessary, to protect the nonbleeding lung, place him in the lateral decubitus position, with the suspected bleeding lung facing down. Perform this maneuver with caution because hypoxemia may worsen with the healthy lung facing up.

Suspect pulmonary embolism in any patient presenting with dyspnea, tachypnea, chest pain, cough, and hemoptysis. Because 10% of patients with a pulmonary embolism die within the first hour, early identification of signs and symptoms is critical.[2]

Prepare the patient for diagnostic tests to determine the cause of bleeding. These may include a complete blood count, a sputum culture and smear, chest X-rays, coagulation studies, bronchoscopy, lung biopsy, pulmonary arteriography, and a lung scan.

Pediatric pointers
Hemoptysis in children may stem from Goodpasture's syndrome, cystic fibrosis, or (rarely) idiopathic primary pulmonary hemosiderosis. Sometimes no cause can be found for pulmonary hemorrhage occurring within the first 2 weeks of life; in such cases, the prognosis is poor.

Geriatric pointers
If the patient is receiving anticoagulants, determine any changes that need to be made in his diet or drug regimen (including over-the-counter drugs and natural supplements) because these factors may affect clotting.

Patient counseling
Hemoptysis usually ceases gradually during treatment of the causative disorder. Many chronic disorders, however, cause recurrent hemoptysis. Instruct the patient to report recurring episodes and to bring a sputum specimen containing blood if he returns for treatment or reevaluation.

REFERENCES
1. Pruitt, W.C. "Why Is This Patient Coughing Up Blood?" *Nursing Made Incredibly Easy!* 3(3):50-53, May/June 2005.
2. Charlebois, D. "Early Recognition of Pulmonary Embolism: The Key to Lowering Mortality." *The Journal of Cardiovascular Nursing* 20(4):254-259, July/August 2005.

● HOMANS' SIGN

Homans' sign is positive when deep calf pain results from strong and abrupt dorsiflexion of the ankle. This pain results from venous thrombosis or inflammation of the calf muscles. However, because a positive Homans' sign appears in only 35% of patients with these conditions, it's an unreliable indicator. (See *Eliciting Homans' sign,* page 238.) Even when accurate, a positive Homans' sign doesn't indicate the extent of the venous disorder.

This elicited sign may be confused with continuous calf pain, which can result from strains, contusions, cellulitis, or arterial occlusion, or with pain in the posterior ankle or

Eliciting Homans' sign

To elicit Homans' sign, first support the patient's thigh with one hand and his foot with the other. Bend his leg slightly at the knee; then firmly and abruptly dorsiflex the ankle. Resulting deep calf pain indicates a positive Homans' sign. (The patient also may resist ankle dorsiflexion or flex the knee involuntarily if Homans' sign is positive.)

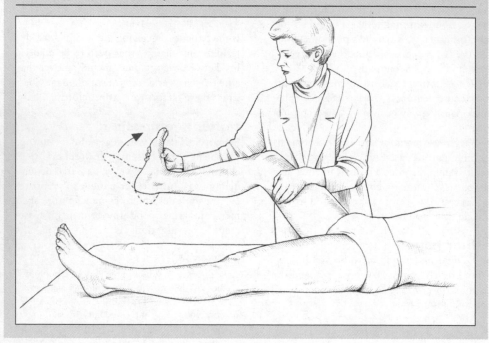

Achilles tendon (for example, in a woman with Achilles tendons shortened from wearing high heels).

History and physical examination

When you detect a positive Homans' sign, focus your patient history on signs and symptoms that can accompany deep vein thrombosis or thrombophlebitis. These include throbbing, aching, heavy, or tight sensations in the calf and leg pain during or after exercise or routine activity. Also, ask about any shortness of breath or chest pain, which may indicate pulmonary embolism. Be sure to ask about predisposing events, such as leg injury, recent surgery, childbirth, use of hormonal contraceptives, associated diseases (cancer, nephrosis, hypercoagulable states), and prolonged inactivity or bed rest.

Next, inspect and palpate the patient's calf for warmth, tenderness, redness, swelling, and a palpable vein. If you strongly suspect deep vein thrombosis, elicit Homans' sign very carefully to avoid dislodging the clot, which could cause a life-threatening pulmonary embolism.

In addition, measure the circumference of both the patient's calves. The calf with the positive Homans' sign may be larger because of edema and swelling.

Medical causes

▶ *Cellulitis (superficial).* This disorder typically affects the legs but can also affect the arms, producing pain, redness, tenderness, and edema. Some patients also experience fever, chills, tachycardia, headache, and hypotension.

Patient compliance using TEDS and SCDs

Question: *How can patient compliance with thromboembolic deterrent stockings (TEDS) and sequential compression devices (SCDs) be increased?*

Research: TEDS and SCDs, both alone and with antithrombolytics, have been shown to be good preventive measures against deep vein thrombosis (DVT). The researchers' goal was to determine whether knee-length or thigh-length TEDS or SCDs were more comfortable, applied correctly, and worn by patients. They also looked to assess reasons for noncompliance. The authors collected data from 137 randomly selected patients with orders for TEDS or SCDs via a patient survey and observational data tool. The survey was used to collect information from the patient about the reason the stockings or devices were being used, whether they were comfortable to wear, and how long they wore them per day. Observations on the fit of the TEDS or SCDs were also performed.

Conclusion: Most patients had thigh-length TEDS and SCDs; however, only 29.2% were wearing them at the time of the survey. The major reasons for noncompliance were discomfort and not reapplying the devices after bathing or ambulating. Discomfort complaints were 50% higher in those wearing thigh-length devices.

Application: Patient preference for knee-length TEDS or SCDs should be considered in order to increase compliance and thereby decrease DVT risk. Be sure to determine appropriate fit for each patient by selecting the correct size and properly securing the Velcro closure. Teach patients how to apply the devices properly and remind them of the importance of reapplying them after bathing or ambulating.

Source: Brady, D., Raingruber, B., Peterson, J., Varnau, W., Denman, J., Resuello, R., De Contreaus, R., and Mahnke, J. "The Use of Knee-Length versus Thigh-Length Compression Stockings and Sequential Compression Devices." *Critical Care Nursing Quarterly*, 30(3):255-262, 2007.

▶ *Deep vein thrombophlebitis.* A positive Homans' sign and calf tenderness may be the only clinical features of this disorder. However, the patient may also have severe pain, heaviness, warmth, and swelling of the affected leg; visible, engorged superficial veins or palpable, cordlike veins; and fever, chills, and malaise.

▶ *Deep vein thrombosis (DVT).* DVT causes a positive Homans' sign along with tenderness over the deep calf veins, slight edema of the calves and thighs, a low-grade fever, and tachycardia. If DVT affects the femoral and iliac veins, you'll notice marked local swelling and tenderness. If DVT causes venous obstruction, you'll notice cyanosis and possibly cool skin in the affected leg. While a positive Homans' sign has been considered a classic assessment finding, the absence of this sign does not rule out DVT.[1]

▶ *Popliteal cyst (ruptured).* Rupture of this synovial cyst may produce a positive Homans' sign as well as sudden onset of calf tenderness, swelling, and redness.

Special considerations

Place the patient on bed rest, with the affected leg elevated above the heart level. Apply warm, moist compresses to the affected area, and administer mild oral analgesics. In addition, prepare the patient for further diagnostic tests, such as Doppler studies and venograms.

Once the patient is ambulatory, advise him to wear elastic support stockings after his discomfort decreases (usually in 5 to 10 days) and to continue wearing them for at least 3 months. Be sure to advise the patient on the importance of wearing the support stockings as directed. (See *Patient compliance using TEDS and SCDs.*) In addition, instruct the patient to keep the affected leg elevated while sitting and to avoid crossing his legs at the knees because this may impair circulation to the popliteal area. (Crossing at the ankles is acceptable.)

Pediatric pointers

Homans' sign is seldom assessed in children, who rarely have DVT or thrombophlebitis.

Patient counseling

If the patient is prescribed long-term anticoagulant therapy, instruct him to report any signs of prolonged clotting time. These include black, tarry stools; brown or red urine; bleeding gums; and bruises. Also, stress the importance of keeping follow-up appointments so that prothrombin time can be monitored.

Instruct the patient to avoid alcohol and restrict his intake of green leafy vegetables (spinach and parsley), which are high in vitamin K. Also instruct him to review all drugs he's taking with his physician because some drugs may enhance or inhibit the effects of the anticoagulant. The patient should also verify with his physician that any future prescription and over-the-counter drugs are safe to take.

REFERENCES
1. Bartley, M. "Keep Venous Thromboembolism at Bay." *Nursing* 36(10):36-41, October 2006.

HYPERPNEA

Hyperpnea indicates increased respiratory effort for a sustained period—a normal rate (at least 12 breaths/minute) with increased depth (a tidal volume greater than 7.5 ml/kg), an increased rate (more than 20 breaths/minute) with normal depth, or increased rate and depth. This sign differs from sighing (intermittent deep inspirations) and may or may not be associated with tachypnea (increased respiratory rate).

The typical patient with hyperpnea breathes at a normal or increased rate and inhales deeply, displaying marked chest expansion. He may complain of shortness of breath if a respiratory disorder is causing hypoxemia, or he may not be aware of his breathing if a metabolic, psychiatric, or neurologic disorder is causing involuntary hyperpnea. Other causes of hyperpnea include profuse diarrhea or dehydration, loss of pancreatic juice or bile from GI drainage, and ureterosigmoidostomy. All these conditions and procedures cause a loss of bicarbonate ions, resulting in metabolic acidosis. Hyperpnea may also accompany strenuous exercise, and voluntary hyperpnea can promote relaxation in patients experiencing stress or pain—for example, women in labor.

Hyperventilation, a consequence of hyperpnea, is characterized by alkalosis (arterial pH above 7.45 and partial pressure of carbon dioxide [Pco_2] below 35 mm Hg). In central neurogenic hyperventilation, brain stem dysfunction (as results from a severe cranial injury) increases the rate and depth of respirations. In acute intermittent hyperventilation, the respiratory pattern may be a response to hypoxemia, anxiety, fear, pain, or excitement. Hyperpnea may also be a compensatory mechanism in metabolic acidosis. Under these conditions, it's known as *Kussmaul's respirations.* (See *Kussmaul's respirations: A compensatory mechanism.*)

History and physical examination

If you observe hyperpnea in a patient whose other signs and symptoms signal a life-threatening emergency, you must intervene quickly and effectively. (See *Managing hyperpnea,* page 242.) However, if the patient's condition isn't grave, first determine his level of consciousness (LOC). If he's alert (and if his hyperpnea isn't interfering with speaking), ask about recent illnesses or infections; ingestion of aspirin or other drugs or chemicals; or inhalation of drugs or chemicals. Find out if the patient has diabetes mellitus, renal disease, or any pulmonary conditions. Is he excessively thirsty or hungry? Has he recently had severe diarrhea or an upper respiratory tract infection?

Next, observe the patient for clues to his abnormal breathing pattern. Is he unable to speak, or does he speak only in brief, choppy phrases? Is his breathing abnormally rapid? Examine the patient for cyanosis (especially the mouth, lips, mucous membranes, and earlobes), anxiety, and restlessness—all signs of decreased tissue oxygenation, as occurs in

Kussmaul's respirations: A compensatory mechanism

Kussmaul's respirations—fast, deep breathing without pauses—characteristically sound labored, with deep breaths that resemble sighs. This breathing pattern develops when respiratory centers in the medulla detect decreased blood pH, thereby triggering compensatory fast and deep breathing to remove excess carbon dioxide and restore pH balance.

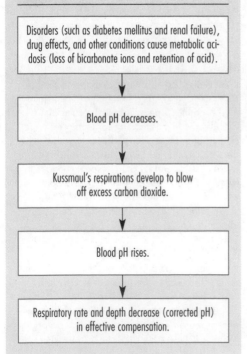

Disorders (such as diabetes mellitus and renal failure), drug effects, and other conditions cause metabolic acidosis (loss of bicarbonate ions and retention of acid).

↓

Blood pH decreases.

↓

Kussmaul's respirations develop to blow off excess carbon dioxide.

↓

Blood pH rises.

↓

Respiratory rate and depth decrease (corrected pH) in effective compensation.

cous membranes for turgor, possibly indicating dehydration. Auscultate the patient's heart and lungs.

Medical causes

▶ *Head injury.* Hyperpnea that results from a severe head injury is called *central neurogenic hyperventilation.* Whether its onset is acute or gradual, this type of hyperpnea indicates damage to the lower midbrain or upper pons. Accompanying signs reflect the site and extent of injury and can include loss of consciousness; soft-tissue injury or bony deformity of the face, head, or neck; facial edema; clear or bloody drainage from the mouth, nose, or ears; raccoon eyes; Battle's sign; an absent doll's eye sign; and motor and sensory disturbances.

Signs of increased intracranial pressure include decreased response to painful stimulation, loss of pupillary reaction, bradycardia, increased systolic pressure, and widening pulse pressure.

▶ *Hyperventilation syndrome.* Acute anxiety triggers episodic hyperpnea, resulting in respiratory alkalosis. Other findings may include agitation, vertigo, syncope, pallor, circumoral and peripheral paresthesia, muscle twitching, carpopedal spasm, weakness, and arrhythmias.

▶ *Hypoxemia.* Many pulmonary disorders that cause hypoxemia—for example, pneumonia, pulmonary edema, chronic obstructive pulmonary disease, and pneumothorax—may cause hyperpnea and episodes of hyperventilation with chest pain, dizziness, and paresthesia. Other effects include dyspnea, cough, crackles, rhonchi, wheezing, and decreased breath sounds.

▶ *Ketoacidosis. Alcoholic ketoacidosis* (occurring most often in women with a history of alcohol abuse) typically follows cessation of drinking after a marked increase in alcohol consumption has caused severe vomiting. Kussmaul's respirations begin abruptly and are accompanied by vomiting for several days, fruity breath odor, slight dehydration, abdominal pain and distention, and absent bowel sounds. The patient is alert and has a normal blood glucose level, unlike the patient with diabetic ketoacidosis.

shock. Also, observe the patient for intercostal and abdominal retractions, use of accessory muscles, and diaphoresis, all of which may indicate deep breathing related to an insufficient supply of oxygen. Next, inspect for draining wounds or signs of infection, and ask about nausea and vomiting. Take the patient's vital signs, including oxygen saturation, noting fever. Also, examine his skin and mu-

Managing hyperpnea

Carefully examine a patient with hyperpnea for related signs of life-threatening conditions, such as increased intracranial pressure (ICP), metabolic acidosis, diabetic ketoacidosis, and uremia. Be prepared for rapid intervention.

INCREASED ICP

If you observe hyperpnea in a patient who has signs of head trauma (soft-tissue injury, edema, or ecchymosis on the face or head) from a recent accident and has lost consciousness, act quickly to prevent further brain stem injury and irreversible deterioration. Then take the patient's vital signs, noting bradycardia, increased systolic blood pressure, and widening pulse pressure—signs of increased ICP.

Examine his pupillary reaction. Elevate the head of the bed 30 degrees (unless you suspect spinal cord injury), and insert an artificial airway. Connect the patient to a cardiac monitor, and continuously observe his respiratory pattern. (Irregular respirations signal deterioration.) Start an I.V. line at a slow infusion rate and prepare to administer an osmotic diuretic, such as mannitol, to decrease cerebral edema. Catheterize the patient to measure urine output, administer supplemental oxygen, and keep emergency resuscitation equipment close by. Obtain arterial blood gas measurements to help guide treatments.

METABOLIC ACIDOSIS

If the patient with hyperpnea doesn't have a head injury, his increased respiratory rate probably indicates metabolic acidosis. If his level of consciousness is decreased, check his chart for history data to help you determine the cause of his metabolic acidosis, and intervene appropriately. Suspect shock if the patient has cold, clammy skin. Palpate for a rapid, thready pulse and take his blood pressure, noting hypotension. Elevate the patient's legs 30 degrees, apply pressure dressings to any obvious hemorrhage, start several large-bore I.V. lines, and

prepare to administer fluids, vasopressors, and blood transfusions.

A patient with hyperpnea who has a history of alcohol abuse, is vomiting profusely, has diarrhea or profuse abdominal drainage, has ingested an overdose of aspirin, or is cachectic and has a history of starvation may also have metabolic acidosis. Inspect his skin for dryness and poor turgor, indicating dehydration. Take his vital signs, looking for low-grade fever and hypotension. Start an I.V. line for fluid replacement. Draw blood for electrolyte studies, and prepare to administer sodium bicarbonate.

DIABETIC KETOACIDOSIS

If the patient has a history of diabetes mellitus, is vomiting, and has a fruity breath odor (acetone breath), suspect diabetic ketoacidosis. Catheterize him to monitor for increased urine output, and infuse saline solution. Perform a fingerstick to estimate blood glucose levels with a reagent strip. Obtain a urine specimen to test for glucose and acetone, and draw blood for glucose and ketone tests. Also, administer fluids, insulin, potassium, and sodium bicarbonate I.V.

UREMIA

If the patient has a history of renal disease, an ammonia breath odor (uremic fetor), and a fine, white powder on his skin (uremic frost), suspect uremia. Start an I.V. line at a slow rate, and prepare to administer sodium bicarbonate. Monitor his electrocardiogram for arrhythmias due to hyperkalemia. Monitor his serum electrolyte, blood urea nitrogen, and creatinine levels as well until hemodialysis or peritoneal dialysis begins.

Diabetic ketoacidosis is potentially life-threatening and typically produces Kussmaul's respirations. The patient usually has polydipsia, polyphagia, and polyuria before the onset of acidosis; he may have a history of diabetes mellitus. Other clinical features include fruity

breath odor; orthostatic hypotension; rapid, thready pulse; generalized weakness; decreased LOC (lethargy to coma); nausea; vomiting; anorexia; and abdominal pain.

Starvation ketoacidosis is also potentially life-threatening and can cause Kussmaul's respirations. Its onset is gradual; typical findings include signs of cachexia and dehydration, decreased LOC, bradycardia, and a history of severely limited food intake.

▶ *Renal failure.* Acute or chronic renal failure can cause life-threatening acidosis with Kussmaul's respirations. Signs and symptoms of severe renal failure include oliguria or anuria, uremic fetor, and yellow, dry, scaly skin. Other cutaneous signs include severe pruritus, uremic frost, purpura, and ecchymosis. The patient may complain of nausea and vomiting, weakness, burning pain in the legs and feet, and diarrhea or constipation.

As acidosis progresses, corresponding clinical features include frothy sputum, pleuritic chest pain, and signs of heart failure and pleural or pericardial effusion. Neurologic signs include altered LOC (lethargy to coma), twitching, and seizures. Hyperkalemia and hypertension, if present, require rapid intervention to prevent cardiovascular collapse.

▶ *Sepsis.* Early or uncomplicated infection may cause mild hyperventilation.[1] A severe infection may cause lactic acidosis, resulting in Kussmaul's respirations. Other findings include tachycardia, fever or a low temperature, chills, headache, lethargy, profuse diaphoresis, anorexia, cough, wound drainage, burning on urination, confusion or change in mental status, and other signs of local infection.

▶ *Shock.* Potentially life-threatening metabolic acidosis produces Kussmaul's respirations, hypotension, tachycardia, narrowed pulse pressure, weak pulse, dyspnea, oliguria, anxiety, restlessness, stupor that can progress to coma, and cool, clammy skin. Other clinical features may include external or internal bleeding (in hypovolemic shock); chest pain, arrhythmias, and signs of heart failure (in cardiogenic shock); high fever, chills and, rarely, hypothermia (in septic shock); or stridor due to laryngeal edema (in anaphylactic shock). Onset is usually acute in hypovolemic, cardiogenic, or anaphylactic shock, but it may be gradual in septic shock.

Other causes

DRUG WATCH *Toxic levels of salicylates, ammonium chloride, acetazolamide, and other carbonic anhydrase inhibitors can cause Kussmaul's respirations.*

So can ingestion of methanol or ethylene glycol, found in antifreeze solutions.

Special considerations

Monitor vital signs, including oxygen saturation, in all patients with hyperpnea, and observe for increasing respiratory distress or an irregular respiratory pattern signaling deterioration. Prepare for immediate intervention to prevent cardiovascular collapse: Start an I.V. line for giving fluids, blood transfusions, and vasopressors for hemodynamic stabilization, as ordered, and prepare to give ventilatory support. Prepare the patient for arterial blood gas analysis and blood chemistry studies.

Monitor patients with hyperpnea for evidence of dehydration. Hyperpnea can increase insensible fluid losses from the respiratory tract.[2]

Pediatric pointers

Hyperpnea in children indicates the same metabolic or neurologic causes as in adults and requires the same prompt intervention. Diabetic ketoacidosis is more common in young children and adults, and is the most common presentation of diabetes in children younger than age four.[2] The most common cause of metabolic acidosis in children is diarrhea, which can cause a life-threatening crisis. In infants, Kussmaul's respirations may accompany acidosis due to inborn errors of metabolism.

Patient counseling

Teach the patient how to monitor his blood sugar level. Stress the importance of compliance with diabetes therapy, if applicable. Provide information on fluids and foods the patient should avoid. Discuss pulmonary hygiene and teach the patient ways to avoid respiratory infections. Emphasize the importance of abstinence from alcohol; refer to support groups or other resources that can assist, if indicated.

REFERENCES

1. Wood, S., Lavieri, M.C., and Durkin, T. "What You Need to Know about Sepsis." *Nursing* 37(3):46-51, March 2007.
2. Steinmann, R. "Pediatric Diabetic Ketoacidosis." *AJN* 107(3):72cc-72kk, March 2007.

HYPERTHERMIA

Hyperthermia, also known as heat syndrome, refers to an elevation of the core body temperature above normal. (See *Signs and symptoms of heat syndromes*.) It results when environmental and internal factors increase heat production or decrease heat loss beyond the body's ability to compensate.[1] Hyperthermia affects both sexes equally; however, incidence increases among elderly patients and neonates during excessively hot days. Risk factors for hyperthermia include obesity, salt and water depletion, alcohol use, poor physical condition, age, and socioeconomic status.

A temperature between 99° and 102° F (37.2° and 38.9° C) is considered mild hyperthermia. A temperature between 102° and 105° F (38.9° and 40.6° C) is considered moderate hyperthermia. A temperature of 105° F (40.6 °C) or above is considered critical hyperthermia and is an emergency, particularly if the temperature rises rapidly or stays elevated for a prolonged period.

For critical hyperthermia, immediate action should include providing supplemental oxygen and preparing the patient for endotracheal intubation and mechanical ventilation, if needed. The goal is to reduce the patient's temperature, but not too rapidly. Rapid reduction can lead to vasoconstriction and then to shivering, which increases metabolic demands and oxygen consumption. Give diazepam or chlorpromazine to control shivering. Continuous cardiac monitoring will be instituted, and the patient will be monitored for arrhythmias. Prepare the patient for pulmonary artery catheter insertion to monitor the body's core temperature. Closely observe the patient's vital signs and level of consciousness. Give fluids and replace electrolytes, as ordered. Remove the patient's clothing, apply cool water to the skin, and then fan the patient with cool air.

In mild and moderate hyperthermia, provide a cool, calm environment and allow the patient to rest. Encourage oral intake and administration of I.V. fluids. Replace electrolytes, as necessary.

History and physical examination

Ask the patient about the onset and duration of the fever. Ask the patient to describe the pattern of the fever. Did the temperature rise progressively or did it rise, disappear, and then reappear? Does he have accompanying symptoms, such as chills, headache, fatigue, diarrhea, or pain? Has the patient recently had an infection or exposure to an organism or someone else who was ill? Ask the patient whether he was exposed to high temperatures for a prolonged time. Ask about his work environment and water consumption while working. Has the patient had unusual physical or emotional stress recently? Ask if he has had any burns or trauma, undergone surgery under general anesthesia, or received a blood transfusion. Does the patient have a history of endocrine dysfunction or malignant hyperthermia? Is he taking thyroid medication? Ask the patient about other drugs that disrupt thermoregulatory function, such as salicylates, and drugs that impair sweating, such as antibiotics, anticholinergics, monoamine oxidase inhibitors, and phenytoin.

Perform a physical examination based on the patient's health history. Note the rate and depth of the patient's breathing and any changes from normal respiratory patterns. Inspect the skin color and temperature. Check the skin turgor and monitor for diaphoresis. Assess for signs of trauma or needle marks on the arms or legs. Inspect for shivering of the body or flushing of the face. Assess his oral mucosa for lesions or signs of dehydration. Assess the patient's mental status and be alert for signs of malaise, fatigue, restlessness, or anxiety. Auscultate lung fields and the abdomen. Monitor vital signs and the cardiac rate, rhythm, and intensity. Keep in mind that palpating the thyroid gland of a patient with hyperthyroidism can induce thyrotoxicosis.

Medical causes

▶ *Infection and inflammatory disorders.* Depending on the specific disorder, the temperature elevation may be insidious or abrupt. It can be a prodromal symptom and is often accompanied by chills, goose bumps, generalized symptoms of fatigue, headache, weakness, anorexia, malaise, and possibly, pain. If

Signs and symptoms of heat syndromes

Hyperthermia, or heat syndrome, can be classified as mild (heat cramps), moderate (heat exhaustion), or critical (heatstroke). This table highlights assessment findings in each classification.

CLASSIFICATION	ASSESSMENT FINDINGS
Mild hyperthermia Heat cramps	• Mild agitation (central nervous system findings otherwise normal) • Mild hypertension • Moist, cool skin and muscle tenderness; involved muscle groups possibly hard and lumpy • Muscle twitching and cramps • Nausea and abdominal cramps • Report of prolonged activity in a very warm or hot environment, without adequate salt intake • Tachycardia • Temperature ranging from 99° to 102° F (37.2° to 38.9° C)
Moderate hyperthermia Heat exhaustion	• Dizziness • Headache • Hypotension • Muscle cramping • Nausea and vomiting • Oliguria • Pale, moist skin • Rapid, thready pulse • Syncope or confusion • Thirst • Weakness • Temperature elevated up to 105° F (40.6° C)
Critical hyperthermia Heatstroke	• Atrial or ventricular tachycardia • Confusion, combativeness, and delirium • Fixed, dilated pupils • Hot, dry, reddened skin • Loss of consciousness • Seizures • Tachypnea • Temperature greater than 106° F (41.1° C)

the temperature is high, you may find that the patient, particularly an elderly patient, is disoriented and confused. Other signs and symptoms depend on the disease and can involve any body system. The patient's history may include exposure to an infectious agent, travel to an endemic area, or exposure to the animal or insect vector of an infectious organism. Or his recent history may include a blood transfusion, surgery, trauma, or burns.

▶ *Malignant hyperthermia.* Rapid temperature increases occur at a rate of about 2° F (1.1° C) every 15 minutes to as high as 109.4° F (43° C). Usually the rise is preceded by skeletal muscle rigidity, cardiac arrhythmia, tachycardia, and tachypnea. The patient's history will include exposure to inhalant anesthesia, particularly halothane, or muscle relaxants, particularly succinylcholine, which can trigger malignant hyperthermia in patients with the inherited trait. Other predicting factors in susceptible persons include trauma, exercise, exposure to high environmental temperatures, and infection.

▶ *Neuroleptic malignant syndrome.* Neuroleptic malignant syndrome is marked by an explosive onset of hyperthermia with muscle rigidity, altered level of consciousness, cardiac arrhythmias, tachycardia, wide fluctuations in blood pressure, postural instability, dyspnea, and tachypnea. The patient history will include use of neuroleptic drugs such as haloperidol, chlorpromazine, thioridazine, or thiothixene.

▶ *Thermoregulatory dysfunction.* With thermoregulatory dysfunction, the patient's temperature rises suddenly and rapidly. The temperature then stays at 105° F to 107° F (40.6° C to 41.7° C). Assessment may reveal vomiting, hot flushed skin, and a decreased level of consciousness. The patient may also experience complications such as tachycardia, tachypnea, or hypotension. Other findings may include mottle cyanosis if the patient has malignant hyperthermia; diarrhea if he is experienceing a thyroid storm; and signs of increased intracranial pressure when the problem is central nervous system trauma or hemorrhage. Heatstroke, brain stem compression, and thyroid storm are common causes of thermoregulatory dysfunction. Toxic doses of amphetamines and salicylates will also disrupt the thermoregulatory centers in the brain.

Other causes

DRUG WATCH *Hyperthermia may be caused by tricyclic antidepressants and drugs that impair sweating, such as anticholinergics, phenothiazines, and monoamine oxidase inhibitors.*

▶ *Impaired heat dissipation.* Impaired heat dissipation occurs with severe dehydration, in which sweat production decreases heat loss by evaporation. It also occurs when the environmental temperature is high and the body can't rid itself of heat as fast as it's being received.

Special considerations

Treat mild to moderate hyperthermia by providing a cool, restful environment. Replace oral or I.V. fluid and electrolyte losses. If the patient has heatstroke, apply cool water to the skin and fan the patient. Apply a hyper-

thermia blanket or ice packs to the groin and axilla. Expect treatment to continue until the patient's body temperature drops to 102.2° F (39° C). Vital signs will require continuous monitoring, especially the core body temperature. Follow measures to avoid shivering. Employ additional external cooling measures, such as cool, wet sheets and tepid baths. Monitor hemodynamic parameters, fluid and electrolyte balance, and laboratory and diagnostic studies. Monitor blood urea nitrogen and serum creatinine levels and assess for signs and symptoms associated with rhabdomyolysis.

Don't reduce the patient's temperature too rapidly, as too rapid a reduction can lead to vasoconstriction, which can cause shivering.

Early identification and treatment of malignant hyperthermia is critical to prevent death. Administration of dantrolene, a skeletal muscle relaxant introduced in 1979, has reduced mortality from 70% to 80% before the drug was used, to less than 5%.[2] These patients will need general anesthesia with nontriggering drugs or local/regional anesthesia, if needed.[2]

Pediatric pointers

Rarely, maternal thyrotoxicosis may be passed to the neonate, resulting in hyperthermia. More commonly, acquired thyrotoxicosis appears between ages 12 and 14, although this too is infrequent. Dehydration also will make a child sensitive to excessive heat.

Geriatric pointers

Older adults are at greater risk for hyperthermia because of a decreased ability to control their body temperature, a chronic state of volume depletion, an impaired ability to increase cardiac output in response to heat, and a decreased ability to sweat.[3]

Patient counseling

Caution the patient to reduce activity, especially outdoor activity, in the hot, humid weather. Advise him to wear light-colored, lightweight, loose-fitting clothing as well as a hat and sunglasses during hot weather. Instruct the patient to drink sufficient fluids, especially water, in hot weather and after vigorous physical activity. Warn him to avoid caffeine and alcohol in hot weather. Advise the patient to use air conditioning or to open windows and use a fan to help circulate air indoors.

Teach at-risk patients the signs and symptoms of malignant hyperthermia so they can recognize the syndrome early and seek prompt treatment.[2]

REFERENCES

1. Henker, R., Carlson, K.K. "Fever: Applying Research to Bedside Practice." *AACN Advanced Critical Care* 18(1):76-87, January/March 2007.
2. Dixon, B.A. and O'Donnell, J.M. "Is Your Patient Susceptible to Malignant Hyperthermia?" *Nursing* 36(12):26-27, December 2006.
3. Lewis, A.M. "Heatstroke in Older Adults: in This Population It's a Short Step from Heat Exhaustion." *AJN* 107(6):52-56, June 2007.

HYPOTENSION, ORTHOSTATIC

In orthostatic hypotension (also called *postural hypotension*) the patient's systolic blood pressure drops at least 20 mm Hg or more or his diastolic blood pressure drops at least 10 mm Hg within 3 minutes of rising from a supine to a sitting or standing position.[1] (Blood pressure should be measured 5 minutes after the patient has changed position.[1]) This common sign indicates failure of compensatory vasomotor responses to adjust to position changes. More specifically, in patients with orthostatic hypotension, heart rate and contractility don't increase and vasoconstriction in the legs doesn't occur in response to position changes, which results in decreased venous blood return to the heart and a rapid decrease in blood pressure.[2] It's typically associated with light-headedness, syncope, or blurred vision, and may occur in a hypotensive, normotensive, or hypertensive patient. Although commonly a nonpathologic sign in the elderly, orthostatic hypotension may result from prolonged bed rest, fluid and electrolyte imbalance, endocrine or systemic disorders, and the effects of drugs.

To detect orthostatic hypotension, take and compare blood pressure readings with the patient supine, sitting, and then standing.

If you detect orthostatic hypotension, quickly check for tachycardia, altered level of consciousness (LOC), and pale, clammy skin. If these signs are present, suspect hypovolemic shock. Insert a large-bore I.V. for fluid or blood replacement. Take the patient's vital signs every 15 minutes, and monitor his intake and output.

History and physical examination

If the patient is in no danger, obtain a history. Ask the patient if he frequently experiences dizziness, weakness, or fainting when he stands. Also ask about associated symptoms, particularly fatigue, orthopnea, impotence, nausea, headache, abdominal or chest discomfort, and GI bleeding. Then obtain a complete drug history.

Begin the physical examination by checking the patient's skin turgor. Palpate peripheral pulses and auscultate the heart and lungs. Finally, test muscle strength and observe the patient's gait for unsteadiness.

Medical causes

▶ *Adrenal insufficiency.* This disorder typically begins insidiously, with progressively severe signs and symptoms. Orthostatic hypotension may be accompanied by fatigue, muscle weakness, poor coordination, anorexia, nausea and vomiting, fasting hypoglycemia, weight loss, abdominal pain, irritability, and a weak, irregular pulse. Another common feature is hyperpigmentation—bronze coloring of the skin—which is especially prominent on the face, lips, gums, tongue, buccal mucosa, elbows, palms, knuckles, waist, and knees. Diarrhea, constipation, decreased libido, amenorrhea, and syncope may also occur along with enhanced taste, smell, and hearing, and cravings for salty food.

▶ *Alcoholism.* Chronic alcoholism can lead to development of peripheral neuropathy, which can present as orthostatic hypotension. Impotence is also a major issue in these patients. Other symptoms include numbness, tingling, nausea, vomiting, changes in bowel habits, and bizarre behavior.

▶ *Amyloidosis.* Orthostatic hypotension is commonly associated with amyloid infiltration of the autonomic nerves. Other signs and symptoms vary widely and include angina, tachycardia, dyspnea, orthopnea, fatigue, and cough.

▶ *Diabetic autonomic neuropathy.* Here, orthostatic hypotension may be accompanied by syncope, dysphagia, constipation or diarrhea, painless bladder distention with overflow incontinence, impotence, and retrograde ejaculation.

▶ *Hyperaldosteronism.* This disorder typically produces orthostatic hypotension with sustained elevated blood pressure. Most other clinical effects of hyperaldosteronism result from hypokalemia, which increases neuromuscular irritability and produces muscle weakness, intermittent flaccid paralysis, fatigue, headache, paresthesia and, possibly, tetany with positive Trousseau's and Chvostek's signs. The patient also may have visual disturbance, nocturia, polydipsia, and personality changes. Diabetes mellitus is a common finding.

▶ *Hyponatremia.* In this disorder, orthostatic hypotension typically is accompanied by headache, profound thirst, tachycardia, nausea and vomiting, abdominal cramps, muscle twitching and weakness, fatigue, oliguria or anuria, cold clammy skin, poor skin turgor, irritability, seizures, and decreased LOC. Cyanosis, thready pulse, and eventually vasomotor collapse may occur in severe sodium deficit. Common causes include adrenal insufficiency, hypothyroidism, syndrome of inappropriate antidiuretic hormone secretion, and use of thiazide diuretics.

▶ *Hypovolemia.* Mild to moderate hypovolemia may cause orthostatic hypotension with apathy, fatigue, muscle weakness, anorexia, nausea, and profound thirst. The patient also may develop dizziness, oliguria, sunken eyeballs, poor skin turgor, and dry mucous membranes.

▶ *Pheochromocytoma.* Although this disorder may produce orthostatic hypotension, its cardinal sign is paroxysmal or sustained hypertension. Typically, the patient is pale or flushed and diaphoretic, and extreme anxiety makes him appear panicky. Other signs and symptoms include tachycardia, palpitations, chest and abdominal pain, paresthesia, tremors, nausea and vomiting, low-grade fever, insomnia, and headache.

▶ *Shy-Drager syndrome.* This neurodegenerative disorder is characterized by an insidious onset of multiple autonomic failure, manifested by orthostatic hypotension, urinary and fecal incontinence, decreased sweating, and impotence. This syndrome is most common in young and middle-aged adults.

Other causes

DRUG WATCH *Certain drugs may cause orthostatic hypotension by reducing circulating blood volume, causing blood vessel dilation, or depressing the sympathetic nervous system. These drugs include antihypertensives (especially the initial dosage of prazosin hydrochloride), tricyclic antidepressants, phenothiazines, levodopa, nitrates, monoamine oxidase inhibitors, morphine, bretylium tosylate, and spinal anesthesia. Large doses of diuretics can also cause orthostatic hypotension.*

▶ *Treatments.* Orthostatic hypotension is commonly associated with prolonged bed rest (24 hours or longer). It may also result from sympathectomy, which disrupts normal vasoconstrictive mechanisms.

Special considerations

Monitor the patient's fluid balance by carefully recording his intake and output and weighing him daily. To help minimize orthostatic hypotension, advise the patient to change his position gradually. Elevate the head of the patient's bed, and help him to a sitting position with his feet dangling over the side of the bed. If he can tolerate this position, have him sit in a chair for brief periods. Immediately return him to bed if he becomes dizzy or pale, or displays other signs of hypotension. Elastic stockings may help to improve blood return to the heart from the legs.[2] Patients who are on bed rest for long periods of time may need to practice sitting for gradually longer intervals of time to prevent orthostatic hypotension.[2]

Always keep the patient's safety in mind. Never leave him unattended while he's sitting or walking; evaluate his need for assistive devices, such as a cane or walker.

Prepare the patient for diagnostic tests, such as hematocrit, serum electrolyte and drug levels, urinalysis, 12-lead electrocardiogram, and chest X-ray.

Pediatric pointers
Because normal blood pressure is lower in children than in adults, familiarize yourself with normal age-specific values to detect orthostatic hypotension. From birth to age 3 months, normal systolic pressure is 40 to 80 mm Hg. From age 3 months to 1 year, it's 80 to 100 mm Hg. From ages 1 to 12, it's 100 mm Hg plus 2 mm Hg for every year over age 1. Diastolic blood pressure is first heard at about age 4; it's normally 60 mm Hg at this age and gradually increases to 70 mm Hg by age 12.

The causes of orthostatic hypotension in children may be the same as those in adults.

Geriatric pointers
Elderly patients commonly experience autonomic dysfunction, which can present as orthostatic hypotension. Postprandial hypotension occurs 45 to 60 minutes after a meal and has been documented in up to one-third of nursing home residents. Orthostatic hypotension is a common risk factor for falls in the elderly.[3]

Patient counseling
Patients with conditions that can lead to autonomic dysfunction should be made aware of the acute drop in blood pressure than can occur with positional changes. This is particularly important in diabetic patients. Once the problem appears, such patients need to avoid volume depletion and perform positional changes gradually instead of suddenly. Tell the patient that sleeping with the head of the bed elevated may help to prevent or minimize orthostatic hypotension.[2]

REFERENCES
1. Rushing, J. "Assessing for Orthostatic Hypotension." Nursing 35(1):30, January 2005.
2. "The Ups and Downs of Orthostatic Hypotension." Nursing Made Incredibly Easy! 3(3):46-49, May/June 2005.
3. Bucher, G.M., Szczerba, P., and Curtin, P.M. "A Comprehensive Fall Prevention Program for Assessment, Intervention, and Referral." Home Healthcare Nurse 25(3):174-183, March 2007.

HYPOTHERMIA

Hypothermia refers to a core body temperature below 95° F (35° C) and affects chemical changes in the body. It may be classified as mild (93.2° to 96.8° F [32° to 35° C]), moderate (86° to 93.2° F [32° to 35° C]), or severe, which may be fatal (less than 86° F [30° C]).[1] Risk factors that contribute to serious cold injury, especially hypothermia, include lack of insulating body fat, wet or inadequate clothing, drug abuse, cardiac disease, smoking, fatigue, malnutrition and depletion of caloric reserves, and excessive alcohol intake. The incidence of hypothermia is highest in children and elderly people.

Hypothermia commonly results from cold-water near drowning and prolonged expsoure to cold temperatures. It can also occur in normal temperatures, if disease or debility alters the patient's homeostasis. Administration of large amounts of cold blood or blood products can also cause hypothermia. A process such as hemodialysis, which circulates the blood outside of the body and then returns it to the body, will result in hypothermia.

Initiate cardiopulmonary resuscitation (CPR), if needed. Hypothermia helps protect the brain from anoxia, which normally accompanies prolonged cardiopulmonary arrest. Therefore, even if the patient has been unresponsive for a long time, CPR may resuscitate him, especially after a cold-water near drowning.

Institute continuous cardiac monitoring, and give supplemental oxygen. Prepare the patient for intubation and mechanical ventilation, if needed. Institute rewarming measures. Prepare the patient for placement of a pulmonary artery catheter to monitor core body temperatuers. Monitor the patient's vital signs closely. Continue warming the patient until the core body temrperature is within 1° to 2° F (0.6° to 1.1° C) of the desired body temperature. If the patient has been hypothermic for longer than 45 minutes, give additional fluids, as ordered, to compensate for the expansion of the vascular space that occurs during vasodilation in warming.

If oxygen therapy is needed, be sure to use warm, humidified oxygen to prevent additional cooling.

History and physical examination

Obtain the patient's history for clues to the causative factor. Was he exposed to cold and, if so, what temperature and for what length of time? Ask whether he has recently undergone hemodialysis. Has he had major surgery, especially a type of surgery that requires cooling of the patient's body? Has he recently received a blood transfusion that may have been administered while the blood was still cold? Does he have a history of thyroid, adrenal, liver, or cerebrovascular disease? Has the patient ingested any substances that result in a lowered body temperature, such as alcohol or barbiturates? If the exposure occurred indoors, determine whether the patient has adequate heat in his home. If the exposure occurred outdoors, determine whether he's homeless and sleeping outside.

Assess level of consciousness; a patient with mild hypothermia is unresponsive, and the patient with severe hypothermia will be comatose. Assess the patient's rectal temperature, a more reliable indicator of body temperature because of the abundant supply of blood to the area.[1] A patient with a body temperature below 86° F (30° C) is at risk for cardiopulmonary arrest. Assess for shivering, slurred speech, and peripheral cyanosis. Assess the patient's neurologic status and presence or absence of deep tendon reflexes. Assess for muscle rigidity that can produce a rigor-mortis-like state.

Medical causes

▶ *Prolonged exposure to extremely low temperatures.* The patient will have severe hypothermia, accompanied by lethargy or coma, depressed respiratory rate and depth, bradycardia, and muscle stiffness. The patient may have been exposed to an extremely low temperature with an excessive wind chill factor. If the patient is elderly or debilitated, he may have been exposed to a low room temperature. The patient may also have recently received a blood transfusion with cold blood or underwent a hemodialysis treatment.

▶ *Disorders.* Hypothermia may be a result of a certain disorder, but may not require immediate intervention. Endocrine disorders, such as hypothyroidism, hypoadrenalism, hypopituitarism, diabetes mellitus, cirrhosis, stroke, and renal failure, also affect the body's ability to regulate temperature.

Other causes

DRUG WATCH *Alchohol ingestion and an overdose of barbiturates can induce mild to moderate hypothermia as a result of vasodilation, lowered metabolism, and central nervous system effects.*

Special considerations

Specific rewarming techniques include passive rewarming (the patient rewarms on his own); active rewarming (using heating blankets, warm-water immersion, heated objects such as water bottles, and radiant heat); and active core warming (using heated I.V. fluids, genitourinary tract irrigation, extracorporeal warming, and lavage).[2] Arrhythmias that develop usually convert to a normal sinus rhythm with rewarming. Administration of oxygen, endotracheal intubation, controlled ventilation, I.V. fluids, and treatment of metabolic acidosis depends upon test results and careful patient monitoring.

Stay alert for signs and symptoms of hyperkalemia. If hyperkalemia occurs, administer calcium chloride, sodium bicarbonate, glucose, and insulin as ordered. Anticipate the need for sodium polysterene sulfonate enemas.

Pediatric pointers

Neonates and young infants are at greater risk for thermoregulation problems than children and adults because of their increased body surface area-to-body mass ratio, higher metabolism with limited energy reserve, and immature thermoregulatory behaviors such as a poorly developed ability to shiver.[3] Hypothermia in neonates may occur as a result of a cool environment, heat loss during bathing, and also from infection or a central nervous system or endocrine abnormality.[3]

Geriatric pointers

Older adults are at greater risk for hypothermia even without exposure to extremely low temperatures.[1] They may have decreased subcutaneous fat for insulation, limited mobility to leave a cold room, or an illness that impairs their ability to thermoregulate.[2]

Patient counseling

Advise the patient, especially if he's elderly, to maintain proper insulation in the home and keep the indoor temperature 70° F (21.1° C) or higher. Caution the patient to wear warm clothing and use warm bedding. Advise the patient of the importance of adequate nutrition, rest, and exercise. When the patient is expected to be out in the cold, especially for prolonged periods, advise him to wear loose-fitting clothing in layers and cover his hands, feet, and head; advise him to wear dry clothing and footwear and wind- and water-resistant outer garments and to avoid the intake of alcohol.

REFERENCES

1. Day, M.P. "Hypothermia: A Hazard for All Seasons." *Nursing* 36(12):44-47, December 2006.
2. Snyder, M. "Learn the Chilling Facts about Hypothermia." *Nursing* 35(2):32hn1-32hn4, February 2005.
3. Galligan, M. "Proposed Guidelines for Skin-to-Skin Treatment of Neonatal Hypothermia." MCN, *The American Journal of Maternal/Child Nursing* 31(5):298-304, September/October 2006.

I

INSOMNIA

Insomnia is the inability to fall asleep, remain asleep, or feel refreshed by sleep. Acute and transient during periods of stress, insomnia may become chronic, causing constant fatigue, extreme anxiety as bedtime approaches, and psychiatric disorders. This common complaint is experienced occasionally by about 35% of Americans[1] and chronically by another 10% to 15%.[2]

Physiologic causes of insomnia include jet lag, arguing, and lack of exercise. Pathophysiologic causes range from medical and psychiatric disorders to pain, adverse effects of a drug, and idiopathic factors. Complaints of insomnia are subjective and require close investigation; for example, the patient may mistakenly attribute his fatigue to an organic cause, such as anemia.

History and physical examination

Take a thorough sleep and health history. Find out when the patient's insomnia began and the circumstances surrounding it. Is the patient trying to stop using a sedative? Does he take a central nervous system (CNS) stimulant, such as an amphetamine, pseudoephedrine, a theophylline derivative, phenylpropanolamine, cocaine, or a drug that contains caffeine, or does he drink caffeinated beverages?

Find out if the patient has a chronic or acute condition, the effects of which may be disturbing his sleep, particularly cardiac or respiratory disease or painful or pruritic conditions. Ask if he has an endocrine or neurologic disorder, or a history of drug or alcohol abuse. Is he a frequent traveler who suffers from jet lag? Does he use his legs a lot during the day and then feel restless at night? Ask about daytime fatigue and regular exercise. Also ask if he often finds himself gasping for air, experiencing apnea, or frequently repositioning his body. If possible, consult the patient's spouse or sleep partner because the patient may be unaware of his own behavior. Ask how many pillows the patient uses to sleep.

Assess the patient's emotional status, and try to estimate his level of self-esteem. Ask about personal and professional problems and psychological stress. Also ask if he experiences hallucinations, and note behavior that may indicate alcohol withdrawal. After reviewing any complaints that suggest an undiagnosed disorder, perform a physical examination. (See *Differential diagnosis: Insomnia.*)

Consider asking the patient to keep a 2-week sleep log or diary with details regarding sleep habits, his description of sleep quality, and any daytime signs or symptoms.[1,3]

Medical causes

▶ *Alcohol withdrawal syndrome.* Abrupt cessation of alcohol intake after long-term use causes insomnia that may persist for up to 2 years. Other early effects of this acute syndrome include excessive diaphoresis, tachycardia, hypertension, tremors, restlessness, irritability, headache, nausea, flushing, and nightmares. Progression to delirium tremens

Differential diagnosis: Insomnia

HISTORY OF PRESENT ILLNESS
Focused physical examination: mental health; respiratory, endocrine, and cardiovascular systems

POSSIBLE CAUSES	SIGNS AND SYMPTOMS	DIAGNOSIS	TREATMENT AND FOLLOW-UP
Generalized anxiety disorder	• Diaphoresis • Palpitations • Shortness of breath • Tachycardia • Fatigue • Restlessness • Dyspepsia • Dry mouth • Light-headedness • Nausea • Diarrhea • Flushes or chills • Excessive worry • Irritability • Trouble concentrating	• Psychological evaluation	• Medication (selective serotonin reuptake inhibitors [SSRIs], antidepressants, beta-adrenergic blockers [for physical symptoms], short-term benzodiazepines), cognitive and behavioral therapies *Follow-up:* Reevaluation every 2 to 3 weeks until stabilized on medication
Thyrotoxicosis	• Diaphoresis • Palpitations • Shortness of breath • Tachycardia • Trouble falling asleep, then sleeping only briefly • Dyspnea • Atrial or ventricular gallop • Inability to concentrate • Emotional lability • Weight loss despite increased appetite • Tremors • Nervousness • Diaphoresis • Hypersensitivity to heat • Enlarged thyroid • Exophthalmos	• Physical examination • Laboratory tests (thyroid-stimulating hormone, T_3, T_4, thyroid resin uptake)	• Medication (antithyroid agents, therapeutic radioiodine, beta-adrenergic blockers) *Follow-up:* Reevaluation of thyroid function every 6 months; reevaluation at 6 weeks and 12 weeks, and then every 6 months, if undergoing radionuclide therapy
Depression	• Chronic insomnia with difficulty falling asleep and early waking • Dysphoria • Decreased or increased appetite	• Beck Depression Inventory • Zung Self-Rating Depression Scale • Geriatric Depression Scale • Laboratory tests (complete blood count, erythrocyte sedi-	• Medication (SSRIs, tricyclic antidepressants) • Cognitive therapy • Support groups • Exercise program

(continued)

Differential diagnosis: Insomnia *(continued)*

POSSIBLE CAUSES	SIGNS AND SYMPTOMS	DIAGNOSIS	TREATMENT AND FOLLOW-UP
Depression *(continued)*	• Psychomotor agitation or retardation • Loss of interest in usual activities • Feelings of worthlessness or guilt • Fatigue • Trouble concentrating • Indecisiveness • Recurrent thoughts of death • Tachycardia • Possible suicidal ideation	mentation rate, Venereal Disease Research Laboratory, electrolytes, thyroid profile, drug screening)	*Follow-up:* Initial reevaluation at 2 weeks, then every 4 to 8 weeks, then every 3 months; referral to psychologist
Sleep apnea syndrome	• Repeated episodes of obstructive apnea and hypopnea during sleep that end with a series of gasps and arousal • Morning headache • Daytime sleepiness • Hypertension • Personality changes	• Polysomnography in a sleep laboratory	• Treatment of underlying cause • Continuous positive airway pressure at night • Oral appliances • Antidepressants • Surgery • Weight loss (if indicated) • Smoking and alcohol cessation • Positional therapy *Follow-up:* Referrals to sleep specialist and pulmonologist

produces confusion, disorientation, paranoia, delusions, hallucinations, and seizures.

▶ *Generalized anxiety disorder.* Anxiety can cause chronic insomnia as well as symptoms of tension, such as fatigue and restlessness; signs of autonomic hyperactivity, such as diaphoresis, dyspepsia, and high resting pulse and respiratory rates; and signs of apprehension.

▶ *Mood (affective) disorders.* Up to 40% of cases of insomnia are related to or caused by depression.[4] Depression commonly causes chronic insomnia with difficulty falling asleep, waking and being unable to fall back to sleep, or waking early in the morning. Related findings include dysphoria (a primary symptom), decreased appetite with weight loss or in-

creased appetite with weight gain, and psychomotor agitation or retardation. The patient has reduced interest in his usual activities, feelings of worthlessness and guilt, fatigue, difficulty concentrating, indecisiveness, and recurrent thoughts of death.

Manic episodes produce a decreased need for sleep with an elevated mood and irritability. Related findings include increased energy and activity, fast speech, speeding thoughts, inflated self-esteem, easy distractibility, and involvement in high-risk activities such as reckless driving.

▶ *Nocturnal myoclonus.* With this seizure disorder, involuntary and fleeting muscle jerks of the legs occur every 20 to 40 seconds, disturbing sleep.

Tips for relieving insomnia

COMMON PROBLEMS	CAUSES	INTERVENTIONS
Acroparesthesia	Improper positioning may compress superficial (ulnar, radial, and peroneal) nerves, disrupting circulation to the compressed nerve. This causes numbness, tingling and stiffness in an arm or leg.	Teach the patient to assume a comfortable position in bed, with his limbs unrestricted. If he tends to awaken with a numb arm or leg, tell him to massage and move it until sensation returns completely and then to assume an unrestricted position.
Anxiety	Physical and emotional stress produces anxiety, which causes autonomic stimulation.	Encourage the patient to discuss his fears and concerns, and teach him relaxation techniques, such as guided imagery and deep breathing. If ordered, administer a mild sedative, such as temazepam or another sedative hypnotic, before bedtime. Emphasize that these drugs should be used only for short-term treatment.
Dyspnea	With many cardiac and pulmonary disorders, a recumbent position and inactivity cause restricted chest expansion, secretion pooling, and pulmonary vascular congestion, leading to coughing and shortness of breath.	Elevate the head of the bed, or provide at least two pillows or a reclining chair to help the patient sleep. Suction him when he awakens, and encourage deep breathing and incentive spirometry every 2 to 4 hours. Also, provide supplementary oxygen by nasal cannula. If the patient is pregnant, encourage her to sleep on her left side at a comfortable elevation to ease dyspnea.
Pain	Chronic or acute pain from any cause can prevent or disrupt sleep.	Administer analgesics, as ordered, 20 minutes before bedtime, and teach deep, even, slow breathing to promote relaxation. If the patient has back pain, help him lie on his side with his legs flexed. If he has epigastric pain, encourage him to take an antacid before bed and to sleep with the head of the bed elevated. If he has incisions, instruct him to splint during coughing or movement.
Pruritus	A localized skin infection or a systemic disorder, such as liver failure, may produce intensely annoying itching, even during the night.	Wash the patient's skin with a mild soap and water, and dry it thoroughly. Apply moisturizing lotion on dry, unbroken skin and an antipruritic such as calamine lotion on pruritic areas. Give diphenhydramine or hydroxyzine, as ordered, to help minimize itching.
Restless leg syndrome	Excessive exercise during the day may cause tired, aching legs at night, requiring movement for relief.	Help the patient exercise his legs gently by slowly walking with him around the room and down the hall. If ordered, give a muscle relaxant such as diazepam.

▶ *Pain.* Almost any condition that causes pain can cause insomnia. Related findings reflect the specific cause.

▶ *Pheochromocytoma.* This rare disorder causes paroxysms of acute hypermetabolic activity, which can prevent or interrupt sleep. Its cardinal sign is severe hypertension, which may be sustained between attacks. Other effects include headache, palpitations, and anxiety.

▶ *Pruritus.* Localized skin infections and systemic disorders, such as liver failure, can cause pruritus, resulting in insomnia.

▶ *Sleep apnea syndrome.* Apneic periods begin with the onset of sleep, continue for 10 to 90 seconds, and end with a series of gasps and arousal. With central sleep apnea, respiratory movement ceases for the apneic period; with obstructive sleep apnea, upper airway obstruction blocks incoming air, although breathing movements continue. Some patients display both types of apnea. Repeated possibly hundreds of times during the night, this cycle alternates with bradycardia and tachycardia. Other findings include morning headache, daytime fatigue, hypertension, ankle edema, and personality changes, such as hostility, paranoia, and agitated depression.

▶ *Thyrotoxicosis.* Difficulty falling asleep and then sleeping for only a brief period is one of the characteristic symptoms of this disorder. Cardiopulmonary features include dyspnea, tachycardia, palpitations, and atrial or ventricular gallop. Other findings include weight loss despite increased appetite, diarrhea, tremors, nervousness, diaphoresis, hypersensitivity to heat, an enlarged thyroid, and exophthalmos.

Other causes

DRUG WATCH *Use of, abuse of, or withdrawal from sedatives or hypnotics may produce insomnia. CNS stimulants—including amphetamines, theophylline derivatives, pseudoephedrine, cocaine, and caffeinated beverages—may also produce insomnia.*

▶ *Herbs.* Herbal remedies, such as ginseng and green tea, can also cause insomnia.

Special considerations

Prepare the patient for tests to evaluate his insomnia, such as blood and urine studies for 17-hydroxycorticosteroids and catecholamines, and sleep EEG. Polysomnography (including an EEG, electro-oculography, and electrocardiography) isn't used routinely, but is appropriate for patients with suspected sleep apnea, narcolepsy, restless leg syndrome, or periodic limb movement.[2,5]

Cognitive-behavioral therapy, which includes techniques such as cognitive therapy, relaxation therapy, sleep-hygiene education, and others, has been shown to be effective for 50% to 75% of patients.[2] Drugs such as intermediate-acting benzodiazepines and the newer non-benzodiazepines are also safe and effective options for insomnia and may be used alone or with behavioral therapies.[1,2,3]

Pediatric pointers

Insomnia in early childhood may develop along with separation anxiety at ages 2 to 3, after a stressful or tiring day, or during illness or teething. In children ages 6 to 11, insomnia usually reflects residual excitement from the day's activities; a few children continue to have bedtime fears. Sleep problems are common in foster children.

Patient counseling

Teach the patient comfort and relaxation techniques to promote natural sleep. (See *Tips for relieving insomnia,* page 255.) Advise him to awaken and retire at the same time each day and to exercise regularly. When he can't sleep, advise him to get up but remain inactive. Urge him to use his bed only for sleeping, not for relaxation or watching television.

Advise the patient to use sleep aids for acute insomnia only when relaxation techniques fail. If appropriate, refer him for counseling or to a sleep disorder clinic for biofeedback training or other interventions.

REFERENCES

1. Turkoski, B.B. "Managing Insomnia." *Orthopaedic Nursing* 25(5):339-345, September/October 2006.
2. Silber, M.H. "Insomnia." *CONTINUUM: Lifelong Learning in Neurology* 13(3) Sleep Disorders:85-100, July 2007.

3. Nadolski, N. "Getting A Good Night's Sleep: Diagnosing and Treating Insomnia." *Plastic Surgical Nursing* 25(4):167-173, October/December 2005.
4. Holcomb, S.S. "Putting Insomnia to Rest." *The Nurse Practitioner* 32(4):28-34, April 2007.
5. Holcomb, S.S. "Recommendations for Assessing Insomnia." *The Nurse Practitioner* 31(2):55-60, February 2006.

INTERMITTENT CLAUDICATION

Most common in the legs, intermittent claudication is cramping limb pain brought on by exercise and relieved within 10 minutes of rest. It is a symptom of limb ischemia, occurring distal to the site of arterial occlusion.[1] This pain may be acute or chronic; when acute, it may signal acute arterial occlusion. Intermittent claudication is most common in men ages 50 to 60 with a history of diabetes mellitus, hyperlipidemia, hypertension, or tobacco use. Without treatment, it may progress to pain at rest. With chronic arterial occlusion, limb loss is uncommon because collateral circulation usually develops.

With occlusive artery disease, intermittent claudication results from an inadequate blood supply. Pain in the calf (the most common area) or foot indicates disease of the femoral or popliteal arteries; pain in the buttocks and upper thigh, disease of the aortoiliac arteries. During exercise, the pain typically results from the release of lactic acid due to anaerobic metabolism in the ischemic segment, secondary to obstruction. When exercise stops, the lactic acid clears and the pain subsides.

Intermittent claudication may also have a neurologic cause: narrowing of the vertebral column at the level of the cauda equina. This condition creates pressure on the nerve roots to the lower limbs. Walking stimulates circulation to the cauda equina, causing increased pressure on those nerves and resultant pain.

Physical findings include pallor on elevation, rubor on dependency (especially the toes and soles), loss of hair on the toes, and diminished arterial pulses.

If the patient has sudden intermittent claudication with severe or aching leg pain at rest, check the leg's temperature and color and palpate femoral, popliteal, posterior tibial, and dorsalis pedis pulses. Ask about numbness and tingling. Suspect acute arterial occlusion if pulses are absent; if the leg feels cold and looks pale, cyanotic, or mottled; and if paresthesia and pain are present. Mark the area of pallor, cyanosis, or mottling, and reassess it frequently, noting an increase in the area.

Don't elevate the leg. Protect it, allowing nothing to press on it. Prepare the patient for preoperative blood tests, urinalysis, electrocardiography, chest X-rays, Doppler studies of the legs, and angiography. Start an I.V. line, and give an anticoagulant and analgesics.

History and physical examination

If the patient has chronic intermittent claudication, gather history data first. Ask how far he can walk before pain occurs and how long he must rest before it subsides. Can he walk less far now than before, or does he need to rest longer? Does the pain-rest pattern vary? Has this symptom affected his lifestyle?

Obtain a history of risk factors for atherosclerosis, such as smoking (the most significant risk factor for arterial disease[2]), diabetes, hypertension, and hyperlipidemia. Next, ask about associated signs and symptoms, such as paresthesia in the affected limb and visible changes in the color of the fingers (white to blue to pink) when he's smoking, exposed to cold, or under stress. If the patient is male, does he experience impotence?

Focus the physical examination on the cardiovascular system. Palpate for femoral, popliteal, dorsalis pedis, and posterior tibial pulses. Note character, amplitude, and bilateral equality. Diminished or absent popliteal and pedal pulses with the femoral pulse present may indicate atherosclerotic disease of the femoral artery. Diminished femoral and distal pulses may indicate disease of the terminal aorta or iliac branches. Absent pedal pulses with normal femoral and popliteal pulses may indicate Buerger's disease.

Listen for bruits over the major arteries. Note color and temperature differences between his legs or compared with his arms; also note where on his leg the changes in temperature and color occur. Elevate the affected leg for 2 minutes; if it becomes pale or white, blood flow is severely decreased. When the leg hangs down, how long does it take for color to return? (Thirty seconds or longer indicates severe disease.) If possible, check the patient's deep tendon reflexes after exercise; note if they're diminished in his lower limbs.

Examine his feet, toes, and fingers for ulceration, and inspect his hands and lower legs for small, tender nodules and erythema along blood vessels. Note the quality of his nails and the amount of hair on his fingers and toes.

If the patient has arm pain, inspect his arms for a change in color (to white) on elevation. Next, palpate for changes in temperature, muscle wasting, and a pulsating mass in the subclavian area. Palpate and compare the radial, ulnar, brachial, axillary, and subclavian pulses to identify obstructed areas.

Medical causes

▶ *Aortic arteriosclerotic occlusive disease.* With this disorder, intermittent claudication occurs in the buttock, hip, thigh, and calf, along with absent or diminished femoral pulses. Bruits can be auscultated over the femoral and iliac arteries. Examination reveals pallor of the affected limb on elevation and profound limb weakness. The leg may be cool to the touch.

▶ *Arterial occlusion (acute).* This disorder produces intense intermittent claudication. A saddle embolus may affect both legs. Associated findings include paresthesia, paresis, and a sensation of cold in the affected limb. The limb is cool, pale, and cyanotic (mottled) with absent pulses below the occlusion. Capillary refill time is increased.

▶ *Arteriosclerosis obliterans.* This disorder usually affects the femoral and popliteal arteries, causing intermittent claudication (the most common symptom) in the calf. Typical associated findings include diminished or absent popliteal and pedal pulses, coolness in the affected limb, pallor on elevation, and profound limb weakness with continuing exercise. Other possible findings include numbness, paresthesia and, in severe disease, pain in the toes or foot while at rest, ulceration, and gangrene.

▶ *Buerger's disease (thromboangiitis obliterans).* This disorder typically produces intermittent claudication of the instep. Men are affected more than women; most affected men smoke and are between ages 20 and 40. It's common in the Orient, southeast Asia, India, and the Middle East and is rare in Blacks. Early signs include migratory superficial nodules and erythema along extremity blood vessels (nodular phlebitis) as well as migratory venous phlebitis. With exposure to cold, the feet initially become cold, cyanotic, and numb; later, they redden, become hot, and tingle. Occasionally, Buerger's disease also affects the hands and can cause painful ulcerations on the fingertips. Other characteristic findings include impaired peripheral pulses, paresthesia of the hands and feet, and migratory superficial thrombophlebitis.

▶ *Cauda equina syndrome.* Spinal stenosis causes pressure on nerve roots resulting in symptoms of claudication from the hip down as with Leriche's syndrome. Diagnosis can be determined by noninvasive exercise studies. With cauda equina syndrome, the pressure doesn't drop when the patient exercises on the treadmill.

▶ *Leriche's syndrome.* Arterial occlusion causes intermittent claudication of the hip, thigh, buttocks, and calf as well as impotence in men. Examination reveals bruits, global atrophy, absent or diminished pulses, and gangrene of the toes. The leg becomes cool and pale when elevated.

▶ *Neurogenic claudication.* Neurospinal disease causes pain from neurogenic intermittent claudication that requires a longer rest time than the 2 to 3 minutes needed in vascular claudication. Associated findings include paresthesia, weakness and clumsiness when walking, and hypoactive deep tendon reflexes after walking. Pulses are unaffected.

▶ *Thoracic outlet syndrome.* Activity that requires raising the hands above the shoulders, lifting a weight, or abducting the arm can cause intermittent pain along the ulnar distribution of the arm and forearm along with paresthesia and weakness. The pain isn't true

Maintaining walking therapy compliance

Question: *What psychosocial variables are associated with walking intentions and exercise among patients with intermittent claudication? Is perceived pain intensity a potential moderator between intention and walking exercise?*

Research: Intermittent claudication is a symptom of leg muscle pain that occurs while walking. It occurs as a result of reduced blood flow that's typically caused by peripheral arterial disease (PAD). The management of intermittent claudication aims to improve walking ability and includes walking exercise as a key therapy.

Study participants were recruited from a diagnostic and treatment center for PAD. To be eligible for the study, patients had to have been previously diagnosed with PAD and had experienced intermittent claudication. Baseline measures were collected and included information regarding attitudes toward walking exercise, subjective norms (such as perceived social pressure), perceived behavioral control, and intentions of walking exercise during the upcoming four weeks. Weekly telephone interviews were conducted and participants were asked to report their walking exercise and perceived pain for the previous seven days.

Conclusion: Overall, initial measures were positive. However, the frequency of walking was less than recommended (at least 30 minutes 3 days per week). Perceived behavioral control was a strong predictor of walking intentions, which was not surprising since patients who suffer from intermittent claudication experience barriers to walking. Both perceived behavioral control and intentions accounted for a significant proportion of variance in walking behavior. Perceived pain intensity didn't affect the relationship between intentions and behavior.

Application: Work with patients who experience intermittent claudication to develop a positive sense of control and strong intentions to perform walking exercise. Inform patients about the benefits of walking and emphasize the long-term outcomes. Also, address concerns about barriers to walking, such as the need to take rest breaks and how to cope with pain.

Source: Galea, M. N. and Bray, S. R. "Determinants of Walking Exercise among Individuals with Intermittent Claudication: Does Pain Play a Role?" *Journal of Cardiopulmonary Rehabilitation and Prevention,* 27(2):107-113, 2007.

claudication pain because it's related to position, not exercise. Signs and symptoms disappear when the arm is lowered. Other features include asymmetrical blood pressure and cool, pale skin.

Special considerations
Encourage the patient to exercise to improve collateral circulation and increase venous return, and advise him to avoid prolonged sitting or standing as well as crossing his legs at the knees. Help him plan ways to maintain compliance with walking therapy. (See *Maintaining walking therapy compliance.*) If intermittent claudication interferes with the patient's lifestyle, he may require diagnostic tests (Doppler flow studies, arteriography, and digital subtraction angiography) to determine the location and degree of occlusion.

Pediatric pointers
Intermittent claudication rarely occurs in children. Although it sometimes develops in patients with coarctation of the aorta, extensive compensatory collateral circulation typically prevents manifestation of this sign. Muscle cramps from exercise and growing pains may be mistaken for intermittent claudication in children.

Geriatric pointers

Although considered a hallmark of peripheral arterial disease, only 30% to 50% of older patients with the disorder report intermittent claudication.[1] Older patients with peripheral arterial disease are more likely to have exertional leg symptoms or to be asymptomatic.[1] Often, older patients may not engage in exercise that is strenuous enough to produce symptoms.[1,2]

Patient counseling

Counsel the patient with intermittent claudication about risk factors. Encourage him to stop smoking, and refer him to a support group, if appropriate. Encourage the patient to keep blood pressure, cholesterol, and blood glucose levels under control.[3] Teach him to inspect his legs and feet for ulcers; to keep his limbs warm, clean, and dry; and to avoid injury.

Urge the patient to immediately report skin breakdown that doesn't heal. Also urge him to report any chest discomfort when circulation is restored to his legs. Increased exercise tolerance may lead to angina if the patient has coronary artery disease that was previously asymptomatic because of exercise limitations.

REFERENCES

1. Oka, R.K. "Peripheral Arterial Disease in Older Adults: Management of Cardiovascular Disease Risk Factors." *The Journal of Cardiovascular Nursing* 21(5) Supplement 1:S15-S20, September/October 2006.
2. Sieggreen, M. "A Contemporary Approach to Peripheral Arterial Disease." *The Nurse Practitioner* 31(7):14-25, July 2006.
3. Morgan, E. "When Critical Limb Ischemia Strikes." *Nursing* 35(8):32cc1-32cc4, August 2005.

JAUNDICE

A yellow discoloration (also called *icterus*) of the skin, mucous membranes, or sclera of the eyes, jaundice indicates excessive levels of conjugated or unconjugated bilirubin in the blood. In fair-skinned patients, it's most noticeable on the face, trunk, and sclera; in dark-skinned patients, on the hard palate, sclera, and conjunctiva.

Jaundice is most apparent in natural sunlight. In fact, it may be undetectable in artificial or poor light. It's commonly accompanied by pruritus (because bile pigment damages sensory nerves), dark urine, and clay-colored stools.

Jaundice may result from any of three pathophysiologic processes. (See *Jaundice: Impaired bilirubin metabolism,* page 262.) It may be the only warning sign of certain disorders such as pancreatic cancer.

History and physical examination

Documenting a history of the patient's jaundice is critical in determining its cause. Begin by asking the patient when he first noticed the jaundice. Does he also have pruritus, clay-colored stools (from decreased bilirubin in the intestinal tract), or dark urine (deep orange and foamy from secretion of bilirubin by the kidneys)? Ask about past episodes or a family history of jaundice. Does he have nonspecific signs or symptoms, such as fatigue, fever, or chills; GI signs or symptoms, such as anorexia, abdominal pain, nausea, weight loss, or vomiting; or cardiopulmonary symptoms, such as shortness of breath or palpitations? Ask about alcohol use and a history of cancer or liver or gallbladder disease. Has the patient lost weight recently? Also, obtain a drug history. Ask about a history of hepatitis, gallstones, or liver or pancreatic disease.

Perform a physical examination in a room with natural light. Make sure that the orange-yellow hue is jaundice and not hypercarotenemia, which is more prominent on the palms and soles and doesn't affect the sclera. Inspect the patient's skin for texture and dryness and for hyperpigmentation and xanthomas. Look for spider angiomas or petechiae, clubbed fingers, and gynecomastia. If the patient has heart failure, auscultate for arrhythmias, murmurs, and gallops. For all patients, auscultate for crackles and abnormal bowel sounds. Palpate the lymph nodes for swelling and the abdomen for tenderness, pain, and swelling. Palpate and percuss the liver and spleen for enlargement, and test for ascites with the shifting dullness and fluid wave techniques. Obtain baseline data on the patient's mental status: Slight changes in sensorium may be an early sign of deteriorating hepatic function. (See *Differential diagnosis: Jaundice,* pages 264 and 265.)

Medical causes

▶ *Agnogenic myeloid metaplasia.* This myeloproliferative disorder of the bone marrow may cause jaundice. Its typical effects, however, are associated with anemia, including fatigue, weakness, anorexia, massive spleno-

Jaundice: Impaired bilirubin metabolism

Jaundice occurs in three forms: prehepatic, hepatic, and posthepatic. In all three, bilirubin levels in the blood increase because of impaired metabolism.

With *prehepatic jaundice,* certain conditions and disorders, such as transfusion reactions and sickle cell anemia, cause massive hemolysis. Red blood cells rupture faster than the liver can conjugate bilirubin, so large amounts of unconjugated bilirubin pass into the blood, causing increased intestinal conversion of this bilirubin to water-soluble urobilinogen for excretion in urine and stools. (Unconjugated bilirubin is insoluble in water, so it can't be directly excreted in urine.)

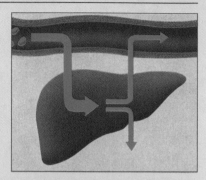

Hepatic jaundice results from the liver's inability to conjugate or excrete bilirubin, leading to increased blood levels of conjugated and unconjugated bilirubin. This occurs with such disorders as hepatitis, cirrhosis, and metastatic cancer and during the prolonged use of drugs metabolized by the liver.

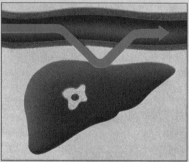

With *posthepatic jaundice,* which occurs in patients with a biliary or pancreatic disorder, bilirubin forms at its normal rate, but inflammation, scar tissue, a tumor, or gallstones block the flow of bile into the intestine. This causes conjugated bilirubin to accumulate in the blood. Water-soluble, conjugated bilirubin is excreted in the urine.

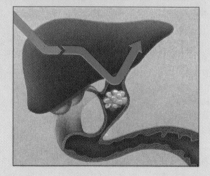

megaly, hepatomegaly, purpura, and bleeding tendencies.

▶ *Carcinoma.* Cancer of the ampulla of Vater initially produces fluctuating jaundice, mild abdominal pain, recurrent fever, and chills. Occult bleeding may be its first sign. Other findings include weight loss, pruritus, and back pain.

Hepatic cancer (primary liver cancer or another cancer that has metastasized to the liver) may cause jaundice by causing obstruction of the bile duct. Even advanced cancer causes nonspecific signs and symptoms, such as right-upper-quadrant discomfort and tenderness, nausea, weight loss, and slight fever. Examination may reveal irregular, nodular, firm hepatomegaly, ascites, peripheral edema, a bruit heard over the liver, and a right-upper-quadrant mass.

With pancreatic cancer, progressive jaundice—possibly with pruritus—may be the only sign. Related early findings are nonspecific, such as weight loss and back or abdominal pain. Other signs and symptoms include anorexia, nausea and vomiting, fever, steatorrhea, fatigue, weakness, diarrhea, pruritus, and skin lesions (usually on the legs).

▶ *Cholangitis.* Obstruction and infection in the common bile duct cause Charcot's triad: jaundice, right-upper-quadrant pain, and high fever with chills.

▶ *Cholecystitis.* This disorder produces nonobstructive jaundice in about 25% of patients. Biliary colic typically peaks abruptly, persisting for 2 to 4 hours. The pain then localizes to the right upper quadrant and becomes constant. Local inflammation or passage of stones to the common bile duct causes jaundice. Other findings include nausea, vomiting (usually indicating the presence of a stone), fever, profuse diaphoresis, chills, tenderness on palpation, a positive Murphy's sign and, possibly, abdominal distention and rigidity.

▶ *Cholelithiasis.* This disorder commonly causes jaundice and biliary colic. It's characterized by severe, steady pain in the right upper quadrant or epigastrium that radiates to the right scapula or shoulder and intensifies over several hours. Other signs and symptoms include nausea and vomiting, tachycardia, and restlessness. Occlusion of the common bile duct causes fever, chills, jaundice, clay-colored stools, and abdominal tenderness. After consuming a fatty meal, the patient may experience vague epigastric fullness and dyspepsia.

▶ *Cholestasis.* With benign, recurrent intrahepatic cholestasis, the patient experiences prolonged attacks of jaundice (sometimes spaced several years apart) accompanied by pruritus. Other signs and symptoms are similar to those of hepatitis—fatigue, nausea, weight loss, anorexia, pale stools, and right-upper-quadrant pain.

▶ *Cirrhosis.* With Laënnec's cirrhosis, mild to moderate jaundice with pruritus usually signals hepatocellular necrosis or progressive hepatic insufficiency. Common early findings include ascites, weakness, leg edema, nausea and vomiting, diarrhea or constipation, anorexia, weight loss, and right-upper-quadrant pain. Massive hematemesis and other bleeding tendencies also may occur. Other findings include an enlarged liver and parotid gland, clubbed fingers, Dupuytren's contracture, mental changes, asterixis, fetor hepaticus, spider angiomas, and palmar erythema. Men may have gynecomastia, scanty chest and axillary hair, and testicular atrophy; women may have menstrual irregularities.

With primary biliary cirrhosis, fluctuating jaundice may appear years after the onset of other signs and symptoms, such as pruritus that worsens at bedtime (commonly the first sign), weakness, fatigue, weight loss, and vague abdominal pain. Itching may lead to skin excoriation. Other findings include hyperpigmentation; indications of malabsorption, such as nocturnal diarrhea, steatorrhea, purpura, and osteomalacia; hematemesis from esophageal varices; ascites; edema; xanthelasmas; xanthomas on the palms, soles, and elbows; and hepatomegaly.

▶ *Dubin-Johnson syndrome.* With this rare, chronic inherited syndrome, fluctuating jaundice that increases with stress is the major sign, appearing as late as age 40. Related findings include slight hepatic enlargement and tenderness, upper abdominal pain, nausea, and vomiting.

▶ *Glucose-6-phosphate dehydrogenase deficiency.* Acute intravascular hemolysis following ingestion of such drugs as quinine or aspirin causes jaundice, pallor, dyspnea, tachycardia, and malaise. Palpation may reveal splenomegaly and hepatomegaly.

▶ *Heart failure.* Jaundice from liver dysfunction occurs in patients with severe right-sided heart failure. Other effects include jugular vein distention, cyanosis, dependent edema of the legs and sacrum, steady weight gain, confusion, hepatomegaly, nausea and vomiting, abdominal discomfort, and anorexia due to visceral edema. Ascites is a late sign. Oliguria, marked weakness, and anxiety also may occur. If left-sided heart failure develops first, other findings may include fatigue, dyspnea, orthopnea, paroxysmal nocturnal dyspnea, tachypnea, arrhythmias, and tachycardia.

Differential diagnosis: Jaundice

Patients with jaundice commonly experience nausea, vomiting, dark urine, clay-colored stools, and pruritus. Additional symptoms can help you differentiate between these common causes.

POSSIBLE CAUSES	ADDITIONAL SYMPTOMS	DIAGNOSIS CONSIDERATIONS
Cholelithiasis	• Biliary colic • Severe, steady pain in right upper quadrant (RUQ) or epigastrium that radiates to the right scapula • Positive Murphy's sign • Tachycardia • Restlessness • Dyspepsia after a fatty meal	• Laboratory tests (complete blood count [CBC], liver function test, electrolytes) • Imaging studies (ultrasound, computed tomography [CT] scan, endoscopic retrograde cholangiopancreatography [ERCP], cholecystogram, hydroxy iminodiacetic acid [HIDA] scan)
Acute hepatitis	• Fatigue • Malaise • Arthralgia • Myalgia • Headache • Anorexia • Photophobia • Cough • Sore throat • Liver and lymph node enlargement	• Hepatitis surface antigen or antibody based testing (A, B, C, D)
Cholestasis	• Prolonged attacks of jaundice • Fatigue • Weight loss • Anorexia • RUQ pain	• History • Liver function tests • Imaging studies (CT scan, magnetic resonance imaging, cholangiography, ultrasound, ERCP)
Acute pancreatitis	• Severe relentless epigastric pain that radiates to the back • Nausea • Persistent vomiting • Abdominal distention • Turner's or Cullen's sign (possibly) • Fever • Tachycardia • Hypoactive bowel sounds • Abdominal rigidity and tenderness • Shock (if severe)	• Laboratory tests (amylase, lipase, CBC, electrolytes, calcium, albumin, liver function test) • Imaging studies (CT scan, ultrasound)

Additional differential diagnoses include agnogenic jaundice, cholangitis, cholecystitis, cirrhosis, Dubin-Johnson syndrome, glucose-6-phosphate dehydrogenase deficiency, hemolytic anemia (acquired), hepatic abscess, hepatic cancer, leptospirosis, myeloid metaplasia, pancreatic cancer, sickle cell anemia, and Zieve syndrome.

Other causes of jaundice include androgenic steroids, erythromycin estolate, HMG-CoA reductase inhibitors, hormonal contraceptives, isoniazid, I.V. tetracycline, mercaptopurine, niacin, phenothiazines, portocaval shunt, sulfonamides, troleandomycin, and upper abdominal surgery.

TREATMENT AND FOLLOW-UP

- Gallstone-solubilizing agent
- Diet modification
- Surgery

Follow-up: Reevaluation every 3 months; referral to surgeon, if acute

---

- Based on symptoms, rest, avoidance of alcohol and hepatotoxic substances, safer sex practices

Follow-up: For hepatitis A and E, reevaluation every 2 to 4 weeks; for hepatitis B, C, D, referral to hepatologist or gastroenterologist

---

- Treatment of causative factor
- Diet modification
- Medication (antibacterial, phenobarbital)
- Surgery

Follow-up: Referral to gastroenterologist

- Based on symptoms, I.V. hydration, medication (analgesics, electrolyte replacement, insulin therapy)

Follow-up: Referral to gastroenterologist

▶ *Hemolytic anemia (acquired).* This disorder may produce prominent jaundice along with dyspnea, fatigue, pallor, tachycardia, and palpitations. Rapid hemolysis causes chills, fever, irritability, headache, and abdominal pain; severe hemolysis causes signs of shock.

▶ *Hepatic abscess.* Multiple abscesses may cause jaundice, but the main effects are persistent fever with chills and sweating. Other findings include steady, severe pain in the right upper quadrant or midepigastrium that may be referred to the shoulder; nausea and vomiting; anorexia; hepatomegaly; elevated right hemidiaphragm; and ascites.

▶ *Hepatitis.* Dark urine and clay-colored stools usually develop before jaundice in the late stages of acute viral hepatitis. Early systemic signs and symptoms vary and include fatigue, nausea, vomiting, malaise, arthralgias, myalgias, headache, anorexia, photophobia, pharyngitis, cough, diarrhea or constipation, and a low-grade fever associated with liver and lymph node enlargement. During the icteric phase (which subsides within 2 to 3 weeks unless complications occur), systemic signs subside, but an enlarged, palpable liver may be present along with weight loss, anorexia, and right-upper-quadrant pain and tenderness.

▶ *Leptospirosis.* Severe leptospirosis (Weil's disease) may cause jaundice. This disorder begins suddenly with a frontal headache, severe muscle aches in the thighs and lumbar area, cutaneous hyperesthesia, abdominal pain, nausea, conjunctival suffusion, and vomiting. Chills and a rapidly rising fever follow. Signs and symptoms of meningeal irritation include drowsiness, decreased mentation, stiff neck, and positive Kernig's and Brudzinski's signs. Right-upper-quadrant tenderness, hepatomegaly, and jaundice indicate hepatic involvement; proteinuria, pyuria, and hematuria indicate renal involvement. Epistaxis, hematemesis, melena, and hemoptysis also may occur.

▶ *Pancreatitis (acute).* Edema of the head of the pancreas and obstruction of the common bile duct can cause jaundice; however, this disorder's primary symptom is usually severe epigastric pain that commonly radiates to the back. Lying with the knees flexed on the chest or sitting up and leaning forward brings relief. Early related signs and symptoms include nausea, persistent vomiting, abdominal distention, and Turner's or Cullen's sign. Other findings include fever, tachycardia, abdominal rigidity and tenderness, hypoactive bowel sounds, and crackles.

Severe pancreatitis produces extreme restlessness; mottled skin; cold, diaphoretic limbs; paresthesia; and tetany—the last two being symptoms of hypocalcemia. Fulminant pancreatitis causes massive hemorrhage.

▶ *Sickle cell anemia.* Hemolysis produces jaundice in patients with this disorder. Other findings include impaired growth and development, increased susceptibility to infection, life-threatening thrombotic complications and, commonly, leg ulcers, (painful) swollen joints, fever, and chills. Bone aches and chest pain also may occur. Severe hemolysis may cause hematuria and pallor, chronic fatigue, weakness, dyspnea (or dyspnea on exertion), and tachycardia. The patient also may have splenomegaly. During a sickle cell crisis, the patient may have severe bone, abdominal, thoracic, and muscular pain; low-grade fever; and increased weakness, jaundice, and dyspnea.

▶ *Zieve syndrome.* Caused by alcohol abuse, this relatively rare disorder produces abdominal pain and a sudden onset of severe jaundice. However, spider angiomas, ascites, and other signs of advanced liver disease are absent.

Other causes

DRUG WATCH *Many drugs can cause hepatic injury and jaundice. Examples include acetaminophen, androgenic steroids, erythromycin estolate, ethanol, HMG-CoA reductase inhibitors (statins), hormonal contraceptives, isoniazid, mercaptopurine, methyldopa, niacin, phenothiazines, phenytoin, rifampin, sulfonamides, and tetracycline (I.V.).*

▶ *Treatments.* Upper abdominal surgery may cause postoperative jaundice, which occurs secondary to hepatocellular damage from the manipulation of organs, leading to edema and obstructed bile flow; from use of halothane; or from prolonged surgery resulting in shock, blood loss, or blood transfusion.

A surgical shunt used to reduce portal hypertension (such as a portacaval shunt) also may produce jaundice.

Special considerations

To help decrease pruritus, bathe the patient often, apply an antipruritic lotion such as calamine, and give antihistamines as ordered. Prepare the patient for diagnostic tests to evaluate gallbladder, pancreas, liver, and biliary function.[1] Laboratory studies include urine and fecal urobilinogen, serum bilirubin, hepatic enzyme, and cholesterol levels; prothrombin time; and a complete blood count. Other tests include ultrasonography, cholangiography, liver biopsy, and exploratory laparotomy.

Pediatric pointers

Physiologic jaundice is common in neonates, developing 3 to 5 days after birth. In infants, obstructive jaundice usually results from congenital biliary atresia. A choledochal cyst—a congenital cystic dilation of the common bile duct—also may cause jaundice in children, particularly those of Japanese descent.

The list of other causes of jaundice is extensive and includes, but isn't limited to, Crigler-Najjar syndrome, Gilbert's disease, Rotor's syndrome, thalassemia major, hereditary spherocytosis, erythroblastosis fetalis, Hodgkin's disease, infectious mononucleosis, Wilson's disease, amyloidosis, and Reye's syndrome.

For an infant who needs phototherapy, make sure that as much skin as possible is exposed to the phototherapy by positioning the lights appropriately, dressing the infant in only a diaper, and repositioning the infant often to expose different areas of skin to the lights. Monitor the irradiance level of the phototherapy with a radiometer at periodic intervals to ensure that it is adequate.[2] Prevent damage to the retina by keeping opaque eye shields in place whenever phototherapy is in use.[2] Check the infant's temperature often because some phototherapy units can increase temperature significantly.[2] Encourage enteral feedings to promote bilirubin excretion in the stool. Monitor bilirubin levels as ordered.[2] Promote parent–infant bonding as much as possible: remove eye shields and allow parents to hold, feed, and care for the infant as possible.[2]

Geriatric pointers
In patients older than age 60, jaundice is usually caused by cholestasis resulting from extrahepatic obstruction.

Patient counseling
Encourage the patient with a hepatic disorder to decrease his protein intake sharply and increase his intake of carbohydrates. If he has obstructive jaundice, encourage a nutritious, balanced diet (avoiding high-fat foods) and frequent small meals.

Provide the patient with strategies to minimize the intense itching he may experience. Tell him to keep his skin well hydrated and lubricated by using fragrance-free lotion or cream.[1] Encourage him to bathe or shower in lukewarm water; hot water can increase itching.[1] Tell him to keep his fingernails short to prevent scratching and to wear cool, lightweight clothing.[1]

REFERENCES
1. McCarron, K. "Jaundice: More Than Meets The Eye," *Nursing Made Incredibly Easy!* 5(3):25-27, May/June 2007.
2. Stokowski, L.A. "Fundamentals of Phototherapy for Neonatal Jaundice," *Advances in Neonatal Care* 6(6):303-312, December 2006.

JAW PAIN

Jaw pain may arise from either of the two bones that hold the teeth in the jaw—the maxilla (upper jaw) and the mandible (lower jaw). Jaw pain also includes pain in the temporomandibular joint (TMJ), where the mandible meets the temporal bone.

Jaw pain may develop gradually or abruptly and may range from barely noticeable to excruciating, depending on its cause. It usually results from disorders of the teeth, soft tissue, or glands of the mouth or throat or from local trauma or infection. Systemic causes include musculoskeletal, neurologic, cardiovascular, endocrine, immunologic, metabolic, and infectious disorders. Life-threatening disorders, such as myocardial infarction (MI) and tetany, also produce jaw pain, as do certain drugs (especially phenothiazines) and dental or surgical procedures.

Jaw pain is seldom a primary indicator of any one disorder; however, some causes are medical emergencies.

Ask the patient when the jaw pain began. Did it arise suddenly or gradually? Is it more severe or frequent now than when it first occurred? Sudden severe jaw pain, especially with chest pain, shortness of breath, or arm pain, requires prompt evaluation because it may herald a life-threatening disorder. Obtain an electrocardiogram and blood samples for cardiac markers. Give aspirin, oxygen, morphine sulfate, and nitroglycerin as indicated.

History and physical examination
Begin the patient history by asking the patient to describe the pain's character, intensity, and frequency. When did he first notice the jaw pain? Where on the jaw does he feel pain? Does the pain radiate to other areas? Sharp or burning pain arises from the skin or subcutaneous tissues. Causalgia, an intense burning sensation, usually results from damage to the fifth cranial, or trigeminal, nerve. This type of superficial pain is easily localized, unlike dull, aching, boring, or throbbing pain, which originates in muscle, bone, or joints. Also ask about aggravating or alleviating factors.

Ask about recent trauma, surgery, or procedures, especially dental work. Ask about associated signs and symptoms, such as joint or chest pain, dyspnea, palpitations, fatigue, headache, malaise, anorexia, weight loss, intermittent claudication, diplopia, and hearing loss. (Keep in mind that jaw pain may accompany more characteristic signs and symptoms of life-threatening disorders, such as chest pain in a patient with an MI.)

Focus your physical examination on the jaw. Inspect the painful area for redness, and palpate for edema or warmth. Facing the patient directly, look for facial asymmetry indicating swelling. Check the TMJs by placing your fingertips just anterior to the external auditory meatus and asking the patient to open and close, and to thrust out and retract his jaw. Note the presence of crepitus, an abnormal scraping or grinding sensation in the joint. (Clicks heard when the jaw is widely spread apart are normal.) How wide can the patient open his mouth? Less than 1⅛″ (3 cm) or more than 2⅜″ (6 cm) between upper and lower teeth is abnormal. Next, palpate the parotid area for pain and swelling, and inspect and palpate the oral cavity for lesions, elevation of the tongue, or masses.

Medical causes

▶ *Angina pectoris.* Angina may produce jaw pain (usually radiating from the substernal area) and left arm pain. Angina is less severe than the pain of an MI. It's commonly triggered by exertion, emotional stress, or ingestion of a heavy meal and usually subsides with rest and the administration of nitroglycerin. Other signs and symptoms include shortness of breath, nausea and vomiting, tachycardia, dizziness, diaphoresis, belching, and palpitations.

▶ *Arthritis.* With osteoarthritis, which usually affects the small joints of the hand, aching jaw pain increases with activity (talking, eating) and subsides with rest. Other features are crepitus heard and felt over the TMJ, enlarged joints with a restricted range of motion, and stiffness on awakening that improves with a few minutes of activity. Redness and warmth are usually absent.

Rheumatoid arthritis causes symmetrical pain in all joints (commonly affecting proximal finger joints first), including the jaw. The joints display limited range of motion and are tender, warm, swollen, and stiff after inactivity, especially in the morning. Myalgia is common. Systemic signs and symptoms include fatigue, weight loss, malaise, anorexia, lymphadenopathy, and mild fever. Painless, movable rheumatoid nodules may appear on the elbows, knees, and knuckles. Progressive disease causes deformities, crepitation with joint rotation, muscle weakness and atrophy around the involved joint, and multiple systemic complications.

▶ *Head and neck cancer.* Many types of head and neck cancer, especially of the oral cavity and nasopharynx, produce aching jaw pain of insidious onset. Other findings include a history of leukoplakia ulcers of the mucous membranes; palpable masses in the jaw, mouth, and neck; dysphagia; bloody discharge; drooling; lymphadenopathy; and trismus.

▶ *Hypocalcemic tetany.* Besides painful muscle contractions of the jaw and mouth, this life-threatening disorder produces paresthesia and carpopedal spasms. The patient may complain of weakness, fatigue, and palpitations. Examination reveals hyperreflexia and positive Chvostek's and Trousseau's signs. Muscle twitching, choreiform movements, and muscle cramps also may occur. With severe hypocalcemia, laryngeal spasm may occur with stridor, cyanosis, seizures, and cardiac arrhythmias.

▶ *Ludwig's angina.* An acute streptococcal infection of the sublingual and submandibular spaces that produces severe jaw pain in the mandibular area with tongue elevation, sublingual edema, and drooling. Fever is a common sign. Progressive disease produces dysphagia, dysphonia, and stridor and dyspnea due to laryngeal edema and obstruction by an elevated tongue.

▶ *Myocardial infarction.* Initially, this life-threatening disorder causes intense, crushing substernal pain that's unrelieved by rest or nitroglycerin. The pain may radiate to the lower jaw, left arm, neck, back, or shoulder blades. (Rarely, jaw pain occurs without chest pain.) Other findings include pallor, clammy skin, dyspnea, excessive diaphoresis, nausea and vomiting, anxiety, restlessness, a feeling of impending doom, low-grade fever, decreased or increased blood pressure, arrhythmias, an atrial gallop, new murmurs (in many cases from mitral insufficiency), and crackles.

▶ *Osteomyelitis.* Bone infection after trauma, sinus infection, dental injury, or surgery (dental or facial) may produce diffuse, aching jaw pain along with warmth, swelling, tenderness, erythema, and restricted jaw movement. Acute osteomyelitis also may cause tachycardia, sudden fever, nausea, and malaise. Chronic osteomyelitis may recur after minor trauma.

▶ *Sialolithiasis.* With this disorder, stones form in the salivary glands, causing painful swelling that makes chewing uncomfortable. Jaw pain occurs in the lower jaw, floor of the mouth, and TMJ. It also may radiate to the ear or neck.

▶ *Sinusitis.* Maxillary sinusitis produces intense boring pain in the maxilla and cheek that may radiate to the eye. This type of sinusitis also causes a feeling of fullness, increased pain on percussion of the first and second molars and, in those with nasal obstruction, the loss of the sense of smell. Sphenoid sinusitis causes scanty nasal discharge and chronic pain at the mandibular ramus and vertex of the head and in the temporal area. Other signs and symptoms of both types of sinusitis include fever, halitosis, headache, malaise, cough, sore throat, and fever.

▶ *Suppurative parotitis.* Bacterial infection of the parotid gland by Staphylococcus aureus tends to develop in debilitated patients with dry mouth or poor oral hygiene. Besides the abrupt onset of jaw pain, high fever, and chills, findings include erythema and edema of the overlying skin; a tender, swollen gland; and pus at the second top molar (Stensen's ducts). Infection may lead to disorientation; shock and death are common.

▶ *Temporal arteritis.* Most common in women older than age 60, this disorder produces sharp jaw pain after chewing or talking. Nonspecific signs and symptoms include low-grade fever, generalized muscle pain, malaise, fatigue, anorexia, and weight loss. Vascular lesions produce jaw pain; throbbing, unilateral headache in the frontotemporal region; swollen, nodular, tender and, possibly, pulseless temporal arteries; and, at times, erythema of the overlying skin.

▶ *Temporomandibular joint syndrome.* This common syndrome produces jaw pain at the TMJ; spasm and pain of the masticating muscle; clicking, popping, or crepitus of the TMJ; and restricted jaw movement. Unilateral, localized pain may radiate to other head and neck areas. The patient typically reports teeth clenching, bruxism, and emotional stress. He also may experience ear pain, headache, deviation of the jaw to the affected side upon opening the mouth, and jaw subluxation or dislocation, especially after yawning.

▶ *Tetanus.* A rare life-threatening disorder caused by a bacterial toxin, tetanus produces stiffness and pain in the jaw and difficulty opening the mouth. Early nonspecific signs and symptoms (commonly unnoticed or mistaken for influenza) include headache, irritability, restlessness, low-grade fever, and chills. Examination reveals tachycardia, profuse diaphoresis, and hyperreflexia. Progressive disease leads to painful, involuntary muscle spasms that spread to the abdomen, back, or face. The slightest stimulus may produce reflex spasms of any muscle group. Ultimately, laryngospasm, respiratory distress, and seizures may occur.

▶ *Trauma.* Injury to the face, head, or neck—particularly fracture of the maxilla or mandible—may produce jaw pain and swelling and decreased jaw mobility. Related findings include hypotension and tachycardia (indicating shock), lacerations, ecchymoses, and hematomas. Rhinorrhea or otorrhea indicates the leakage of cerebrospinal fluid; blurred vision indicates orbital involvement.

▶ *Trigeminal neuralgia.* This disorder is marked by paroxysmal attacks of intense unilateral jaw pain (stopping at the midline of the face) or rapid-fire shooting sensations in one division of the trigeminal nerve (usually the mandibular or maxillary division). This superficial pain, felt mainly over the lips and chin and in the teeth, lasts from 1 to 15 minutes. Mouth and nose areas may be hypersensitive. Involvement of the ophthalmic branch of the trigeminal nerve causes a diminished or absent corneal reflex on the same side. Attacks can be triggered by mild stimulation of the nerve (for example, lightly touching the cheeks), exposure to heat or cold, or consumption of hot or cold foods or beverages.

Other causes

DRUG WATCH *Some drugs, such as phenothiazines, affect the extrapyramidal tract, causing dyskinesias. Drugs used to treat pulmonary arterial hypertension, such as iloprost, treprostinil, and epoprostenol, also may cause jaw pain.*[1]

Special considerations

If the patient is in severe pain, withhold food, liquids, and oral drugs until the diagnosis is confirmed. Give an analgesic. Prepare the patient for diagnostic tests, such as jaw X-rays. Apply an ice pack if the jaw is swollen, and discourage the patient from talking or moving his jaw.

Pediatric pointers

Be alert for nonverbal signs of jaw pain, such as rubbing the affected area or wincing while talking or swallowing. In infants, initial signs of tetany from hypocalcemia include episodes of apnea and generalized jitteriness progressing to facial grimaces and generalized rigidity. Finally, seizures may occur.

Jaw pain in children sometimes stems from disorders uncommon in adults. Mumps, for example, causes unilateral or bilateral swelling from the lower mandible to the zygomatic arch. Parotiditis due to cystic fibrosis also causes jaw pain. When trauma causes jaw pain in children, always consider the possibility of abuse.

Patient counseling

To avoid delay in seeking treatment, instruct patients at risk for acute MI (especially women and older adults, who most commonly experience atypcial symptoms) to recognize jaw pain as a possible symptom of the condition.[2,3]

Instruct the patient on measures to relieve jaw discomfort, depending on the source of the pain.

REFERENCES

1. Murali, S. "Pulmonary Arterial Hypertension," *Current Opinion in Critical Care* 12(3):228-234, June 2006.
2. Tullmann, D.F., and Dracup, K. "Knowledge of Heart Attack Symptoms in Older Men and Women at Risk for Acute Myocardial Infarction," *Journal of Cardiopulmonary Rehabilitation* 25(1):33-39, January/February 2005.
3. Lackey, S.A. "Suppressing the Scourge of AMI," *Nursing* 36(5):36-41, May 2006.

● JUGULAR VEIN DISTENTION

Jugular vein distention is the abnormal fullness and height of the pulse waves in the internal or external jugular veins. For a patient in a supine position with his head elevated 45 degrees, a pulse wave height greater than 1¼″ to 1½″ (3 to 4 cm) above the angle of Louis indicates distention. Engorged, distended veins reflect increased venous pressure in the right side of the heart, which in turn, indicates an increased central venous pressure. This common sign characteristically occurs in heart failure and other cardiovascular disorders, such as constrictive pericarditis, tricuspid stenosis, and obstruction of the superior vena cava.

Evaluating jugular vein distention involves visualizing and assessing venous pulsations. (See *Evaluating jugular vein distention*.) If you detect jugular vein distention in a patient with pale, clammy skin who suddenly appears anxious and dyspneic, take his blood pressure. If you note hypotension and paradoxical pulse, suspect cardiac tamponade. Elevate the foot of the bed 20 to 30 degrees, give supplemental oxygen, and monitor cardiac status and rhythm, oxygen saturation, and mental status. Start an I.V. line for drug administration, and keep cardiopulmonary resuscitation equipment close by. Assemble the needed equipment for emergency pericardiocentesis (to relieve pressure on the heart.) Throughout the procedure, monitor the patient's blood pressure, heart rhythm, and respirations.

History and physical examination

If the patient isn't in severe distress, obtain a personal history. Has he recently gained weight? Does he have difficulty putting on shoes? Are his ankles swollen? Ask about chest pain, shortness of breath, paroxysmal nocturnal dyspnea, anorexia, nausea or vomiting, and a history of cancer or cardiac, pulmonary, hepatic, or renal disease. Obtain a drug history noting diuretic use and dosage. Is the patient taking drugs as prescribed? Ask the patient about his regular diet patterns, noting a high sodium intake.

Next, perform a physical examination, beginning with vital signs. Tachycardia, tachypnea, and increased blood pressure indicate fluid overload that's stressing the heart. Inspect and palpate the patient's limbs and face for edema. Then weigh the patient and compare that weight to his baseline.

Auscultate his lungs for crackles and his heart for gallops, a pericardial friction rub, and muffled heart sounds. Inspect his abdomen for distention, and palpate and percuss for an enlarged liver. Finally monitor urine output and note any decrease.

Evaluating jugular vein distention

Place the patient in a supine position so you can see his jugular vein pulsations reflected from the right atrium. Elevate the head of the bed 45 to 90 degrees. (In a normal patient, veins distend only when the patient lies flat.)

Next, locate the angle of Louis (sternal notch)—the reference point for measuring venous pressure. To do so, palpate the clavicles where they join the sternum (the suprasternal notch). Place your first two fingers on the suprasternal notch. Then, without lifting them from the skin, slide them down the sternum until you feel a bony protuberance—this is the angle of Louis.

Find the internal jugular vein (which indicates venous pressure more reliably than the external jugular vein). Shine a flashlight across the patient's neck to create shadows that highlight his venous pulse. Be sure to distinguish jugular vein pulsations from carotid artery pulsations. One way to do this is to palpate the vessel: Arterial pulsations continue despite light finger pressure, whereas venous pulsations disappear. Also, venous pulsations increase or decrease with changes in body position; arterial pulsations remain constant.

Next, locate the highest point along the vein where you can see pulsations. Using a centimeter ruler, measure the distance between that high point and the sternal notch. Record this finding as well as the angle at which the patient was lying. A finding greater than 1¼" to 1½" (3 to 4 cm) above the sternal notch, with the head of the bed at a 45-degree angle, indicates jugular vein distention.

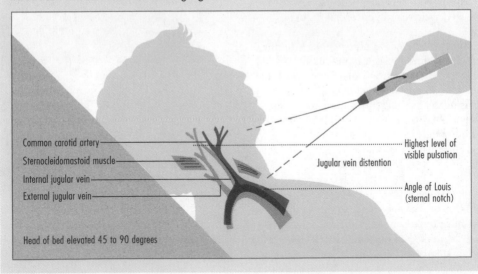

Common carotid artery
Sternocleidomastoid muscle
Internal jugular vein
External jugular vein

Jugular vein distention

Highest level of visible pulsation

Angle of Louis (sternal notch)

Head of bed elevated 45 to 90 degrees

Medical causes

▶ *Cardiac tamponade*. This life-threatening condition produces jugular vein distention along with hypotension and muffled heart sounds (known as Beck's triad).[1] It also causes tachycardia, tachypnea, a pericardial friction rub, weak or absent peripheral pulses or pulses that decrease during inspiration (pulsus paradoxus), anxiety, restlessness, cyanosis, chest pain, dyspnea, clammy skin, and hepatomegaly. The patient may sit upright or lean forward to ease breathing.

▶ *Heart failure*. Sudden or gradual development of right-sided heart failure commonly causes jugular vein distention, ascites, dependent edema of the legs and sacrum, and liver engorgement.[2] Other findings include weakness, anxiety, confusion, cyanosis, steady weight gain, hepatomegaly, nausea and vomiting, abdominal discomfort, and anorexia due to visceral edema. Ascites is a late sign. Massive right-sided heart failure may produce anasarca and oliguria.

If left-sided heart failure precedes right-sided heart failure, jugular vein distention is a late sign. Other signs and symptoms include fatigue, dyspnea, orthopnea, paroxysmal nocturnal dyspnea, tachypnea, tachycardia, and arrhythmias. Auscultation reveals crackles and a ventricular gallop.

▶ *Hypervolemia.* Markedly increased intravascular fluid volume causes jugular vein distention, along with rapid weight gain, elevated blood pressure, bounding pulse, peripheral edema, dyspnea, and crackles.

▶ *Pericarditis (chronic constrictive).* Progressive signs and symptoms of restricted heart filling include jugular vein distention that's more prominent on inspiration (Kussmaul's sign).[1] The patient usually complains of chest pain. Other signs and symptoms include fluid retention with dependent edema, hepatomegaly, ascites, and pericardial friction rub.

▶ *Superior vena cava obstruction.* A tumor or, rarely, thrombosis may gradually lead to jugular vein distention when the veins of the head, neck, and arms fail to empty effectively, causing facial, neck, and upper arm edema. Metastasis of a malignant tumor to the mediastinum may cause dyspnea, cough, substernal chest pain, and hoarseness.

Special considerations

If the patient has cardiac tamponade, prepare him for pericardiocentesis.[1] If he doesn't have cardiac tamponade, restrict fluids and monitor his intake and output. Insert an indwelling urinary catheter if needed. If the patient has heart failure, give a diuretic. Weigh the patient daily, and monitor intake and output strictly.[2] Routinely change his position to avoid skin breakdown from peripheral edema. Prepare the patient for a central venous or Swan-Ganz catheter insertion in order to measure right- and left-sided heart pressure.

Pediatric pointers

Jugular vein distention is difficult (sometimes impossible) to evaluate in most infants and toddlers because of their short, thick necks. Even in school-age children, measurement of jugular vein distention can be unreliable because the sternal angle may not be the same distance (2″ to 2¾″ [5 to 7 cm]) above the right atrium as it is in adults.

Patient counseling

Teach the patient with heart failure about appropriate treatments, including dietary restrictions (such as a low-sodium, fluid-restricted diet).

REFERENCES

1. Carter, T. and Brooks, C.A. "Pericarditis: Inflammation or Infarction?" *The Journal of Cardiovascular Nursing* 20(4):239-244, July/August 2005.
2. Riggs, J.M. "Manage Heart Failure," *Men in Nursing* 1(2):18-26, April 2006.

K

KERNIG'S SIGN

A reliable early indicator and tool used to diagnose meningeal irritation, Kernig's sign elicits both resistance and hamstring muscle pain when the examiner attempts to extend the knee while the hip and knee are both flexed 90 degrees. However, when the patient's thigh isn't flexed on the abdomen, he's usually able to completely extend his leg. (See *Eliciting Kernig's sign,* page 274.) This sign usually appears in meningitis or subarachnoid hemorrhage. With these potentially life-threatening disorders, hamstring muscle resistance results from stretching the blood- or exudate-irritated meninges surrounding spinal nerve roots.

Kernig's sign can also indicate a herniated disk or spinal tumor. With these disorders, sciatic pain results from disk or tumor pressure on spinal nerve roots.

History and physical examination

If you elicit a positive Kernig's sign and suspect life-threatening meningitis or subarachnoid hemorrhage, immediately prepare for emergency intervention. (See *When Kernig's sign signals CNS crisis,* page 275.)

If you don't suspect meningeal irritation, ask the patient if he feels any back pain that radiates down one or both legs. Does he also feel leg numbness, tingling, or weakness? Ask about other signs and symptoms, and find out if he has a history of cancer or back injury.

Then perform a physical examination, concentrating on motor and sensory function.

Medical causes

▶ *Lumbosacral herniated disk.* A positive Kernig's sign may appear in patients with this disorder, but the cardinal and earliest feature is sciatic pain on the affected side or on both sides. Other findings include postural deformity (lumbar lordosis or scoliosis), paresthesia, hypoactive deep tendon reflexes in the involved leg, and dorsiflexor muscle weakness.

▶ *Meningitis.* A positive Kernig's sign usually occurs early with meningitis, along with fever and, possibly, chills. Other signs and symptoms of meningeal irritation include nuchal rigidity, hyperreflexia, Brudzinski's sign, and opisthotonos. As intracranial pressure (ICP) increases, headache and vomiting may occur. In severe meningitis, the patient may experience stupor, coma, and seizures. Cranial nerve involvement may produce ocular palsies, facial weakness, deafness, and photophobia. An erythematous maculopapular rash may occur in viral meningitis; a purpuric rash may be seen in those with meningococcal meningitis.

▶ *Spinal cord tumor.* Kernig's sign can be elicited occasionally, but the earliest symptom is typically pain felt locally or along the spinal nerve, commonly in the leg. Associated findings include weakness or paralysis distal to the tumor, paresthesia, urine retention, urinary or fecal incontinence, and sexual dysfunction.

▶ *Subarachnoid hemorrhage.* Kernig's sign and Brudzinski's sign can both be elicited

Eliciting Kernig's sign

To elicit Kernig's sign, place the patient in a supine position. Flex her leg at the hip and knee, as shown here. Then try to extend the leg while you keep the hip flexed. If the patient feels pain and possibly spasm in the hamstring muscle and resists further extension, you can assume she has meningeal irritation.

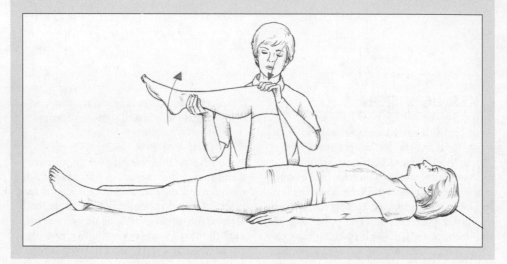

within minutes after the initial bleed. The patient has a sudden onset of severe headache that begins in a localized area and then spreads; pupillary inequality, nuchal rigidity, and decreased level of consciousness are associated findings. Photophobia, fever, nausea and vomiting, dizziness, and seizures are possible. Focal signs include hemiparesis or hemiplegia, aphasia, and sensory or vision disturbances. Increasing ICP may produce bradycardia, increased blood pressure, respiratory pattern change, and rapid progression to coma.

Special considerations

Prepare the patient for diagnostic tests, such as a computed tomography scan, magnetic resonance imaging, spinal X-ray, myelography, and lumbar puncture. Closely monitor his vital signs, ICP, and cardiopulmonary and neurologic status. Ensure bed rest, quiet, and minimal stress.

If the patient has meningitis, institute seizure precautions.[1] Give acetaminophen as ordered to control fever and relieve neck pain and stiffness.[1] Dexamethasone may be ordered to reduce cerebral edema in patients with bacterial meningitis; it should be given either before or with the first dose of antibiotics.[1,2] Mannitol may be ordered to decrease intracranial hypertension.[1]

If the patient has a subarachnoid hemorrhage, keep the environment quiet, dim the lights, and elevate the head of the bed at least 30 degrees to reduce ICP.[3] Give nimodipine as ordered to decrease cerebral vasospasm, which causes 40% to 50% of deaths from subarachnoid hemorrhage.[3]

If the patient has a herniated disk or spinal tumor, he may require pelvic traction.

Pediatric pointers

Kernig's sign is considered ominous in children because of their greater potential for rapid deterioration.

When Kernig's sign signals CNS crisis

Because Kernig's sign may signal meningitis or subarachnoid hemorrhage—each a life-threatening central nervous system (CNS) disorder—take the patient's vital signs at once to obtain baseline information. Then test for Brudzinski's sign to obtain further evidence of meningeal irritation. Next, ask the patient or his family to describe the onset of illness. Typically, a progressive onset of headache, fever, nuchal rigidity, and confusion suggests meningitis. Conversely, a sudden onset of severe headache, nuchal rigidity, photophobia and, possibly, loss of consciousness usually indicates subarachnoid hemorrhage.

MENINGITIS

If a diagnosis of meningitis is suspected, ask about recent infections, especially tooth abscesses. Ask about exposure to infected persons or places where meningitis is endemic. Meningitis usually is a complication of another bacterial infection, so draw blood for culture studies to determine the causative organism. Prepare the patient for a lumbar puncture (if a tumor or abscess can be ruled out). Also, find out if the patient has a history of I.V. drug abuse, an open-head injury, or endocarditis. Insert an I.V. line, and immediately start an antibiotic.

SUBARACHNOID HEMORRHAGE

If subarachnoid hemorrhage is the suspected diagnosis, ask about a history of hypertension, cerebral aneurysm, head trauma, or arteriovenous malformation. Also ask about sudden withdrawal of an antihypertensive.

Check the patient's pupils for dilation, and assess him for signs of increasing intracranial pressure, such as bradycardia, increased systolic blood pressure, and widened pulse pressure. Insert an I.V. line, and give supplemental oxygen.

Patient counseling

Explain the signs and symptoms of meningitis, and ways to prevent it. Give the patient information about appropriate vaccines, such as the pneumococcal vaccine, meningococcal vaccine, and *Haemophilus influenzae* type b vaccine.

Explain the activities that a patient with a herniated disk should avoid. Teach the patient how to apply a back brace or cervical collar, as needed.

REFERENCES

1. Matthews, C., Miller, L., and Mott, M. "Getting Ahead of Acute Meningitis and Encephalitis," *Nursing* 37(11):36-39, November 2007.
2. Roos, K.L. "Acute Meningitis," *CONTINUUM: Lifelong Learning in Neurology. Infectious Diseases* 12(2):13-26, April 2006.
3. Reddy, L.C.S. "Heads Up on Cerebral Bleeds," *Nursing* 36(5) ED Insider: 4-9, Spring 2006.

LEVEL OF CONSCIOUSNESS, DECREASED

A decrease in level of consciousness (LOC), from lethargy to stupor to coma, usually results from a neurologic disorder and may signal a life-threatening complication, such as hemorrhage, trauma, or cerebral edema. It also can indicate disease progression of conditions such as encephalitis and meningitis.[1] However, this sign can also result from a metabolic, GI, musculoskeletal, urologic, or cardiopulmonary disorder; severe nutritional deficiency; the effects of toxins; or drug use. LOC can deteriorate suddenly or gradually and can remain altered temporarily or permanently.

Consciousness is affected by the reticular activating system (RAS), an intricate network of neurons with axons extending from the brain stem, thalamus, and hypothalamus to the cerebral cortex. A disturbance in any part of this integrated system prevents the intercommunication that makes consciousness possible. Loss of consciousness can result from a bilateral cerebral disturbance, an RAS disturbance, or both. Cerebral dysfunction characteristically produces the least dramatic decrease in a patient's LOC. In contrast, dysfunction of the RAS produces the most dramatic decrease in LOC: coma.

The most sensitive indicator of decreased LOC is a change in the patient's mental status. The Glasgow Coma Scale, which measures a patient's ability to respond to verbal, sensory, and motor stimulation, can be used to quickly evaluate a patient's LOC.

After evaluating the patient's airway, breathing, and circulation, use the Glasgow Coma Scale to quickly determine his LOC and to obtain baseline data. (See *Using the Glasgow Coma Scale*.) If the patient scores 13 or less, emergency surgery may be needed. Insert an artificial airway, elevate the head of the bed 30 degrees and, if spinal cord injury has been ruled out, turn the patient's body to either side. (Turning the head only could decrease venous outflow and lead to an increase in intracranial pressure.[2]) Prepare to suction the patient if needed. You may need to hyperventilate him to reduce carbon dioxide levels and decrease intracranial pressure (ICP). (See *Key note about hyperventilation*, page 278.) Then determine the rate, rhythm, and depth of spontaneous respirations. Support his breathing with a handheld resuscitation bag, if needed. If the patient's Glasgow Coma Scale score is 7 or less, intubation and resuscitation may be needed.

Continue to monitor the patient's vital signs, staying alert for signs of increasing ICP, such as bradycardia and widening pulse pressure. When his airway, breathing, and circulation are stabilized, perform a neurologic examination.

History and physical examination

Try to obtain history information from the patient, if he's lucid, and from his family. Did the patient complain of headache, dizziness,

Using the Glasgow Coma Scale

The Glasgow Coma Scale describes a patient's baseline mental status and helps to detect and interpret changes from baseline findings. When using the Glasgow Coma Scale, test the patient's ability to respond to verbal, motor, and sensory stimulation, and grade your findings according to the scale. A score of 15 indicates that the patient is alert, can follow simple commands, and is oriented to time, place, and person. A decreased score in one or more categories may signal an impending neurologic crisis. A score of 7 or less indicates severe neurologic damage.

TEST	SCORE	RESPONSE
Eye-opening response		
Spontaneous	4	Opens eyes spontaneously
To speech	3	Opens eyes when told to
To pain	2	Opens eyes only to painful stimulus
None	1	Doesn't open eyes in response to stimuli
Motor response		
Obeys	6	Shows two fingers when asked
Localizes	5	Reaches toward painful stimulus and tries to remove it
Withdraws	4	Moves away from painful stimulus
Abnormal flexion	3	Assumes a decorticate posture (shown below)
Abnormal extension	2	Assumes a decerebrate posture (shown below)
None	1	No response; just lies flaccid (an ominous sign)
Verbal response (to question, "What year is this?")		
Oriented	5	Tells correct year
Confused	4	Tells incorrect year
Inappropriate words	3	Replies randomly with incorrect words
Incomprehensible	2	Moans or screams
No response	1	No response
Total score	(3 to 15)	

Key note about hyperventilation

Hyperventilation that lowers arterial carbon dioxide levels below 35 mm Hg will cause vasoconstriction and may worsen cerebral ischemia.[2] Keep arterial carbon dioxide levels at 35 to 40 mm Hg.

nausea, vision or hearing disturbances, weakness, fatigue, or any other problems before his LOC decreased? Has his family noticed any changes in the patient's behavior, personality, memory, or temperament? Also ask about a history of neurologic disease, cancer, or recent trauma or infections; drug and alcohol use; and the development of other signs and symptoms.

Because decreased LOC can result from a disorder affecting virtually any body system, tailor the remainder of your evaluation according to the patient's associated symptoms.

Medical causes

▶ *Adrenal crisis.* Decreased LOC, ranging from lethargy to coma, may develop within 8 to 12 hours of onset. Early associated findings include progressive weakness, irritability, anorexia, headache, nausea and vomiting, diarrhea, abdominal pain, and fever. Later signs and symptoms include hypotension; rapid, thready pulse; oliguria; cool, clammy skin; and flaccid extremities. The patient with chronic adrenocortical hypofunction may have hyperpigmented skin and mucous membranes.

▶ *Brain abscess.* Decreased LOC varies from drowsiness to deep stupor, depending on abscess size and site. Early signs and symptoms—constant intractable headache, nausea, vomiting, and seizures—reflect increasing ICP. Typical later features include ocular disturbances (nystagmus, vision loss, and pupillary inequality) and signs of infection such as fever. Other findings may include personality changes, confusion, abnormal behavior, dizziness, facial weakness, aphasia, ataxia, tremor, and hemiparesis.

▶ *Brain tumor.* LOC decreases slowly, from lethargy to coma. It's often caused by the shifting of cerebral structures due to increased intracranial pressure.[3] The patient also may experience apathy, behavior changes, memory loss, decreased attention span, morning headache, dizziness, vision loss, ataxia, and sensorimotor disturbances. Aphasia and seizures are possible, along with signs of hormonal imbalance, such as fluid retention or amenorrhea. Signs and symptoms vary with the location and size of the tumor. In later stages, papilledema, vomiting, bradycardia, and widening pulse pressure also appear. In the final stages, the patient may have a decorticate or decerebrate posture.

▶ *Cerebral aneurysm (ruptured).* Somnolence, confusion and, at times, stupor characterize a moderate bleed; deep coma occurs with severe bleeding, which can be fatal. Onset is usually abrupt, with sudden, severe headache, nausea, and vomiting. Nuchal rigidity, back and leg pain, fever, restlessness, irritability, occasional seizures, and blurred vision point to meningeal irritation. The type and severity of other findings vary with the site and severity of the hemorrhage and may include hemiparesis, hemisensory defects, dysphagia, and visual defects.

▶ *Cerebral contusion.* Usually unconscious for a prolonged period, the patient may develop dilated, nonreactive pupils and decorticate or decerebrate posture. If he's conscious or recovers consciousness, he may be drowsy, confused, disoriented, agitated, or even violent. Other findings include blurred or double vision, fever, headache, pallor, diaphoresis, tachycardia, altered respirations, aphasia, and hemiparesis. Residual effects include seizures, impaired mental status, slight hemiparesis, and vertigo.

▶ *Diabetic ketoacidosis.* This disorder produces a rapid decrease in LOC, ranging from lethargy to coma, commonly preceded by polydipsia, polyphagia, and polyuria. The patient may complain of weakness, anorexia, abdominal pain, nausea, and vomiting. He also may have orthostatic hypotension; fruity breath odor; Kussmaul's respirations; warm, dry skin; and a rapid, thready pulse. Untreated, this condition invariably leads to coma and death.

▶ *Encephalitis.* Within 24 to 48 hours after onset, the patient may develop LOC changes ranging from lethargy to coma. Other findings may include abrupt onset of fever, headache, nuchal rigidity, nausea, vomiting, irritability, personality changes, seizures, aphasia, ataxia, hemiparesis, nystagmus, photophobia, myoclonus, and cranial nerve palsies.

▶ *Encephalomyelitis (postvaccinal).* This life-threatening disorder produces rapid LOC deterioration from drowsiness to coma. The patient also has rapid onset of fever, headache, nuchal rigidity, back pain, vomiting, and seizures.

▶ *Encephalopathy.* With *hepatic encephalopathy,* signs and symptoms develop in four stages: in the prodromal stage, slight personality changes (disorientation, forgetfulness, slurred speech) and slight tremor; in the impending stage, tremor progressing to asterixis (the hallmark of hepatic encephalopathy), lethargy, aberrant behavior, and apraxia; in the stuporous stage, stupor and hyperventilation, with the patient noisy and abusive when aroused; in the comatose stage, coma with decerebrate posture, hyperactive reflexes, positive Babinski's reflex, and fetor hepaticus.

With life-threatening *hypertensive encephalopathy,* LOC progressively decreases from lethargy to stupor to coma. Besides markedly elevated blood pressure, the patient may experience severe headache, vomiting, seizures, vision disturbances, transient paralysis, and eventually Cheyne-Stokes respirations.

With *hypoglycemic encephalopathy,* LOC rapidly deteriorates from lethargy to coma. Early signs and symptoms include nervousness, restlessness, agitation, and confusion; hunger; alternate flushing and cold sweats; and headache, trembling, and palpitations. Blurred vision progresses to motor weakness, hemiplegia, dilated pupils, pallor, decreased pulse rate, shallow respirations, and seizures. Flaccidity and decerebrate posture appear late.

Depending on its severity, *hypoxic encephalopathy* produces a sudden or gradual decrease in LOC, leading to coma and brain death. Early on, the patient appears confused and restless, with cyanosis and increased heart and respiratory rates and blood pressure. Later, his respiratory pattern becomes abnormal, and assessment reveals decreased pulse, blood pressure, and deep tendon reflexes (DTRs); Babinski's reflex; absent doll's eye sign; and fixed pupils.

With *uremic encephalopathy,* LOC decreases gradually from lethargy to coma. Early on, the patient may appear apathetic, inattentive, confused, and irritable and may complain of headache, nausea, fatigue, and anorexia. Other findings include vomiting, tremors, edema, papilledema, hypertension, cardiac arrhythmias, dyspnea, crackles, oliguria, and Kussmaul's and Cheyne-Stokes respirations.

▶ *Epidural hemorrhage (acute).* This life-threatening posttraumatic disorder produces momentary loss of consciousness, sometimes followed by a lucid interval. While lucid, the patient has a severe headache, nausea, vomiting, and bladder distention. Rapid deterioration in consciousness follows, possibly leading to coma. Other findings include irregular respirations, seizures, decreased and bounding pulse, increased pulse pressure, hypertension, unilateral or bilateral fixed and dilated pupils, unilateral hemiparesis or hemiplegia, decerebrate posture, and Babinski's reflex.

▶ *Heatstroke.* As body temperature increases, LOC gradually decreases from lethargy to coma. Early signs and symptoms include malaise, tachycardia, tachypnea, orthostatic hypotension, muscle cramps, rigidity, and syncope. The patient may be irritable, anxious, and dizzy and may report a severe headache. At the onset of heatstroke, the patient's skin is hot, flushed, and diaphoretic with blotchy cyanosis; later, when his fever exceeds 105° F (40.5° C), his skin becomes hot, flushed, and anhidrotic. Pulse and respiratory rate increase markedly, and blood pressure drops precipitously. Other findings include vomiting, diarrhea, dilated pupils, and Cheyne-Stokes respirations.

▶ *Hypercapnia with pulmonary syndrome.* LOC decreases gradually from lethargy to coma (usually not prolonged). The patient becomes confused or drowsy and develops asterixis and muscle twitching. He may complain of headache and display mental dullness, papilledema, and small, reactive pupils.

▶ *Hypernatremia.* This disorder, life-threatening if acute, causes LOC to deteriorate from lethargy to coma. The patient is irritable and has twitches progressing to seizures. Other signs and symptoms include a weak, thready pulse; nausea; malaise; fever; thirst; flushed skin; and dry mucous membranes.

▶ *Hyperosmolar hyperglycemic nonketotic syndrome.* LOC decreases rapidly from lethargy to coma. Early findings include polyuria, polydipsia, weight loss, and weakness. Later, the patient may develop hypotension, poor skin turgor, dry skin and mucous membranes, tachycardia, tachypnea, oliguria, and seizures.

▶ *Hyperventilation syndrome.* Brief episodes of unconsciousness follow stress-induced deep, rapid breathing with anxiety and agitation. Other findings include dizziness, circumoral and peripheral paresthesia, twitching, carpopedal spasm, and arrhythmias.

▶ *Hypokalemia.* LOC gradually decreases to lethargy; coma is rare. Other findings include confusion, nausea, vomiting, diarrhea, and polyuria; weakness, decreased reflexes, and malaise; and dizziness, hypotension, arrhythmias, and abnormal electrocardiogram results.

▶ *Hyponatremia.* This disorder, life-threatening if acute, produces decreased LOC in late stages. Early nausea and malaise may progress to behavior changes, confusion, lethargy, incoordination and, eventually, seizures and coma.

▶ *Hypothermia.* With severe hypothermia (temperature below 90° F [32.2° C]), LOC decreases from lethargy to coma.[4] DTRs disappear, and ventricular fibrillation occurs, possibly followed by cardiopulmonary arrest. With mild to moderate hypothermia, the patient may experience memory loss and slurred speech as well as shivering, weakness, fatigue, and apathy.[4] Other early signs and symptoms include ataxia, muscle stiffness, and hyperactive DTRs; diuresis; tachycardia and decreased respiratory rate and blood pressure; and cold, pale skin. Later, muscle rigidity and decreased reflexes may develop, along with

peripheral cyanosis, bradycardia, arrhythmias, severe hypotension, decreased respiratory rate with shallow respirations, and oliguria.

▶ *Intracerebral hemorrhage.* This life-threatening disorder produces a rapid, steady loss of consciousness within hours, commonly accompanied by severe headache, dizziness, nausea, and vomiting. Related signs and symptoms vary and may include increased blood pressure, irregular respirations, Babinski's reflex, seizures, aphasia, decreased sensations, hemiplegia, decorticate or decerebrate posture, and dilated pupils.

▶ *Listeriosis.* If this serious infection spreads to the nervous system and causes meningitis, signs and symptoms include decreased LOC, fever, headache, and nuchal rigidity. Early signs and symptoms of listeriosis include fever, myalgias, abdominal pain, nausea, vomiting, and diarrhea.

▶ *Meningitis.* Confusion and irritability are expected; however, stupor, coma, and seizures may occur in those with severe meningitis. Fever develops early, possibly accompanied by chills. Associated findings include severe headache, nuchal rigidity, hyperreflexia and, possibly, opisthotonos. The patient has Kernig's and Brudzinski's signs and may have ocular palsies, photophobia, facial weakness, and hearing loss.

▶ *Myxedema crisis.* The patient may have a swift decline in LOC. Other findings include severe hypothermia, hypoventilation, hypotension, bradycardia, hypoactive reflexes, periorbital and peripheral edema, impaired hearing and balance, and seizures.

▶ *Pontine hemorrhage.* A sudden, rapid decrease in LOC to the point of coma occurs within minutes and death within hours. The patient also may have total paralysis, decerebrate posture, Babinski's reflex, absent doll's eye sign, and bilateral miosis (however, the pupils remain reactive to light).

▶ *Seizure disorders.* A *complex partial seizure* produces decreased LOC, manifested as a blank stare, purposeless behavior (picking at clothing, wandering, lip smacking or chewing motions), and unintelligible speech. The seizure may be heralded by an aura and followed by several minutes of mental confusion.

An *absence seizure* usually involves a brief change in LOC, indicated by blinking or eye rolling, blank stare, and slight mouth movements.

A *generalized tonic-clonic seizure* typically begins with a loud cry and sudden loss of consciousness. Muscle spasm alternates with relaxation. Tongue biting, incontinence, labored breathing, apnea, and cyanosis also may occur. Consciousness returns after the seizure, but the patient remains confused and may have difficulty talking. He may complain of drowsiness, fatigue, headache, muscle aching, and weakness and may fall into deep sleep.

An *atonic seizure* produces sudden unconsciousness for a few seconds.

Status epilepticus, rapidly recurring seizures without intervening periods of physiologic recovery and return of consciousness, can be life threatening.

▶ *Shock.* Decreased LOC—lethargy progressing to stupor and coma—occurs late in shock. Other findings include confusion, anxiety, and restlessness; hypotension; tachycardia; weak pulse with narrowing pulse pressure; dyspnea; oliguria; and cool, clammy skin.

Hypovolemic shock is typically the result of massive or insidious bleeding, either internally or externally. *Cardiogenic shock* may produce chest pain or arrhythmias and signs of heart failure, such as dyspnea, cough, edema, jugular vein distention, and weight gain. *Septic shock* may be accompanied by high fever and chills. *Anaphylactic shock* usually involves stridor.

▶ *Stroke.* Decreased LOC will occur if the stroke affects the patient's brainstem or cerebellum, although it may vary in degree and onset.[5] A *thrombotic stroke* usually follows multiple transient ischemic attacks (TIAs). LOC changes may be abrupt or take several minutes, hours, or days. An *embolic stroke* occurs suddenly, and deficits reach their peak almost at once. Deficits in a *hemorrhagic stroke* usually develop over minutes or hours.

Additional findings vary with stroke type and severity and may include disorientation; intellectual deficits, such as memory loss and poor judgment; personality changes; and emotional lability. Other possible findings include dysarthria, dysphagia, ataxia, aphasia, apraxia, agnosia, unilateral sensorimotor loss, and visual disturbances. In addition, urine retention, incontinence, constipation, headache, vomiting, and seizures may occur.

▶ *Subdural hematoma (chronic).* LOC deteriorates slowly. Other signs and symptoms include confusion, decreased ability to concentrate, personality changes, headache, lightheadedness, seizures, and a dilated ipsilateral pupil with ptosis.

▶ *Subdural hemorrhage (acute).* With this potentially life-threatening disorder, agitation and confusion are followed by progressively decreasing LOC from somnolence to coma. The patient also may have headache, fever, unilateral pupil dilation, decreased pulse and respiratory rates, widening pulse pressure, seizures, hemiparesis, and Babinski's reflex.

▶ *Thyroid storm.* LOC decreases suddenly and can progress to coma. Irritability, restlessness, confusion, and psychotic behavior precede the deterioration. Other signs and symptoms include tremors and weakness; vision disturbances; tachycardia, arrhythmias, angina, and acute respiratory distress; warm, moist, flushed skin; and vomiting, diarrhea, and fever to 105° F (40.5° C).

▶ *Transient ischemic attack.* LOC decreases abruptly (with varying severity) and gradually returns to normal within 24 hours. Site-specific findings may include vision loss, nystagmus, dizziness, dysarthria, unilateral hemiparesis or hemiplegia, tinnitus, paresthesia, staggering or incoordinated gait, aphasia, or dysphagia.

▶ *West Nile encephalitis.* This brain infection is caused by the West Nile virus, a mosquito-borne flavivirus commonly found in Africa, West Asia, and the Middle East and, less commonly, in the United States. Mild infection is common. Signs and symptoms include fever, headache, and body aches, commonly with skin rash and swollen lymph glands. More severe infection is marked by high fever, headache, neck stiffness, stupor, disorientation, coma, tremors, occasional seizures, paralysis and, rarely, death.

Other causes

▶ *Alcohol use.* Alcohol use causes varying degrees of sedation, irritability, and incoordination; intoxication commonly causes stupor.

DRUG WATCH *Sedation and other degrees of decreased LOC can result from an overdose of aspirin, a barbiturate, or a central nervous system depressant.*

▶ *Poisoning.* Toxins, such as lead, carbon monoxide, and snake venom, can cause varying degrees of decreased LOC. Ethylene glycol and methanol poisoning also can cause decreased LOC.[6] Confusion is common, as are headache, nausea, and vomiting. Other general features include hypotension, cardiac arrhythmias, dyspnea, sensorimotor loss, and seizures.

Special considerations

Reassess the patient's LOC and neurologic status at least hourly. Carefully monitor ICP and intake and output. Ensure airway patency and proper nutrition. Take precautions to help ensure the patient's safety. Keep him on bed rest with the side rails up and maintain seizure precautions. Keep emergency resuscitation equipment at the patient's bedside. Prepare the patient for a computed tomography scan of the head, magnetic resonance imaging of the brain, EEG, and lumbar puncture. Maintain an elevation of the head of the bed to at least 30 degrees. Don't administer an opioid or sedative because either may further decrease the patient's LOC and hinder an accurate, meaningful neurologic examination. Apply restraints only if necessary because their use may increase his agitation and confusion. Talk to the patient even if he appears comatose; your voice may help reorient him to reality.

Pediatric pointers

The main cause of decreased LOC in children is head trauma, which often results from physical abuse or a motor vehicle accident. Other causes include accidental poisoning, hydrocephalus, and meningitis or brain abscess following an ear or respiratory infection. To reduce the parents' anxiety, include them in the child's care. Offer them support and realistic explanations of their child's condition.

Patient counseling

Explain the treatments and procedures the patient needs. Teach safety and seizure precautions. Provide referrals to sources of support. Discuss quality of life issues with the patient and his family, as indicated.

REFERENCES

1. Matthews, C., Miller, L., and Mott, M. "Getting Ahead of Acute Meningitis and Encephalitis," *Nursing* 37(11):36-39, November 2007.
2. Ahrens, T.S., Prentice, D., and Kleinpell, R.M. *Critical Care Nursing Certification,* 5th Ed. New York: McGraw-Hill, 2007.
3. Palmieri, R.L. "Responding to Primary Brain Tumour," *Nursing* 37(1):36-42, January 2007.
4. Day, M.P. "Hypothermia: A Hazard for All Seasons," *Nursing* 36(12):44-47, December 2006.
5. Harvey, J. "Countering 'Brain Attacks," *Nursing* 37(ED Insider):7-10, Fall 2007.
6. Emory, S.L. "Slow the Ticking Clock of Toxicity," *Nursing Management* 38(9):33-39, September 2007.

LYMPHADENOPATHY

Lymphadenopathy—enlargement of one or more lymph nodes—may result from increased production of lymphocytes or reticuloendothelial cells, or from infiltration of cells that aren't normally present. This sign may be generalized (involving three or more node groups) or localized. Generalized lymphadenopathy may be caused by an inflammatory process, such as bacterial or viral infection, connective tissue disease, an endocrine disorder, or neoplasm. Localized lymphadenopathy most commonly results from infection or trauma affecting a specific area. (See *Causes of localized lymphadenopathy.*)

Normally, lymph nodes are discrete, mobile, soft, nontender and, except in children, nonpalpable. (However, palpable nodes may be normal in adults.) Nodes that are more than ⅜″ (1 cm) in diameter are cause for concern. They may be tender and the skin overlying the lymph node may be erythematous, suggesting a draining lesion. Or, they may be

Causes of localized lymphadenopathy

Although lymphadenopathy usually results from infection or trauma affecting a specific area, many disorders can cause it. Here are some common causes of lymphadenopathy, listed according to the area affected.

Occipital
- Infection
- Roseola
- Scalp infection
- Seborrheic dermatitis
- Tick bite
- Tinea capitis

Auricular
- Erysipelas
- Herpes zoster ophthalmicus
- Infection
- Rubella
- Squamous cell carcinoma
- Styes or chalazion
- Tularemia

Cervical
- Cat-scratch fever
- Facial or oral cancer

- Infection
- Mononucleosis
- Monocutaneous lymph node syndrome
- Rubella
- Rubeola
- Thyrotoxicosis
- Tonsillitis
- Tuberculosis
- Varicella

Submaxillary and submental
- Cystic fibrosis
- Dental infection
- Gingivitis
- Glossitis
- Infection

Supraclavicular
- Infection
- Neoplastic disease

Axillary
- Breast cancer
- Infection
- Lymphoma
- Mastitis

Inguinal and femoral
- Carcinoma
- Chancroid
- Infection
- Lymphogranuloma venereum
- Syphilis

Popliteal
- Infection

hard and fixed, tender or nontender, suggesting a malignant tumor.

History and physical examination

Ask the patient when he first noticed the swelling, and whether it's located on one side of his body or both. Are the swollen areas sore, hard, or red? Ask the patient if he has recently had an infection or other health problem. Also ask if a biopsy has ever been done on any node because this may indicate a previously diagnosed cancer. Find out if the patient has a family history of cancer.

Palpate the entire lymph node system to determine the extent of lymphadenopathy and to detect any other areas of local enlargement. Use the pads of your index and middle fingers to move the skin over underlying tissues at the nodal area. If you detect enlarged nodes, note their size in centimeters and whether they're fixed or mobile, tender or nontender, and ery-

thematous or not. Note their texture: Is the node discrete, or does the area feel matted? If you detect tender, erythematous lymph nodes, check the area drained by that part of the lymph system for signs of infection, such as erythema and swelling. Also, palpate for and percuss the spleen.

Medical causes

▶ *Acquired immunodeficiency syndrome.* Besides lymphadenopathy, findings include a history of fatigue, night sweats, afternoon fevers, diarrhea, weight loss, and cough with several concurrent infections appearing soon afterward.

▶ *Anthrax (cutaneous).* Lymphadenopathy, malaise, headache and fever may develop along with a lesion that progresses into a painless, necrotic-centered ulcer.[1]

▶ *Brucellosis.* Generalized lymphadenopathy usually affects cervical and axillary lymph nodes, making them tender. This disease usually begins insidiously with easy fatigability, malaise, headache, backache, anorexia, weight loss, and arthralgias; it also may begin abruptly with chills, fever that usually rises in the morning and subsides during the day, and diaphoresis.

▶ *Chronic fatigue syndrome.* Lymphadenopathy may occur with incapacitating fatigue, sore throat, low-grade fevers, myalgia, cognitive dysfunction, and sleep disturbances. The diagnosis is one of exclusion and the cause of this syndrome is unknown.

▶ *Cytomegalovirus infection.* Generalized lymphadenopathy occurs in the immunocompromised patient and is accompanied by fever, malaise, rash, and hepatosplenomegaly.

▶ *Hodgkin's disease.* Lymphadenopathy is a hallmark of this disorder.[2] The extent of lymphadenopathy reflects the stage of malignancy—from stage I involvement of a single lymph node region to stage IV generalized lymphadenopathy. Common early signs and symptoms include pruritus and, in older patients, fatigue, weakness, night sweats, malaise, weight loss, and unexplained fever (usually to 101° F [38.3° C]). Also, if mediastinal lymph nodes enlarge, tracheal and esophageal pressure produces dyspnea and dysphagia.

▶ *Kawasaki syndrome.* Cervical lymphadenopathy is a characteristic sign of this potentially life-threatening illness. Affected people present with high, spiking fever, along with other diagnostic signs including erythema, bilateral conjunctival injection, and swelling in the peripheral extremities. Kawasaki syndrome isn't contagious, however the cause remains unknown and typically affects children under age 5. Prompt detection and treatment with I.V. gamma globulin is essential in preventing serious complications, such as coronary artery dilations and aneurysms.

▶ *Leptospirosis.* Lymphadenopathy occurs infrequently in this rare disease. More common findings include sudden onset of fever and chills, malaise, myalgia, headache, nausea and vomiting, and abdominal pain.

▶ *Leukemia (acute lymphocytic).* Generalized lymphadenopathy is accompanied by fatigue, malaise, pallor, and low fever. The patient also experiences prolonged bleeding time, swollen gums, weight loss, bone or joint pain, and hepatosplenomegaly.

▶ *Leukemia (chronic lymphocytic).* Generalized lymphadenopathy appears early, along with fatigue, malaise, and fever. As the disease progresses, hepatosplenomegaly, severe fatigue, and weight loss occur. Other late findings include bone tenderness, edema, pallor, dyspnea, tachycardia, palpitations, bleeding, anemia, and macular or nodular lesions.

▶ *Lyme disease.* Spread by the bite of certain ticks, Lyme disease begins with a skin lesion called *erythema chronicum migrans*. As the disease progresses, the patient may suffer from lymphadenopathy, constant malaise and fatigue, and intermittent headache, fever, chills, and aches. He may go on to develop arthralgias and, eventually, neurologic and cardiac abnormalities.

▶ *Monkeypox.* Lymphadenopathy is the one symptom that clearly distinguishes monkeypox from smallpox. Humans infected with monkeypox usually develop cervical or inguinal lymphadenopathy, along with other characteristic symptoms such as fever, chills, throat pain, muscle aches, and rash. This rare viral disease acquired its name after being discovered in laboratory monkeys; however, many other animals can carry this disease. Although the monkeypox virus is similar to smallpox, the smallpox vaccine is only used in limited circumstances to protect certain at-risk individuals against the disease.

▶ *Mononucleosis (infectious).* Characteristic, painful lymphadenopathy involves cervical, axillary, and inguinal nodes. Posterior cervical adenopathy is also common. Prodromal symptoms, such as malaise, fatigue, and headache, typically occur 3 to 5 days before the appearance of the classic triad of lymphadenopathy, sore throat, and temperature fluctuations with an evening peak of about 102° F (38.9° C). Hepatosplenomegaly may develop, along with findings of stomatitis, exudative tonsillitis, or pharyngitis.

▶ *Mycosis fungoides.* Lymphadenopathy occurs in stage III of this rare, chronic malignant lymphoma and is accompanied by ulcerated brownish red tumors that are painful and itchy.

▶ *Non-Hodgkin's lymphoma.* Painless enlargement of one or more peripheral lymph nodes is the most common sign of this disease, with generalized lymphadenopathy characterizing stage IV.[2] Dyspnea, cough, and hepatosplenomegaly occur, along with systemic complaints of fever to 101° F (38.3° C), night sweats, fatigue, malaise, and weight loss.

▶ *Plague.* Signs and symptoms of the bubonic form of this bacterial (*Yersinia pestis*) infection include lymphadenopathy, fever, and chills.

▶ *Rheumatoid arthritis.* Lymphadenopathy is an early, nonspecific finding associated with fatigue, malaise, continuous low fever, weight loss, and vague arthralgias and myalgias. Later, the patient develops joint tenderness, swelling, and warmth; joint stiffness after inactivity (especially in the morning); and subcutaneous nodules on the elbows. Eventually joint deformity, muscle weakness, and atrophy may occur.

▶ *Sarcoidosis.* Generalized, bilateral hilar and right paratracheal forms of lymphadenopathy (seen on chest X-ray) with splenomegaly are common. Initial findings are arthralgia, fatigue, malaise, weight loss, and pulmonary symptoms. Other findings vary with the site and extent of fibrosis. Typical cardiopulmonary findings include breathlessness, cough, substernal chest pain, and arrhythmias. About 90% of patients have an abnormal chest X-ray at sometime during their illness. Musculoskeletal and cutaneous features may include muscle weakness and pain, phalangeal and nasal mucosal lesions, and subcutaneous skin nodules. Common ophthalmic findings include eye pain, photophobia, and nonreactive pupils. Central nervous system involvement may produce cranial or peripheral nerve palsies and seizures.

▶ *Sjögren's syndrome.* Lymphadenopathy of the parotid and submaxillary nodes may occur in this rare disorder. Assessment reveals cardinal signs of dry mouth, eyes, and mucous membranes, possibly with photosensitivity, poor vision, eye fatigue, nasal crusting, and epistaxis.

▶ *Syphilis (primary).* Localized lymphadenopathy and a painless ulcer (canker) with an indurated border and relatively smooth base at the site of sexual exposure characterize this infection. The ulcer usually is single but more than one may be present.

▶ *Syphilis (secondary).* Generalized lymphadenopathy occurs in the second stage and may be accompanied by a macular, papular, pustular, or nodular rash on the arms, trunk, palms, soles, face, and scalp. A palmar rash is a significant diagnostic sign. Headache, malaise, anorexia, weight loss, nausea, vomiting, sore throat, and low fever may occur.

▶ *Systemic lupus erythematosus.* Generalized lymphadenopathy typically accompanies the hallmark butterfly rash, photosensitivity, Raynaud's phenomenon, and joint pain and stiffness. Pleuritic chest pain and cough may appear with systemic findings, such as fever, anorexia, and weight loss.

▶ *Tuberculous lymphadenitis.* Lymphadenopathy may be generalized or restricted to superficial lymph nodes. Affected lymph nodes may become fluctuant and drain to surrounding tissue. They may be accompanied by fever, chills, weakness, and fatigue.

▶ *Waldenström's macroglobulinemia.* Lymphadenopathy may appear along with hepatosplenomegaly. Associated findings include retinal hemorrhage, pallor, and signs of heart failure, such as jugular vein distention and crackles. The patient shows decreased level of consciousness, abnormal reflexes, and signs of peripheral neuritis. Weakness, fatigue, weight loss, epistaxis, and GI bleeding also may occur. Circulatory impairment occurs because of an increased viscosity of the blood.

Other causes

▶ *Body piercing.* Lymphadenopathy can be a local complication of body piercings.[3]

 DRUG WATCH *Phenytoin may cause generalized lymphadenopathy.*

▶ *Immunizations.* Typhoid vaccination may cause generalized lymphadenopathy.

Special considerations

If the patient has fever above 101° F (38.3° C), don't automatically assume that the temperature should be lowered. A patient with a bacterial or viral infection must tolerate the fever, which may assist recovery. Provide an antipyretic if the patient is uncomfortable. Tepid sponge baths or a hypothermia blanket also may be used.

Expect to obtain blood for routine blood work, platelet and white blood cell counts, liver and renal function studies, erythrocyte sedimentation rate, and blood cultures. Prepare the patient for other scheduled diagnostic tests, such as chest X-ray, liver and spleen scan, lymph node biopsy, or lymphography, to visualize the lymphatic system. If tests reveal infection, check your facility's policy regarding infection control.

Pediatric pointers
Infection is the most common cause of lymphadenopathy in children. The condition is commonly associated with otitis media and pharyngitis.

Provide an antipyretic if the child has a history of febrile seizures.

Patient counseling
Explain the treatments and procedures the patient needs. Teach safety and seizure precautions. Provide referrals to sources of support.

REFERENCES
1. Godyn, J.J., Reyes, L., Siderits, R., and Hazra, A. "Cutaneous Anthrax: Conservative or Surgical Treatment?" *Advances in Skin & Wound Care* 18(3):146-150, April 2005.
2. Rogers, B. "Looking at Lymphoma and Leukemia," *Nursing* 35(7):56-63, July 2005.
3. Beers, M.S., Meires, J., and Loriz, L. "Body Piercing: Coming to a Patient Near You," *The Nurse Practitioner* 32(2):55-60, February 2007.

M

MELENA

A common sign of upper GI bleeding, melena is the passage of black, tarry stools containing digested blood. Characteristic color results from bacterial degradation and hydrochloric acid acting on the blood as it travels through the GI tract. At least 60 ml of blood is needed to produce this sign. (See *Comparing melena to hematochezia,* page 288.)

Severe melena can signal acute bleeding and life-threatening hypovolemic shock. Usually, melena indicates bleeding from the esophagus, stomach, or duodenum, although it also may indicate bleeding from the jejunum, ileum, or ascending colon. This sign also may result from swallowing blood, as in epistaxis; from taking certain drugs; or from ingesting alcohol. Because false melena may be caused by ingestion of lead, iron, bismuth, or licorice (which produces black stools without the presence of blood), all black stools should be tested for occult blood.

If your patient has severe melena, quickly take orthostatic vital signs to detect hypovolemic shock. A decline of 10 mm Hg or more in systolic pressure or an increase of 10 beats/minute or more in pulse rate indicates volume depletion. Quickly examine the patient for other signs of shock, such as tachycardia, tachypnea, and cool, clammy skin. Insert a large-bore I.V. line for replacement fluids and blood transfusion. Obtain hematocrit, prothrombin time, international normalized ratio, and partial thromboplastin time. Place the patient flat with his head turned to the side and his feet elevated. Give supplemental oxygen as needed.

History and physical examination

If the patient's condition permits, ask when he discovered his stools were black and tarry. Ask about the frequency and quantity of bowel movements. Has he had melena before? Ask about other signs and symptoms, notably hematemesis or hematochezia, and about use of anti-inflammatories, alcohol, or other GI irritants. Also, find out if he has a history of GI lesions. Ask if the patient takes iron supplements, which also may cause black stools. Obtain a drug history, noting the use of warfarin or other anticoagulants.

Next, inspect the patient's mouth and nasopharynx for evidence of bleeding. Perform an abdominal examination that includes auscultation, palpation, and percussion.

Medical causes

▶ *Colon cancer.* On the right side of the colon, early tumor growth may cause melena with abdominal aching, pressure, or cramps. As the disease progresses, weakness, fatigue, and anemia develop. Eventually, the patient also will have diarrhea or obstipation, anorexia, weight loss, vomiting, and other signs and symptoms of intestinal obstruction.

With a tumor on the left side, melena is rare until late in the disease. Early tumor growth commonly causes rectal bleeding with intermittent abdominal fullness or cramping and rectal pressure. As the disease progresses, the patient may develop obstipation, diarrhea,

Comparing melena to hematochezia

With GI bleeding, the site, amount, and rate of blood flow through the GI tract determine if a patient will develop melena (black, tarry stools) or hematochezia (bright red, bloody stools). Usually, melena indicates upper GI bleeding and hematochezia indicates lower GI bleeding. However, with some disorders, melena and hematochezia may alternate. This table helps differentiate these two commonly related signs.

SIGN	SITES	CHARACTERISTICS
Melena	• Esophagus, stomach, duodenum • Rarely jejunum, ileum, ascending colon	• Black, loose, tarry stools • Delayed or minimal passage of blood through GI tract
Hematochezia	• Usually distal to or affecting the colon • Esophagus, stomach, or duodenum with rapid hemorrhage of 1 L or more	• Bright red or dark, mahogany-colored stools, pure blood, blood mixed with formed stool, or bloody diarrhea • Reflects lower GI bleeding or rapid blood loss and passage of undigested blood through GI tract

or pencil-shaped stools. At this stage, bleeding from the colon is signaled by melena or bloody stools.

▶ *Ebola virus.* Melena, hematemesis, and bleeding from the nose, gums, and vagina may occur later with this disorder. Patients usually report abrupt onset of headache, malaise, myalgia, high fever, diarrhea, abdominal pain, dehydration, and lethargy on the fifth day of illness. Pleuritic chest pain, dry hacking cough, and pharyngitis have also been noted. A maculopapular rash develops between days 5 and 7 of the illness.

▶ *Esophageal cancer.* Melena is a late sign of this malignant neoplastic disease that's three times more common in men than women. Increasing obstruction first produces painless dysphagia, then rapid weight loss. The patient may have steady chest pain with substernal fullness, nausea, vomiting, and hematemesis. Other findings include hoarseness, persistent cough (possibly hemoptysis), hiccups, sore throat, and halitosis. In the later stages, signs and symptoms include painful dysphagia, anorexia, and regurgitation.

▶ *Esophageal varices (ruptured).* This life-threatening disorder can produce melena, hematochezia, and hematemesis. Melena is preceded by signs of shock, such as tachycardia, tachypnea, hypotension, and cool, clammy skin. Agitation or confusion signals developing hepatic encephalopathy.

▶ *Gastric cancer.* Melena and altered bowel habits may occur late with this uncommon cancer. More common findings include insidious onset of upper abdominal or retrosternal discomfort and chronic dyspepsia, which are unrelieved by antacids and worsened by food. Anorexia and slight nausea often occur, along with hematemesis, pallor, fatigue, weight loss, and a feeling of abdominal fullness.

▶ *Gastritis.* Melena and hematemesis are common. The patient also may experience mild epigastric or abdominal discomfort that's worsened by eating; belching; nausea; vomiting; and malaise.

▶ *Malaria.* Melena may accompany persistent high fever and orthostatic hypotension in severe malaria. Other features include hemoptysis, vomiting, abdominal pain, diarrhea, oliguria, and headache, seizures, delirium, or coma. These findings are interspersed throughout the malarial paroxysm—chills, then high fever, and then profuse diaphoresis.

▶ *Mallory-Weiss syndrome.* This condition is characterized by massive bleeding from the upper GI tract due to a tear in the mucous membrane of the esophagus or the junction of the esophagus and the stomach. Melena and hematemesis follow vomiting. Severe upper abdominal bleeding leads to signs and symptoms of shock, such as tachycardia, tachypnea, hypotension, and cool, clammy skin. The patient also may report epigastric or back pain.

▶ *Mesenteric vascular occlusion.* This life-threatening disorder produces slight melena with 2 to 3 days of persistent, mild abdominal pain. Later, abdominal pain becomes severe and may be accompanied by tenderness, distention, guarding, and rigidity. The patient also may experience anorexia, vomiting, fever, and profound shock.

▶ *Peptic ulcer.* Melena may signal life-threatening hemorrhage from vascular penetration. The patient also may develop decreased appetite, nausea, vomiting, hematemesis, hematochezia, and left epigastric pain that's gnawing, burning, or sharp and may be described as heartburn or indigestion. With hypovolemic shock come tachycardia, tachypnea, hypotension, dizziness, syncope, and cool, clammy skin.

▶ *Small-bowel tumors.* These tumors may bleed and produce melena. Other signs and symptoms include abdominal pain, distention, and increasing frequency and pitch of bowel sounds.

▶ *Stress-related mucosal disease (SRMD).* SRMD refers to gastric damage caused by physiologic stress in critically ill patients, which can result in ulcers, erosions, and gastritis.[1] Melena signals overt bleeding, and may be associated with tachycardia, hypotension, and a decrease in hemoglobin level of more than 2 g/dl.[1,2] Hematemesis, hematochezia, or gross blood or coffee-ground-like material in nasogastric aspirates also may occur.

▶ *Thrombocytopenia.* Melena or hematochezia may accompany other manifestations of bleeding tendency: hematemesis, epistaxis, petechiae, ecchymoses, hematuria, vaginal bleeding, and characteristic blood-filled oral bullae. Typically, the patient has malaise, fatigue, weakness, and lethargy.

▶ *Typhoid fever.* Melena or hematochezia occurs late in this disorder and may occur with hypotension and hypothermia. Other late findings include mental dullness or delirium, marked abdominal distention and diarrhea, marked weight loss, and profound fatigue.

▶ *Yellow fever.* Melena, hematochezia, and hematemesis are ominous signs of hemorrhage, a classic feature, which occurs along with jaundice. Other findings include fever, headache, nausea, vomiting, epistaxis, albuminuria, petechiae and mucosal hemorrhage, and dizziness.

Other causes

DRUG WATCH *Ethanol and non-steroidal anti-inflammatory drugs (NSAIDs) (including aspirin) can cause melena as a result of gastric irritation.*

Special considerations

Monitor vital signs, and look closely for signs of hypovolemic shock. For general comfort, encourage bed rest, and keep the patient's perianal area clean and dry to prevent skin irritation and breakdown. A nasogastric tube may be necessary to assist with drainage of gastric contents and decompression. Prepare him for diagnostic tests, including blood studies, gastroscopy or other endoscopic studies, barium swallow, and upper GI series. Prepare the patient for blood transfusions as indicated by his hematocrit.

Monitor patients receiving anticoagulation therapy for signs of bleeding, such as melena, hematuria, epistaxis, bleeding gums, and bruising. The dose may need to be decreased or the drug stopped if these signs appear.[3]

Critically ill patients may receive stress ulcer prophylaxis with proton pump inhibitors or histamine blockers to prevent SRMD.[1,2]

Pediatric pointers

Neonates may have melena neonatorum from extravasation of blood into the alimentary canal. In older children, melena usually results from peptic ulcer, gastritis, or Meckel's diverticulum. It also may result from iron poisoning.[4]

Geriatric pointers

In elderly patients with recurrent intermittent GI bleeding without a clear etiology, angiography or exploratory laparotomy should be considered once the risk from continued anemia is deemed to outweigh the risk associated with the procedures.

Patient counseling

Explain the changes in bowel elimination that are important for the patient to recognize and report. Stress the importance of undergoing colorectal cancer screening. Explain to the patient the need to avoid aspirin, other NSAIDs, anticoagulants, and alcohol if he is experiencing melena.

Instruct patients taking anticoagulant therapy to notify their physician if they should recognize any signs of bleeding, such as blood in the urine, blood in the stool, bleeding gums, nosebleeds, or bruising.[3]

REFERENCES
1. Sester, J.M. "Stress-Related Mucosal Disease in the Intensive Care Unit: An Update on Prophylaxis," *AACN Advanced Critical Care* 18(2):119-126, April/June 2007.
2. Ziegler, A.B. "The Role of Proton Pump Inhibitors in Acute Stress Ulcer Prophylaxis in Mechanically Ventilated Patients," *Dimensions of Critical Care Nursing* 24(3):109-114, May/June 2005.
3. Lamarche, K., and Heale, R. "Communicating the Safety Essentials of Oral Anticoagulant Therapy," *Home Healthcare Nurse* 25(7):448-458, July/August 2007.
4. Aldridge, M.D. "Acute Iron Poisoning: What Every Pediatric Intensive Care Unit Nurse Should Know," *Dimensions of Critical Care Nursing* 26(2):43-48, March/April 2007.

MOUTH LESIONS

Mouth lesions include ulcers (the most common type), cysts, firm nodules, hemorrhagic lesions, papules, vesicles, bullae, and erythematous lesions. They may occur anywhere on the lips, cheeks, hard and soft palate, salivary glands, tongue, gingivae, or mucous membranes. Many are painful and can be readily detected. Some, however, are asymptomatic; when they occur deep in the mouth, they may be discovered only through a complete oral examination. Mouth lesions can result from trauma, infection, systemic disease, drug use, or radiation therapy. (See *Common mouth lesions.*)

History and physical examination

Begin your evaluation with a thorough history. Ask the patient when the lesions appeared and whether he has noticed any pain, odor, or drainage. Also ask about associated complaints, particularly skin lesions. Obtain a complete drug history, including drug allergies and antibiotic use, and a complete medical history. Note especially any malignancy, sexually transmitted disease, I.V. drug use, recent infection, or trauma. Ask about his dental history, including oral hygiene habits, frequency of dental examinations, and the date of his most recent dental visit.

Next, perform a complete oral examination, noting lesion sites and character. Examine the patient's lips for color and texture. Inspect and palpate the buccal mucosa and tongue for color, texture, and contour; note especially any painless ulcers on the sides or base of the tongue. Hold the tongue with a piece of gauze, lift it, and examine its underside and the floor of the mouth. Depress the tongue with a tongue blade, and examine the oropharynx. Inspect the teeth and gums, noting missing, broken, or discolored teeth; dental caries; excessive debris; and bleeding, inflamed, swollen, or discolored gums.

Palpate the neck for adenopathy, especially in patients who smoke tobacco or use alcohol excessively.

Medical causes

▶ *Acquired immunodeficiency syndrome (AIDS).* Oral lesions may be an early indication of the immunosuppression that's characteristic of this disease. Fungal infections can occur, with oral candidiasis being the most common. Bacterial or viral infections of oral mucosa, tongue, gingivae, and periodontal tissue also may occur.

The primary oral neoplasm in AIDS is Kaposi's sarcoma. The tumor usually is found on the hard palate and may appear initially as an asymptomatic, flat or raised lesion, ranging in color from red to blue to purple. As these tumors grow, they may ulcerate and become painful.

Common mouth lesions

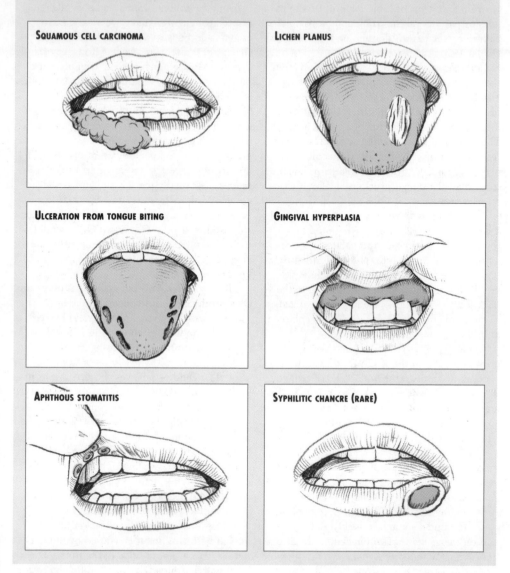

SQUAMOUS CELL CARCINOMA

LICHEN PLANUS

ULCERATION FROM TONGUE BITING

GINGIVAL HYPERPLASIA

APHTHOUS STOMATITIS

SYPHILITIC CHANCRE (RARE)

▶ *Actinomycosis (cervicofacial)*. This chronic fungal infection typically produces small, firm, flat, usually painless swellings on the oral mucosa and under the skin of the jaw and neck. Swellings may indurate and abscess, producing fistulas and sinus tracts with a characteristic purulent yellow discharge.

▶ *Aphthous ulcer*. Aphthous ulcer, also known as a *canker sore, aphthous stomatitis,* or *Sutton's disease,* presents as a painful open sore caused by a break in the mucous membrane. The exact cause is unknown; however, factors that may contribute to their development include stress, illness, fatigue, injury, and weight loss.[1]

▶ *Behçet's syndrome*. This chronic, progressive syndrome that typically affects young men produces small, painful ulcers on the lips, gums, buccal mucosa, and tongue. In severe cases, ulcers also develop on the palate, pharynx, and esophagus. The ulcers typically have a red border and are covered with a gray or yellow exudate. Similar lesions appear on the scrotum and penis or labia majora; small pustules or papules on the trunk and limbs; and painful erythematous nodules on the shins. Ocular lesions also may develop.

▶ *Candidiasis.* This common fungal infection characteristically produces soft, elevated plaques on the buccal mucosa, tongue, and sometimes the palate, gingivae, and floor of the mouth; the plaques may be wiped away. The lesions of acute atrophic candidiasis are red and painful. The lesions of chronic hyperplastic candidiasis are white and firm. Localized areas of redness, pruritus, and foul odor may be present.

▶ *Discoid lupus erythematosus.* Oral lesions are common, typically appearing on the tongue, buccal mucosa, and palate as erythematous areas with white spots and radiating white striae. Associated findings include skin lesions on the face, possibly extending to the neck, ears, and scalp; if the scalp is involved, alopecia may result. Hair follicles are enlarged and filled with scale.

▶ *Epulis (giant cell).* This rare tumor or growth occurs on the gingival or alveolar process, anterior to the molars. Dark red, pedunculated or sessile, and 0.5 to 1.5 cm in diameter, it commonly ulcerates to produce a concave defect in the underlying bone. Gingivae bleed easily with slight trauma.

▶ *Erythema multiforme.* This acute inflammatory skin disease produces sudden onset of vesicles and bullae on the lips and buccal mucosa. Also, erythematous macules and papules form symmetrically on the hands, arms, feet, legs, face, and neck and, possibly, in the eyes and on the genitalia. Lymphadenopathy also may occur. With visceral involvement, other findings include fever, malaise, cough, throat and chest pain, vomiting, diarrhea, myalgias, arthralgias, fingernail loss, blindness, hematuria, and signs of renal failure.

▶ *Gingivitis (acute necrotizing ulcerative).* This recurring periodontal condition causes a sudden onset of gingival ulcers covered with a grayish white pseudomembrane. Other findings include tender or painful gingivae, intermittent gingival bleeding, halitosis, enlarged lymph nodes in the neck, and fever.

▶ *Gonorrhea.* Painful lip ulcerations may occur, along with rough, reddened, bleeding gingivae (possibly necrotic and covered by a yellowish pseudomembrane), and a swollen, ulcerated tongue. Related effects vary. Most men develop dysuria, purulent urethral discharge, and a reddened, edematous urinary meatus. Most women remain asymptomatic, but others develop inflammation and a greenish yellow cervical discharge.

▶ *Herpes simplex 1.* With primary infection, a brief period of prodromal tingling and itching, which is accompanied by fever and pharyngitis, is followed by eruption of small and irritating vesicles on any part of the oral mucosa, especially the tongue, gums, and cheeks. Vesicles form on an erythematous base and then rupture, leaving a painful ulcer, followed by a yellowish crust. Other findings include submaxillary lymphadenopathy, increased salivation, halitosis, anorexia, and keratoconjunctivitis.

▶ *Herpes zoster.* This common viral infection may produce painful vesicles on the buccal mucosa, tongue, uvula, pharynx, and larynx. Small red nodules often erupt unilaterally around the thorax or vertically on the arms and legs, and rapidly become vesicles filled with clear fluid or pus; vesicles dry and form scabs about 10 days after eruption. Fever and general malaise accompany pruritus, paresthesia or hyperesthesia, and tenderness along the course of the involved sensory nerve.

▶ *Inflammatory fibrous hyperplasia.* This painless nodular swelling of the buccal mucosa typically results from cheek trauma or irritation and is characterized by pink, smooth, pedunculated areas of soft tissue.

▶ *Kaposi's sarcoma.* Mouth lesions are involved with this disorder, caused by human herpesvirus 8, about 30% of the time.[2] The hard palate is mostly affected, followed by the gums. Lesions in the mouth may be damaged by chewing, bleed, and have a high rate of secondary infections.

▶ *Leukoplakia, erythroplakia.* Leukoplakia is a white lesion that can't be removed simply by rubbing the mucosal surface—unlike candidiasis. It may occur in response to chronic irritation from dentures or tobacco or pipe smoking, or it may represent dysplasia or early squamous cell carcinoma.

Erythroplakia is red and edematous and has a velvety surface. About 90% of erythroplakia cases are either dysplasia or cancer.

▶ *Lichen planus.* Oral lesions develop on the buccal mucosa or, less commonly, on the tongue as painless, white or gray, velvety, threadlike papules. These precede the eruption of violet papules with white lines or spots, usually on the genitalia, lower back, ankles, and anterior lower legs; pruritus; nails with longitudinal ridges; and alopecia.

▶ *Mucous duct obstruction.* Obstruction produces a ranula—a painless, slow-growing mucocele on the floor of the mouth near the ducts of the submandibular and sublingual glands.

▶ *Pemphigoid (benign mucosal).* This rare autoimmune disease is characterized by thick-walled vesicles on the oral mucous membranes, the conjunctiva and, less often, the skin. Mouth lesions typically develop months or even years before other manifestations and may occur as desquamative patchy gingivitis or as a vesicobullous eruption. Secondary fibrous bands may lead to dysphagia, hoarseness, and blindness. Recurrent skin lesions include vesicobullous eruptions, usually on the inguinal area and extremities, and an erythematous, vesicobullous plaque on the scalp and face near the affected mucous membranes.

▶ *Pemphigus.* This chronic skin disease is characterized by thin-walled vesicles and bullae that appear in cycles on skin or mucous membranes that otherwise appear normal. On the oral mucosa, bullae rupture, leaving painful lesions and raw patches that bleed easily. Other findings include bullae anywhere on the body, denudation of the skin, and pruritus.

▶ *Pyogenic granuloma.* Commonly the result of injury, trauma, or irritation, this soft, tender nodule, papule, or polypoid mass of excessive granulation tissue usually appears on the gingivae but can also erupt on the lips, tongue, or buccal mucosa. The lesions bleed easily because they contain many capillaries. The affected area may be smooth or have a warty surface; erythema develops in the surrounding mucosa. The lesions may ulcerate, producing a purulent exudate.

▶ *Squamous cell carcinoma.* This is typically a painless ulcer with an elevated, indurated border. It may erupt in areas of leukoplakia and is most common on the lower lip, but it also may occur on the edge of the tongue or the floor of the mouth. High risk factors include chronic smoking and alcohol intake.

▶ *Stomatitis (aphthous).* This common disease is characterized by painful ulcerations of the oral mucosa, usually on the dorsum of the tongue, gingivae, and hard palate.

With recurrent *aphthous stomatitis minor,* the ulcer begins as one or more erosions covered by a gray membrane and surrounded by a red halo. It's commonly found on the buccal and lip mucosa and junction, tongue, soft palate, pharynx, gingivae, and all places not bound to the periosteum.

With recurrent *aphthous stomatitis major,* large, painful ulcers commonly occur on the lips, cheek, tongue, and soft palate; they may last up to 6 weeks and leave a scar.

▶ *Syphilis.* Primary syphilis typically produces a solitary painless, red ulcer (chancre) on the lip, tongue, palate, tonsil, or gingivae. The ulcer appears as a crater with undulated, raised edges and a shiny center; lip chancres may develop a crust. Similar lesions may appear on the fingers, breasts, or genitals, and regional lymph nodes may become enlarged and tender.

During the secondary stage, multiple painless ulcers covered by a grayish white plaque may erupt on the tongue, gingivae, or buccal mucosa. A macular, papular, pustular, or nodular rash appears, usually on the arms, trunk, palms, soles, face, and scalp; genital lesions usually subside. Other findings include generalized lymphadenopathy, headache, malaise, anorexia, weight loss, nausea, vomiting, sore throat, low fever, metrorrhagia, and postcoital bleeding.

At the tertiary stage, lesions (often chronic, painless, superficial nodules or deep granulomatous lesions, called *gummas*) develop on the skin and mucous membranes, especially the tongue and palate.

▶ *Systemic lupus erythematosus.* Oral lesions are common and appear as erythematous areas associated with edema, petechiae, and superficial ulcers with a red halo and a tendency to bleed. Primary effects include nondeforming arthritis, butterfly rash across the nose and cheeks, and photosensitivity.

▶ *Trauma.* The most common cause of oral lesions, trauma can produce ulcers anywhere in the mouth, especially on the tongue and buccal mucosa.

▶ *Tuberculosis (oral mucosal).* This rare disorder produces a painless ulcer (usually on the tongue) and, sometimes, caseation. Other findings include lymphadenopathy, fatigue, weakness, anorexia, weight loss, cough, low fever, and night sweats.

Other causes

DRUG WATCH *Chemotherapy drugs may produce stomatitis. Also, allergic reactions to aspirin, barbiturates, penicillin, phenytoin, quinine, streptomycin, and sulfonamides commonly cause lesions to develop and erupt. Inhaled steroids used for pulmonary disorders also may cause oral lesions.*

▶ *Orthodontics.* The rubbing of orthodontic equipment or prosthesis on the buccal mucosa may cause eroded, tender areas.

▶ *Radiation therapy.* Radiation therapy may cause oral lesions.

Special considerations

If the patient's mouth ulcers are painful, provide a coating agent, such as viscous lidocaine or sucralfate.[3] Avoid the use of triple mouthwash mixes (such as the combination of viscous lidocaine, diphenhydramine, and loperamide), because they may cause further ulceration.[3]

Pediatric pointers

Causes of mouth ulcers in children include chickenpox, measles, scarlet fever, diphtheria, and hand-foot-and-mouth disease. In neonates, mouth ulcers can result from candidiasis or congenital syphilis.

Patient counseling

Instruct the patient to avoid irritants, such as highly seasoned foods, citrus fruits, foods that contain salt or vinegar, alcohol, and tobacco. For mouth care, warn against using lemonglycerin swabs because these can dry and irritate the lesions.

As appropriate, teach the patient proper oral hygiene. If toothbrushing is contraindicated, instruct him to use a mouth rinse, such as normal saline solution or half-strength hydrogen peroxide, and to avoid commercial mouthwashes that contain alcohol. Stress the importance of frequently changing to a new toothbrush and of using the softest toothbrush available. If the patient uses an inhaled steroid, instruct him to rinse his mouth after each use. Also, tell him to report mouth lesions that don't heal within 2 weeks.

REFERENCES
1. Chattopadhyay, A.K., and Chatterjee, S. "Risk Indicators for Recurrent Aphthous Ulcers Among Adults in the U.S.," *Community Dentistry and Oral Epidemiology* 35(2):152-159, April 2007.
2. Yarchoan, R., et al. "Therapy Insight: AIDS-Related Malignancies—The Influence of Antiviral Therapy on Pathogenesis and Management," *Nature Clinical Practice. Oncology* 2(8):406-415, August 2005.
3. Dahlin, C. "Oral Complications At The End of Life," *Home Healthcare Nurse* 23(1):39-46, January 2005.

● MURMURS

Murmurs are auscultatory sounds heard in the heart chambers or major arteries. They're classified by their timing and duration in the cardiac cycle, auscultatory location, loudness, configuration, pitch, and quality.

Timing can be characterized as systolic (between S_1 and S_2), holosystolic (continuous throughout systole), diastolic (between S_2 and S_1), or continuous throughout systole and diastole; systolic and diastolic murmurs can be further characterized as early, middle, or late.

Location refers to the area of maximum loudness, such as the apex, the lower left sternal border, or an intercostal space. *Loudness* is graded on a scale of 1 to 6. A grade 1 murmur is very faint, only detected after careful auscultation. A grade 2 murmur is a soft, evident murmur. Murmurs considered to be grade 3 are moderately loud. A grade 4 murmur is a loud murmur with a possible intermittent thrill. Grade 5 murmurs are loud and associated with a palpable precordial thrill. Grade 6 murmurs are loud and, like grade 5 murmurs, are associated with a thrill. A grade 6 murmur is audible even when the stethoscope is lifted from the thoracic wall.[1]

Configuration, or shape, refers to the nature of loudness—crescendo (grows louder), decrescendo (grows softer), crescendo-decrescendo (first rises, then falls), decrescendo-crescendo (first falls, then rises), plateau (even intensity), or variable (uneven intensity). The murmur's *pitch* may be high or low. Its *quality* may be described as harsh, rumbling, blowing, scratching, buzzing, musical, or squeaking.

Murmurs can reflect accelerated blood flow through normal or abnormal valves; forward blood flow through a narrowed or irregular valve or into a dilated vessel; blood backflow through an incompetent valve, septal defect, or patent ductus arteriosus; or decreased blood viscosity. Commonly the result of organic heart disease, murmurs occasionally may signal an emergency situation—for example, a loud holosystolic murmur after an acute myocardial infarction (MI) may signal papillary muscle rupture or ventricular septal defect. Murmurs also may result from surgical implantation of a prosthetic valve. (See *When murmurs mean emergency.*)

Some murmurs are innocent, or functional. An *innocent systolic murmur* is generally soft, medium-pitched, and loudest along the left sternal border at the second or third intercostal space. It's worsened by physical activity, excitement, fever, pregnancy, anemia, or thyrotoxicosis. Examples include Still's murmur in children and mammary souffle, often heard over either breast during late pregnancy and early postpartum. (See *Detecting congenital murmurs,* pages 296 and 297.)

History and physical examination

If you discover a murmur, try to determine its type through careful auscultation. (See *Identifying common murmurs,* page 298.) Use the bell of your stethoscope for low-pitched murmurs and the diaphragm for high-pitched murmurs. A diastolic murmur is an abnormal finding and may indicate a cardiac problem;

When murmurs mean emergency

Although not normally a sign of an emergency, murmurs—especially newly developed ones—may signal a serious complication in patients with bacterial endocarditis or a recent acute myocardial infarction (MI).

When caring for a patient with known or suspected bacterial endocarditis, carefully auscultate for any new murmurs. Their development, along with crackles, distended jugular veins, orthopnea, and dyspnea, may signal heart failure.

Regular auscultation is also important in a patient with an acute MI. A loud decrescendo holosystolic murmur at the apex that radiates to the axilla and left sternal border or throughout the chest is significant, particularly with a widely split S_2 and an atrial gallop (S_4). This murmur, when accompanied by signs of acute pulmonary edema, usually indicates acute mitral insufficiency from rupture of the chordae tendineae—a medical emergency.

midsystolic murmurs are commonly associated with benign murmurs in children and young adults.[1]

Next, obtain a patient history. Ask if the murmur is a new discovery, or if it has been known since birth or childhood. Find out if the patient has experienced any associated symptoms, particularly palpitations, dizziness, syncope, chest pain, dyspnea, and fatigue. (See *Differential diagnosis: Murmurs,* pages 300 and 301.) Explore the patient's medical history, noting especially any incidence of rheumatic fever, recent dental work, heart disease, or heart surgery, particularly prosthetic valve replacement.

Perform a systematic physical examination. Note especially the presence of cardiac arrhythmias, jugular vein distention, and such pulmonary signs and symptoms as dyspnea, orthopnea, and crackles. Is the patient's liver tender or palpable? Does he have peripheral edema?

Detecting congenital murmurs

HEART DEFECT	TYPE OF MURMUR
Aortopulmonary septal defect	*Small defect:* A continuous rough or crackling murmur best heard at the upper left sternal border and below the left clavicle, possibly accompanied by a systolic ejection click. *Large defect:* A harsh systolic murmur heard at the left sternal border.
Atrial septal defect	A midstystolic, spindle-shaped murmur of grade II or III intensity heard at the upper left sternal border, with a fixed splitting of S_2. Large shunts may also produce a low- to medium-pitched early diastolic murmur over the lower left sternal border.
Bicuspid aortic valve	An early systolic, loud, high-pitched ejection sound or click that's best heard at the apex and is commonly accompanied by a soft, early or midsystolic murmur at the upper right sternal border. The aortic component of S_2 is usually accentuated at the apex. This murmur may not be recognized until early childhood.
Coarctation of the aorta	Usually a systolic ejection click at the base of the heart, at the apex, and occasionally over the carotid arteries, often accompanied by a systolic ejection murmur at the base. This disorder may also produce a blowing diastolic murmur of aortic insufficiency or an apical pansystolic murmur of unknown origin.
Common atrioventricular canal defects (endocardial cushion defect)	*With a competent mitral valve:* A midsystolic, spindle-shaped murmur of grade II or III intensity heard at the upper left sternal border, with a fixed splitting of S_2; may be accompanied by a low- to medium-pitched early diastolic murmur over the lower left sternal border. *With an incompetent mitral valve:* An early systolic or holosystolic decrescendo murmur at the apex, along with a widely split S_2 and often an S_4.
Ebstein's anomaly	A soft, high-pitched holosystolic blowing murmur that increases with inspiration (Carvallo's sign); best heard over the lower left sternal border and the xiphoid area; possibly accompanied by a low-pitched diastolic rumbling murmur at the apex. Fixed splitting of S_2 and a loud split S_4 also occur.
Left ventricular–right atrial communication	A holosystolic, decrescendo murmur of grades II and IV intensity heard along the lower left sternal border, accompanied by a normal S_2; large shunts also produce a diastolic rumbling murmur over the apex.
Mitral atresia	A nonspecific systolic murmur and a diastolic flow rumble at the lower left sternal border, with one loud S_2.
Partial anomalous pulmonary venous connection	A midsystolic, spindle-shaped grade II to III murmur at the upper left sternal border, possibly accompanied by a low- to medium-pitched early diastolic murmur over the lower left sternal border.
Patent ductus arteriosus	A continuous rough or crackling murmur best heard at the upper left sternal border and below the left clavicle. The murmur is accentuated late in systole.
Pulmonic insufficiency	An early to middiastolic, soft, medium-pitched crescendo-decrescendo murmur best heard at the second or third right intercostal space.

Detecting congenital murmurs (continued)

HEART DEFECT	TYPE OF MURMUR
Pulmonic stenosis	An early systolic, harsh, crescendo-decrescendo murmur of grades IV to VI intensity heard at the second left intercostal space, possibly radiating along the left sternal border.
Single atrium	A holosystolic regurgitant murmur at the apex, accompanied by a fixed splitting of S_2.
Supravalvular aortic stenosis	A systolic ejection murmur best heard over the second right intercostal space or higher in the episternal notch or over the lower right side of the neck. The aortic closure sound is usually preserved, and no ejection clicks are heard.
Tetralogy of Fallot	A midsystolic murmur with a systolic thrill palpable at the left midsternal border; softer murmurs occurring earlier in systole generally indicate a more severe obstruction.
Tricuspid atresia	Variable, depending on associated defects.
Trilogy of Fallot	A systolic, harsh, crescendo-decrescendo murmur, best heard at the upper left sternal border with radiation toward the left clavicle. The pulmonic component of S_2 becomes progressively softer with increasing degrees of obstruction.
Ventricular septal defect	*Small defect:* Usually a holosystolic (but may be limited to early or midsystole), grades II to IV decrescendo murmur heard along the lower left sternal border, accompanied by a normal S_2. *Large defect:* A holosystolic murmur at the lower left sternal border and a midsystolic rumbling murmur at the apex, accompanied by an increased S_1 at the lower left sternal border and an increased pulmonic component of S_2.

Medical causes

▶ *Aortic insufficiency.* Acute aortic insufficiency typically produces a soft, short diastolic murmur over the left sternal border that's best heard when the patient sits and leans forward and at the end of a forced held expiration. S_2 may be soft or absent. Sometimes, a soft, short midsystolic murmur also may be heard over the second right intercostal space. Associated findings include tachycardia, dyspnea, jugular vein distention, crackles, increased fatigue, and pale, cool limbs.

Chronic aortic insufficiency causes a high-pitched, blowing, decrescendo diastolic murmur that's best heard over the second or third right intercostal space or the left sternal border with the patient sitting, leaning forward, and holding his breath after deep expiration. An Austin Flint murmur—a rumbling, mid-to-late diastolic murmur best heard at the apex—also may occur. Complications may

not develop until ages 40 to 50; then, typical findings include palpitations, tachycardia, angina, increased fatigue, dyspnea, orthopnea, and crackles.

▶ *Aortic stenosis.* With this valvular disorder, the murmur is systolic, beginning after S_1 and ending at or before aortic valve closure. It's harsh and grating, medium-pitched, and crescendo-decrescendo. Loudest over the second right intercostal space when the patient is sitting and leaning forward, this murmur also may be heard at the apex, at the suprasternal notch (Erb's point), and over the carotid arteries.

If the patient has advanced disease, S_2 may be heard as a single sound, with inaudible aortic closure. An early systolic ejection click at the apex is typical but is absent when the valve is severely calcified. Associated signs and symptoms usually don't appear until age 30 in congenital aortic stenosis, ages 30 to 65

Identifying common murmurs

The timing and configuration of a murmur can help you identify its underlying cause. Learn to recognize the characteristics of these common murmurs.

AORTIC INSUFFICIENCY (CHRONIC)
Thickened valve leaflets fail to close correctly, permitting backflow of blood into the left ventricle.

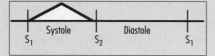

AORTIC STENOSIS
Thickened, scarred, or calcified valve leaflets impede ventricular systolic ejection.

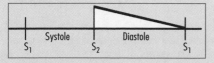

MITRAL PROLAPSE
Incompetent mitral valve bulges into the left atrium because of an enlarged posterior leaflet and elongated chordae tendineae.

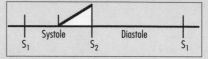

MITRAL INSUFFICIENCY (CHRONIC)
Incomplete mitral valve closure permits backflow of blood into the left atrium.

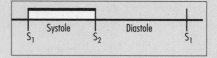

MITRAL STENOSIS
Thickened or scarred valve leaflets cause valve stenosis and restrict blood flow.

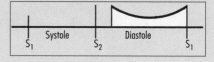

in stenosis due to rheumatic disease, and after age 65 in calcific aortic stenosis. They may include dizziness, syncope, dyspnea on exertion, paroxysmal nocturnal dyspnea, fatigue, and angina.

▶ *Cardiomyopathy (hypertrophic)*. The obstructive form of this disorder causes a harsh, crescendo-decrescendo, systolic murmur.[2] Best heard over the left sternal border and at the apex, the murmur is commonly accompanied by an audible S_3 or S_4. The murmur decreases with squatting and increases with sitting down. Other major symptoms are dyspnea and chest pain; palpitations, dizziness, and syncope also may occur.

▶ *Mitral insufficiency*. Acute mitral insufficiency is characterized by a medium-pitched blowing, early systolic or holosystolic decrescendo murmur at the apex, along with a widely split S_2 and commonly an S_4. This murmur doesn't get louder on inspiration as with tricuspid insufficiency. Other findings typically include tachycardia and signs of acute pulmonary edema.

Chronic mitral insufficiency produces a high-pitched, blowing, holosystolic plateau murmur that's loudest at the apex and usually radiates to the axilla or back. Fatigue, dyspnea, and palpitations also may occur.

▶ *Mitral prolapse*. This disorder generates a midsystolic to late-systolic click with a high-pitched late-systolic crescendo murmur, best heard at the apex. Occasionally, multiple clicks may be heard, with or without a systolic murmur. Other findings include cardiac awareness, migraine headaches, dizziness, weakness, syncope, palpitations, chest pain, dyspnea, severe episodic fatigue, mood swings, and anxiety.

▶ *Mitral stenosis.* With this valvular disorder, the murmur is soft, low-pitched, rumbling, crescendo-decrescendo, and diastolic, accompanied by a loud S_1 or an opening snap—a cardinal sign. It's best heard at the apex with the patient in the left lateral position. Mild exercise will help make this murmur audible.

With severe stenosis, the murmur of mitral insufficiency also may be heard. Other findings include hemoptysis, exertional dyspnea and fatigue, and signs of acute pulmonary edema.

▶ *Myxomas.* A *left atrial myxoma* (most common) usually produces a middiastolic murmur and a holosystolic murmur that's loudest at the apex, with an S_4, an early diastolic thudding sound (tumor plop), and a loud, widely split S_1. Related features include dyspnea, orthopnea, chest pain, fatigue, weight loss, and syncope.

A *right atrial myxoma* causes a late diastolic rumbling murmur, a holosystolic crescendo murmur, and tumor plop, best heard at the lower left sternal border. Other findings include fatigue, peripheral edema, ascites, and hepatomegaly.

A *left ventricular myxoma* (rare) produces a systolic murmur, best heard at the lower left sternal border, arrhythmias, dyspnea, and syncope.

A *right ventricular myxoma* commonly generates a systolic ejection murmur with delayed S_2 and a tumor plop, best heard at the left sternal border. It's accompanied by peripheral edema, hepatomegaly, ascites, dyspnea, and syncope.

▶ *Papillary muscle rupture.* With this life-threatening complication of an acute MI, a loud holosystolic murmur can be auscultated at the apex. Related findings include severe dyspnea, chest pain, syncope, hemoptysis, tachycardia, and hypotension.

▶ *Rheumatic fever with pericarditis.* A pericardial friction rub along with murmurs and gallops are heard best with the patient leaning forward on his hands and knees during forced expiration. The most common murmurs heard are the systolic murmur of mitral insufficiency, a midsystolic murmur due to swelling of the leaflet of the mitral valve, and the diastolic murmur of aortic insufficiency. Other signs and symptoms include fever, joint and sternal pain, edema, and tachypnea.

▶ *Tricuspid insufficiency.* This valvular abnormality is characterized by a soft, high-pitched, holosystolic blowing murmur that increases with inspiration (Carvallo's sign), decreases with exhalation and Valsalva's maneuver, and is best heard over the lower left sternal border and the xiphoid area. Following a lengthy asymptomatic period, exertional dyspnea and orthopnea may develop, along with jugular vein distention, ascites, peripheral cyanosis and edema, muscle wasting, fatigue, weakness, and syncope.

▶ *Tricuspid stenosis.* This valvular disorder produces a diastolic murmur similar to that of mitral stenosis, but louder with inspiration and decreased with exhalation and Valsalva's maneuver. S_1 also may be louder. Other signs and symptoms include fatigue, syncope, peripheral edema, jugular vein distention, ascites, hepatomegaly, and dyspnea.

Other causes
▶ *Treatments.* Prosthetic valve replacement may cause variable murmurs, depending on the location, valve composition, and method of operation.

Special considerations
Prepare the patient for diagnostic tests, such as electrocardiography, echocardiography, and angiography. Give an antibiotic and an anticoagulant as appropriate. Because any cardiac abnormality is frightening to the patient, provide emotional support.

Pediatric pointers
Innocent murmurs, such as Still's murmur, are commonly heard in young children and typically disappear in puberty. A harsh murmur, persistent tachypnea, an unusual heart rhythm, and additional heart sounds are strong indicators of infant cardiac disease when they occur together.[3] A loud, harsh, blowing murmur may indicate coarctation of the aorta, but is absent in about one-half of infants with the disorder.[3] Other murmurs can be acquired, as with rheumatic heart disease.

Differential diagnosis: Murmurs

POSSIBLE CAUSE	SIGNS AND SYMPTOMS	DIAGNOSIS
Mitral insufficiency	• Arrhythmias • Palpitations • Crackles • Shortness of breath • Fatigue • Tachycardia • Jugular vein distention ***Acute*** • Early systolic or holosystolic decrescendo murmur at the apex • Widely split S_2 • S_4 ***Chronic*** • High-pitched, blowing, holosystolic murmur at the apex that radiates to the axilla or back • Weight loss • Nocturia	• Physical examination • Angiography • Echocardiogram
Aortic insufficiency	• Arrhythmias • Palpitations • Crackles • Shortness of breath • Fatigue • Tachycardia • Jugular vein distention ***Acute*** • Short diastolic murmur over the left sternal border • Soft or absent S_2 • Soft, midsystolic murmur over the second right intercostal space (possibly) ***Chronic*** • High-pitched, blowing, decrescendo diastolic murmur that's best heard over the second or third right intercostal space	• Physical examination • Imaging studies (ultrasound, angiography, echocardiogram) • Cardiac catheterization
Aortic stenosis	• Angina • Dyspnea • Arrhythmias • Fatigue • Dizziness • Hypotension • Harsh, grating systolic murmur over the second right intercostal space, the apex, Erb's point, or the carotid arteries	• Physical examination • Imaging studies (angiography, Doppler ultrasound, chest X-ray)
Cardiomyopathy	• Angina • Dyspnea • Arrhythmias • Fatigue • Dizziness • Hypotension • Harsh, late systolic murmur that ends at S_2 • Murmur located over the left sternal border and apex • S_3 or S_4 (possibly) • Palpitations • Sudden cardiac death	• Physical examination • Imaging studies (chest X-ray, computed tomography scan, magnetic resonance imaging, angiography) • Echocardiogram

Additional differential diagnoses for murmurs include mitral prolapse, mitral stenosis, myxomas, papillary muscle rupture, tricuspid insufficiency, and tricuspid stenosis.

Other causes of murmurs include prosthetic valve replacement.

TREATMENT AND FOLLOW-UP

- Medication (antibiotics [if infection is present], anticoagulants [if atrial fibrillation is present], diuretics)
  Follow-up: Referral to cardiologist

- As needed (based on the severity of symptoms)
- Medications (diuretics, digoxin)
  Follow-up: Referral to cardiologist

- Avoidance of strenuous activity
- Medication (diuretics, digoxin)
  Follow-up: Reevaluation every 6 to 12 months

- Symptomatic treatment
- Oxygen therapy
  Follow-up: Referral to cardiologist

Geriatric pointers

Aortic systolic murmurs are commonly heard in older adults, especially those age 85 and over.[4] Older adults also have an increased risk for a systolic murmur associated with mitral valve regurgitation.[4]

Patient counseling

Tell patient to contact his physician before undergoing invasive procedures or dental work; prophylactic antibiotics may be necessary.

REFERENCES

1. Quigley, P. "Valve Jobs Aren't Just for '57 Chevys: Expertly Sorting Through The Various Types of Valvular Disorders," *Nursing Made Incredibly Easy!* 3(3):20-35, May/June 2005.
2. Bruce, J. "Getting to the Heart of Cardiomyopathies," *Nursing* 36(Cardiac Insider):16-20, Spring 2006.
3. Taylor, M.L. "Coarctation of the Aorta: A Critical Catch for Newborn Well-Being," *The Nurse Practitioner* 30(12):34-43, December 2005.
4. Neal-Boylan, L. "Health Assessment of the Very Old Person at Home," *Home Healthcare Nurse* 25(6):388-98, June 2007.

● MUSCLE WEAKNESS

Muscle weakness is detected by observing and measuring the strength of a muscle or muscle group. It can result from a malfunction in the cerebral hemispheres, brain stem, spinal cord, nerve roots, peripheral nerves, or myoneural junctions and within the muscle itself. Muscle weakness occurs with certain neurologic, musculoskeletal, metabolic, endocrine, and cardiovascular disorders; as a response to certain drugs; and after prolonged immobilization.

History and physical examination

Begin by determining the location of the patient's muscle weakness. Ask if he has trouble with specific movements, such as rising from a chair. Find out when he first noticed the weakness; ask him if it worsens with exercise or as the day progresses. Also ask about relat-

(Text continues on page 304.)

Testing muscle strength

Obtain an overall picture of your patient's motor function by testing strength in 10 selected muscle groups. Ask the patient to attempt normal range-of-motion movements against your resistance. If the muscle group is weak, vary the amount of resistance to permit accurate assessment. If needed, position the patient so his limbs don't have to resist gravity, and repeat the test.

ARM MUSCLES

Biceps. With your hand on the patient's hand, have him flex his forearm against your resistance. Watch for biceps contraction.

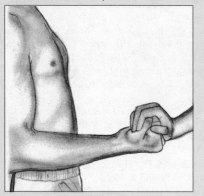

Deltoid. With the patient's arm fully extended, place one hand over his deltoid muscle and the other on his wrist. Ask him to abduct his arm to a horizontal position against your resistance; as he does so, palpate for deltoid contraction.

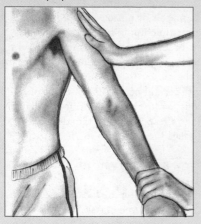

Triceps. Have the patient abduct and hold his arm midway between flexion and extension. Hold and support his arm at the wrist, and ask him to extend it against your resistance. Watch for triceps contraction.

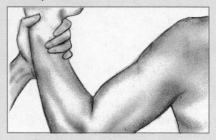

Dorsal interossei. Have the patient extend and spread his fingers, and tell him to try to resist your attempt to squeeze them together.

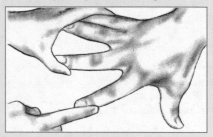

Forearm and hand (grip). Have the patient grasp your middle and index fingers and squeeze as hard as he can. To prevent pain or injury to the examiner, the examiner should cross his fingers.

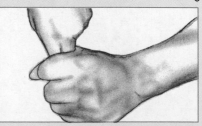

Rate muscle strength on a scale from 0 to 5:
0 = No evidence of muscle contraction; no movement
1 = Visible or palpable contraction, but no movement
2 = Full muscle movement with force of gravity eliminated
3 = Full muscle movement against gravity, but no movement against resistance
4 = Full muscle movement against gravity; partial movement against resistance
5 = Full muscle movement against both gravity and resistance—normal strength.

LEG MUSCLES

Anterior tibial. With the patient's leg extended, place your hand on his foot and ask him to dorsiflex his ankle against your resistance. Palpate for anterior tibial contraction.

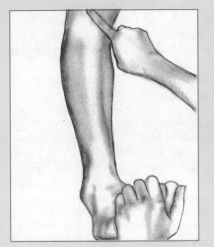

Psoas. While you support his leg, have the patient raise his knee and then flex his hip against your resistance. Watch for psoas contraction.

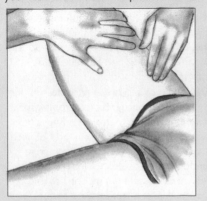

Extensor hallucis longus. With your finger on the patient's great toe, have him dorsiflex the toe against your resistance. Palpate for extensor hallucis contraction.

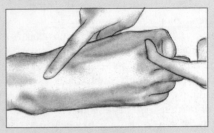

Quadriceps. Have the patient bend his knee slightly while you support his lower leg. Then ask him to extend the knee against your resistance; as he's doing so, palpate for quadriceps contraction.

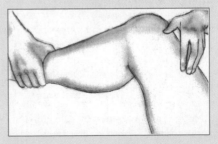

Gastrocnemius. With the patient on his side, support his foot and ask him to plantarflex his ankle against your resistance. Palpate for gastrocnemius contraction.

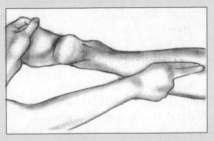

ed symptoms, especially muscle or joint pain, altered sensory function, and fatigue.

Obtain a medical history, noting especially chronic disease such as hyperthyroidism; musculoskeletal or neurologic problems, including recent trauma; family history of chronic muscle weakness, especially in males; and alcohol and drug use.

Focus your physical examination on evaluating muscle strength. Test all major muscles bilaterally. (See *Testing muscle strength,* pages 302 and 303.) When testing, make sure the patient's effort is constant; if it isn't, suspect pain or other reluctance to make the effort. If the patient complains of pain, ease or discontinue testing and have him try the movements again. Remember that the patient's dominant arm, hand, and leg are somewhat stronger than their nondominant counterparts. Besides testing individual muscle strength, test for range of motion at all major joints (shoulder, elbow, wrist, hip, knee, and ankle). Also test sensory function in the involved areas, and test deep tendon reflexes bilaterally.

Medical causes

▶ *Amyotrophic lateral sclerosis.* This disorder typically begins with muscle weakness and atrophy in one hand that rapidly spread to the arm and then to the other hand and arm.[1] Eventually, these effects spread to the trunk, neck, tongue, larynx, pharynx, and legs; progressive respiratory muscle weakness leads to respiratory insufficiency.

▶ *Anemia.* Varying degrees of muscle weakness and fatigue are worsened by exertion and temporarily relieved by rest. Other signs and symptoms include pallor, tachycardia, paresthesia, and bleeding tendencies.

▶ *Brain tumor.* Signs and symptoms of muscle weakness vary with the location and size of the tumor. Other findings include headache, vomiting, diplopia, decreased visual acuity, decreased level of consciousness, pupillary changes, decreased motor strength, hemiparesis, hemiplegia, diminished sensations, ataxia, seizures, and behavioral changes.

▶ *Guillain-Barré syndrome.* Rapidly progressive, symmetrical weakness and pain ascends from the feet to the arms and facial nerves and may progress to total motor paralysis and respiratory failure.[2] Other findings include

sensory loss or paresthesia, muscle flaccidity, loss of deep tendon reflexes, tachycardia or bradycardia, fluctuating hypertension and orthostatic hypotension, diaphoresis, bowel and bladder incontinence, facial diplegia, dysphagia, dysarthria, and hypernasality.

▶ *Head trauma.* Severe head injury can cause varying degrees of muscle weakness. Other findings include decreased level of consciousness, otorrhea or rhinorrhea, raccoon eyes and Battle's sign, sensory disturbances, and signs of increased intracranial pressure.

▶ *Herniated disk.* Pressure on nerve roots leads to muscle weakness, disuse and, ultimately, atrophy. The primary symptom is severe lower back pain, possibly radiating to the buttocks, legs, and feet—usually on one side. Diminished reflexes and sensory changes also may occur.

▶ *Hodgkin's lymphoma.* Muscle weakness may accompany the classic sign of painless, progressive lymphadenopathy. Other findings include paresthesia, fatigue, and weight loss.

▶ *Hypercortisolism.* This disorder may cause limb weakness and eventually atrophy. Other cushingoid features include buffalo hump, moon face, truncal obesity, purple striae, thin skin, acne, elevated blood pressure, fatigue, hyperpigmentation, easy bruising, poor wound healing, and diaphoresis. Men may be impotent; women may have hirsutism and menstrual irregularities.

▶ *Hypothyroidism.* Reversible weakness and atrophy of proximal limb muscles may occur in hypothyroidism. Other findings commonly include muscle cramps; cold intolerance; weight gain despite anorexia; mental dullness; dry, pale, doughy skin; puffy face, hands, and feet; impaired hearing and balance; and bradycardia.

▶ *Multiple sclerosis.* Muscle weakness in one or more limbs may progress to atrophy, spasticity, and contractures. Other findings come and go and may include diplopia and blurred vision, vision loss, nystagmus, hyperactive deep tendon reflexes, sensory loss or paresthesia, dysarthria, dysphagia, incoordination, ataxic gait, intention tremors, emotional lability, impotence, and urinary dysfunction.

▶ *Myasthenia gravis.* Gradually progressive skeletal muscle weakness and fatigue are the cardinal symptoms of this disorder. Typically, weakness is mild upon awakening but worsens during the day. Early signs include weak eye closure, ptosis, and diplopia; a blank, masklike face; difficulty chewing and swallowing; nasal regurgitation of fluid with hypernasality; and a hanging jaw and bobbing head. Respiratory muscle involvement may eventually lead to respiratory failure.

▶ *Osteoarthritis.* This chronic disorder causes progressive muscle disuse and weakness that lead to atrophy.

▶ *Paget's disease.* As this disease progresses, muscle weakness or paralysis may develop, along with paresthesia and pain. The patient also may have bowed tibias, frequent fractures, and kyphosis.

▶ *Parkinson's disease.* Muscle weakness accompanies rigidity in this degenerative disorder. Related findings include a unilateral pill-rolling tremor, propulsive gait, dysarthria, bradykinesia, drooling, dysphagia, masklike face, and a high-pitched, monotonic voice.

▶ *Peripheral nerve trauma.* Prolonged pressure on or injury to a peripheral nerve causes muscle weakness and atrophy. Other findings include paresthesia or sensory loss, pain, and loss of reflexes due to the damaged nerve.

▶ *Peripheral neuropathy.* With this disorder, muscle weakness progresses slowly to flaccid paralysis, generally affecting distal limbs first. It may be accompanied by loss of vibration sense; paresthesia, hyperesthesia, or anesthesia in the hands and feet; hypoactive or absent deep tendon reflexes; mild-to-sharp burning pain; anhidrosis; and glossy red skin.

▶ *Poliomyelitis.* Rapidly developing asymmetrical muscle weakness, progressing to flaccid paralysis, occurs with paralytic poliomyelitis. Other signs and symptoms include moderate fever, headache, vomiting, lethargy, irritability, and widespread pain. As the disorder progresses, it may cause loss of superficial and deep reflexes, paresthesia, hyperalgesia, urine retention, constipation, abdominal distention, nuchal rigidity, and Hoyne's, Kernig's, and Brudzinski's signs. Bulbar paralytic poliomyelitis produces symptoms of encephalitis, along with facial weakness, dysphasia, dysphagia, and respiratory abnormalities.

▶ *Polymyositis.* This disorder produces insidious or acute onset of symmetrical limb and trunk muscle weakness and tenderness. Weakness may progress to facial, neck, pharyngeal, and laryngeal muscles. Associated findings include hypoactive deep tendon reflexes, dysphagia, and dysphonia.

▶ *Potassium imbalance.* With *hypokalemia,* temporary generalized muscle weakness may be accompanied by nausea, vomiting, diarrhea, decreased mentation, leg cramps, diminished reflexes, malaise, polyuria, dizziness, hypotension, and arrhythmias.

With *hyperkalemia,* weakness may progress to flaccid paralysis accompanied by irritability and confusion, hyperreflexia, paresthesia or anesthesia, oliguria, anorexia, nausea, diarrhea, abdominal cramps, tachycardia or bradycardia, and arrhythmias.

▶ *Protein deficiency.* Prolonged protein deficiency may lead to muscle weakness and wasting, chronic fatigue, apathy, anorexia, lethargy, dry skin, and dull, sparse, dry hair.

▶ *Rhabdomyolysis.* Signs and symptoms include muscle weakness or pain, fever, nausea, vomiting, malaise, and dark urine. Acute renal failure, due to renal structure obstruction and injury from the kidneys' attempt to filter the myoglobin from the bloodstream, is a common complication.[3]

▶ *Rheumatoid arthritis.* With this disease, symmetric muscle weakness may accompany increased warmth, swelling, and tenderness in involved joints; pain; and stiffness, restricting motion.

▶ *Seizure disorder.* Temporary generalized muscle weakness may occur after a generalized tonic-clonic seizure; other postictal findings include headache, muscle soreness, and profound fatigue.

▶ *Spinal trauma and disease.* Trauma can cause severe muscle weakness, leading to flaccidity or spasticity and, eventually, paralysis. Infection, tumor, and cervical spondylosis or stenosis can also cause muscle weakness.

▶ *Stroke.* Depending on the site and extent of damage, a stroke may produce contralateral or bilateral weakness of the arms, legs, face, and tongue, possibly progressing to hemiplegia and atrophy. Associated effects include dysarthria, aphasia, ataxia, apraxia, agnosia, ipsilateral paresthesia or sensory loss, visual disturbance, altered level of consciousness, amnesia and poor judgment, personality changes, bowel and bladder dysfunction, headache, vomiting, and seizures.

▶ *Thyrotoxicosis.* This disorder may produce insidious, generalized muscle weakness and atrophy. Other effects include anxiety, fatigue, heat intolerance, diaphoresis, tremors, tachycardia, palpitations, ventricular or atrial gallop, dyspnea, weight loss, an enlarged thyroid, and warm, flushed skin. Exophthalmos may be present.

▶ *Vitamin D deficiency.* Muscle weakness of the spine, rib cage, shoulders, and hips occur with this deficiency, along with muscle and bone pain and back pain. Treatment will show a marked increase in muscle strength and will diminish pain.[4]

Other causes

DRUG WATCH *Generalized muscle weakness can result from prolonged corticosteroid use, digoxin, and excessive doses of dantrolene sodium. Aminoglycoside antibiotics may worsen weakness in patients with myasthenia gravis.*

▶ *Immobility.* Immobilization in a cast, a splint, or traction can lead to muscle weakness in the involved extremity; prolonged bed rest or inactivity results in generalized muscle weakness.

Special considerations

Provide assistive devices as needed, and protect the patient from injury. If he has sensory loss, guard against pressure ulcer formation and thermal injury. With chronic weakness, provide range-of-motion exercises or splint limbs as necessary. Arrange therapy sessions to allow for adequate rest periods, and administer drugs for pain as needed. Prepare the patient for blood tests, muscle biopsy, electromyography, nerve conduction studies, and X-rays or computed tomography scans.

Pediatric pointers

Muscular dystrophy, usually the Duchenne type, is a major cause of muscle weakness in children.

Geriatric pointers

Older patients with diabetes may experience severe muscle weakness that may result in permanent disability as a result of neuropathy. [5]

Patient counseling

Encourage the patient to comply with regular physical therapy and range of motion exercises to reduce loss of muscle strength and prevent joint contractures.[2]

REFERENCES

1. Valente, S.M., and Karp, J.R. "Life with Lou Gehrig's Disease: Managing ALS Symptoms," *The Nurse Practitioner* 32(12):26-33, December 2007.
2. Atkinson, S.B., et al. "The Challenges of Managing and Treating Guillain-Barre Syndrome During the Acute Phase," *Dimensions of Critical Care Nursing* 25(6):256-263, November/December 2006.
3. Spradling, K. "Protect Your Patient from Rhabdomyolysis," *Nursing* 37(10):56hn4-56hn6, October 2007.
4. Heath, K.M., and Elovic, E.P. "Vitamin D Deficiency: Implications in the Rehabilitation Setting," *American Journal of Physical Medicine and Rehabilitation* 85(11):916-923, November 2006.
5. Haas, L. "Functional Decline in Older Adults with Diabetes," *AJN* 107(6):Supplement 50-54, June 2007.

NAUSEA

Nausea is a sensation of profound revulsion to food or of impending vomiting. It's a subjective experience determined by the patient.[1] Often accompanied by autonomic signs, such as hypersalivation, diaphoresis, tachycardia, pallor, and tachypnea, it's closely associated with both anorexia and vomiting.

Nausea, a common symptom of GI disorders, also occurs with fluid and electrolyte imbalance; infection; and metabolic, endocrine, labyrinthine, and cardiac disorders; and as a result of drug therapy, surgery, and radiation. Often present during the first trimester of pregnancy, nausea also may arise from severe pain, anxiety, alcohol intoxication, overeating, or ingestion of distasteful food or liquids.

History and physical examination

Begin by obtaining a complete medical history. Focus on GI, endocrine, and metabolic disorders; recent infections; and cancer and its treatment. Ask about drug use and alcohol consumption. If the patient is a female of childbearing age, ask if she is or could be pregnant. Have the patient describe the onset, duration, and intensity of the nausea, as well as what causes or relieves it. Ask about related complaints, particularly vomiting (color, amount), abdominal pain, anorexia and weight loss, changes in bowel habits or stool character, excessive belching or flatus, and a sensation of bloating.

Inspect the skin for jaundice, bruises, and spider angiomas, and assess skin turgor. Next, inspect the abdomen for distention, auscultate for bowel sounds and bruits, palpate for rigidity and tenderness, and test for rebound tenderness. Palpate and percuss the liver for enlargement. Assess other body systems as appropriate.

Medical causes

▶ *Adrenal insufficiency.* Common GI findings in this endocrine disorder include nausea, vomiting, anorexia, and diarrhea. Other findings include weakness; fatigue; weight loss; bronze skin; hypotension; a weak, irregular pulse; vitiligo; and depression.

▶ *Anthrax (GI).* Initial signs and symptoms include nausea, vomiting, loss of appetite, and fever. Signs and symptoms may progress to abdominal pain, severe bloody diarrhea, and hematemesis.

▶ *Appendicitis.* With acute appendicitis, a brief period of nausea may accompany onset of abdominal pain. Pain typically begins as vague epigastric or periumbilical discomfort and rapidly progresses to severe stabbing pain localized in the right lower quadrant (McBurney's sign). Associated findings usually include abdominal rigidity and tenderness, cutaneous hyperalgesia, fever, constipation or diarrhea, tachycardia, anorexia, moderate malaise, and positive psoas (increased abdominal pain occurs when the examiner places his hand above the patient's right knee and the patient flexes his right hip against resistance) and obturator signs (internal rotation of the right leg with the leg flexed to 90 degrees at the hip and knee with a resulting tightening of the internal obturator muscle that causes abdominal discomfort).

▶ *Cholecystitis (acute).* With this disease, nausea often follows severe right-upper-quadrant pain that may radiate to the back or shoulders, often following meals. Associated findings include mild vomiting, flatulence, abdominal tenderness and, possibly, rigidity and distention, fever with chills, diaphoresis, and a positive Murphy's sign.

▶ *Cholelithiasis.* With this disease, nausea accompanies attacks of severe right-upper-quadrant or epigastric pain after ingestion of fatty foods. Other associated findings include vomiting, abdominal tenderness and guarding, flatulence, belching, epigastric burning, tachycardia, and restlessness. Occlusion of the common bile duct may cause jaundice, clay-colored stools, fever, and chills.

▶ *Cirrhosis.* Insidious early signs and symptoms of cirrhosis typically include nausea and vomiting, anorexia, abdominal pain, and constipation or diarrhea. As the disease progresses, jaundice and hepatomegaly may occur with abdominal distention, spider angiomas, palmar erythema, severe pruritus, dry skin, fetor hepaticus, enlarged superficial abdominal veins, mental changes, and bilateral gynecomastia and testicular atrophy or menstrual irregularities.

▶ *Diverticulitis.* Besides nausea, diverticulitis causes intermittent crampy abdominal pain, constipation or diarrhea, low-grade fever, and often a palpable, tender, firm, fixed mass.

▶ *Ectopic pregnancy.* Nausea, vomiting, vaginal bleeding, and lower abdominal pain occur in this potentially life-threatening disorder. Suspect ectopic pregnancy in a female of childbearing age with a 1- to 2-month history of amenorrhea.

▶ *Electrolyte imbalances.* Such disturbances as hyponatremia or hypernatremia, hypokalemia, and hypercalcemia commonly cause nausea and vomiting. Other effects include cardiac arrhythmias, tremors or seizures, anorexia, malaise, and weakness.

▶ *Escherichia coli O157:H7.* Signs and symptoms include nausea, watery or bloody diarrhea, vomiting, fever, and abdominal cramps. In children younger than age 5 and in the elderly, hemolytic uremic syndrome may develop in which red blood cells are destroyed, which may ultimately lead to acute renal failure.

▶ *Gastric cancer.* This rare cancer may produce vague GI symptoms, such as mild nausea, anorexia, upper abdominal discomfort, and chronic dyspepsia. Fatigue, weight loss, weakness, hematemesis, melena, and altered bowel habits are also common.

▶ *Gastritis.* Nausea is common with this disorder, especially after ingestion of alcohol, aspirin, spicy foods, or caffeine. Vomiting of mucus or blood, epigastric pain, belching, fever, and malaise also may occur.

▶ *Gastroenteritis.* Usually viral, this disorder causes nausea, vomiting, diarrhea, and abdominal cramping. Fever, malaise, hyperactive bowel sounds, abdominal pain and tenderness, and possible dehydration and electrolyte imbalances also may develop.

▶ *Heart failure.* This disorder may produce nausea and vomiting, particularly with right-sided heart failure. Associated findings include tachycardia, ventricular gallop, profound fatigue, dyspnea, crackles, peripheral edema, jugular vein distention, ascites, nocturia, and diastolic hypertension.

▶ *Hepatitis.* Nausea is an insidious early symptom of viral hepatitis. Vomiting, fatigue, myalgia and arthralgia, headache, anorexia, photophobia, pharyngitis, cough, and fever also occur early in the preicteric phase.

▶ *Hyperemesis gravidarum.* Unremitting nausea and vomiting that persist beyond the first trimester are characteristic of this pregnancy disorder. Vomitus ranges from undigested food, mucus, and bile early in the disorder to a coffee-ground appearance in later stages. Other findings include weight loss, signs of dehydration, headache, and delirium.

▶ *Infection.* Acute localized or systemic infection typically produces nausea. Other common findings include fever, headache, fatigue, and malaise.

▶ *Inflammatory bowel disease.* The most common symptom is recurrent diarrhea with blood, pus, and mucus. Nausea, vomiting, abdominal pain, and anorexia also may occur.

▶ *Intestinal obstruction.* Nausea commonly occurs, especially with obstruciton of the high small intestine. Vomiting may be bilious or fecal; abdominal pain is usually episodic and colicky but can become severe and steady with strangulation. Constipation occurs early in large-intestine obstruction and later in small-intestine obstruction; obstipation may signal complete obstruction. Bowel sounds typically are hyperactive in partial obstruction and hypoactive or absent in complete obstruction. Abdominal distention and tenderness occur, possibly with visible peristaltic waves and a palpable abdominal mass.

▶ *Irritable bowel syndrome.* Nausea, dyspepsia, and abdominal distention may occur with this syndrome, especially during periods of increased stress. Other findings include lower abdominal pain and abdominal tenderness, which is generally relieved by moving the bowels; diurnal diarrhea alternating with constipation or normal bowel function; and small stools with visible mucus and a feeling of incomplete evacuation.

▶ *Labyrinthitis.* Nausea and vomiting commonly occur with this acute inner ear inflammation. More significant findings include severe vertigo, progressive hearing loss, nystagmus, tinnitus and, possibly, otorrhea.

▶ *Lactose intolerance.* Signs and symptoms vary but may include nausea, diarrhea, cramps, bloating, and gas. They occur after eating dairy products.

▶ *Listeriosis.* Signs and symptoms include nausea, vomiting, diarrhea, fever, myalgias, and abdominal pain. If the infection spreads to the nervous system and causes meningitis, signs and symptoms include fever, headache, nuchal rigidity, and change in level of consciousness.

▶ *Ménière's disease.* This disease causes sudden, brief, recurrent attacks of nausea, vomiting, vertigo, tinnitus, diaphoresis, and nystagmus. It also causes hearing loss and ear fullness.

▶ *Mesenteric artery ischemia.* With this condition, nausea and vomiting may accompany severe cramping abdominal pain, especially after meals. Other findings include diarrhea or constipation, abdominal tenderness and bloating, anorexia, weight loss, and abdominal bruits.

▶ *Mesenteric venous thrombosis.* Insidious or acute onset of nausea, vomiting, and abdominal pain occurs, with diarrhea or constipation, abdominal distention, hematemesis, and melena.

▶ *Metabolic acidosis.* This acid-base imbalance may produce nausea and vomiting, anorexia, diarrhea, Kussmaul's respirations, and decreased level of consciousness.

▶ *Migraine headache.* Nausea and vomiting may occur in the prodromal stage, along with photophobia, light flashes, increased sensitivity to noise, light-headedness and, possibly, partial vision loss and paresthesia of the lips, face, and hands.

▶ *Motion sickness.* With this disorder, nausea and vomiting are brought on by motion or rhythmic movement. Headache, dizziness, fatigue, diaphoresis, hypersalivation, and dyspnea also may occur.

▶ *Myocardial infarction.* Nausea and vomiting may occur, but the cardinal symptom is severe substernal chest pain that may radiate to the left arm, jaw, or neck. Dyspnea, pallor, clammy skin, diaphoresis, altered blood pressure, and arrhythmias also occur.

▶ *Norovirus infection.* Acute gastroenteritis from noroviruses commonly causes infected individuals to experience nausea. Often, other symptoms include vomiting, diarrhea, and abdominal pain or cramping. Less often, low-grade fever, headache, chills, muscle aches, and generalized tiredness may develop. Noroviruses are carried in the stool or vomit of infected people and often are spread through contaminated food or water. Duration of illness is brief, with healthy people recovering in 24 to 60 hours.

▶ *Pancreatitis (acute).* Nausea, usually followed by vomiting, is an early symptom of pancreatitis. Other common findings include steady, severe pain in the epigastrium or left upper quadrant that may radiate to the back; abdominal tenderness and rigidity; anorexia; diminished bowel sounds; and fever. Tachycardia, restlessness, hypotension, skin mottling, and cold, sweaty limbs may occur in severe cases.

▶ *Peptic ulcer.* With this disorder, nausea and vomiting may follow attacks of sharp or gnawing, burning epigastric pain. Attacks typically occur when the stomach is empty, or after ingestion of alcohol, caffeine, or aspirin; they're relieved by eating food or taking an antacid or an antisecretory. Hematemesis or melena also may occur.

▶ *Peritonitis.* Nausea and vomiting usually accompany acute abdominal pain localized to the area of inflammation. Other findings include high fever with chills; tachycardia; hypoactive or absent bowel sounds; abdominal distention, rigidity, and tenderness (including rebound tenderness); positive obturator sign and obturator weakness; pale, cold skin; diaphoresis; hypotension; shallow respirations; and hiccups.

▶ *Preeclampsia.* Nausea and vomiting commonly occur with this disorder of pregnancy, along with rapid weight gain, epigastric pain, oliguria, severe frontal headache, hyperreflexia, and blurred or double vision. The classic diagnostic triad of signs include hypertension, proteinuria, and edema.

▶ *Q Fever.* Signs and symptoms include nausea, vomiting, diarrhea, fever, chills, severe headache, malaise, and chest pain. Fever may last up to 2 weeks, and in severe cases, the patient may develop hepatitis or pneumonia.

▶ *Renal and urologic disorders.* Cystitis, pyelonephritis, calculi, uremia, and other disorders of the renal system can cause nausea. Related findings reflect the specific disorder.

▶ *Rhabdomyolysis.* Signs and symptoms include nausea, vomiting, muscle weakness or pain, fever, malaise, and dark urine. Acute renal failure is the most commonly reported complication of the disorder. It results from renal structure obstruction and injury during the kidneys' attempt to filter the myoglobin from the bloodstream.

▶ *Thyrotoxicosis.* With this disorder, nausea and vomiting may accompany the classic findings of severe anxiety, heat intolerance, weight loss despite increased appetite, diaphoresis, diarrhea, tremor, tachycardia, and palpitations. Other signs include exophthalmos, ventricular or atrial gallop, and an enlarged thyroid gland.

▶ *Typhus.* An abrupt onset of nausea, vomiting, fever, and chills follows the initial symptoms of headache, myalgia, arthralgia, and malaise.

Other causes

DRUG WATCH *Common nausea-producing drugs include anesthetics, antibiotics, antineoplastics, cardiac glycosides, estrogens, ferrous sulfate, levodopa, nonsteroidal anti-inflammatories, opioids, potassium chloride replacements (oral), quinidine, sulfasalazine, and theophylline (overdose).*

▶ *Herbs.* Herbal remedies, such as ginkgo biloba and St. John's wort, can produce adverse reactions, including nausea.

▶ *Radiation and surgery.* Radiation therapy can cause nausea and vomiting. Postoperative nausea and vomiting are common, especially after abdominal surgery.

Special considerations

If your patient is experiencing severe nausea, prepare him for blood tests to determine fluid and electrolyte status, and acid-base balance. Have him breathe deeply to ease his nausea; keep his room air fresh and clean-smelling by removing bedpans and emesis basins promptly after use and by providing adequate ventilation. Because he could easily aspirate vomitus when in a supine position, elevate his head or position him on his side.

Because pain can cause or worsen nausea, give analgesics promptly, as needed. If possible, give them by injection or suppository to avoid worsening nausea, and use nonopioid analesics to reduce the risk of opioid-induced nausea.[2] Be alert for abdominal distention and hypoactive bowel sounds when you give an antiemetic: These signs may indicate gastric retention. If you detect them, immediately insert a nasogastric tube, as needed.

Prepare the patient for such procedures as computed tomography scan, ultrasound, endoscopy, and colonoscopy. Consult a nutritionist to determine the patient's metabolic needs, such as total or partial parenteral nutrition. Evaluate the patient's response to treatments and interventions continuously.[2]

Pediatric pointers

Nausea, commonly described as stomachache, is one of the most common childhood complaints. Often the result of overeating, it can also occur as part of diverse disorders, ranging from acute infections to a conversion reaction caused by fear.

Geriatric pointers

Elderly patients have increased dental caries; tooth loss; decreased salivary gland function,

Lessening chemotherapy nausea with progressive muscle relaxation

Question: *What's the effect of progressive muscle relaxation intervention on nausea and vomiting associated with anticancer chemotherapy?*

Research: Nausea and vomiting are common adverse drug reactions associated with chemotherapy. Progressive muscle relaxation is a non-pharmacological intervention used by nurses to alleviate chemotherapy-induced nausea and vomiting. Thirty hospitalized cancer patients took part in this study. All had experienced nausea and vomiting at the time of data collection. Data were collected before and after the 25-minute relaxation session.

Prerelaxation data collected included demographic information, physiologic indicators of nausea and vomiting, muscle reactions, nausea and vomiting levels using an adaptive version of Huskisson's visual analogue scale, and comments by participants. After the progressive muscle relaxation session, data on physiologic indicators of nausea and vomiting, muscle reactions, and levels of nausea and vomiting were again collected.

Conclusion: After progressive muscle relaxation, the intensity of nausea and vomiting levels was reduced. Physiologic indicators such as arterial pressure and pulse, respiratory rate, and body temperature were also significantly reduced after the intervention.

Application: Incorporate relaxation techniques into the care plan for patients receiving chemotherapy. Educate patients about progressive muscle relaxation and teach them how to perform the technique. In using the technique, the patient retracts a specific set of muscles and experiences feelings of lightness, tension, or pain in these muscles. Then the person relaxes the muscles and focuses on feelings of relaxation. The process is completed systematically for each set of muscles.

Source: De Carvalho, E.C., Martins, F. T. M., and dos Santos, C. B. "A Pilot Study of a Relaxation Technique for Management of Nausea and Vomiting in Patients Receiving Cancer Chemotherapy," *Cancer Nursing*, 30(2):163-167, 2007.

which causes mouth dryness; reduced gastric acid output and motility; and decreased senses of taste and smell—any of which can contribute to nonpathologic nausea.

Patient counseling

Instruct the patient to avoid fatty foods and carbonated beverages.[2] Urge the patient to move slowly and deliberately to minimize nausea.[2] Teach about nondrug therapies to help minimize or prevent nausea, such as acupressure, acupuncture, aromatherapy, music therapy, relaxation training, and distraction.[2] (See *Lessening chemotherapy nausea with progressive muscle relaxation*.)

REFERENCES

1. Baker, P.D., Morzorati, S.L., and Ellet, M.L. "The Pathophysiology of Chemotherapy-Induced Nausea and Vomiting," *Gastroenterology Nursing* 28(6):469-480, November/December 2005.
2. Steele, A., and Carlson, K.K. "Nausea and Vomiting: Applying Research to Bedside Practice," *AACN Advanced Critical Care* 18(1):61-73, January/March 2007.

NIPPLE DISCHARGE

Nipple discharge is the third most common breast complaint by women after breast pain and breast mass.[1] It's relatively common and may occur in up to 50% of women of reproductive age.[1] Nipple discharge can occur spontaneously or in response to nipple stimulation. It's characterized as intermittent or constant, unilateral or bilateral, and by color, consistency, and composition. It most often results from a benign process.[1] This sign rarely occurs (and is more likely to be pathologic) in men and in nulligravid, regularly menstruating women. A thick, grayish discharge—benign epithelial debris from inactive ducts—often can be elicited in middle-aged parous women. Colostrum—a thin, yellowish or milky discharge—often occurs in the last weeks of pregnancy.

Especially when accompanied by other breast changes, nipple discharge may signal a serious underlying disease. Significant causes include endocrine disorders, cancer, certain drugs, and blocked lactiferous ducts.

History and physical examination

Ask the patient when she first noticed the discharge, and determine its duration, extent, quantity, color, consistency, and smell, if any. Has she had other nipple and breast changes, such as pain, tenderness, itching, warmth, changes in contour, and lumps? If she reports a lump, ask about its onset, location, size, and consistency.

Obtain a complete gynecologic and obstetric history, and determine her normal menstrual cycle and the date of her last menses. Ask if she experiences breast swelling and tenderness, bloating, irritability, headaches, abdominal cramping, nausea, or diarrhea before or during menses. Note the number, date, and outcome of her pregnancies and, if she breastfed, the approximate time of her last lactation. Also, check for any risk factors of breast cancer—family history, previous or current malignancies, nulliparity or first pregnancy after age 30, early menarche, or late menopause. Ask about recent trauma to the chest region.

Start your physical examination by characterizing the discharge. If the discharge isn't frank, try to elicit it. (See *Eliciting nipple discharge.*) Then examine the nipples and breasts with the patient in four different positions: sitting with her arms at her sides; with her arms overhead; with her hands pressing on her hips; and leaning forward so her breasts are suspended. Check for nipple deviation, flattening, retraction, redness, asymmetry,

thickening, excoriation, erosion, or cracking. Inspect the breasts for asymmetry, irregular contours, dimpling, erythema, and peau d'orange. With the patient in a supine position, palpate the breasts and axillae for lumps, giving special attention to the areolae. Note the size, location, delineation, consistency, and mobility of any lump you find.

Is the patient taking hormones (hormonal contraceptives or hormone replacement therapy)? Is the discharge spontaneous, or does it have to be expressed?

Medical causes

▶ *Breast abscess.* This disorder, most common in breast-feeding women, may produce a thick, purulent discharge from a cracked nipple or infected duct. Other findings include abrupt onset of high fever with chills; breast pain, tenderness, and erythema; a palpable soft nodule or generalized induration; and possibly, nipple retraction.

▶ *Breast cancer.* This may cause bloody, watery, or purulent discharge from a normal-appearing nipple. About 75% to 80% of cases of bloody nipple discharge stem from malignancy.[2] Characteristic findings include a hard, irregular, fixed lump; erythema; dimpling; peau d'orange; changes in contour; nipple deviation, flattening, or retraction; axillary lymphadenopathy; and, possibly, breast pain.

▶ *Choriocarcinoma.* Galactorrhea (a white or grayish milky discharge) may result from this highly malignant neoplasm, which can follow pregnancy. Other characteristics include persistent uterine bleeding and bogginess after delivery or curettage, and vaginal masses.

▶ *Herpes zoster.* This virus can stimulate the thoracic nerves, causing bilateral, spontaneous, intermittent galactorrhea. Other characteristics include shooting or burning pain, eruption of small red nodules or vesicles on the thorax and possibly the arms and legs, pruritus and paresthesia or hyperesthesia in affected areas, headache, and fever and malaise.

▶ *Hypothyroidism.* This disorder occasionally causes galactorrhea. Related findings include bradycardia; weight gain despite anorexia; decreased mentation; periorbital edema; menorrhagia; constipation; puffy face,

Eliciting nipple discharge

If your patient has a history or evidence of nipple discharge, you can attempt to elicit it during your examination. Help the patient into a supine position, and gently squeeze her nipple between your thumb and index finger; note any discharge through the nipple. Then place your fingers on the areola, as shown, and palpate the entire areolar surface, watching for any discharge through areolar ducts.

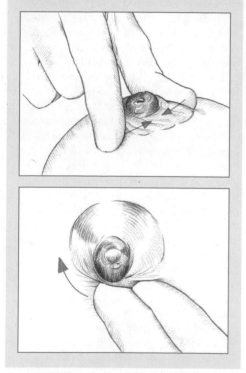

hands, and feet; brittle, sparse hair; and dry, doughy, pale, cool skin.

▶ *Intraductal papilloma.* This disorder is the primary cause of nipple discharge in women who aren't pregnant or breast-feeding.[1] Unilateral serous, serosanguineous, or bloody nipple discharge—usually from only one duct—is its predominant sign. Discharge may be intermittent or profuse and constant, and can often be stimulated by gentle pressure around the areola. Subareolar nodules, breast pain, and tenderness may occur.

▶ *Mammary duct ectasia.* A thick, sticky, grayish discharge from multiple ducts may be the first sign of this disorder. The discharge may be bilateral and is usually spontaneous. Other findings include a rubbery, poorly delineated lump beneath the areola, with a blue-green discoloration of the overlying skin; nipple retraction; and redness, swelling, tenderness, and burning pain in the areola and nipple.

▶ *Paget's disease.* With this disorder, serous or bloody discharge emits from denuded skin on the nipple, which is red, intensely itchy and, possibly, eroded or excoriated. The discharge is usually unilateral.

▶ *Prolactin-secreting pituitary tumor.* Bilateral galactorrhea may occur with this tumor. Other findings include amenorrhea, infertility, decreased libido and vaginal secretions, headaches, and blindness.

▶ *Proliferative (fibrocystic) breast disease.* This benign disorder occasionally causes a bilateral clear, milky, or straw-colored discharge, which is rarely purulent or bloody. Multiple round, soft, tender nodules are usually palpable in both breasts, although they may occur singly. Usually, nodules are mobile and are located in the upper outer quadrant. Nodule size, tenderness, and discharge increase during the luteal phase of the menstrual cycle. Symptoms then regress after menses.

▶ *Trauma.* Bilateral galactorrhea can result from trauma to the breasts.

Other causes

DRUG WATCH *Galactorrhea may be caused by antihypertensives (reserpine, methyldopa), cimetidine, hormonal contraceptives, metoclopramide, psychotropic drugs (particularly phenothiazines and tricyclic antidepressants), and verapamil.*

▶ *Surgery.* Chest wall surgery may stimulate the thoracic nerves, causing intermittent bilateral galactorrhea.

Special considerations

Although nipple discharge is usually insignificant, it can be frightening to the patient. Help relieve the patient's anxieties by clearly explaining the nature and origin of her discharge. Apply a breast binder, which may reduce discharge by eliminating nipple stimulation.

Diagnostic tests may include mammography, cytologic study of the discharge, ductal aspiration, ductoscopy, magnetic resonance imaging, and serum prolactin.[1]

Pediatric pointers

Infants of both sexes may have a milky breast discharge beginning 3 days after birth and lasting up to 2 weeks; it results from maternal hormonal influences. Nipple discharge in children and adolescents is rare. When it does occur, it's almost always nonpathologic, as in the bloody discharge that sometimes accompanies onset of menarche.

Geriatric pointers

In postmenopausal women, consider breast changes malignant until proven otherwise. Duct ectasia, a benign breast lesion that affects mainly elderly women, may produce a green or black nipple discharge.[3]

Patient counseling

Counsel your patient to be aware of discharge characteristics, such as its consistency (thick or thin), odor, origin in single or multiple ducts, and relation to the menstrual cycle. If the discharge becomes bloody, instruct the patient to seek medical evaluation. Urge her to perform breast self-examinations and maintain appointments for breast examinations by a physician and mammograms as recommended.

REFERENCES
1. Hussain, A.N., Policarpio, C., and Miriam, T. "Evaluating Nipple Discharge," *Obstetrical & Gynecological Survey* 61(4):278-83, April 2006.
2. Barron, M.A., and Fishel, R.S. "Talk to Your Patients About Breast Disease," *The Nurse Practitioner* 32(10):22-32, October 2007.
3. Moroney, J.W., and Zahn, C.M. "Common Gynecologic Problems in Geriatric-Aged Women," *Clinical Obstetrics and Gynecology* 50(3):687-708, September 2007.

NUCHAL RIGIDITY

Commonly an early sign of meningeal irritation, nuchal rigidity refers to stiffness of the neck that prevents flexion. To elicit this sign, attempt to passively flex the patient's neck and touch his chin to his chest. If nuchal rigidity is present, this maneuver triggers pain and muscle spasms. (Be sure that there is no cervical spinal misalignment, such as a fracture or dislocation, before testing for nuchal rigidity. Severe spinal cord damage could result.) The patient also may notice nuchal rigidity when he attempts to flex his neck during daily activities. This sign isn't reliable in children and infants.

Nuchal rigidity may herald life-threatening subarachnoid hemorrhage or meningitis. It also may be a late sign of cervical arthritis, in which joint mobility is gradually lost.

After eliciting nuchal rigidity, check for Kernig's and Brudzinski's signs. Quickly evaluate level of consciousness (LOC). Take vital signs. If you note signs of increased intracranial pressure (ICP), such as increased systolic pressure, bradycardia, and widened pulse pressure, start an I.V. line for drug administration and deliver oxygen as needed. Keep the head of the bed at no more than 30 degrees. Draw a specimen for routine blood studies such as a complete blood count with a white blood cell count and electrolyte levels.

History and physical examination

Obtain a patient history, relying on family members if altered LOC prevents the patient from responding. Ask about the onset and duration of neck stiffness. Did anything cause it? Also ask about associated signs and symptoms, such as headache, fever, nausea and vomiting, and motor and sensory changes. Check for a history of hypertension, head trauma, cerebral aneurysm or arteriovenous malformation, endocarditis, recent infection (such as sinusitis or pneumonia), or recent dental work. Then, obtain a complete drug history.

If the patient has no other signs of meningeal irritation, ask about a history of arthritis or neck trauma. Can the patient recall pulling a muscle in his neck? Inspect the patient's hands for swollen, tender joints, and palpate the neck for pain or tenderness.

Medical causes

▶ *Cervical arthritis*. With this disorder, nuchal rigidity develops gradually. Initially, the patient may complain of neck stiffness in the early morning or after a period of inactivity. Stiffness then becomes increasingly severe and frequent. Pain on movement, especially with lateral motion or head turning, is common. Typically, arthritis also affects other joints, especially those in the hands.

▶ *Encephalitis*. This viral infection may cause nuchal rigidity accompanied by other signs of meningeal irritation, such as positive Kernig's and Brudzinski's signs. Usually, nuchal rigidity appears abruptly and accompanies the two other hallmarks of this disorder, headache and fever.[1] The patient may have a rapidly decreasing LOC, progressing from lethargy to coma within 24 to 48 hours of onset. Other findings include vomiting, seizures, ataxia, hemiparesis, nystagmus, and cranial nerve palsies, such as dysphagia and ptosis.

▶ *Listeriosis*. If this bacterial infection spreads to the nervous system, meningitis may develop. Signs and symptoms include nuchal rigidity, fever, headache, and change in LOC. Initial signs and symptoms include fever, myalgias, abdominal pain, nausea, vomiting, and diarrhea.

▶ *Meningitis*. Nuchal rigidity is part of the classic symptom triad of this disorder, along with fever and changes in LOC.[2] It's accompanied by other signs of meningeal irritation, such as positive Kernig's and Brudzinski's signs, hyperreflexia and, possibly opisthotonos. Other early features include headache, photophobia, and vomiting. Initially, the patient is confused and irritable; later, he may become stuporous and seizure-prone or may slip into coma. Cranial nerve involvement may cause ocular palsies, facial weakness, and hearing loss. An erythematous papular rash occurs in some forms of viral meningitis; a purpuric rash may occur in meningococcal meningitis.

▶ *Subarachnoid hemorrhage*. Nuchal rigidity develops immediately after bleeding into the subarachnoid space. The patient may have positive Kernig's and Brudzinski's signs, severe headache of abrupt onset, photophobia, fever, nausea and vomiting, dizziness, cranial nerve palsies, and focal neurologic signs, such as hemiparesis or hemiplegia. His LOC deteriorates rapidly, possibly progressing to coma. Signs of increased ICP, such as bradycardia and altered respirations, also may occur.

Special considerations

Prepare the patient for diagnostic tests, such as computed tomography scans, magnetic resonance imaging, and cervical spinal X-rays.

Monitor vital signs, intake and output, and neurologic status closely. Avoid routine use of opioid analgesics because they may mask signs of increasing ICP. Enforce strict bed rest, and keep the head of the bed elevated at 30 degrees to help minimize ICP. Maintain a dark, quiet environment to reduce photophobia and headache.[2] Implement seizure precautions, if needed.

Pediatric pointers

Tests for nuchal rigidity are less reliable in children, especially infants. In younger children, move the head gently in all directions, noting resistance. In older children, ask the child to sit upright and touch his chin to his chest. Resistance to this movement may indicate meningeal irritation.

Patient counseling

Help the patient find a comfortable position so he can get adequate rest. Teach the patient about warning signs and symptoms to report. Provide emotional support to the patient and his family.

REFERENCES

1. DeBiasi, R.L., and Tyler, K.L. "Viral Meningitis and Encephalitis," *CONTINUUM: Lifelong Learning in Neurology. Infectious Diseases.* 12(2):58-94, April 2006.
2. Lawes, R. "Uncovering the Layers of Meningitis and Encephalitis," *Nursing Made Incredibly Easy!* 5(4):26-35, July/August 2007.

OLIGURIA

A cardinal sign of renal and urinary tract disorders, oliguria is clinically defined as urine output of less than 400 ml/24 hours.[1] Typically, this sign occurs abruptly and may herald serious—possibly life-threatening—hemodynamic instability. Its causes can be classified as prerenal (decreased renal blood flow), intrarenal (intrinsic renal damage), or postrenal (urinary tract obstruction); the pathophysiology differs for each classification. (See *How oliguria develops.*) Oliguria from a prerenal or postrenal cause usually is promptly reversible with treatment, although it may lead to intrarenal damage if untreated. However, oliguria from an intrarenal cause is usually more persistent and may be irreversible.

History and physical examination

Begin by asking the patient about his usual daily voiding pattern, including frequency and amount. When did he first notice changes in this pattern and in the color, odor, or consistency of his urine? Ask about pain or burning on urination. Has the patient had a fever? Note his normal daily fluid intake. Has he recently been drinking more or less than usual? Has his intake of caffeine or alcohol changed drastically? Has he had recent episodes of diarrhea or vomiting that might cause fluid loss? Next, explore associated complaints, especially fatigue, loss of appetite, thirst, dyspnea, chest pain, or recent weight gain or loss (in dehydration).

Check for a history of renal, urinary tract, or cardiovascular disorders. Note recent traumatic injury or surgery associated with significant blood loss, as well as recent blood transfusions. Was the patient exposed to nephrotoxic agents, such as heavy metals, organic solvents, anesthetics, or radiographic contrast media? Next, obtain a drug history.

Begin the physical examination by taking the patient's vital signs and weighing him. Assess his overall appearance for edema. Palpate both kidneys for tenderness and enlargement, and percuss for costovertebral angle (CVA) tenderness. Also, inspect the flank area for edema or erythema. Auscultate the heart and lungs for abnormal sounds, and the flank area for renal artery bruits. Assess the patient for edema or signs of dehydration such as dry mucous membranes.

Obtain a urine sample and inspect it for abnormal color, odor, or sediment. Use reagent strips to test for glucose, protein, and blood. Also, use a urinometer to measure specific gravity.

Medical causes

▶ *Acute tubular necrosis (ATN).* An early sign of ATN, oliguria may occur abruptly (in shock) or gradually (in nephrotoxicity). Usually, it persists for about 2 weeks, followed by polyuria. Related features include signs of hyperkalemia (muscle weakness and cardiac arrhythmias); uremia (anorexia, confusion, lethargy, twitching, seizures, pruritus, and Kussmaul's respirations); and heart failure (edema, jugular vein distention, crackles, and dyspnea).

How oliguria develops

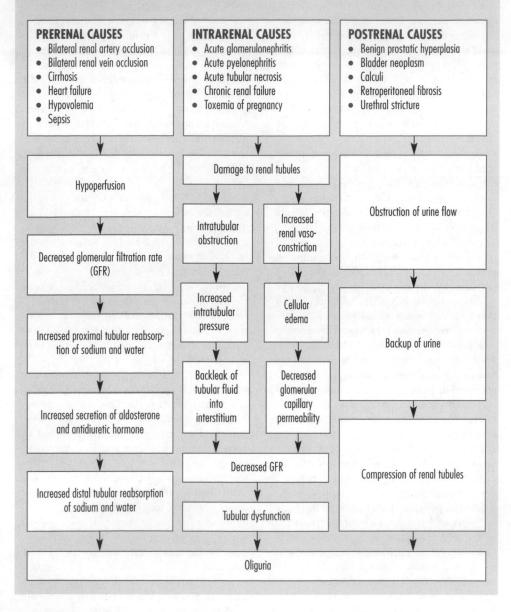

PRERENAL CAUSES
- Bilateral renal artery occlusion
- Bilateral renal vein occlusion
- Cirrhosis
- Heart failure
- Hypovolemia
- Sepsis

INTRARENAL CAUSES
- Acute glomerulonephritis
- Acute pyelonephritis
- Acute tubular necrosis
- Chronic renal failure
- Toxemia of pregnancy

POSTRENAL CAUSES
- Benign prostatic hyperplasia
- Bladder neoplasm
- Calculi
- Retroperitoneal fibrosis
- Urethral stricture

Hypoperfusion

Decreased glomerular filtration rate (GFR)

Increased proximal tubular reabsorption of sodium and water

Increased secretion of aldosterone and antidiuretic hormone

Increased distal tubular reabsorption of sodium and water

Damage to renal tubules

Intratubular obstruction

Increased renal vaso-constriction

Increased intratubular pressure

Cellular edema

Backleak of tubular fluid into interstitium

Decreased glomerular capillary permeability

Decreased GFR

Tubular dysfunction

Obstruction of urine flow

Backup of urine

Compression of renal tubules

Oliguria

▶ *Benign prostatic hyperplasia.* This disorder, which is common in men older than age 50, in rare cases may cause oliguria resulting from bladder outlet obstruction. More common symptoms include urinary frequency or hesitancy, urge or overflow incontinence, decrease in the force of the urine stream or inability to stop the stream, nocturia and, possibly, hematuria.

▶ *Bladder neoplasm.* Uncommonly, this disorder may produce oliguria if the tumor obstructs the bladder outlet. The cardinal signs of such obstruction include urinary frequency and urgency, as well as gross hematuria, which may lead to clot retention and flank pain.

▶ *Calculi.* Oliguria or anuria may result from stones lodging in the kidneys, ureters, bladder outlet, or urethra. Other signs and symptoms include urinary frequency and urgency, dysuria, and hematuria or pyuria. Usually, the patient has renal colic—excruciating pain that radiates from the CVA to the flank, the suprapubic region, and the genitals. He also may have nausea, vomiting, hypoactive bowel sounds, abdominal distention and, occasionally, fever and chills.

▶ *Cholera.* In this bacterial infection, severe water and electrolyte loss lead to oliguria, thirst, weakness, muscle cramps, decreased skin turgor, tachycardia, hypotension, and abrupt watery diarrhea and vomiting. Death may occur in hours without treatment.

▶ *Cirrhosis.* In severe cirrhosis, hepatorenal syndrome may develop with oliguria, in addition to ascites, edema, fatigue, weakness, jaundice, hypotension, tachycardia, gynecomastia, testicular atrophy, and signs of GI bleeding such as hematemesis.

▶ *Glomerulonephritis (acute).* This disorder produces oliguria or anuria. Other features are mild fever, fatigue, gross hematuria, proteinuria, generalized edema, elevated blood pressure, headache, nausea and vomiting, flank and abdominal pain, and signs of pulmonary congestion (dyspnea and productive cough).

▶ *Heart failure.* Oliguria may occur in left ventricular failure as a result of low cardiac output and decreased renal perfusion. Other signs and symptoms include dyspnea, fatigue, weakness, peripheral edema, distended jugular veins, tachycardia, tachypnea, crackles, and a dry or productive cough. In advanced heart failure, the patient also may develop orthopnea, cyanosis, clubbing, ventricular gallop, diastolic hypertension, cardiomegaly, and hemoptysis.

▶ *Hypovolemia.* Any disorder that decreases circulating fluid volume can produce oliguria. Associated findings include orthostatic hypotension, apathy, lethargy, fatigue, gross muscle weakness, anorexia, nausea, profound thirst, dizziness, sunken eyeballs, poor skin turgor, and dry mucous membranes.

▶ *Pyelonephritis (acute).* Accompanying the sudden onset of oliguria in this disorder are high fever with chills, fatigue, flank pain, CVA tenderness, weakness, nocturia, dysuria, hematuria, urinary frequency and urgency, and tenesmus. The urine may appear cloudy. Occasionally, the patient also experiences anorexia, nausea, diarrhea, and vomiting.

▶ *Renal artery occlusion (bilateral).* This disorder may produce oliguria or, more commonly, anuria. Other features include severe, constant upper abdominal and flank pain, nausea and vomiting, and hypoactive bowel sounds. The patient also develops a fever 1 to 2 days after the occlusion, as well as diastolic hypertension.

▶ *Renal failure (chronic).* Oliguria is a major sign of end-stage chronic renal failure. Associated findings reflect progressive uremia and include fatigue, weakness, irritability, uremic fetor, ecchymoses and petechiae, peripheral edema, elevated blood pressure, confusion, emotional lability, drowsiness, coarse muscle twitching, muscle cramps, peripheral neuropathies, anorexia, metallic taste in the mouth, nausea and vomiting, constipation or diarrhea, stomatitis, pruritus, pallor, and yellow- or bronze-tinged skin. Eventually, seizures, coma, and uremic frost may develop.

▶ *Renal vein occlusion (bilateral).* This disorder occasionally causes oliguria accompanied by acute low back and flank pain, CVA tenderness, fever, pallor, hematuria, enlarged and palpable kidneys, edema and, possibly, signs of uremia.

▶ *Retroperitoneal fibrosis.* Oliguria may result from bilateral ureteral obstruction by dense fibrous tissue. Other effects include hematuria, diffuse lower back pain, anorexia, weight loss, nausea and vomiting, fatigue, malaise, low-grade fever, and elevated blood pressure.

▶ *Sepsis.* Any condition that results in sepsis may produce oliguria, along with fever, chills, restlessness, confusion, diaphoresis, anorexia, vomiting, diarrhea, pallor, hypotension, and tachycardia. The patient may have signs of local infection, such as dysuria and wound drainage. In severe infection, he may develop lactic acidosis marked by Kussmaul's respirations.

▶ *Toxemia of pregnancy.* In severe pre-eclampsia, oliguria may be accompanied by elevated blood pressure, dizziness, diplopia, blurred vision, epigastric pain, nausea and vomiting, irritability, and severe frontal headache. Typically, the oliguria is preceded by generalized edema and sudden weight gain of more than 3 lb (1.4 kg) per week during the second trimester, or more than 1 lb (0.5 kg) per week during the third trimester. If preeclampsia progresses to eclampsia, the patient develops seizures and may slip into coma.

▶ *Urethral stricture.* This disorder produces oliguria accompanied by chronic urethral discharge, urinary frequency and urgency, dysuria, pyuria, and diminished urine stream. As obstruction worsens, urine extravasation may lead to formation of urinomas and urosepsis.

Other causes

▶ *Diagnostic studies.* Radiographic studies that use contrast media may cause nephrotoxicity and oliguria.[2]

DRUG WATCH *Oliguria may result from drugs that decrease renal perfusion (such as diuretics), drugs that cause nephrotoxicity (most notably, aminoglycosides and chemotherapy drugs), drugs that cause urine retention (adrenergics, anticholinergics), and drugs that cause urinary obstruction from precipitation of urinary crystals (acyclovir, sulfonamides).*

Special considerations

Monitor vital signs, intake and output, and daily weight. Depending on the cause of the oliguria, fluids are normally restricted to between 600 ml and 1 L more than the patient's urine output for the previous day. Provide a diet low in sodium, potassium, and protein.

Laboratory tests may be needed to determine if the oliguria is reversible. Such tests include serum blood urea nitrogen and creatinine levels, urea and creatinine clearance, urine sodium levels, and urine osmolality. Abdominal X-rays, ultrasonography, computed tomography scan, cystography, and a renal scan may be required.

Pediatric pointers

In the neonate, oliguria may result from edema or dehydration. Major causes include congenital heart disease, respiratory distress syndrome, sepsis, congenital hydronephrosis, acute tubular necrosis, and renal vein thrombosis. Common causes of oliguria in children between ages 1 and 5 are acute poststreptococcal glomerulonephritis and hemolytic-uremic syndrome. After age 5, causes of oliguria are similar to those in adults.

Geriatric pointers

In elderly patients, oliguria may result from gradual progression of an underlying disorder. It also may result from overall poor muscle tone secondary to inactivity, poor fluid intake, and infrequent voiding attempts.

Instruct the patient to report signs such as weight gain or edema.[1] If needed, teach him about restricting fluids.[1]

REFERENCES

1. Ward, K. "Kidneys, Don't Fail Me Now!" *Nursing Made Incredibly Easy!* 3(2):18-26, March/April 2005.
2. Kohtz, C., and Thompson, M. "Preventing Contrast Medium-Induced Nephropathy," *AJN* 107(9):40-49, September 2007.

● ORTHOPNEA

O rthopnea—trouble breathing in the supine position—is a common symptom of cardiopulmonary disorders that produce dyspnea. It's often a subtle symptom; the patient may complain that he can't catch his breath when lying down, or he may mention that he sleeps most comfortably in a reclining chair or propped up by pillows. Derived from this complaint is the common classification of two- or three-pillow orthopnea.

Orthopnea presumably results from increased hydrostatic pressure in the pulmonary vasculature related to gravitational effects in the supine position. It's a sensitive indicator of volume overload, along with jugular vein distention and an S_3 heart sound.[1] It may be aggravated by obesity or pregnancy, which restrict diaphragmatic excursion. Assuming the upright position relieves orthopnea by placing much of the pulmonary vasculature above the left atrium, which reduces mean hydrostatic pressure, and by enhancing diaphragmatic excursion, which increases inspiratory volume.

History and physical examination

Begin by asking about a history of cardiopulmonary disorders, such as myocardial infarction, rheumatic heart disease, valvular disease, asthma, emphysema, or chronic bronchitis. Does the patient smoke? If so, how much? Explore related symptoms, noting especially complaints of cough, nocturnal or exertional dyspnea, fatigue, weakness, loss of appetite, or chest pain. Does the patient use alcohol or have a history of heavy alcohol use?

When examining the patient, check for other signs of increased respiratory effort, such as accessory muscle use, shallow respirations, and tachypnea. Also note barrel chest. Inspect the patient's skin for pallor or cyanosis, and the fingers for clubbing. Observe and palpate for edema, and check for neck vein distention. Auscultate the lungs and heart. Monitor the patient's oxygen saturation.

Medical causes

▶ *Chronic obstructive pulmonary disease.* This disorder typically produces orthopnea and other dyspneic complaints, accompanied by accessory muscle use, tachypnea, tachycardia, and paradoxical pulse.[2] Auscultation may reveal diminished breath sounds, rhonchi, crackles, and wheezing. The patient also may have a dry or productive cough with copious sputum. Other features include anorexia, weight loss, and edema. Barrel chest, cyanosis, and clubbing are usually late signs.

▶ *Left-sided heart failure.* Orthopnea occurs late in this disorder. If heart failure is acute, orthopnea may begin suddenly; if chronic, it may become constant. The earliest symptom of this disorder is progressively severe dyspnea. Other common early symptoms include Cheyne-Stokes respirations, paroxysmal nocturnal dyspnea, fatigue, weakness, and a cough that may occasionally produce clear or blood-tinged sputum. Tachycardia, tachypnea, and crackles also may occur.

Other late findings include cyanosis, clubbing, ventricular gallop, and hemoptysis. Left-sided heart failure also may lead to signs of shock, such as hypotension, thready pulse, and cold, clammy skin.

▶ *Mediastinal tumor.* Orthopnea is an early sign of this disorder, resulting from pressure of the tumor against the trachea, bronchus, or lung when the patient lies down. However, many patients are asymptomatic until the tumor enlarges. Then, it produces retrosternal chest pain, dry cough, hoarseness, dysphagia, stertorous respirations, palpitations, and cyanosis. Examination reveals suprasternal retractions on inspiration, bulging of the chest wall, tracheal deviation, dilated jugular and superficial chest veins, and edema of the face, neck, and arms.

▶ *Valve disorders.* Orthopnea, paroxysmal nocturnal dyspnea, and fatigue may occur with aortic or mitral valve stenosis or regurgitation.[3,4]

Special considerations

To relieve orthopnea, place the patient in semi-Fowler's or high Fowler's position; if this doesn't help, have the patient lean over a bedside table with his chest forward. If needed, give oxygen by nasal cannula. A diuretic may be needed to reduce lung fluid. Monitor electrolyte levels closely after giving diuretics. Unless contraindicated, use angiotensin-converting enzyme inhibitors for patients with left-sided heart failure. Monitor intake and output closely.

An electrocardiogram, chest X-ray, pulmonary function test, and an arterial blood gas test may be necessary for further evaluation.

A central venous line or pulmonary artery catheter may be inserted to help measure central venous pressure and wedge and cardiac output, respectively.

Pediatric pointers

Common causes of orthopnea in children include heart failure, croup syndrome, cystic fibrosis, and asthma. Sleeping in an infant seat may improve symptoms for a young child.

Children with a mediastinal mass who experience orthopnea shouldn't receive general anesthesia due to the risk of total airway obstruction. These patients should be kept calm and maintained in an upright or prone position. They are candidates for only light sedation or local anesthesia, which won't impair spontaneous breathing.[5]

Geriatric pointers

If the elderly patient is using more than one pillow at night, consider noncardiogenic pulmonary reasons for this, such as gastroesophageal reflux disease, sleep apnea, arthritis, or simply the need for greater comfort.

Patient counseling

Instruct the patient to notify the physician if he's using additional pillows regularly, or if dyspnea worsens at night.

REFERENCES

1. Wingate, S. "Caring for Persons with Advanced Heart Failure," *Home Healthcare Nurse* 25(8):511-520, September 2007.
2. Mulroy, J. "Chronic Obstructive Pulmonary Disease in Women," *Dimensions of Critical Care Nursing* 24(1):1-18, January/February 2005.
3. Todd, B.A., and Higgins, K. "Recognizing Aortic Mitral Valve Disease," *Nursing* 35(6):58-63, June 2005.
4. Aronow, W.S. "Valvular Aortic Stenosis in the Elderly," *Cardiology in Review* 15(5):217-225, September/Octoboer 2007.
5. Sakakeeny-Zaal, K. "Pediatric Orthopnea and Total Airway Obstruction," *AJN* 107(4):40-43, April 2007.

PALLOR

Pallor is abnormal paleness or loss of skin color, which may develop suddenly or gradually. Although generalized pallor affects the entire body, it's most apparent on the face, conjunctiva, oral mucosa, and nail beds. Localized pallor commonly affects a single limb.

How easily pallor is detected varies with skin color and the thickness and vascularity of underlying subcutaneous tissue. At times, it's merely a subtle lightening of skin color that may be difficult to detect in dark-skinned people; sometimes it's evident only on the conjunctiva and oral mucosa.

Pallor may result from decreased peripheral oxyhemoglobin or decreased total oxyhemoglobin. The former reflects diminished peripheral blood flow associated with peripheral vasoconstriction or arterial occlusion or with low cardiac output. (Transient peripheral vasoconstriction may occur with exposure to cold, causing nonpathologic pallor.) The latter usually results from anemia, the chief cause of pallor. (See *How pallor develops.*)

If generalized pallor develops suddenly, quickly look for signs of shock, such as tachycardia, hypotension, oliguria, and decreased level of consciousness. Prepare to rapidly infuse fluids or blood. Keep emergency resuscitation equipment nearby.

History and physical examination

If the patient's condition permits, take a complete history. Does the patient or anyone in his family have a history of anemia or of a chronic disorder that might lead to pallor, such as renal failure, heart failure, or diabetes? Ask about the patient's diet, particularly his intake of green vegetables.

Explore the pallor more fully. Find out when the patient first noticed it. Is pallor constant or intermittent? Does it occur when he's exposed to the cold? Does it occur when he's under emotional stress? Explore associated signs and symptoms, such as dizziness, fainting, orthostasis, weakness and fatigue on exertion, dyspnea, chest pain, palpitations, menstrual irregularities, or loss of libido. If the pallor is confined to one or both legs, ask the patient if walking is painful. Do his legs feel cold or numb? If the pallor is confined to his fingers, ask about tingling and numbness.

Start the physical examination by taking the patient's vital signs. Be sure to check for orthostatic hypotension. Auscultate the heart for gallops and murmurs and the lungs for crackles. Check the patient's skin temperature—cold limbs are common with vasoconstriction or arterial occlusion. Note skin ulceration. Examine the abdomen for splenomegaly. Palpate peripheral pulses. An absent pulse in a pale limb may indicate arterial occlusion, whereas a weak pulse may indicate low cardiac output.

Medical causes

▶ *Anemia.* Typically, pallor develops gradually with this disorder. Pallor may also appear in the conjunctivae and oral mucus membranes.[1] The patient's skin may also appear sallow or grayish. Other effects include fa-

How pallor develops

Pallor may result from decreased peripheral oxyhemoglobin or decreased total oxyhemoglobin. This flowchart illustrates the progression to pallor.

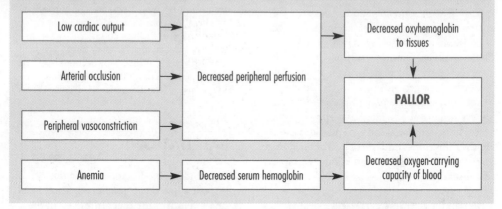

tigue, dyspnea, tachycardia, bounding pulse, atrial gallop, systolic bruit over the carotid arteries and, possibly, crackles and bleeding tendencies.

▶ *Arterial occlusion (acute).* Pallor develops abruptly in the limb with the occlusion, which usually results from an embolism or aneurysm. Pallor is also part of the six P's that describe the sequence of acute arterial occlusion: pain, pallor, pulselessness, poikilothermia, paresthesia, and paralysis.[2] A line of demarcation develops, separating the cool, pale, cyanotic, and mottled skin below the occlusion from the normal skin above it.

▶ *Arterial occlusive disease (chronic).* With this disorder, pallor is specific to a limb—usually one leg, but occasionally both legs or an arm. It develops gradually from obstructive arteriosclerosis or a thrombus and is aggravated by elevating the limb. Other findings include intermittent claudication, weakness, cool skin, diminished pulses in the limb and, possibly, ulceration and gangrene.

▶ *Cardiac arrhythmias.* Cardiac arrhythmias that seriously reduce cardiac output, such as complete heart block and attacks of tachyarrhythmia, may cause acute onset of pallor. Other features include irregular, rapid, or slow pulse; dizziness; weakness and fatigue; hypotension; confusion; palpitations; di-

aphoresis; oliguria; and, possibly, loss of consciousness.

▶ *Frostbite.* Pallor is localized to the frostbitten area, such as the feet, hands, or ears. Typically, the area feels cold, waxy and, perhaps, hard in deep frostbite. The skin doesn't blanch and sensation may be absent. As the area thaws, the skin turns purplish blue. Blistering and gangrene may then follow if the frostbite was severe.

▶ *Orthostatic hypotension.* With this condition, pallor occurs abruptly on rising from a recumbent position to a sitting or standing position. An abrupt drop in blood pressure, an increase in heart rate, and dizziness are also characteristic. At times, the patient loses consciousness for several minutes.

▶ *Raynaud's disease.* Pallor of the fingers upon exposure to cold or stress is a hallmark of this disease. Typically, the fingers abruptly turn pale, then cyanotic; with rewarming, they become red and paresthetic. With chronic disease, ulceration may occur.

▶ *Shock.* Two forms of shock initially cause acute onset of pallor and cool, clammy skin. With *hypovolemic shock,* other early signs and symptoms include restlessness, thirst, slight tachycardia, and tachypnea. As shock progresses, the skin becomes increasingly clammy, pulse becomes more rapid and thready, and hypotension develops with narrowing pulse pressure. Other signs and symptoms include oliguria, subnormal body temperature, and decreased level of consciousness. With *cardiogenic shock,* the signs and symptoms are similar, but usually more profound.

▶ *Vasopressor syncope.* Sudden onset of pallor immediately precedes or accompanies loss of consciousness during syncopal attacks. These common fainting spells may be triggered by emotional stress or pain and usually last only a few seconds or minutes. Before loss of consciousness, the patient may exhibit diaphoresis, nausea, yawning, hyperpnea, weakness, confusion, tachycardia, and dim vision. He then develops bradycardia, hypotension, a few clonic jerks, and dilated pupils with loss of consciousness.

Special considerations

If the patient has chronic generalized pallor, prepare him for blood studies and, possibly, bone marrow biopsy. If the patient has localized pallor, he may require arteriography or other diagnostic studies to accurately determine the cause.

When pallor results from low cardiac output, administer blood and fluids and as well as a diuretic, a cardiotonic, and an antiarrhythmic, as needed. Frequently monitor the patient's vital signs, intake and output, electrocardiogram results, and hemodynamic status.

Pediatric pointers

In children, pallor stems from the same causes as it does in adults. It also can stem from a congenital heart defect or chronic lung disease.

Patient counseling

If the patient's pallor is related to anemia, explain the importance of an iron-rich diet and rest.[1] If he has pallor due to frostbite or Raynaud's disease, inform him about cold protection measures. Patients with Raynaud's disease should also avoid tobacco, limit their intake of caffeine and alcohol, and exercise regularly to prevent vasoconstriction.[3] If pallor is related to orthostatic hypotension, explain the need to stand up slowly and to sit down when dizziness occurs.

REFERENCES

1. Holcomb, S.S. "Recognizing and Managing Anemia," *The Nurse Practitioner* 30(12):16-31, December 2005.
2. Sieggreen, M. "A Contemporary Approach to Peripheral Arterial Disease," *The Nurse Practitioner* 31(7):14-25, July 2006.
3. Reilly, A., and Snyder, B. "Raynaud Phenomenon: Whether It's Primary or Secondary, There Is No Cure, But Treatment Can Alleviate Symptoms," *AJN* 105(8):56-65. August 2005.

⦿ PALPITATIONS

Defined as a conscious awareness of one's heartbeat, palpitations are usually felt over the precordium or in the throat or neck. The patient may describe them as pounding, jumping, turning, fluttering, or flopping, or as missing or skipping beats. Palpitations may be regular or irregular, fast or slow, paroxysmal or sustained.

Although usually insignificant, palpitations may result from a cardiac or metabolic disorder and from the effects of certain drugs. Nonpathologic palpitations may occur with a newly implanted prosthetic valve because the valve's clicking sound heightens the patient's awareness of his heartbeat. Transient palpitations may accompany emotional stress (such as fright, anger, or anxiety) or physical stress (such as exercise and fever). They can also accompany use of stimulants, such as tobacco and caffeine.

To help characterize the palpitations, ask the patient to simulate their rhythm by tapping his finger on a hard surface. An irregular "skipped beat" rhythm points to premature ventricular contractions, whereas an episodic racing rhythm that ends abruptly suggests paroxysmal atrial tachycardia.

If the patient complains of palpitations, ask him about dizziness and shortness of breath. Inspect for pale, cool, clammy skin. Take the patient's vital signs, noting hypotension and irregular or abnormal pulse. If these signs are present, suspect cardiac arrhythmia. Prepare to begin cardiac monitoring and, if necessary, to deliver electroshock therapy. Start an I.V. line to give an antiarrhythmic, if needed.

History and physical examination

If the patient isn't in distress, perform a complete cardiac history and physical examination. Ask if he has a cardiovascular or pulmonary disorder, which may produce arrhythmias. Does the patient have a history of hypertension or hypoglycemia? Be sure to obtain a drug history. Has the patient recently started cardiac glycoside therapy? Ask about caffeine, tobacco, and alcohol consumption.

Explore related symptoms, such as weakness, fatigue, and angina. Auscultate for gallops, murmurs, and abnormal breath sounds.

Medical causes

▶ *Anemia.* Palpitations may occur with anemia, especially on exertion. Pallor, fatigue, and dyspnea are also common. Other signs include a systolic ejection murmur, bounding pulse, tachycardia, crackles, an atrial gallop, and a systolic bruit over the carotid arteries.

▶ *Anxiety attack (acute).* Anxiety is the most common cause of palpitations in children and adults. With this disorder, palpitations may be accompanied by diaphoresis, facial flushing, trembling, and an impending sense of doom. Almost invariably, the patient hyperventilates, which may lead to dizziness, weakness, and syncope. Other typical findings include tachycardia, precordial pain, shortness of breath, restlessness, and insomnia.

▶ *Cardiac arrhythmias.* Paroxysmal or sustained palpitations may be accompanied by dizziness, weakness, and fatigue. The patient also may have an irregular, rapid, or slow pulse rate; decreased blood pressure; confusion; pallor; oliguria; and diaphoresis.

▶ *Hypertension.* With this disorder, the patient may be asymptomatic or may complain of sustained palpitations alone or with headache, dizziness, tinnitus, and fatigue. His blood pressure typically exceeds 140/90 mm Hg. He also may have nausea and vomiting, seizures, and decreased level of consciousness (LOC).

▶ *Hypocalcemia.* Typically, this disorder produces palpitations, weakness, and fatigue. It progresses from paresthesia to muscle tension and carpopedal spasms. The patient may also have muscle twitching, hyperactive deep tendon reflexes, chorea, and positive Chvostek's and Trousseau's signs.

▶ *Hypoglycemia.* When blood glucose levels drop significantly, the sympathetic nervous system triggers adrenaline production. This may cause sustained palpitations, which may be accompanied by fatigue, irritability, hunger, cold sweats, tremors, tachycardia, anxiety, and headache. Eventually the patient may develop central nervous system reactions. These include blurred or double vision, muscle weakness, hemiplegia, and altered LOC.

▶ *Mitral prolapse.* The most common symptoms of this valvular disorder are palpitations, chest discomfort, and dyspnea.[1] The hallmark of this disorder is a midsystolic click followed by an apical systolic murmur. Other signs and symptoms may include dizziness, severe fatigue, migraine headache, anxiety, paroxysmal tachycardia, crackles, and peripheral edema.

▶ *Mitral stenosis.* Early features of this valvular disorder typically include sustained palpitations accompanied by exertional dyspnea and fatigue. Auscultation also reveals a loud S_1 or opening snap, and a rumbling diastolic murmur at the apex. Patients also may have other signs and symptoms, such as an atrial gallop and, with advanced mitral stenosis, orthopnea, dyspnea at rest, paroxysmal nocturnal dyspnea, peripheral edema, jugular vein distention, ascites, hepatomegaly, and atrial fibrillations.

▶ *Pheochromocytoma.* This rare adrenal medulla tumor causes episodic hypermetabolism, commonly associated with paroxysmal palpitations. The cardinal sign of pheochromocytoma is dramatically elevated blood pressure, which may be sustained or paroxysmal. Other signs and symptoms include tachycardia, headache, chest or abdominal pain, diaphoresis, warm and pale or flushed skin, paresthesia, tremors, insomnia, nausea and vomiting, and anxiety.

▶ *Seizures.* Although rare, palpitations may be caused by seizures with autonomic features. Autonomic signs and symptoms may occur in complex partial or generalized tonic-clonic seizures with associated signs and symptoms including confusion, loss of consciousness, incontinence, and involuntary movements.[2] Simple partial seizures may also cause palpitations, but occur without accompanying changes in mental status and motor/sensory disturbances.[2]

▶ *Sick sinus syndrome.* A patient with this disorder may have palpitations, bradycardia, tachycardia, chest pain, syncope, and heart failure.

▶ *Thyrotoxicosis.* A characteristic symptom of this disorder, sustained palpitations may be accompanied by tachycardia, dyspnea, weight loss despite increased appetite, diarrhea, tremors, nervousness, diaphoresis, heat intolerance and, possibly, exophthalmos and an enlarged thyroid. The patient also may have an atrial or ventricular gallop.

▶ *Wolff-Parkinson-White syndrome.* Seen in children and adolescents, this disorder results in recurrent palpitations and frequent episodes of paroxysmal tachycardia.

Other causes

DRUG WATCH *Palpitations may be caused by atropine, beta blockers, calcium channel blockers, drugs that cause cardiac arrhythmias or increase cardiac output (such as cardiac glycosides), ganglionic blockers, minoxidil, and sympathomimetics (such as cocaine).*

▶ *Exercise.* Exercise can normally cause palpitations, as well as in patients with coronary heart disease, hypertension, mitral valve prolapse, and cardiomegaly.

▶ *Herbs.* Herbal remedies such as ginseng and ephedra (banned by the Food and Drug Administration) may cause adverse reactions, including palpitations and an irregular heartbeat.

Special considerations

Prepare the patient for diagnostic tests, such as an electrocardiogram and Holter monitoring. Remember that even mild palpitations can cause the patient much concern. Maintain a quiet, comfortable environment to minimize anxiety and perhaps decrease palpitations.

Pediatric pointers

Palpitations in children commonly result from fever and congenital heart defects, such as patent ductus arteriosus and septal defects. Because many children can't describe this complaint, focus your attention on objective measurements, such as cardiac monitoring, physical examination, and laboratory tests.

Geriatric pointers

Age-related changes in the coronary arteries predispose older adults to heart disease that may cause palpitations.[3] Menopausal women may also experience heart palpitations.[3]

Patient counseling

If the patient's palpitations are related to anxiety, provide information about anxiety and stress management. Refer him to community support services for stress management and therapy. Reinforce the need to avoid caffeine and provide information on alcohol and smoking cessation programs, as appropriate.

REFERENCES

1. Sims, J.M., and Miracle, V.A. "An Overview of Mitral Valve Prolapse," *Dimensions of Critical Care Nursing* 26(4):145-149, July/August 2007.
2. Gandelman-Marton, R., Segev, Y., Theitler, J., Rabey, J.M., and Pollak, L. "Palpitations: Could They Be Neurogenic? A Case Report," *The Neurologist* 12(3):160-162, May 2006.
3. Thompson, J. "Psychological and Physical Etiologies of Heart Palpitations," *The Nurse Practitioner* 31(2):14-23, February 2006.

● PAPULAR RASH

A papular rash consists of small, raised, circumscribed—and perhaps discolored (red to purple)—lesions that measure up to 1 cm known as papules.[1] It may erupt anywhere on the body in various configurations and may be acute or chronic. Papular rashes characterize many cutaneous disorders; they may also result from allergy and from infectious, neoplastic, and systemic disorders. (To compare papules with other skin lesions, see *Recognizing common skin lesions,* pages 328 and 329.)

History and physical examination

Your first step is to fully evaluate the papular rash: Note its color, configuration, and location on the patient's body. Find out when it erupted. Has the patient noticed any changes in the rash since then? Is it itchy or burning, or painful or tender? Have him describe other signs and symptoms, such as fever, headache, and GI distress.

Next, obtain a medical history, including allergies, previous rashes or skin disorders, infections, childhood diseases, sexual history, including any sexually transmitted infections (STIs), and cancers. Has the patient recently been bitten by an insect or rodent or been exposed to anyone with an infectious disease? Finally, obtain a complete drug history including prescription and nonprescription drugs and herbal remedies.[2]

Medical causes

▶ *Acne vulgaris.* Acne affects more than 50 million Americans.[3] With this disorder, rupture of enlarged comedones produces inflamed—and sometimes painful and pruritic—papules, pustules, nodules, or cysts on the face and sometimes the shoulders, chest, and back.

▶ *Anthrax (cutaneous).* Anthrax is an acute infectious disease caused by the gram-positive, spore-forming bacterium *Bacillus anthracis.* The disease can occur in humans exposed to infected animals, tissue from infected animals, or biological warfare. Cutaneous anthrax occurs when the bacterium enters a cut or abrasion on the skin. The infection begins as a small, painless, or pruritic macular or papular lesion resembling an insect bite. Within 1 to 2 days it develops into a vesicle and then a painless ulcer with a characteristic black, necrotic center. Lymphadenopathy, malaise, headache, or fever may develop.

▶ *Dermatitis (perioral).* This inflammatory disorder causes an erythematous eruption of discrete, tiny papules and pustules on the nasolabial fold, chin, and upper lip area. The lesions may be pruritic and painful.

▶ *Dermatomyositis.* Gottron's papules—flat, violet-colored lesions on the dorsa of the finger joints and the nape of the neck and shoulders—are pathognomonic of this disorder, as is the dusky lilac discoloration of periorbital tissue and lid margins (heliotrope edema). These signs may be accompanied by a transient, erythematous, macular rash in a malar distribution on the face and sometimes on the scalp, forehead, neck, upper torso, and arms. This rash may be preceded by symmetrical muscle soreness and weakness in the pelvis, upper limbs, shoulders, neck and, possibly, the face (polymyositis).

▶ *Erythema migrans.* Transmitted through a tick bite, this systemic disorder is characterized by a papular or macular rash starting from a single lesion (usually on the leg) that spreads at the margins while clearing centrally. The rash commonly appears on the thighs, trunk, or upper arms. It's the classic early sign of Lyme disease, but about 25% of patients don't develop it. The patient also may have fever, chills, headache, malaise, nausea, vomiting, fatigue, backache, knee pain, and stiff neck.

▶ *Follicular mucinosis.* With this cutaneous disorder, perifollicular papules or plaques are accompanied by prominent alopecia.

▶ *Fox-Fordyce disease.* This chronic disorder is marked by pruritic papules on the axillae, pubic area, and areolae associated with apocrine sweat gland inflammation. Sparse hair growth in these areas is also common.

▶ *Gonococcemia.* With this chronic STI, sporadic eruption of an erythematous macular rash is characteristic, although fistulas and petechiae may appear. The rash typically affects the distal limbs (palms and soles) and rapidly becomes maculopapular, vesiculopustular and, commonly, hemorrhagic. Bullae may form. The mature lesion is raised; has a gray, necrotic center; and is surrounded by erythema. Typically, it heals in 3 to 4 days. Eruptions are commonly accompanied by fever and joint pain.

▶ *Granuloma annulare.* This benign, chronic disorder produces papules that usually coalesce to form plaques. The papules spread peripherally to form a ring with a normal or slightly depressed center. They usually appear

Recognizing common skin lesions

MACULE

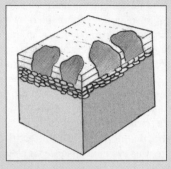

A small (usually less than 1 cm in diameter), flat blemish or discoloration that can be brown, tan, red, or white and has same texture as surrounding skin

VESICLE

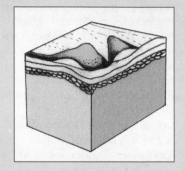

A small (less than 0.5 cm in diameter), thin-walled, raised blister containing clear, serous, purulent, or bloody fluid

BULLA

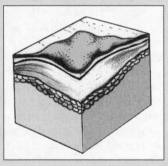

A raised, thin-walled blister greater than 0.5 cm in diameter, containing clear or serous fluid

PUSTULE

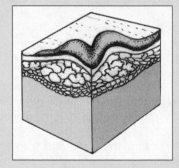

A circumscribed, pus- or lymph-filled, elevated lesion that varies in diameter and may be firm or soft, and white or yellow

on the feet, legs, hands, or fingers, and may be pruritic or asymptomatic.

▶ *Human immunodeficiency virus (HIV) infection.* Acute infection with the HIV retrovirus typically causes a generalized maculopapular rash. Other signs and symptoms include fever, malaise, sore throat, and headache. Lymphadenopathy and hepatosplenomegaly may also occur. Most patients don't recall these symptoms of acute infection.

▶ *Insect bites.* Salivary secretions from insect bites—especially ticks, lice, flies, and mosqui-toes—may produce an allergic reaction associated with a papular, macular, or petechial rash. The rash usually is accompanied by non-specific signs and symptoms, such as fever, myalgia, headache, lymphadenopathy, nausea, and vomiting.

▶ *Kaposi's sarcoma.* This neoplastic disorder is characterized by purple or blue papules or macules of vascular origin on the skin, mucous membranes, and viscera. These lesions decrease in size with firm pressure and then return to their original size within 10 to 15

WHEAL

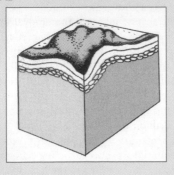

A slightly raised, firm lesion of variable size and shape, surrounded by edema; skin may be red or pale

PAPULE

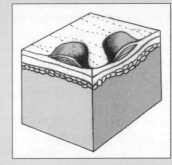

A small, solid, raised lesion less than 1 cm in diameter, with red to purple skin discoloration

NODULE

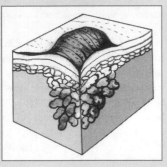

A small, firm, circumscribed, elevated lesion 1 to 2 cm in diameter with possible skin discoloration

TUMOR

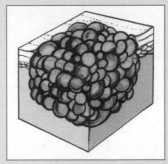

A solid, raised mass usually larger than 2 cm in diameter with possible skin discoloration

seconds. They may become scaly and ulcerate with bleeding.

Kaposi's sarcoma has multiple variants; most people who have it are immunocompromised, as from HIV or acquired immunodeficiency syndrome. Human herpes virus-8 has been strongly implicated as a cofactor in the development of Kaposi's sarcoma.

▶ *Leprosy.* This chronic infectious disorder produces various skin lesions. Early papular or macular lesions are erythematous, hypopigmented, and symmetrical (with lepromatous leprosy) or asymmetrical (with tuberculoid leprosy). The lesions may spread over the entire skin surface. Later, plaques and nodules form, especially on the ear lobes, nose, eyebrows, and forehead. Other findings include hypoesthesia or anesthesia, anhidrosis, and dry, scaly skin in affected areas; enlarged, palpable peripheral nerves with severe neuralgia; and muscle atrophy and contractures.

▶ *Lichen amyloidosis.* This idiopathic cutaneous disorder produces discrete, firm, hemispherical, pruritic papules on the anterior tibiae. Papules may be brown or yellow, smooth or scaly.

▶ *Lichen planus.* Discrete, flat, angular or polygonal, violet papules, commonly marked with white lines or spots, are characteristic of this disorder. The papules may be linear or coalesce into plaques and usually appear on the lumbar region, genitalia, ankles, anterior tibiae, and wrists. Lesions usually develop first on the buccal mucosa as a lacy network of white or gray threadlike papules or plaques. Pruritus, distorted fingernails, and atrophic alopecia are common.

▶ *Monkeypox.* Usually preceded 1 to 3 days by a fever, a papular rash is a characteristic sign of monkeypox. The rash is often blister-like and can follow these stages: vesiculation, postulation, umbilication, and crusting. Often starting on the face and spreading to the trunk and limbs, the rash may be either localized or generalized. Other accompanying symptoms in humans include lymphadenopathy, chills, throat pain, and muscle aches. Most humans recover within 2 to 4 weeks.

▶ *Mononucleosis (infectious).* A maculopapular rash that resembles rubella is an early sign of this infection in 10% of patients. The rash is typically preceded by headache, malaise, and fatigue. It may be accompanied by sore throat, cervical lymphadenopathy, and fluctuating temperature with an evening peak of 101° to 102° F (38.3° to 38.9° C). Splenomegaly and hepatomegaly may also develop.

▶ *Mycosis fungoides.* Stage I (premycotic stage) of this rare, cutaneous T-cell lymphoma is marked by the eruption of erythematous, pruritic macules on the trunk and limbs. In stage II, these lesions coalesce into pruritic papules and plaques, and nodes become irregular. Stage III is evidenced by large, irregular, brown to red tumors that ulcerate and are painful and itchy.

▶ *Necrotizing vasculitis.* With this systemic disorder, crops of purpuric, but otherwise asymptomatic, papules are typical. Some patients also develop low-grade fever, headache, myalgia, arthralgia, and abdominal pain.

▶ *Parapsoriasis (chronic).* This disorder mimics psoriasis, producing small to moderately sized asymptomatic papules with a thin, adherent scale, primarily on the trunk, hands, and feet.

▶ *Pityriasis rosea.* This disorder starts with an erythematous "herald patch"—a slightly raised, oval lesion about 2 to 6 cm in diameter that may appear anywhere on the body. A few days to weeks later, yellow to tan or erythematous patches with scaly edges appear on the trunk, arms, and legs, commonly erupting along body cleavage lines in a characteristic "pine tree" pattern. These patches may be asymptomatic or slightly pruritic, are 0.5 to 1 cm in diameter, and typically improve with moderate skin exposure to sunlight. This treatment should be used cautiously, however, to avoid sunburn.

▶ *Pityriasis rubra pilaris.* This rare chronic disorder initially produces scaling seborrhea on the scalp that spreads to the face and ears. Scaly red patches then develop on the palms and soles; these patches thicken, become keratotic, and may develop painful fissures. Later, follicular papules erupt on the hands and forearms and then spread over wide areas of the trunk, neck, and limbs. These papules coalesce into large, scaly, erythematous plaques. Striated fingernails may appear.

▶ *Polymorphic light eruption.* Abnormal reactions to light may produce papular, vesicular, or nodular rashes on sun-exposed areas. Other symptoms include pruritus, headache, and malaise.

▶ *Psoriasis.* This common chronic disorder begins with small, erythematous papules on the scalp, chest, elbows, knees, back, buttocks, and genitalia. These papules are sometimes pruritic and painful. Eventually they enlarge and coalesce, forming elevated, red, scaly plaques covered by characteristic silver scales, except in moist areas such as the genitalia. These scales may flake off easily or thicken, covering the plaque. Other features include pitted fingernails and arthralgia.

▶ *Rat bite fever.* A maculopapular or petechial rash develops on the palms and soles several weeks after a bite from an infected rodent. Other findings typically include pain, redness, and swelling at the bite site; tender regional lymph nodes; fever with chills; malaise; headache; and myalgia.

▶ *Rosacea.* This hyperemic disorder is characterized by persistent erythema, telangiectasia, and recurrent eruption of papules and pustules on the forehead, malar areas, nose, and chin. Eventually, eruptions occur more frequently and erythema deepens. Rhinophyma may occur in severe cases.

▶ *Sarcoidosis.* This multisystem granulomatous disorder may produce crops of small, erythematous or yellow-brown papules around the eyes and mouth and on the nose, nasal mucosa, and upper back. Other findings include dyspnea with a nonproductive cough, fatigue, arthralgia, weight loss, lymphadenopathy, vision loss, and dysphagia.

▶ *Seborrheic keratosis.* With this cutaneous disorder, benign skin tumors begin as small, yellow-brown papules on the chest, back, or abdomen, eventually enlarging and becoming deeply pigmented. However, in blacks, these papules may remain small and affect only the malar part of the face (dermatosis papulosa nigra).

▶ *Smallpox (variola major).* Initial signs and symptoms include high fever, malaise, prostration, severe headache, backache, and abdominal pain. A maculopapular rash develops on the mucosa of the mouth, pharynx, face, and forearms and then spreads to the trunk and legs. Within 2 days the rash becomes vesicular and later pustular. The lesions develop at the same time, appear identical, and are more prominent on the face and limbs. The pustules are round, firm, and deeply embedded in the skin. After 8 to 9 days the pustules form a crust, and later the scab separates from the skin leaving a pitted scar. In fatal cases, death results from encephalitis, extensive bleeding, or secondary infection.

▶ *Syphilis.* A discrete, reddish brown, mucocutaneous rash and general lymphadenopathy herald the onset of secondary syphilis. The rash may be papular, macular, pustular, or nodular. It typically erupts between rolls of fat on the trunk and proximally on the arms, palms, soles, face, and scalp. Lesions in warm, moist areas enlarge and erode, producing highly contagious, pink or grayish white condylomata lata. The patient also may have mild headache, malaise, anorexia, weight loss, nausea and vomiting, sore throat, low-grade fever, temporary alopecia, and brittle, pitted nails.

▶ *Syringoma.* With this disorder, adenoma of the sweat glands produces a yellowish or erythematous papular rash on the face (especially the eyelids), neck, and upper chest.

▶ *Systemic lupus erythematosus (SLE).* SLE is characterized by a "butterfly rash" of erythematous maculopapules or discoid plaques that appears in a malar distribution across the nose and cheeks. Similar rashes may appear elsewhere, especially on exposed body areas. Other cardinal features include photosensitivity and nondeforming arthritis, especially in the hands, feet, and large joints. Common effects are patchy alopecia, mucous membrane ulceration, low-grade or spiking fever, chills, lymphadenopathy, anorexia, weight loss, abdominal pain, diarrhea or constipation, dyspnea, tachycardia, hematuria, headache, and irritability.

DRUG WATCH *Drug-induced lupus can be triggered by hydralazine, isoniazid, methyldopa, minocycline, phenytoin, and procainamide, and may occur months or years after continuous drug therapy.[4]*

▶ *Typhus.* Typhus is a rickettsial disease transmitted to humans by fleas, mites, or body louse. Initial symptoms include headache, myalgia, arthralgia, and malaise, followed by an abrupt onset of chills, fever, nausea, and vomiting. A maculopapular rash may be present in some cases.

Other causes

DRUG WATCH *Transient maculopapular rashes, usually on the trunk, may result from many drugs, including allopurinol, antibiotics (ampicillin, cephalosporins, sulfonamides, tetracycline), benzodiazepines (such as diazepam), gold salts, isoniazid, lithium, and salicylates.*

Special considerations

Apply cool compresses or an antipruritic lotion. Give an antihistamine for allergic reactions and an antibiotic for infection.

Pediatric pointers

Common causes of papular rashes in children are infectious diseases, such as molluscum contagiosum and scarlet fever; scabies; insect bites; allergies and drug reactions; and miliaria, which occurs in three forms, depending on the depth of sweat gland involvement.

Geriatric pointers
In bedridden elderly patients, the first sign of pressure ulcers is commonly an erythematous area, sometimes with firm papules. If not properly managed, these lesions progress to deep ulcers and can lead to death.

Patient counseling
Advise the patient to keep his skin clean and dry, to wear loose-fitting, nonirritating clothing, and to avoid scratching the rash. Instruct him to promptly report changes in the rash's color, size, or configuration as well as the onset of itching or bleeding. Tell him to avoid excessive exposure to direct sunlight and to apply a protective sunscreen before going outdoors.

Warn patients with chronic conditions (such as SLE, psoriasis, or sarcoidosis) about the typical skin rashes that can develop. Tell them that these rashes can be an early sign of disease flare-up and that they should seek prompt treatment to prevent serious complications.

Encourage patients with acne to comply with treatment. Educate the patient on his drug regimen, and teach proper application of topical drugs. Discuss potential short-term adverse effects to therapy. Tell the patient that he should start to see improvement 4 to 6 weeks after starting therapy.[3]

REFERENCES
1. Pullen, R.L. "Assessing Skin Lesions: Learn to Identify the Different Types and Document Their Characteristics," *Nursing* 37(8):44-45, August 2007.
2. Anderson, J., Langemo, D., Hanson, D., Thompson, P., and Hunter, S. "What You Can Learn from A Comprehensive Skin Assessment," *Nursing* 37(4):65-66, April 2007.
3. Roebuck, H.L. "Acne: Intervene Early," *The Nurse Practitioner* 31(10:24-43, October 2006.
4. Hayden, M.L. "Did That Medication Cause This Rash?" *Nursing* 35(9):62-64, September 2005.

PARALYSIS

Paralysis, the total loss of voluntary motor function, results from severe cortical or pyramidal tract damage. It can occur with a cerebrovascular disorder, degenerative neuromuscular disease, trauma, tumor, or central nervous system infection. Acute paralysis may be an early indicator of a life-threatening disorder, such as Guillain-Barré syndrome.

Paralysis can be local or widespread, symmetrical or asymmetrical, transient or permanent, and spastic or flaccid. It's commonly classified according to location and severity as paraplegia (sometimes transient paralysis of the legs), quadriplegia (permanent paralysis of the arms, legs, and body below the level of the spinal lesion), or hemiplegia (unilateral paralysis of varying severity and permanence). Incomplete paralysis with profound weakness (paresis) may precede total paralysis in some patients.

If paralysis has developed suddenly, suspect trauma or an acute vascular insult. After ensuring that the patient's spine is properly immobilized, quickly determine his level of consciousness (LOC) and take his vital signs. Elevated systolic blood pressure, widening pulse pressure, and bradycardia may signal increasing intracranial pressure (ICP). If possible, elevate the patient's head 30 degrees to decrease ICP.

Evaluate respiratory status, and be prepared to give oxygen, insert an artificial airway, or provide intubation and mechanical ventilation, as needed. To help determine the nature of the patient's injury, ask him what happened. If he can't respond, try to find an eyewitness.

History and physical examination
If the patient is in no immediate danger, perform a complete neurologic assessment. Start with the history, relying on family members for information if needed. Ask about the onset, duration, intensity, and progression of paralysis and about the events preceding its development. Focus medical history questions on the incidence of degenerative neurologic or neuromuscular disease, recent infectious ill-

ness, sexually transmitted disease, cancer, or recent injury. Explore related signs and symptoms, noting fever, headache, vision disturbances, dysphagia, nausea and vomiting, bowel or bladder dysfunction, muscle pain or weakness, and fatigue.

Next, perform a complete neurologic examination, testing cranial nerve, motor, and sensory function and deep tendon reflexes. Assess strength in all major muscle groups, and note any muscle atrophy. (See *Testing muscle strength,* pages 302 and 303.) Document all findings to serve as a baseline.

Medical causes

▶ *Amyotrophic lateral sclerosis.* This invariably fatal disorder produces spastic or flaccid paralysis in the body's major muscle groups, eventually progressing to total paralysis. Earlier findings include progressive muscle weakness, fasciculations, and muscle atrophy, usually beginning in the arms and hands. Cramping and hyperreflexia are also common. Involvement of respiratory muscles and the brain stem produces dyspnea and possibly respiratory distress. Progressive cranial nerve paralysis causes dysarthria, dysphagia, drooling, choking, and difficulty chewing.

▶ *Bell's palsy.* Bell's palsy, a disease of cranial nerve VII, causes transient, unilateral facial muscle paralysis that develops over 2 to 5 days.[1] The affected muscles sag and eyelid closure is impossible. Other signs include increased tearing, drooling, and a diminished or absent corneal reflex.

▶ *Botulism.* This bacterial toxin infection can cause rapidly descending muscle weakness that progresses to paralysis within 2 to 4 days after the ingestion of contaminated food. Respiratory muscle paralysis leads to dyspnea and respiratory arrest. Nausea, vomiting, diarrhea, blurred or double vision, bilateral mydriasis, dysarthria, and dysphagia are some early findings.

▶ *Brain abscess.* Advanced abscess in the frontal or temporal lobe can cause hemiplegia accompanied by other late findings, such as ocular disturbances, unequal pupils, decreased LOC, ataxia, tremors, and signs of infection.

▶ *Brain tumor.* A tumor affecting the motor cortex of the frontal lobe may cause con-

tralateral hemiparesis that progresses to hemiplegia. Onset is gradual, but paralysis is permanent without treatment. In early stages, frontal headache and behavioral changes may be the only indicators. Eventually, seizures, aphasia, and signs of increased ICP (decreased LOC and vomiting) develop.

▶ *Conversion disorder.* Hysterical paralysis, a classic symptom of conversion disorder, is characterized by the loss of voluntary movement with no obvious physical cause. It can affect any muscle group, appears and disappears unpredictably, and may occur with histrionic behavior (manipulative, dramatic, vain, irrational) or a strange indifference.

▶ *Encephalitis.* Variable paralysis develops in the late stages of this disorder. Earlier signs and symptoms include rapidly decreasing LOC (possibly coma), fever, headache, photophobia, vomiting, signs of meningeal irritation (nuchal rigidity, positive Kernig's and Brudzinski's signs), aphasia, ataxia, nystagmus, ocular palsies, myoclonus, and seizures.

▶ *Guillain-Barré syndrome.* This syndrome is characterized by a rapidly developing, but reversible, ascending paralysis. It commonly begins as leg muscle weakness and progresses symmetrically, sometimes affecting even the cranial nerves, producing dysphagia, nasal speech, and dysarthria. Respiratory muscle paralysis may be life-threatening. Other effects include transient paresthesia, orthostatic hypotension, tachycardia, diaphoresis, and bowel and bladder incontinence.

▶ *Head trauma.* Cerebral injury can cause paralysis due to cerebral edema and increased intracranial pressure. Onset is usually sudden. Location and extent vary, depending on the injury. Associated findings also vary but include decreased LOC; sensory disturbances, such as paresthesia and loss of sensation; headache; blurred or double vision; nausea and vomiting; and focal neurologic disturbances.

▶ *Migraine headache.* Hemiparesis, scotomas, paresthesia, confusion, dizziness, photophobia, or other transient symptoms may precede the onset of a throbbing unilateral headache and may persist after it subsides.

▶ *Multiple sclerosis.* With this disorder, paralysis commonly waxes and wanes until the later stages, when it may become permanent. Its extent can range from monoplegia to quadriplegia. In most patients, vision and sensory disturbances (paresthesia) are the earliest symptoms. Later findings are widely variable and may include muscle weakness and spasticity, nystagmus, hyperreflexia, intention tremor, gait ataxia, dysphagia, dysarthria, impotence, and constipation. Urinary frequency, urgency, and incontinence may also occur.

▶ *Myasthenia gravis.* With this neuromuscular disease, profound muscle weakness and abnormal fatigability may produce paralysis of certain muscle groups. Paralysis is usually transient in early stages but becomes more persistent as the disease progresses. Associated findings depend on the areas of neuromuscular involvement; they include weak eye closure, ptosis, diplopia, lack of facial mobility, dysphagia, nasal speech, and frequent nasal regurgitation of fluids. Neck muscle weakness may cause the patient's jaw to drop and his head to bob. Respiratory muscle involvement can lead to respiratory distress—dyspnea, shallow respirations, and cyanosis.

▶ *Neurosyphilis.* Irreversible hemiplegia may occur in the late stages of neurosyphilis. Dementia, cranial nerve palsies, tremors, and abnormal reflexes are other late findings.

▶ *Parkinson's disease.* Tremors, bradykinesia, and lead-pipe or cogwheel rigidity are the classic signs of Parkinson's disease. Extreme rigidity can progress to paralysis, particularly in the limbs. In most cases, paralysis resolves with prompt treatment of the disease.

▶ *Peripheral nerve trauma.* Severe injury to a peripheral nerve or group of nerves results in the loss of motor and sensory function in the innervated area. Muscles become flaccid and atrophied, and reflexes are lost. If transection isn't complete, paralysis may be temporary.

▶ *Peripheral neuropathy.* Typically, this syndrome produces muscle weakness that may lead to flaccid paralysis and atrophy. Related effects include paresthesia, loss of vibration sensation, hypoactive or absent deep tendon reflexes, neuralgia, and skin changes such as anhidrosis.

▶ *Poliomyelitis.* This disorder can produce insidious, permanent flaccid paralysis and hyporeflexia. Sensory function remains intact, but the patient loses voluntary muscle control.

▶ *Rabies.* This acute disorder produces progressive flaccid paralysis, vascular collapse, coma, and death within 2 weeks of contact with an infected animal. Prodromal signs and symptoms—fever; headache; hyperesthesia; paresthesia, coldness, and itching at the bite site; photophobia; tachycardia; shallow respirations; and excessive salivation, lacrimation, and perspiration—develop almost immediately. Within 2 to 10 days, a phase of excitement begins, marked by agitation, cranial nerve dysfunction (pupil changes, hoarseness, facial weakness, ocular palsies), tachycardia or bradycardia, cyclic respirations, high fever, urine retention, drooling, and hydrophobia.

▶ *Seizure disorders.* Seizures, particularly focal seizures, can cause transient local paralysis (Todd's paralysis). Any part of the body may be affected, although paralysis tends to occur contralateral to the side of the irritable focus.

▶ *Spinal cord injury.* Complete spinal cord transection results in permanent spastic paralysis below the level of injury. Reflexes may return after spinal shock resolves. Partial transection causes variable paralysis and paresthesia, depending on the location and extent of injury. (See *Understanding spinal cord syndromes.*)

▶ *Spinal cord tumors.* Paresis, pain, paresthesia, and variable sensory loss may occur along the nerve distribution pathway served by the affected cord segment. Eventually, these symptoms may progress to spastic paralysis with hyperactive deep tendon reflexes (unless the tumor is in the cauda equina, which produces hyporeflexia) and, perhaps, bladder and bowel incontinence. Paralysis is permanent without treatment.

▶ *Stroke.* A stroke involving the motor cortex can produce contralateral paresis or paralysis. Onset may be sudden or gradual, and paralysis may be transient or permanent. Other signs and symptoms vary widely and may include headache, vomiting, seizures, decreased LOC and mental acuity, dysarthria, dysphagia, ataxia, contralateral paresthesia or sensory loss, apraxia, agnosia, aphasia, vision disturbances, emotional lability, and bowel and bladder dysfunction.

▶ *Subarachnoid hemorrhage.* This potentially life-threatening disorder can produce sudden

Understanding spinal cord syndromes

When a patient's spinal cord is incompletely severed, he develops partial motor and sensory loss. Most incomplete cord lesions fit into one of the syndromes described below.

Anterior cord syndrome, usually resulting from a flexion injury, causes motor paralysis and loss of pain and temperature sensation below the level of injury. Touch, proprioception, and vibration sensation usually are preserved.

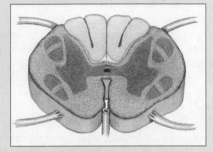

Central cord syndrome is caused by hyperextension or flexion injury. Motor loss is variable and greater in the arms than in the legs; sensory loss is usually slight.

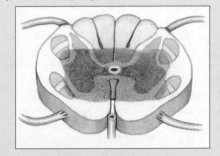

Brown-Séquard syndrome can result from flexion, rotation, or penetration injury. It's characterized by unilateral motor paralysis ipsilateral to the injury and loss of pain and temperature sensation contralateral to the injury.

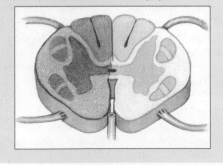

Posterior cord syndrome, produced by a cervical hyperextension injury, causes only a loss of proprioception and loss of light touch sensation. Motor function remains intact.

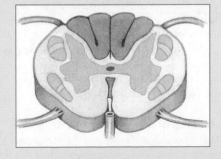

paralysis. The condition may be temporary, resolving with decreasing edema, or permanent, if tissue destruction has occurred. Other acute effects are severe headache, mydriasis, photophobia, aphasia, sharply decreased LOC, nuchal rigidity, vomiting, and seizures.

▶ *Syringomyelia.* This degenerative spinal cord disease produces segmental paresis, leading to flaccid paralysis of the hands and arms. Reflexes are absent, and loss of pain and tem-

perature sensation is distributed over the neck, shoulders, and arms in a capelike pattern.

▶ *Thoracic aortic aneurysm.* Occlusion of spinal arteries by a ruptured thoracic aortic aneurysm may cause sudden onset of transient bilateral paralysis. Severe chest pain radiating to the neck, shoulders, back, and abdomen and a sensation of tearing in the thorax are prominent symptoms. Related findings include syncope, pallor, diaphoresis, dyspnea, tachycardia, cyanosis, diastolic heart murmur, and abrupt loss of radial and femoral pulses or wide variations in pulses and blood pressure between arms and legs. Ironically, the patient appears to be in shock, and his systolic blood pressure is either normal or elevated.

▶ *Transient ischemic attack (TIA)*. Episodic TIAs may cause transient unilateral paresis or paralysis accompanied by paresthesia, blurred or double vision, dizziness, aphasia, dysarthria, decreased LOC, and other site-dependent effects.

▶ *West Nile encephalitis*. This brain infection is caused by West Nile virus, a mosquito-borne flavivirus endemic to Africa, the Middle East, western Asia, and the United States. Mild infections are common and include fever, headache, and body aches, which are sometimes accompanied by skin rash and swollen lymph glands. More severe infections are marked by headache, high fever, neck stiffness, stupor, disorientation, coma, tremors, occasional convulsions, paralysis and, rarely, death.

Other causes

DRUG WATCH *Therapeutic use of neuromuscular blockers, such as pancuronium, produces paralysis.*

▶ *Electroconvulsive therapy*. This therapy can produce acute, but transient, paralysis.

Special considerations

Because a paralyzed patient is particularly susceptible to complications of prolonged immobility, provide frequent position changes, meticulous skin care, and frequent chest physiotherapy. He may benefit from passive range-of-motion exercises to maintain muscle tone, application of splints to prevent contractures, and the use of footboards or other devices to prevent footdrop. Because prolonged immobilization raises the risk of deep vein thrombosis; preventive therapy may include enoxaparin, thromboembolic deterrent support hose, or sequential compression devices.[2]

If his cranial nerves are affected, the patient will have trouble chewing and swallowing. Provide a liquid or soft diet, and keep suction equipment on hand in case of aspiration.

Feeding tubes or total parenteral nutrition may be needed in severe paralysis. Paralysis and accompanying vision disturbances may make ambulation hazardous; provide a call light, and show the patient how to call for help.

As appropriate, arrange for physical, speech, or occupational therapy and wound care. Stroke rehabilitation may include therapies aimed at recovering motor function.[3]

Pediatric pointers

Although children may develop paralysis from an obvious cause—such as trauma, infection, or tumor—they also may develop it from a hereditary or congenital disorder, such as Tay-Sachs disease, Werdnig-Hoffmann disease, spina bifida, or cerebral palsy.

Geriatric pointers

Although most patients with Guillain-Barré Syndrome recover over a period of months to years, being age 60 or older is a predictor of poor outcome.[2]

Patient counseling

Provide information and referrals to home care and other support services. Assess the home environment, and provide information to the family about safety measures and physical alterations that may be needed to allow wheelchair access and maneuverability. Provide teaching on equipment that may be needed and used at home.

REFERENCES

1. Carlson, D.S., and Pfadt, E. "When Your Patient Has Acute Facial Paralysis," *Nursing* 35(4):54-55, April 2005.
2. Atkinson, S.B., Carr, R.L., Maybee, P., and Haynes, D. "The Challenges of Managing and Treating Guillain-Barre Syndrome During The Acute Phase," *Dimensions of Critical Care Nursing* 25(6):256-263, November/December 2006.
3. Alverzo, J.P., Brigante, M.A., and McNish, M. "Improving Stroke Outcomes," *AJN* 72A-72G, November 2007.

PARESTHESIA

Paresthesia is an abnormal sensation or combination of sensations—commonly described as numbness, prickling, or tingling—felt along peripheral nerve pathways. These sensations generally aren't painful; unpleasant or painful sensations are called *dysesthesias*. Paresthesia may develop suddenly or gradually and may be transient or permanent.

A common symptom of many neurologic disorders, paresthesia may also result from a systemic disorder or from a particular drug. It may reflect damage or irritation of the parietal lobe, thalamus, spinothalamic tract, or spinal or peripheral nerves—the neural circuit that transmits and interprets sensory stimuli.

History and physical examination

First, explore the paresthesia. When did the abnormal sensations begin? Have the patient describe their character and distribution. Ask about associated signs and symptoms, such as sensory loss and paresis or paralysis. Next, take a medical history, including neurologic, cardiovascular, metabolic, renal, and chronic inflammatory disorders, such as arthritis or lupus. Has the patient recently sustained a traumatic injury or had surgery or an invasive procedure that may have damaged peripheral nerves?

Focus the physical examination on the patient's neurologic status. (See *Differential diagnosis: Paresthesia,* pages 338 and 339.) Assess his level of consciousness (LOC) and cranial nerve function. Test muscle strength and deep tendon reflexes (DTRs) in limbs affected by paresthesia. Systematically evaluate light touch, pain, temperature, vibration, and position sensation. Note skin color and temperature, and palpate pulses.

Medical causes

▶ *Arterial occlusion (acute).* With this disorder, sudden paresthesia and coldness may develop in one or both legs with a saddle embolus. Paresis, intermittent claudication, and aching pain at rest are also characteristic. The limb becomes mottled with a line of temperature and color demarcation at the level of occlusion. Pulses are absent below the occlusion, and capillary refill time is increased.

▶ *Arteriosclerosis obliterans.* This disorder produces paresthesia, intermittent claudication (most common symptom), diminished or absent popliteal and pedal pulses, pallor, paresis, and coldness in the affected leg.

▶ *Arthritis.* Rheumatoid or osteoarthritic changes in the cervical spine may cause paresthesia in the neck, shoulders, and arms. The lumbar spine occasionally is affected, causing paresthesia in one or both legs and feet.

▶ *Brain tumor.* Tumors affecting the sensory cortex in the parietal lobe may cause progressive contralateral paresthesia accompanied by agnosia, apraxia, agraphia, homonymous hemianopsia, and loss of proprioception.

▶ *Buerger's disease.* With this smoking-related inflammatory occlusive disorder, exposure to cold makes the feet cold, cyanotic, and numb; later, they redden, become hot, and tingle. Intermittent claudication, which is aggravated by exercise and relieved by rest, is also common. Other findings include weak peripheral pulses, migratory superficial thrombophlebitis and, later, ulceration, muscle atrophy, and gangrene.

▶ *Diabetes mellitus.* Diabetic neuropathy can cause paresthesia with a burning sensation in the hands and legs. Other findings include insidious, permanent anosmia, fatigue, polyuria, polydipsia, weight loss, and polyphagia.

▶ *Guillain-Barré syndrome.* With this syndrome, transient paresthesia may precede muscle weakness, which usually begins in the legs and ascends to the arms and facial nerves.[1] Weakness may progress to total paralysis. Other findings include dysarthria, dysphagia, nasal speech, orthostatic hypotension, bladder and bowel incontinence, diaphoresis, tachycardia and, possibly, signs of life-threatening respiratory muscle paralysis.

▶ *Head trauma.* Unilateral or bilateral paresthesia may occur when head trauma causes a concussion or contusion; however, sensory loss is more common. Other findings include variable paresis or paralysis, decreased LOC, headache, blurred or double vision, nausea and vomiting, dizziness, and seizures.

Differential diagnosis: Paresthesia

POSSIBLE CAUSE	SIGNS AND SYMPTOMS	DIAGNOSIS
Arterial occlusion (acute)	• Sudden paresthesia and coldness in one or both legs • Abrupt pallor in leg • Paresis • Intermittent claudication • Aching pain at rest • Mottled skin with line of demarcation at level of occlusion • Absent pulses below the occlusion	• Physical examination • Imaging studies (Doppler ultrasound, angiography)
Transient ischemic attack	• Transient unilateral paralysis • Vision disturbances • Dizziness • Aphasia • Dysarthria • Decreased level of consciousness • Carotid bruit	• Physical examination • Imaging studies (carotid ultrasound, computed tomography scan) • Electrocardiogram
Vitamin B deficiency (chronic)	• Paresthesia and weakness in the arms and legs • Burning leg pain • Hypoactive deep tendon reflexes (DTRs) • Variable sensory loss • Mental changes • Impaired vision	• Diet history • Laboratory test results (complete blood count, B_{12}, serum cobalamin levels; serum B_2 activity; 24-hour urine testing for thiamine, riboflavin, niacin, and pyridoxine)
Multiple sclerosis	• Progressive muscle weakness and atrophy • Muscle spasticity • Hyperactive DTRs • Dysarthria • Dysphagia • Waxing and waning signs and symptoms • Vision disturbances • Ataxic gait • Diplopia • Intention tremors • Emotional lability • Urinary and sexual dysfunction	• Cerebrospinal fluid analysis • Magnetic resonance imaging • EEG • Evoked response testing
Migraine headache	• Paresthesia of the lips, face, and hands • Light flashes • Aura • Severe, throbbing, unilateral headache • Dizziness • Photophobia • Nausea and vomiting	• History of headache • Physical examination

TREATMENT AND FOLLOW-UP

- Medication (anticoagulants, analgesics, thrombolytics)
- Surgery

Follow-up: Referral to vascular surgeon

- Diet modification
- Exercise program
- Reduction of risk factors for stroke
- Medication (anticoagulants, platelet inhibitors, antihypertensives, antiarrhythmics)
- Surgery (if carotid stenosis is the cause)

Follow-up: Referral to neurologist or neurosurgeon

- Diet modification
- Supplementary vitamins

Follow-up: Reevaluation of vitamin levels within 3 to 6 months

- Symptomatic treatment
- Medication (antispasmotics, antidepressants, cholinergics, corticosteroids)
- Physical, speech, and occupational therapy

Follow-up: Referral to neurologist

- Rest during headache
- Cold compresses
- Medication (serotonin agonists, ergotamines, antiemetics, analgesics)
- Lifestyle or diet modification (if the trigger is identified)

Follow-up: Referral to headache clinic if uncontrolled, referral to neurologist

▶ *Heavy metal or solvent poisoning.* Exposure to industrial or household products containing lead, mercury, thallium, or organophosphates may cause paresthesia of acute or gradual onset. Mental status changes, tremors, weakness, seizures, and GI distress are also common.

▶ *Herniated disk.* Herniation of a lumbar or cervical disk may cause acute or gradual onset of paresthesia along the distribution pathways of affected spinal nerves. Other neuromuscular effects include severe pain, muscle spasms, and weakness that may progress to atrophy unless herniation is relieved.

▶ *Herpes zoster.* An early symptom of this disorder, paresthesia occurs in the dermatome supplied by the affected spinal nerve. Within several days, this dermatome is marked by a pruritic, erythematous, vesicular rash associated with sharp, shooting, or burning pain. Postherpetic neuralgia, which occurs in 40% of patients who don't receive antiviral therapy and 20% of those who do, may involve paresthesia and other forms of pain that begin 1 to 6 months after the initial herpes zoster eruption.[2]

▶ *Hyperventilation syndrome.* Usually triggered by acute anxiety, this syndrome may produce transient paresthesia in the hands, feet, and perioral area, accompanied by agitation, vertigo, syncope, pallor, muscle twitching and weakness, carpopedal spasm, and cardiac arrhythmias.

▶ *Hypocalcemia.* Asymmetrical paresthesia usually occurs in the fingers, toes, and circumoral area early in this disorder. Other signs and symptoms are muscle weakness, twitching, or cramps; palpitations; hyperactive DTRs; carpopedal spasm; and positive Chvostek's and Trousseau's signs.

▶ *Migraine headache.* Paresthesia in the hands, face, and perioral area may herald an impending migraine headache. Other prodromal symptoms include scotomas, hemiparesis, confusion, dizziness, and photophobia. These effects may persist during the characteristic throbbing headache and continue after it subsides.

▶ *Multiple sclerosis (MS).* With MS, demyelination of the sensory cortex or spinothalamic tract may produce paresthesia—typically one of the earliest symptoms. Like other effects of

MS, paresthesia commonly waxes and wanes until the later stages, when it may become permanent. Associated findings include muscle weakness, spasticity, and hyperreflexia.

▶ *Peripheral nerve trauma.* Injury to any major peripheral nerve can cause paresthesia—often dysesthesia—in the area supplied by that nerve. Paresthesia begins shortly after trauma and may be permanent. Other findings are flaccid paralysis or paresis, hyporeflexia, and variable sensory loss.

▶ *Peripheral neuropathy.* This syndrome can cause progressive paresthesia in all limbs. The patient also commonly displays muscle weakness, which may lead to flaccid paralysis and atrophy, loss of vibration sensation, diminished or absent DTRs, neuralgia, and cutaneous changes, such as glossy, red skin and anhidrosis.

▶ *Rabies.* Paresthesia, coldness, and itching at the site of an animal bite herald the prodromal stage of rabies. Other prodromal signs and symptoms are fever, headache, photophobia, hyperesthesia, tachycardia, shallow respirations, and excessive salivation, lacrimation, and perspiration.

▶ *Raynaud's disease.* Exposure to cold or stress makes the fingers turn pale, cold, and cyanotic; with rewarming, they become red and paresthetic. Ulceration may occur in chronic cases.

▶ *Seizure disorders.* Seizures originating in the parietal lobe usually cause paresthesia of the lips, fingers, and toes. The paresthesia may act as auras that precede tonic-clonic seizures.

▶ *Spinal cord injury.* Paresthesia may occur in partial spinal cord transection, after spinal shock resolves. It may be unilateral or bilateral, occurring at or below the level of the lesion. Associated sensory and motor loss is variable. (See *Understanding spinal cord syndromes,* page 335.) Spinal cord disorders may be associated with paresthesia on head flexion (Lhermitte's sign).

▶ *Spinal cord tumors.* Paresthesia, paresis, pain, and sensory loss along nerve pathways served by the affected cord segment result from such tumors. Eventually, paresis may cause spastic paralysis with hyperactive DTRs (unless the tumor is in the cauda equina,

which produces hyporeflexia) and, possibly, bladder and bowel incontinence.

▶ *Stroke.* Although contralateral paresthesia may occur with stroke, sensory loss is more common. Associated features vary with the artery affected and may include contralateral hemiplegia, decreased LOC, and homonymous hemianopsia.

▶ *Systemic lupus erythematosus.* This disorder may cause paresthesia, but its primary signs and symptoms include nondeforming arthritis (usually of hands, feet, and large joints), photosensitivity, and a "butterfly rash" across the nose and cheeks.

▶ *Tabes dorsalis.* With this disorder, paresthesia—especially of the legs—is a common, but late, symptom. Other findings include ataxia, loss of proprioception and pain and temperature sensation, absent DTRs, Charcot's joints, Argyll Robertson pupils, incontinence, and impotence.

▶ *Thoracic outlet syndrome.* Paresthesia occurs suddenly in this syndrome when the affected arm is raised and abducted. The arm also becomes pale and cool with diminished pulses. Unequal blood pressure between arms may be noted.

▶ *Transient ischemic attack (TIA).* Paresthesia typically occurs abruptly with a TIA and is limited to one arm or another isolated part of the body. It usually lasts about 10 minutes and is accompanied by paralysis or paresis. Other findings include decreased LOC, dizziness, unilateral vision loss, nystagmus, aphasia, dysarthria, tinnitus, facial weakness, dysphagia, and ataxic gait.

▶ *Vitamin B deficiency.* Chronic thiamine or vitamin B_{12} deficiency may cause paresthesia and weakness in the arms and legs. Burning leg pain, hypoactive DTRs, and variable sensory loss are common in thiamine deficiency; vitamin B_{12} deficiency also produces mental status changes and impaired vision. About 15% to 25% of older adults have vitamin B_{12} deficiency.[3]

Other causes

DRUG WATCH *Phenytoin, chemotherapy drugs (such as vincristine, vinblastine, and procarbazine), chloroquine, D-penicillamine, isoniazid, nitrofurantoin,*

Lessening symptoms of RLS

Question: *Does a conditioning program improve the symptoms of restless legs syndrome (RLS)?*

Research: RLS affects about 10% of adults. Criteria for diagnosis include a compelling urge to move the limbs, usually accompanied by paresthesias and dysesthesias; motor restlessness; symptoms worse or exclusively present at rest, possibly relieved by activity; and symptoms worse in the evening or at night. Currently, RLS is mainly treated with drugs.

This randomized controlled trial consisted of 12 weeks of aerobic and resistance training at a hospital-based wellness center. After recruitment, participants were prescreened with questions based on the diagnostic criteria for RLS. Other eligibility requirements included willingness to travel to the study site, acceptance of randomization into the exercise or control group, and no other involvement in another research project. The study physician then confirmed the RLS diagnosis, ruled out secondary causes, and ensured the absence of exclusion criteria.

The intervention consisted of lower body resistance exercises three times per week for 12 weeks, and walking on a treadmill. The exercise program was individualized and weights were increased when progress was demonstrated. The walking component of the program included instructions to walk for 30 minutes, with a 5-minute warm-up and 5-minute cool-down. The intensity of the walking was determined by heart rate and the Borg rating of perceived exertion scale.

Conclusion: Twenty-three participants completed the trial, 11 in the exercise group and 12 in the control group. At baseline, the 2 groups didn't differ significantly in RLS severity determined by the International RLS Study Group severity scale and an ordinal scale of RLS severity. However, at 6 weeks, severity scores dropped by 39% in the exercise group compared to less than 8% in the control group. The reductions were maintained during the 3-month study period, but didn't change significantly after the first 6 weeks.

Application: Assess patients for RLS using specific questions targeting the diagnostic criteria. Educate patients about lifestyle interventions thought to improve symptoms, including cigarette and alcohol cessation, caffeine avoidance, and proper sleep. Become educated about proper exercise techniques and walking to improve RLS symptoms and provide proper referrals, such as to an exercise physiologist, as indicated. Support lifestyle changes including the incorporation of aerobic and lower-body resistance training.

Source Aukerman, M. M., et al. "Exercise and Restless Legs Syndrome: A Randomized Controlled Trial," *Journal of the American Board of Family Medicine*, 19(5):487-493, 2006.

---

and parenteral gold therapy may produce transient paresthesia that disappears when the drug is discontinued.

▶ *Radiation therapy.* Long-term radiation therapy eventually may cause peripheral nerve damage, resulting in paresthesia.

Special considerations

Interventions to relieve paresthesia may include passive range of motion exercises, massage, and application of heat. (See *Lessening symptoms of RLS.*)

Pediatric pointers

Although children may experience paresthesia associated with the same causes as adults, many are unable to describe this symptom. Nevertheless, hereditary polyneuropathies are usually first recognized in childhood.

Patient counseling

Because paresthesia is commonly accompanied by patchy sensory loss, teach the patient safety measures. For example, have him test bath water with a thermometer.

REFERENCES

1. Atkinson, S.B., Carr, R.L., Maybee, P., and Haynes, D. "The Challenges of Managing and Treating Guillain-Barre Syndrome During The Acute Phase," *Dimensions of Critical Care Nursing* 25(6):256-263, November/December 2006.
2. D'Arcy, Y. "Heading Off the Pain of Postherpetic Neuralgia," *Nursing* 36(9):25-26, September 2006.
3. Pacholok, S. "Simple Steps to Stamp Out Vitamin B_{12} Deficiency," *Nursing* 37(1):67-69, January 2007.

PLEURAL FRICTION RUB

Commonly resulting from a pulmonary disorder or trauma, this loud, coarse, grating, creaking, or squeaking sound may be auscultated over one or both lungs during late inspiration or early expiration. It's heard best over the low axilla or the anterior, lateral, or posterior bases of the lung fields with the patient upright. Sometimes intermittent, it may resemble crackles or a pericardial friction rub. (See *Comparing auscultation findings,* pages 344 and 345.)

A pleural friction rub indicates inflammation of the visceral and parietal pleural lining, which causes congestion and edema. The resultant fibrinous exudate covers both pleural surfaces, displacing the fluid that's normally between them and causing the surfaces to rub together.

When you detect a pleural friction rub, quickly look for signs of respiratory distress, such as shallow or decreased respirations; crowing, wheezing, or stridor; dyspnea; increased accessory muscle use; intercostal or suprasternal retractions; cyanosis; and nasal flaring. Check for hypotension, tachycardia, and a decreased level of consciousness.

If you detect signs of distress, open and maintain an airway. Endotracheal intubation and supplemental oxygen may be needed. Insert a large-bore I.V. line to deliver drugs and fluids. Elevate the patient's head 30 degrees. Monitor cardiac status constantly, and check vital signs often.

History and physical examination

If the patient isn't in severe distress, explore related symptoms. Find out if he has had chest pain. If so, ask him to describe its location and severity. How long does the pain last? Does it radiate to his shoulder, neck, or upper abdomen? Does it worsen with breathing, movement, coughing, or sneezing? Does it abate if he splints his chest, holds his breath, or exerts pressure or lies on the affected side?

Because pain is subjective and worsened by anxiety, patients who are highly emotional may complain more readily of pleuritic pain than those who are habitually stoic about symptoms of illness.

Ask the patient about a history of rheumatoid arthritis, a respiratory or cardiovascular disorder, recent trauma, asbestos exposure, or radiation therapy. If he smokes, obtain a history in pack-years.

To distinguish a pleural friction rub from a pericardial friction rub, ask the patient to hold his breath. If the rub continues while the patient isn't breathing, it's a pericardial friction rub.[1] Characterize the pleural friction rub by auscultating the lungs with the patient sitting upright and breathing deeply and slowly through his mouth. Is the friction rub unilateral or bilateral? Listen for absent or diminished breath sounds, noting their location and timing in the respiratory cycle. Do abnormal breath sounds clear with coughing? Observe the patient for clubbing and pedal edema, which may indicate a chronic disorder. Then palpate for decreased chest motion and percuss for flatness or dullness.

Medical causes

▶ *Asbestosis.* Besides a pleural friction rub, this disorder may cause exertional dyspnea, cough, chest pain, and crackles. Clubbing is a late sign.

▶ *Lung cancer.* A pleural friction rub may be heard in the affected area of the lung. Other effects include a cough (with possible hemoptysis), dyspnea, chest pain, weight loss, anorexia, fatigue, clubbing, fever, and wheezing.

▶ *Pleurisy.* A pleural friction rub occurs early in this disorder. However, the cardinal symptom is sudden, intense chest pain that's usually unilateral and located in lower, lateral parts of the chest. Deep breathing, coughing, or thoracic movement aggravates the pain. Decreased breath sounds and inspiratory crackles may be heard over the painful area. Other findings include dyspnea, tachypnea, tachycardia, cyanosis, fever, and fatigue.

▶ *Pneumonia (bacterial).* A pleural friction rub occurs with this disorder, which usually starts with a dry, painful, hacking cough that rapidly becomes productive. Related effects develop suddenly; these include shaking chills, high fever, headache, dyspnea, pleuritic chest pain, tachypnea, tachycardia, grunting respirations, nasal flaring, dullness to percussion, and cyanosis. Auscultation reveals decreased breath sounds and fine crackles.

▶ *Pulmonary embolism.* An embolism can cause a pleural friction rub over the affected area of the lung.[2,3] Usually, the first symptom is sudden dyspnea, which may be accompanied by angina or unilateral pleuritic chest pain. Other clinical features include a nonproductive cough or a cough that produces blood-tinged sputum, tachycardia, tachypnea, low-grade fever, restlessness, and diaphoresis. Less-common findings include massive hemoptysis, chest splinting, leg edema and, with a large embolus, cyanosis, syncope, and jugular vein distention. Crackles, diffuse wheezing, decreased breath sounds, and signs of circulatory collapse may also occur.

▶ *Rheumatoid arthritis.* This disorder occasionally causes a unilateral pleural friction rub, but more typical early findings include fatigue, persistent low-grade fever, weight loss, and vague arthralgias and myalgias. Later findings include warm, swollen, painful joints; joint stiffness after inactivity; subcutaneous nodules on the elbows; joint deformity; and muscle weakness and atrophy.

▶ *Systemic lupus erythematosus.* Pulmonary involvement can cause a pleural friction rub, hemoptysis, dyspnea, pleuritic chest pain, and crackles. More characteristic effects include a butterfly rash, nondeforming joint pain and stiffness, and photosensitivity. Fever, anorexia, weight loss, and lymphadenopathy may also occur.

▶ *Tuberculosis (pulmonary).* With this disorder, a pleural friction rub may occur over the affected part of the lung. Early signs and symptoms include weight loss, night sweats, low-grade fever in the afternoon, malaise, dyspnea, anorexia, and easy fatigability. Progression of the disorder usually produces pleuritic pain, fine crackles over the upper lobes, and a productive cough with blood-streaked sputum. Advanced tuberculosis can cause chest retraction, tracheal deviation, and dullness to percussion.

Other causes
▶ *Treatments.* Thoracic surgery and radiation therapy can cause pleural friction rub.

Special considerations
Continue to monitor the patient's respiratory status and vital signs. If the patient's persistent dry, hacking cough tires him, give an antitussive. (Avoid giving an opioid, which can further depress respirations.) Give oxygen and an antibiotic. Prepare the patient for diagnostic tests such as chest X-rays.

Pediatric pointers
Auscultate for a pleural friction rub in a child who has grunting respirations, reports chest pain, or protects his chest by holding it or lying on one side. A pleural friction rub in a child is usually an early sign of pleurisy.

Geriatric pointers
In elderly patients, the intensity of pleuritic chest pain may mimic that of cardiac chest pain.

Patient counseling
Because pleuritic pain commonly accompanies a pleural friction rub, teach the patient splinting maneuvers to increase his comfort. Apply a heating pad over the affected area and administer an analgesic for pain relief. Although coughing may be painful, instruct the patient not to suppress it because coughing and deep breathing help prevent respiratory complications. Inform the patient that the pain associated with a pleural friction rub may persist even after the cause of the rub has been resolved.

(Text continues on page 346.)

Comparing auscultation findings

During auscultation, you may detect a pleural friction rub, a pericardial friction rub, or crackles—three abnormal sounds that are commonly confused. Here's help to clarify auscultation findings.

Parietal pleura
Pleural space
Visceral pleura

Pleural friction rub
Caused by inflamed visceral and parietal pleural surfaces rubbing against each other

Quality
Loud and grating, creaking, or squeaking

Location
Best heard over the low axilla or the anterior, lateral, or posterior base of the lung

Timing
Occurs in late inspiration and early expiration but ceases when the patient holds his breath; persists during coughing

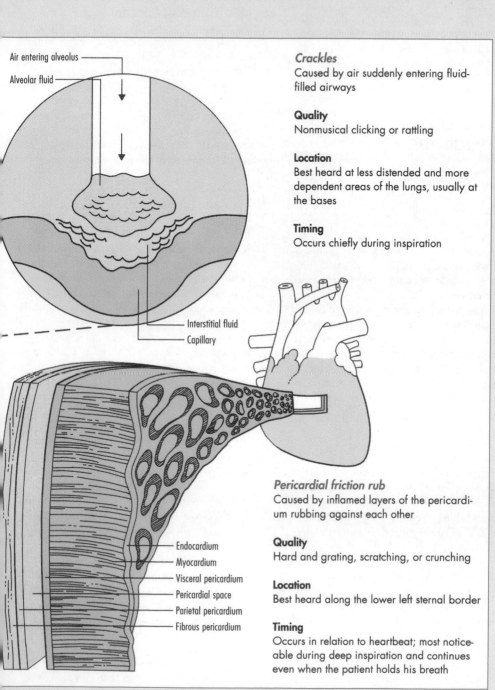

Crackles
Caused by air suddenly entering fluid-filled airways

Quality
Nonmusical clicking or rattling

Location
Best heard at less distended and more dependent areas of the lungs, usually at the bases

Timing
Occurs chiefly during inspiration

Air entering alveolus
Alveolar fluid
Interstitial fluid
Capillary

Pericardial friction rub
Caused by inflamed layers of the pericardium rubbing against each other

Quality
Hard and grating, scratching, or crunching

Location
Best heard along the lower left sternal border

Timing
Occurs in relation to heartbeat; most noticeable during deep inspiration and continues even when the patient holds his breath

Endocardium
Myocardium
Visceral pericardium
Pericardial space
Parietal pericardium
Fibrous pericardium

REFERENCES

1. McCormick, M. "Every Breath You Take: Making Sense of Breath Sounds," *Nursing Made Incredibly Easy!* 5(1):7-11, January/February 2007.
2. Sims, J.M. "An Overview of Pulmonary Embolism," *Dimensions of Critical Care Nursing* 26(5):182-186, September/October 2007.
3. Charlebois, D. "Early Recognition of Pulmonary Embolism: The Key to Lowering Mortality," *Journal of Cardiovascular Nursing* 20(4):254-259, July/August 2005.

● PRURITUS

Commonly provoking scratching to gain relief, this unpleasant itching sensation affects the skin, certain mucous membranes, and the eyes. Often more troublesome at night, pruritus may be worsened by increased skin temperature, skin dryness, local vasodilation, stress, and mechanical stimulation (such as by rubbing from clothing or scratching).

The most common symptom of dermatologic disorders, pruritus may result from a local or systemic disorder. It also may stem from psychological disorders such as compulsive, impulsive, or delusional disorders. Or a patient may have psychogenic pruritus, which is a dermatologic condition with a psychological component to the skin symptoms.[1]

History and physical examination

If the patient reports pruritus, have him describe its onset, frequency, and intensity. If it occurs at night, ask whether it keeps him from falling asleep or wakes him after he falls asleep. (Typically, pruritus related to dermatoses prevents—but doesn't disturb—sleep.) Is the itching localized or generalized? When is it most severe? How long does it last? Has it occurred in the past? Is there a relationship to activities (physical exertion, bathing, applying makeup, or use of perfumes)? Has he been scratching the area? Has he applied any topical treatment or taken any drugs for the itching?

Ask the patient how he cleans his skin. In particular, look for excessive bathing, harsh soaps, contact allergy, and excessively hot water. Does he have exposure to known skin irritants? Ask about the patient's general health and the drugs he takes (new drugs are suspect). Has he recently traveled abroad? Does he have any pets? Does anyone else in the house report itching? Does exercise, stress, fear, depression, or illness seem to aggravate the itching? Ask about contact with skin irritants, previous skin disorders, and related symptoms. Obtain a complete drug history.

Examine the affected skin area as well as the entire body for primary or secondary skin lesions, dryness, increased temperature, erythema, or other changes. Look for signs of scratching, such as excoriation, purpura, scabs, scars, or lichenification.

Medical causes

▶ *Anemia (iron deficiency).* This disorder occasionally produces pruritus. Initially asymptomatic, anemia can later cause exertional dyspnea, fatigue, listlessness, pallor, irritability, headache, tachycardia, poor muscle tone and, possibly, murmurs. Chronic anemia causes spoon-shaped (koilonychia) and brittle nails (cheilosis), cracked mouth corners, a smooth tongue (glossitis), and dysphagia.

▶ *Anthrax (cutaneous).* Anthrax is an acute infectious disease caused by the gram-positive, spore-forming bacterium *Bacillus anthracis*. It can occur in humans who are exposed to infected animals, tissue from infected animals, or biological warfare. Cutaneous anthrax occurs when the bacterium enters a cut or abrasion on the skin. The infection begins as a small, painless or pruritic macular or papular lesion resembling an insect bite. Within 1 to 2 days it develops into a vesicle and then a painless ulcer with a characteristic black, necrotic center. Lymphadenopathy, malaise, headache, or fever may develop.

▶ *Conjunctivitis.* All forms of conjunctivitis cause eye itching, burning, and pain along with photophobia, conjunctival injection, a foreign-body sensation, excessive tearing, and a feeling of fullness around the eye. Allergic conjunctivitis may also cause milky redness and a stringy eye discharge. Bacterial conjunctivitis typically causes brilliant redness and a mucopurulent, discharge that may make the eyelids stick together. Fungal conjunctivitis produces a thick, purulent discharge and crusting and sticking of the eyelid. Viral conjunctivitis may cause copious tearing—but little discharge—and preauricular lymph node enlargement.

▶ *Dermatitis.* Several types of dermatitis can cause pruritus accompanied by a skin lesion. *Atopic dermatitis* is characterized by flare-ups and remissions. A flare-up begins with intense, severe pruritus and an erythematous rash on dry skin at flexion points (antecubital fossa, popliteal area, neck). Scratching may produce edema, scaling, and pustules, and may worsen pruritus. With *chronic atopic dermatitis,* lesions may progress to dry, scaly skin with white dermatographia, blanching, and lichenification.

Mild irritants and allergic substances can cause *contact dermatitis,* with itchy small vesicles that may ooze and scale and are surrounded by redness. A severe reaction can produce marked localized edema.

Dermatitis herpetiformis, most common in men between ages 20 and 50, initially causes intense pruritus and stinging. Between 8 and 12 hours later, symmetrically distributed lesions form on the buttocks, shoulders, elbows, and knees. Sometimes, they also form on the neck, face, and scalp. These lesions are erythematous and papular, bullous, or pustular.

▶ *Enterobiasis.* Also known as *pinworm* or *seatworm,* this benign intestinal disease results from infection by *Enterobius vermicularis.* Adult worms live in the intestine; females migrate to the perianal region to deposit their eggs, causing intense perianal pruritus.

▶ *Hemorrhoids.* Anal pruritus may occur in patients with hemorrhoids along with rectal pain and constipation. External hemorrhoids may be seen outside the external anal sphincter; internal hemorrhoids are less obvious and less painful but more likely to cause rectal bleeding.

▶ *Hepatobiliary disease.* An important diagnostic clue to liver and gallbladder disease, pruritus commonly occurs with jaundice caused by non-metabolized compounds deposited in the skin; it may be generalized or localized to the palms and soles. Other characteristics include right-upper-quadrant pain,

clay-colored stools, chills and fever, flatus, belching and a bloated feeling, epigastric burning, and bitter fluid regurgitation. Later, liver disease may produce mental changes, ascites, bleeding tendencies, spider angiomas, palmar erythema, dry skin, fetor hepaticus, enlarged superficial abdominal veins, bilateral gynecomastia, testicular atrophy or menstrual irregularities, and hepatomegaly.

Pruritus gravidarum involves itching during the third trimester and probably results from gallbladder dysfunction. Jaundice is rare with this condition.

▶ *Herpes zoster.* Within 2 to 4 days of fever and malaise, pruritus, paresthesia or hyperesthesia, and severe, deep pain from cutaneous nerve involvement develop on the trunk or the arms and legs in a dermatome distribution. Up to 2 weeks after initial symptoms, red, nodular skin eruptions appear on the painful areas and become vesicular. About 10 days later, the vesicles rupture and form scabs.

▶ *Hodgkin's disease.* This disease, which is most common in young adults, occasionally causes severe and unexplained itching. As the disease progresses, pruritus may become severe and unresponsive to treatment. Early nonspecific findings include persistent fever (occasionally, cyclic fever and chills), night sweats, fatigue, weight loss, malaise, and painless swelling of a cervical lymph node. Other lymph nodes may enlarge rapidly and cause pain, or they may enlarge slowly and be painless. Later findings include retroperitoneal node enlargement, hepatomegaly, splenomegaly, dyspnea, dysphagia, dry cough, hyperpigmentation, jaundice, and pallor.

▶ *Leukemia (chronic lymphocytic).* Pruritus is an uncommon finding in this disorder. More characteristic signs and symptoms include fatigue, malaise, generalized lymphadenopathy, fever, hepatomegaly, splenomegaly, weight loss, pallor, bleeding, and palpitations.

▶ *Lichen planus.* This uncommon skin disease can cause moderate to severe pruritus that's aggravated by stress. Characteristic oral lesions (white or gray, velvety, lacy, threadlike papules) develop on the buccal mucosa and may cause pain. Violet papules with white lines or spots develop later, usually on the genitalia, lower back, ankles, and shins. Nail distortion and atrophic alopecia may also occur.

▶ *Lichen simplex chronicus.* Persistent rubbing and scratching cause localized pruritus and a circumscribed scaling patch with sharp margins. Later, the skin thickens and papules form.

▶ *Mastocytosis.* With this disorder, reddish brown macules or papules (urticaria pigmentosa), along with patchy erythema and telangiectasia occur. Other signs and symptoms include pruritus, flushing, tachycardia, hypotension, and nausea.

▶ *Multiple myeloma.* Infrequently, this disorder produces pruritus. Other findings include severe, constant back pain that increases with exercise; achiness; joint swelling and tenderness; fever; malaise; slight peripheral neuropathy; and purpura.

▶ *Mycosis fungoides.* Pruritus may precede other symptoms of this neoplastic disease by 10 years. It may persist into the first, or pre-mycotic, stage, accompanied by erythematous lesions.

▶ *Myringitis (chronic).* This disorder produces pruritus in the affected ear, along with a purulent discharge and gradual hearing loss.

▶ *Pediculosis.* A prominent symptom, pruritus occurs in the area of infestation. *Pediculosis capitis* (head lice) also may cause scalp excoriation from scratching; occipital and cervical lymphadenopathy; and oval, gray-white nits on hair shafts.

Pediculosis corporis (body lice) initially causes small red papules (usually on the shoulders, trunk, or buttocks), which become urticarial from scratching. Later, rashes or wheals may develop. Untreated, pediculosis corporis produces dry, discolored, thickly encrusted, scaly skin with bacterial infection and scarring. In severe cases, it also produces headache, fever, and malaise.

With *pediculosis pubis* (pubic lice), scratching commonly produces skin irritation. Nits or adult lice and erythematous, itching papules may appear in pubic hair or hair around the anus, abdomen, or thighs.

▶ *Pityriasis rosea.* This disorder occasionally produces mild pruritus that's aggravated by a hot bath or shower. It usually begins with an erythematous herald patch—a slightly raised, oval lesion about 2 to 6 cm in diameter. After a few days or weeks, scaly yellow-tan or erythematous patches erupt on the trunk and limbs and persist for 2 to 6 weeks. Occasionally, these patches are macular, vesicular, or urticarial.

▶ *Polycythemia vera.* This hematologic disorder can produce pruritus that's generalized or localized to the head, neck, face, and limbs. The itching is typically aggravated by a hot bath or shower and can last from a few minutes to an hour. The patient's oral mucosa may be deep purplish red, especially on the gingivae and tongue. His engorged gingivae ooze blood with even slight trauma.

Related findings include headache, dizziness, fatigue, dyspnea, paresthesia, impaired mentation, tinnitus, double or blurred vision, scotoma, hypotension, intermittent claudication, urticaria, ruddy cyanosis, and ecchymosis. GI effects include gastric distress, weight loss, and hepatosplenomegaly.

▶ *Psoriasis.* Pruritus and pain are common in psoriasis. This chronic skin disorder typically begins with small erythematous papules that enlarge or coalesce to form red elevated plaques with silver scales on the scalp, chest, elbows, knees, back, buttocks, and genitals. Nail pitting may occur.

▶ *Psychogenic pruritus.* Localized or generalized pruritus occurs without symptoms of dermatologic or systemic disease. Anxiety or emotional lability may be evident.

▶ *Renal failure (chronic).* Pruritus may develop gradually or suddenly. It may be accompanied by ammonia breath odor, oliguria or anuria, lassitude, fatigue, irritability, decreased mental acuity, seizures, coarse muscular twitching, muscle cramps, peripheral neuropathies, and coma. Renal failure also causes diverse GI signs and symptoms, such as anorexia, constipation or diarrhea, nausea, and vomiting.

▶ *Scabies.* Typically, scabies causes localized pruritus that awakens the patient. It may become generalized and persist up to 2 weeks after treatment. Threadlike lesions several millimeters long appear with a swollen nodule or red papule. The lesions have a predilection for skin folds. Crusty excoriated lesions form on the wrists, elbows, axillae, waistline, behind the knees and ankles. Excoriation from scratching is common.

▶ *Thyrotoxicosis.* Generalized pruritus may precede or accompany the characteristic signs and symptoms of this disorder: tachycardia, palpitations, weight loss despite increased appetite, diarrhea, tremors, an enlarged thyroid, dyspnea, nervousness, diaphoresis, heat intolerance and, possibly, exophthalmos.

▶ *Tinea pedis.* This fungal infection causes severe foot pruritus, pain with walking, scales and blisters between the toes, and a dry, scaly squamous inflammation on the entire sole.

▶ *Urticaria.* Extreme pruritus and stinging occur as transient erythematous or whitish wheals form on the skin or mucous membranes. Prickly sensations typically precede the wheals, which may affect any part of the body and may range from pinpoint to palm-sized or larger.

▶ *Vaginitis.* This disorder commonly causes localized pruritus and foul-smelling vaginal discharge that may be purulent, white or gray, and curdlike. Perineal pain and urinary dysfunction may also occur.

Other causes

▶ *Bedbug bites.* Typically, bedbug bites produce itching and burning over the ankles and lower legs, along with clusters of purpuric spots.

⏱ DRUG WATCH *When mild and localized, an allergic reaction to such drugs as sulfonamides and penicillin can cause pruritus, erythema, an urticarial rash, and edema. However, with a severe drug reaction, anaphylaxis may occur.*

▶ *Herbs.* Ingestion of fruit pulp from the ginkgo tree can cause rapid formation of vesicles, resulting in severe itching.

Special considerations

Administer a topical or oral corticosteroid, and an antihistamine, as ordered. Cooling agents, such as menthol or camphor, may also provide relief.[2] If the patient doesn't have a localized infection or skin lesions, suspect a systemic disease and prepare him for a complete blood count and differential, erythrocyte sedimentation rate, protein electrophoresis, and radiologic studies. Patients without evidence of a dermatologic or systemic condition as a cause for their pruritus may obtain relief with an antidepressant, antipsychotic, or a mild sedative.[1]

Controlling itching

Teach your patient these simple steps to reduce itching and increase comfort.

● Avoid scratching or rubbing the itchy areas. Ask your family to let you know if you're scratching because you may be unaware of it. Keep your fingernails short to avoid skin damage from unconscious scratching.

● Wear cool, light, loose bedclothes. Avoid wearing rough clothing—particularly wool—over the itchy area.

● Take tepid baths, using little soap and rinsing thoroughly. Try a skin-soothing oatmeal or cornstarch bath for a change.

● Apply an emollient lotion after bathing to soften and cool the skin.

● Apply cold compresses to the itchy area.

● Use topical ointments, and take prescribed drugs as directed.

● Avoid prolonged exposure to excessive heat and humidity. For maximum comfort, keep room temperatures at 68° to 70° F (20° to 21.1° C) and humidity at 30% to 40%.

● Take up an enjoyable hobby that distracts you from the itching during the day and leaves you tired enough to sleep at night.

Pediatric pointers

Many adult disorders also cause pruritus in children, but they may affect different parts of the body. For instance, scabies may affect the head in infants, but not in adults. Pityriasis rosea may affect the face, hands, and feet of adolescents.

Many childhood diseases, such as measles, chickenpox, and a variety of generalized infections are associated with skin rashes or lesions and pruritus.

Geriatric pointers

Older adults are more likely to have systemic illness or malignancy, use multiple drugs, and have dry skin, which may trigger pruritus.[3]

Patient counseling

Suggest ways to control pruritus. (See *Controlling itching.*)

REFERENCES

1. Shaw, R.J., Dayal, S., Good, J., Bruckner, A.L., and Joshi, S.V. "Psychiatric Medications for the Treatment of Pruritus," *Psychosomatic Medicine* 69(9):970-978, November/December 2007.
2. Roebuck, H.L. "For Pruritus, Combination Therapy Works Best," *The Nurse Practitioner* 31(3):12-13, March 2006.
3. "Wound and skin care: Managing Pruritus," *Nursing* 36(7):17, July 2006.

PULSE PRESSURE, WIDENED

Pulse pressure is the difference between systolic and diastolic blood pressures. Normally, systolic pressure is about 40 mm Hg higher than diastolic pressure. Widened pulse pressure—a difference of more than 50 mm Hg—commonly occurs as a physiologic response to fever, hot weather, exercise, anxiety, anemia, or pregnancy. However, it also can result from certain neurologic disorders—especially life-threatening increased intracranial pressure (ICP)—or from cardiovascular disorders that cause backflow of blood into the heart with each contraction, such as aortic insufficiency. Widened pulse pressure can be identified easily by monitoring arterial blood pressure and commonly is detected during routine sphygmomanometric recordings. (See *The predictive value of pulse pressure.*)

If the patient's level of consciousness (LOC) is decreased and you suspect that his widened pulse pressure results from increased ICP, check his vital signs and oxygen saturation. Maintain a patent airway. Provide supplemental oxygen and ventilatory support to keep partial pressure of arterial oxygen above 90 mm Hg or oxygen saturation above 95%. Perform a neurologic examination. Use the Glasgow Coma Scale to evaluate LOC. Check cranial nerve function—especially cranial nerves III, IV, and VI—and assess papillary reactions, reflexes, and muscle tone. Continue ICP monitoring. If you don't suspect increased ICP, ask about other symptoms, such as chest pain, shortness of breath, weakness, fatigue, or syncope. Check for edema, and auscultate for murmurs.

Medical causes

▶ *Aortic insufficiency.* With acute aortic insufficiency, pulse pressure widens progressively as the valve deteriorates, and a bounding pulse and an atrial gallop or ventricular gallop develop. These signs may be accompanied by chest pain; palpitations; pallor; strong, abrupt carotid pulsations; pulsus bisferiens; and signs of heart failure, such as crackles, dyspnea, and jugular vein distention. Auscultation may reveal several murmurs, such as an early diastolic murmur (common) and an apical diastolic rumble (Austin Flint murmur).

▶ *Arteriosclerosis.* With this disorder, reduced arterial compliance causes progressive widening of pulse pressure, which becomes permanent without treatment of the underlying disorder. This sign is preceded by moderate hypertension and accompanied by signs of vascular insufficiency, such as claudication, angina, and speech and vision disturbances.

▶ *Febrile disorders.* Fever can cause widened pulse pressure. Accompanying symptoms vary depending on the specific disorder.

▶ *Increased intracranial pressure.* Widening pulse pressure is an intermediate to late sign of increased ICP. Although decreased LOC is the earliest and most sensitive indicator of this life-threatening condition, the onset and progression of widening pulse pressure also parallel rising ICP. (A gap of only 50 mm Hg can signal a rapid deterioration in the patient's condition.) Assessment reveals Cushing's triad: bradycardia, hypertension, and widened pulse pressures.[5] Other findings include headache, vomiting, and impaired or unequal motor movement. The patient may also exhibit vision disturbances, such as blurring or photophobia, and pupillary changes.

Special considerations

If the patient displays increased ICP, continually reevaluate his neurologic status and compare your findings carefully with those of previous evaluations. Be alert for restlessness, confusion, unresponsiveness, or decreased LOC. Keep in mind, however, that increasing ICP is commonly signaled by subtle changes in the patient's condition, rather than the abrupt development of any one sign or symptom.

The predictive value of pulse pressure

Recent study results, such as those listed here, suggest that widened pulse pressure may be useful in predicting certain health conditions.
• In patients younger than age 60 with type 2 diabetes, pulse pressure widened for more than 24 hours is a better predictor of cardiovascular events than either systolic or diastolic blood pressure.[1]
• Widened pulse pressure is linked to an increased risk of atrial fibrillation.[2]

• After an acute stroke, pulse pressure widened for more than 24 hours is linked to an increased long-term risk of stroke recurrence.[3]
• In patients with Alzheimer's disease, widened pulse pressure is significantly related to changes in cerebral white matter.[4]

Further research is needed to determine whether altering or controlling blood pressure measurements will reduce the risk of these conditions.

Pediatric pointers

Increased ICP causes widened pulse pressure in children. Patent ductus arteriosus (PDA) also can cause it, but this sign may not be evident at birth. An older child with PDA will have exertional dyspnea with pulse pressure that widens even further on exertion.

Widened pulse pressures with bounding pulses indicate a high cardiac output state; children with these assessment findings should be monitored closely for types of distributive shock, such as septic shock or anaphylactic shock.[6]

Geriatric pointers

The aging process increases arterial stiffness, which increases systolic blood pressure and results in a widened pulse pressure.[7] Recently, widened pulse pressure has been found to be a more powerful predictor of cardiovascular events in elderly patients than either increased systolic or diastolic blood pressure.

Patient counseling

Explain needed dietary changes, such as restrictions on sodium and saturated fats. Stress the importance of planning rest periods. If the patient has a decreased LOC, discuss specific safety measures. If the condition is related to body temperature, discuss fever management, proper cooling measures if exposed to excessive heat for long periods, and proper fluid consumption with the patient.

REFERENCES

1. Nakano, S., Konishi, K., Furuya, K., Uehara, K., Nishizawa, M., Nakagawa, A., Kigoshi, T., and Uchida, K. "A Prognostic Role of Mean 24-H Pulse Pressure Level for Cardiovascular Events in Type 2 Diabetic Subjects Under 60 Years of Age," *Diabetes Care* 28(1):95-100, January 2005.
2. Mitchell, G.F., Vasan, R.S., Keyes, M.J., et al. "Pulse Pressure and Risk of New Onset Atrial Fibrillation," *JAMA* 297(7):709-715, February 2007.
3. Tsigoulis, G., Spengas, K., Zakopoulos, N., Manios, E., Xinas, K., Vassilopoulos, D., and Vennons, K.N. "Twenty-Four Hour Pulse Pressure Predicts Long-Term Recurrence in Acute Stroke Patients," *Journal of Neurology, Neurosurgery, and Psychiatry* 76(10):1360-1365, October 2005.
4. Lee, A.Y., Jeong, S., Choi, B.H., Sohn, E.H., and Chui, H. "Pulse Pressure Correlates with Leukoaraiosis in Alzheimer Disease," *Archives of Gerontology and Geriatrics* 42(2):157-166, March/April 2006.
5. Frizzell, J.P. "Acute Stroke: Pathophysiology, Diagnosis, and Treatment," *AACN Clinical Issues: Advanced Practice in Acute and Critical Care* 16(4):421-440, October/December 2005.
6. Mecham, N. "Early Recognition and Treatment of Shock in the Pediatric Patient," *Journal of Trauma Nursing* 13(1):17-21, January/March 2006.
7. Aronow, W.S., Frishman, W.H., and Cheng-Lai, A. "Cardiovascular Drug Therapy in the Elderly," *Cardiology in Review* 15(4):195-215, July/August 2007.

(Text continues on page 356.)

Abnormal pulse rhythm:
A clue to cardiac arrhythmias

An abnormal pulse rhythm may be your only clue that your patient has a cardiac arrhythmia, but this sign doesn't help you pinpoint the specific type of arrhythmia. For that, you need a cardiac monitor or an electrocardiogram (ECG) machine. These devices record the electrical current generated by the heart's conduction system and display this information on an oscilloscope screen or a strip-chart

ARRHYTHMIA

Sinus arrhythmia

Premature atrial contractions (PACs)

Paroxysmal atrial tachycardia

Atrial fibrillation

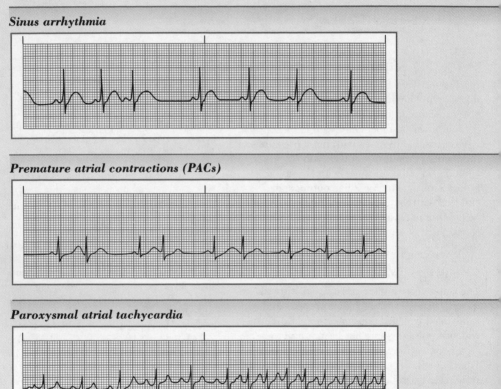

recorder. Besides rhythm disturbances, they can identify conduction defects and electrolyte imbalances.

The ECG strips below show some common cardiac arrhythmias that can cause abnormal pulse rhythms.

PULSE RHYTHM AND RATE	CLINICAL IMPLICATIONS
Irregular rhythm; fast, slow, or normal rate	• Reflex vagal tone inhibition (heart rate increases with inspiration and decreases with expiration) related to normal respiratory cycle. • May result from drugs, as in digoxin toxicity • Occurs most often in children and young adults
Irregular rhythm during PACs; fast, slow, or normal rate	• Occasional PAC may be normal • Isolated PACs indicate atrial irritation—for example, from anxiety or excessive caffeine intake. Increasing PACs may herald other atrial arrhythmias. • May result from heart failure, chronic obstructive pulmonary disease (COPD), or use of cardiac glycosides, aminophylline, or adrenergic
Regular rhythm with abrupt onset and termination of arrhythmia; heart rate exceeding 140 beats/minute	• May occur in otherwise normal, healthy persons who are suffering from physical or psychological stress, hypoxia, or digoxin toxicity; who use marijuana; or who consume excessive amounts of caffeine or other stimulants • May precipitate angina or heart failure
Irregular rhythm; atrial rate exceeding 400 beats/minute; ventricular rate varies	• May result from heart failure, COPD, hypertension, sepsis, pulmonary embolus, mitral valve disease, digoxin toxicity (rarely), atrial irritation, postcoronary bypass, or valve replacement surgery • Because atria don't contract, preload isn't consistent, so cardiac output changes with each beat. Emboli may also result.

(continued)

Abnormal pulse rhythm:
A clue to cardiac arrhythmias *(contintued)*

ARRHYTHMIA

Premature junctional contractions (PJCs)

Second-degree atrioventricular heart block, Mobitz Type I (Wenckebach)

Second-degree atrioventricular heart block, Mobitz Type II

Premature ventricular contractions (multifocal)

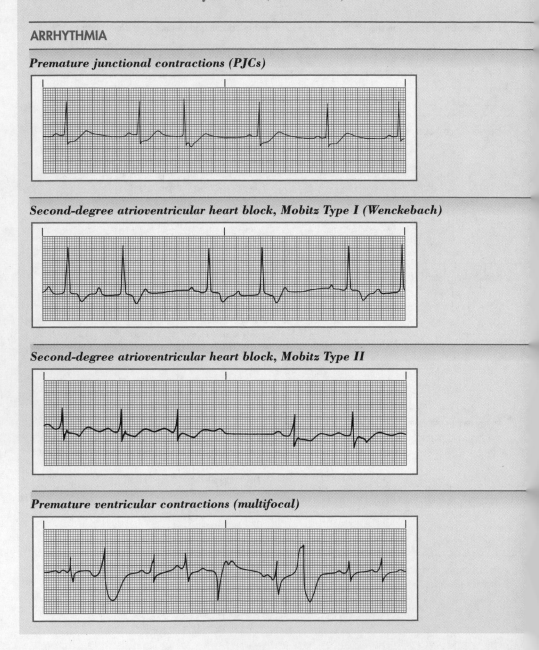

PULSE RHYTHM AND RATE	CLINICAL IMPLICATIONS
Irregular rhythm during PJCs; fast, slow, or normal rate	● May result from myocardial infarction (MI) or ischemia, excessive caffeine intake, and most commonly digoxin toxicity (from enhanced automaticity)
Irregular ventricular rhythm; fast, slow, or normal rate	● Commonly transient; may progress to complete heart block ● May result from inferior wall MI, digoxin or quinidine toxicity, vagal stimulation, electrolyte imbalance, or arteriosclerotic heart disease
Irregular ventricular rhythm; slow or normal rate	● May progress to complete heart block ● May result from degenerative disease of conduction system, ischemia of AV node in an anterior MI, anteroseptal infarction, electrolyte imbalance, or digoxin or quinidine toxicity
Usually irregular rhythm with a long pause after the premature beat; fast, slow, or normal rate	● Arise from different ventricular sites or from the same site with changing patterns of conduction ● May result from caffeine or stress, alcohol ingestion, myocardial ischemia or infarction, myocardial irritation by pacemaker electrodes, hypocalcemia, hypercalcemia, digoxin toxicity, or exercise

PULSE RHYTHM ABNORMALITY

An abnormal pulse rhythm is an irregular expansion and contraction of the peripheral arterial walls. It may be persistent or sporadic, and rhythmic or arrhythmic. Detected by palpating the radial or carotid pulse, an abnormal rhythm is typically reported first by the patient, who complains of feeling palpitations. This important finding reflects an underlying cardiac arrhythmia, which may range from benign to life-threatening.[1] Arrhythmias are commonly associated with cardiovascular, renal, respiratory, metabolic, and neurologic disorders as well as the effects of drugs, diagnostic tests, and treatments. (See *Abnormal pulse rhythm: A clue to cardiac arrhythmias*, pages 352 to 355.)

Quickly look for signs of reduced cardiac output, such as decreased level of consciousness (LOC), hypotension, or dizziness.

Promptly obtain an electrocardiogram (ECG) and, possibly, a chest X-ray, and start cardiac monitoring to identify the cardiac arrhythmia and guide treatment options.[2] Insert an I.V. line for giving emergency cardiac drugs, and immediately flush each drug with 20 ml of normal saline solution.[2] Give oxygen by nasal cannula or mask. Closely monitor vital signs, pulse quality, and cardiac rhythm because bradycardia or tachycardia may reduce tolerance of the abnormal rhythm and cause further deterioration of cardiac output. Keep emergency intubation, cardioversion, and suction equipment handy.

History and physical examination

If the patient's condition permits, ask if he's in pain. If so, find out about onset and location. Does the pain radiate? Ask about a history of heart disease and treatments for arrhythmias. Obtain a drug history and check compliance. Also, ask about caffeine or alcohol intake. Digoxin toxicity, cessation of an antiarrhythmic, and use of quinidine, a sympathomimetic (such as epinephrine), caffeine, or alcohol may cause arrhythmias.

Next, check the patient's apical and peripheral arterial pulses. An apical rate exceeding a peripheral arterial rate indicates a pulse deficit, which may also cause associated signs and symptoms of low cardiac output. Evaluate heart sounds: A long pause between S_1 (*lub*) and S_2 (*dub*) may indicate a conduction defect. A faint or absent S_1 and an easily audible S_2 may indicate atrial fibrillation or flutter. You may hear the two heart sounds close together on certain beats—possibly indicating premature atrial contractions—or other variations in heart rate or rhythm. Take the patient's radial pulses while you listen for heart sounds. With some arrhythmias, such as premature ventricular contractions, you may hear the beat with your stethoscope but not feel it over the radial artery. This indicates an ineffective contraction that failed to produce a peripheral pulse. Next, count the apical pulse for 60 seconds, noting the frequency of skipped peripheral beats. Report your findings to the physician.

Medical causes

▶ *Arrhythmias.* An abnormal pulse rhythm may be the only sign of a cardiac arrhythmia. The patient may complain of palpitations, a fluttering heartbeat, or weak and skipped beats. Pulses may be weak and rapid or slow. Depending on the specific arrhythmia, dull chest pain or discomfort and hypotension may occur. Related findings, if any, reflect decreased cardiac output. Neurologic findings, for example, include confusion, dizziness, light-headedness, decreased LOC and, sometimes, seizures. Other findings include decreased urine output, dyspnea, tachypnea, pallor, and diaphoresis.

Special considerations

The patient may need to be sedated before cardioversion therapy. Also give antiarrhythmics, as ordered.[3] Prepare the patient for transfer to a cardiac or intensive care unit, if indicated. If the patient remains in your care, he may require bed rest or help with ambulation, depending on his condition. To prevent falls and injury, raise the side rails of his bed and don't leave him unattended while he's sitting or walking. Check vital signs often to detect bradycardia, tachycardia, hypertension or hypotension, tachypnea, and dyspnea. Also monitor intake, output, and daily weight.

Collect blood samples for serum electrolyte, cardiac enzyme, and drug level studies. Prepare the patient for a chest X-ray and a 12-lead ECG. If possible, obtain a previous ECG to compare with current findings. Prepare the patient for 24-hour Holter monitoring.

Pediatric pointers
Arrhythmias also produce pulse rhythm abnormalities in children.

Patient counseling
Instruct the patient to keep a diary of activities and symptoms to correlate with the occurrence of arrhythmias. Explain the importance of avoiding tobacco and caffeine, both of which increase arrhythmias. Provide information on smoking cessation programs. Discuss strategies to improve drug compliance.

Teach the patient how to take his pulse rate, and advise him to notify his physician if he detects an abnormality. Explain the signs and symptoms he should report to his physician immediately as well as those that warrant emergency care.

REFERENCES
1. "Take note when hearts march to a different beat," *Nursing Critical Care* 1(1):8-9, January 2006.
2. Fugate, J.H. "Pharmacologic Management of Cardiac Emergencies," *Journal of Infusion Nursing* 29(3):147-150, May/June 2006.
3. Palatnik, A. "And The Beat Goes On..." *Nursing Made Incredibly Easy!* 3(1):30-41, January/February 2005.

RESPIRATIONS, GRUNTING

Characterized by a deep, low-pitched grunting sound at the end of each breath, grunting respirations are a chief sign of respiratory distress in infants and children. They may be soft and heard only on auscultation, or loud and clearly audible without a stethoscope. Typically, the intensity of grunting respirations reflects the severity of respiratory distress. The grunting sound coincides with closure of the glottis, an effort to increase end-expiratory pressure in the lungs and prolong alveolar gas exchange, thereby enhancing ventilation and perfusion.[1]

Grunting respirations indicate intrathoracic disease with lower respiratory involvement. Although most common in children, they sometimes occur in adults in severe respiratory distress. Whether they occur in children or adults, grunting respirations demand immediate medical attention. (See *Positioning an infant for chest physical therapy,* pages 360 and 361.)

If the patient has grunting respirations, quickly place him in a comfortable position and check for signs of respiratory distress, such as wheezing; tachypnea (at least 60 breaths/minute in infants, 40 breaths/minute in children ages 1 to 5, 30 breaths/minute in children older than age 5, or 20 breaths/minute in adults); accessory muscle use; substernal, subcostal, or intercostal retractions; nasal flaring; tachycardia (at least 160 beats/minute in infants, 120 to 140 beats/minute in children ages 1 to 5, 120 beats/minute in children older than age 5, or 100 beats/minute in adults); cyanotic lips or nail beds; hypotension (less than 80/40 mm Hg in infants, less than 80/50 mm Hg in children ages 1 to 5, less than 90/55 mm Hg in children older than age 5, or less than 90/60 mm Hg in adults); and decreased level of consciousness.

If you detect any of these signs, monitor oxygen saturation, and give oxygen and prescribed drugs, such as a bronchodilator. Have emergency equipment available, and prepare to intubate the patient if needed. Obtain arterial blood gas (ABG) analysis to determine oxygenation status.

History and physical examination

After addressing the child's respiratory status, ask his parents when the grunting respirations began. If the patient is a premature infant, find out his gestational age. Ask the parents if anyone in the home has had an upper respiratory tract infection recently. Has the child had signs and symptoms of such an infection, such as a runny nose, cough, low-grade fever, or anorexia? Does he have a history of frequent colds or upper respiratory tract infections? Does he have a history of respiratory syncytial virus? Ask the parents to describe changes in the child's activity level or feeding pattern to determine if the child is lethargic or less alert than usual.

Begin the physical examination by auscultating the lungs, especially the lower lobes. Note diminished or abnormal sounds, such as crackles or sibilant rhonchi, which may indicate mucus or fluid buildup. Characterize the color, amount, and consistency of any discharge or sputum. Note the characteristics of the cough, if any.

Medical causes

▶ *Asthma.*Grunting respirations may occur during a severe asthma attack, usually triggered by a upper respiratory tract infection or an allergic response. As the attack progresses, the patient may have dyspnea, audible wheezing, chest tightness, and coughing. He may have a silent chest if air movement is poor. Immediate bronchodilator therapy is needed.

▶ *Heart failure.* A late sign of left-sided heart failure, grunting respirations accompany increasing pulmonary edema. Other features include a productive cough, crackles, jugular vein distention, and chest wall retractions. Cyanosis also may be evident, depending on the underlying congenital cardiac defect.

▶ *Pneumonia.* Life-threatening bacterial pneumonia is common after an upper respiratory tract infection or cold. *Pneumocystis jiroveci* (formerly *carinii*) pneumonia commonly affects children infected with human immunodeficiency virus. It causes grunting respirations with high fever, tachypnea, a productive cough, anorexia, and lethargy. Auscultation reveals diminished breath sounds, scattered crackles, and sibilant rhonchi over the affected lung. As the disorder progresses, the patient also may develop severe dyspnea, substernal and subcostal retractions, nasal flaring, cyanosis, and increasing lethargy. Some infants have GI signs, such as vomiting, diarrhea, and abdominal distention.

▶ *Respiratory distress syndrome.* The result of lung immaturity in a premature infant (less than 37 weeks' gestation) usually of low birth weight, this syndrome initially causes audible expiratory grunting along with intercostal, subcostal, or substernal retractions; tachycardia; and tachypnea. Later, as respiratory distress tires the infant, apnea or irregular respirations replace the grunting. Severe respiratory distress is characterized by cyanosis, frothy sputum, dramatic nasal flaring, lethargy, bradycardia, and hypotension. Eventually, the infant becomes unresponsive. Auscultation reveals harsh, diminished breath sounds and crackles over the base of the lungs on deep inspiration. Oliguria and peripheral edema also may occur.

▶ *Respiratory syncytial virus (RSV) infection.* This virus can cause bronchiolitis or pneumonia, usually in infants and children less than age 2 years.[2] RSV pneumonia may cause grunting respirations, retractions, tachypnea, and, possibly, vomiting and dehydration.

Special considerations

Closely monitor the patient's condition. Keep emergency equipment nearby in case respiratory distress worsens. Prepare to give oxygen using an oxygen hood or tent. Continually monitor ABG levels, and deliver the minimum amount of oxygen possible to avoid causing retinopathy of prematurity from high oxygen levels.

Begin inhalation therapy with a bronchodilator, and give an I.V. antimicrobial if the patient has pneumonia (or, in some cases, status asthmaticus). Follow these measures with chest physical therapy as needed.

Prepare the patient for chest X-rays. Because sedatives are contraindicated during respiratory distress, resrain a restless child during testing, if needed. To prevent exposure to radiation, wear a lead apron and cover the child's genital area with a lead shield. If a blood culture is ordered, be sure to record on the laboratory slip any current antibiotic use.

Remember to explain all procedures to the patient's parents and to provide emotional support.

Patient counseling

Teach the patient's parents how to perform respiratory care and therapy in the home. Instruct them in the proper use of prescribed drugs. Explain signs and symptoms that need immediate attention. If the grunting is related to asthma, teach the parents measures to assist them in managing the condition and reducing allergens in the home environment.

REFERENCES

1. McCaskey, M.S. "Pediatric Assessment: The Little Differences," *Home Healthcare Nurse* 25(1):20-24, January 2007.
2. Pruitt, B. "Keeping Respiratory Syncytial Virus At Bay," *Nursing* 35(11):62-64, November 2005.

Positioning an infant for chest physical therapy

An infant with grunting respirations may need chest physical therapy to mobilize and drain excess lung secretions. Auscultate first to locate congested areas, and review the illustrations here to determine the best drainage position and where to place your hands for percussion. When you percuss the infant, use the fingers of one hand. Vibrate these fingers and move them toward the infant's head to facilitate drainage.

Hold the infant upright and about 30 degrees forward to percuss and drain the apical segments of the upper lobes.

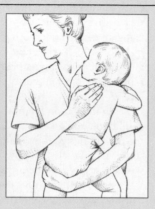

Place the infant in a supine position to percuss and drain the anterior segments of the upper lobes.

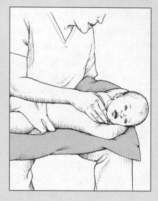

Use this position to percuss and drain the posterior segments of the upper lobes.

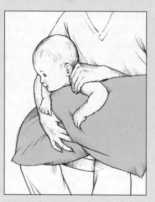

Hold the infant at a 45-degree angle on his side with his head down about 15 degrees to percuss and drain the right middle lobe.

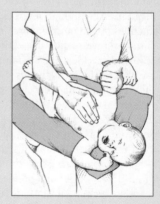

● RESPIRATIONS, SHALLOW

Respirations are shallow when a reduced volume of air enters the lungs during inspiration. To obtain enough air, a patient with shallow respirations usually breathes at an increased rate. However, as he tires or as his muscles weaken, this compensatory increase in respirations declines, leading to inadequate gas exchange and such signs as dyspnea, cyanosis, confusion, agitation, loss of consciousness, and tachycardia.

Shallow respirations may develop suddenly or gradually and may last briefly or become chronic. They're a key sign of respiratory distress and neurologic deterioration. Causes include inadequate central respiratory control over breathing, neuromuscular disorders, increased resistance to airflow into the lungs, respiratory muscle fatigue or weakness, vol-

Place the infant in a supine position with his head 30 degrees lower than his feet to percuss and drain the anterior segments of the lower lobes.

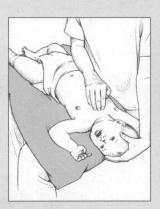

Place the infant in a prone position with his head down 30 degrees to percuss and drain the posterior basal segments of the lower lobes.

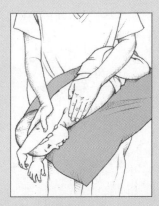

Place the infant on his side with his head down 30 degrees to percuss and drain the lateral basal segments of the lower lobes. Repeat this on the other side.

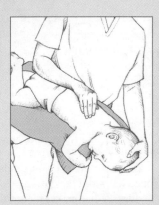

Use a prone position to percuss and drain the superior segments of the lower lobes.

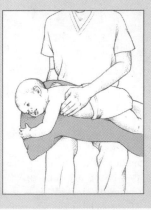

untary alterations in breathing, decreased activity from prolonged bed rest, and pain.

If you observe shallow respirations, be alert for impending respiratory failure or arrest. Is the patient severely dyspneic? Agitated or frightened? Look for signs of airway obstruction. If the patient is choking, perform four back blows and then four abdominal thrusts, to try to expel the foreign object. Use suction if secretions occlude the patient's airway.

If the patient is also wheezing, check for stridor, nasal flaring, and use of accessory muscles. Give oxygen with a face mask or a handheld resuscitation bag. Attempt to calm the patient. Give epinephrine I.V.

If the patient loses consciousness, insert an artificial airway and prepare for endotracheal intubation and ventilatory support. Measure his tidal volume and minute volume with a Wright respirometer to determine the need for mechanical ventilation. (See *Measuring lung*

Measuring lung volumes

Use a Wright respirometer to measure tidal volume (the amount of air inspired with each breath) and minute volume (the volume of air inspired in a minute—or tidal volume multiplied by respiratory rate). You can connect the respirometer to an intubated patient's airway via an endotracheal tube (shown here) or a tracheostomy tube. If the patient isn't intubated, connect the respirometer to a face mask, making sure the seal over the patient's mouth and nose is airtight.

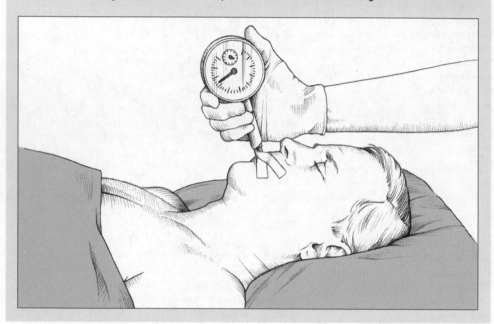

volumes.) Check arterial blood gas (ABG) levels, heart rate, blood pressure, and oxygen saturation. Tachycardia, increased or decreased blood pressure, poor minute volume, and deteriorating ABGs or oxygen saturation signal the need for intubation and mechanical ventilation.

History and physical examination

If the patient isn't in severe respiratory distress, start with the history. Ask about chronic illness and any surgery or trauma. Has he had a tetanus booster in the past 10 years? Does he have asthma, allergies, or a history of heart failure or vascular disease? Does he have a chronic respiratory disorder or respiratory tract infection, tuberculosis, or a neurologic or neuromuscular disease? Does he smoke?

Obtain a drug history, too, and explore the possibility of drug abuse.

Ask about the patient's shallow respirations: When did they begin? How long do they last? What makes them subside? What aggravates them? Ask about changes in appetite, weight, activity level, and behavior.

Begin the physical examination by assessing the patient's level of consciousness and his orientation to time, person, and place. Observe spontaneous movements, and test muscle strength and deep tendon reflexes. Next, inspect the chest for deformities or abnormal movements such as intercostal retractions. Inspect the limbs for cyanosis and digital clubbing.

Palpate for expansion and diaphragmatic tactile fremitus, and percuss for hyperresonance or dullness. Auscultate for reduced, absent, or adventitious breath sounds and for abnormal or distant heart sounds. Do you note any peripheral edema? Finally, examine the abdomen for distention, tenderness, or masses.

Medical causes

▶ *Acute respiratory distress syndrome.* Initially, this life-threatening syndrome produces rapid, shallow respirations and dyspnea, at times after the patient appears stable.[1] Hypoxemia leads to intercostal and suprasternal retractions, diaphoresis, and fluid accumulation, causing rhonchi and crackles. As hypoxemia worsens, the patient has more trouble breathing, restlessness, apprehension, decreased level of consciousness, cyanosis and, possibly, tachycardia.

▶ *Amyotrophic lateral sclerosis (ALS).* Respiratory muscle weakness in this disorder causes progressive shallow respirations. Exertion may result in increased weakness and respiratory distress. ALS initially produces weakness and wasting of arm muscles, which in several years affects the trunk, neck, tongue, and muscles of the larynx, pharynx, and legs. Other signs and symptoms include muscle cramps and atrophy, hyperreflexia, slight spasticity of the legs, coarse fasciculations of the affected muscle, impaired speech, and difficulty chewing and swallowing.

▶ *Asthma.* During an acute attack, bronchospasm and hyperinflation of the lungs cause rapid, shallow respirations. Related respiratory effects include wheezing, rhonchi, a dry cough, dyspnea, prolonged expirations, intercostal and supraclavicular retractions on inspiration, nasal flaring, and use of accessory muscles. Chest tightness, tachycardia, diaphoresis, and flushing or cyanosis may occur.

▶ *Atelectasis.* Decreased lung expansion or pleuritic pain causes sudden onset of rapid, shallow respirations. Other signs and symptoms include a dry cough, dyspnea, tachycardia, anxiety, cyanosis, and diaphoresis. Examination reveals dullness to percussion, decreased breath sounds and vocal fremitus, inspiratory lag, and substernal or intercostal retractions.

▶ *Botulism.* With this disorder, progressive muscle weakness and paralysis initially cause shallow respirations. Within 4 days, the patient develops respiratory distress from respiratory muscle paralysis. Early signs and symptoms include bilateral mydriasis and nonreactive pupils, anorexia, nausea, vomiting, diarrhea, dry mouth, blurred vision, diplopia, ptosis, strabismus, and extraocular muscle palsies. Others quickly follow, including vertigo, deafness, hoarseness, constipation, nasal voice, dysarthria, and dysphagia.

▶ *Bronchiectasis.* Increased secretions obstruct airflow in the lungs, leading to shallow respirations and a productive cough with copious, foul-smelling, mucopurulent sputum (a classic finding). Other findings include hemoptysis, wheezing, rhonchi, coarse crackles during inspiration, and late-stage clubbing. The patient may complain of weight loss, fatigue, exertional weakness and dyspnea, fever, malaise, and halitosis.

▶ *Chronic bronchitis.* Airway obstruction causes chronic shallow respirations. This disorder may start with a nonproductive, hacking cough that later becomes productive. It also may cause prolonged expirations, wheezing, dyspnea, accessory muscle use, barrel chest, cyanosis, tachypnea, scattered rhonchi, coarse crackles, and clubbing (a late sign).

▶ *Coma.* Rapid, shallow respirations result from neurologic dysfunction or restricted chest movement.

▶ *Emphysema.* Increased breathing effort causes muscle fatigue, leading to chronic shallow respirations. The patient also may have dyspnea, anorexia, malaise, tachypnea, reduced breath sounds, cyanosis, pursed-lip breathing, accessory muscle use, barrel chest, chronic productive cough, and clubbing (a late sign).

▶ *Flail chest.* With this disorder, decreased air movement results in rapid, shallow respirations, paradoxical chest wall motion from rib instability, tachycardia, hypotension, ecchymoses, cyanosis, and pain over the affected area.

▶ *Fractured ribs.* Pain on inspiration and possibly expiration may cause shallow respirations.

▶ *Guillain-Barré syndrome.* Progressive ascending paralysis causes rapid or progressive onset of shallow respirations. Muscle weakness begins in the lower limbs and extends finally to the face. Other findings include paresthesia, dysarthria, diminished or absent corneal reflex, nasal speech, dysphagia, ipsilateral loss of facial muscle control, and flaccid paralysis.

▶ *Kyphoscoliosis.* Skeletal cage distortion eventually can cause rapid, shallow respirations from reduced lung capacity. It also causes back pain, fatigue, tracheal deviation, and dyspnea.

▶ *Multiple sclerosis.* Muscle weakness causes progressive shallow respirations. Early features include diplopia, blurred vision, and paresthesia. Other possible findings are nystagmus, constipation, paralysis, spasticity, hyperreflexia, intention tremor, ataxic gait, dysphagia, dysarthria, urinary dysfunction, impotence, and emotional lability.

▶ *Muscular dystrophy.* With progressive thoracic deformity and muscle weakness, shallow respirations may occur along with waddling gait, contractures, scoliosis, lordosis, and muscle atrophy or hypertrophy.

▶ *Myasthenia gravis.* Progression of this disorder causes respiratory muscle weakness marked by shallow respirations, dyspnea, and cyanosis.[2] Other effects include fatigue, weak eye closure, ptosis, diplopia, and difficulty chewing and swallowing.

▶ *Obesity.* Morbid obesity may cause shallow respirations due to the work of breathing associated with movement of the chest wall. Heart and breath sounds may be distant.

▶ *Parkinson's disease.* Fatigue and weakness lead to progressive shallow respirations. Typically, this disorder slowly progresses to increased rigidity (lead-pipe or cogwheel), masklike facies, stooped posture, shuffling gait, dysphagia, drooling, dysarthria, and pill-rolling tremor.

▶ *Pleural effusion.* With this disorder, restricted lung expansion causes shallow respirations, starting suddenly or gradually. Other findings include nonproductive cough, weight loss, dyspnea, and pleuritic chest pain. Examination reveals pleural friction rub, tachycardia, tachypnea, decreased chest motion, flatness to percussion, egophony, decreased or absent breath sounds, and decreased tactile fremitus.

▶ *Pneumonia.* Pulmonary consolidation results in rapid, shallow respirations. The patient may experience dyspnea, fever, shaking chills, chest pain, cough, tachycardia, decreased breath sounds, crackles, and rhonchi. He also may develop myalgias, fatigue, anorexia, headache, abdominal pain, cyanosis, and diaphoresis.

▶ *Pneumothorax.* This disorder causes a sudden onset of shallow respirations and dyspnea. Related effects include tachycardia; tachypnea; sudden sharp, severe chest pain (commonly unilateral) worsening with movement; nonproductive cough; cyanosis; accessory muscle use; asymmetrical chest expansion; anxiety; restlessness; hyperresonance or tympany on the affected side; subcutaneous crepitation; decreased vocal fremitus; and diminished or absent breath sounds on the affected side.

▶ *Pulmonary edema.* Pulmonary vascular congestion causes rapid, shallow respirations. Early signs and symptoms include exertional dyspnea, paroxysmal nocturnal dyspnea, nonproductive cough, tachycardia, tachypnea, dependent crackles, and a ventricular gallop. Severe pulmonary edema produces more rapid, labored respirations; widespread crackles; a productive cough with frothy, bloody sputum; worsening tachycardia; arrhythmias; cold, clammy skin; cyanosis; hypotension; and thready pulse.

▶ *Pulmonary embolism.* This disorder causes sudden, rapid, shallow respirations and severe dyspnea with angina or pleuritic chest pain. Other clinical features include tachycardia, tachypnea, a nonproductive cough or a productive cough with blood-tinged sputum, low-grade fever, restlessness, diaphoresis, pleural friction rub, crackles, diffuse wheezing, dullness to percussion, decreased breath sounds, and signs of circulatory collapse. Less-common findings are massive hemoptysis, chest splinting, leg edema, and (with a large embolism) cyanosis, syncope, and jugular vein distention.

▶ *Spinal injury.* Diaphragmatic breathing and shallow respirations may occur in injury to the C5 to C8 area. Other findings include quadriplegia with flaccidity followed by spastic paralysis, areflexia, hypotension, sensory loss below the level of injury, and bowel and bladder incontinence.

▶ *Tetanus.* With this now-rare disorder, spasm of the intercostal muscles and the diaphragm causes shallow respirations. Late findings typically include jaw pain and stiffening, difficulty opening the mouth, tachycardia, profuse diaphoresis, hyperactive deep tendon reflexes, and opisthotonos.

▶ *Upper airway obstruction.* Partial airway obstruction causes acute shallow respirations with sudden gagging and dry, paroxysmal coughing; hoarseness; stridor; and tachycardia. Other findings include dyspnea, decreased breath sounds, wheezing, and cyanosis.

Other causes

DRUG WATCH *Anesthetics, hypnotics, magnesium sulfate, neuromuscular blockers, opioids, sedatives, and tranquilizers can produce slow, shallow respirations.*

▶ *Surgery.* After abdominal or thoracic surgery, pain linked to chest splinting and decreased chest wall motion may cause shallow respirations.

Special considerations

Prepare the patient for diagnostic tests: ABG analysis, pulmonary function tests, chest X-rays, or bronchoscopy.

Position the patient as nearly upright as possible to ease his breathing. (Help a postoperative patient splint his incision while coughing.) If he's taking a drug that depresses respirations, follow all precautions, and monitor him closely. Ensure adequate hydration, and use humidification as needed to thin secretions and to relieve inflamed, dry, or irritated airway mucosa. Give humidified oxygen, a bronchodilator, a mucolytic, an expectorant, or an antibiotic, as ordered.

Turn the patient often. He may need chest physiotherapy, incentive spirometry, or intermittent positive-pressure breathing. Watch for increasing lethargy, which may indicate rising carbon dioxide levels. Have emergency equipment at the patient's bedside.

If your patient is obese, proper positioning is important to promote ventilation. Reverse Trendelenberg positioning improves ventilatory mechanics by shifting weight off the diaphragm and chest area. The reverse Trende-lengerg position at 45 degrees increases arterial oxygenation and tidal volumes and to decrease the respiratory rate.[3]

Pediatric pointers

In children, shallow respirations commonly indicate a life-threatening condition. Airway obstruction can occur rapidly because of the narrow passageways; if it does, administer back blows or chest thrusts but not abdominal thrusts, which can damage internal organs.

Causes of shallow respirations in infants and children include idiopathic (infant) respiratory distress syndrome, acute epiglottiditis, diphtheria, aspiration of a foreign body, croup, acute bronchiolitis, cystic fibrosis, and bacterial pneumonia.

Observe the child to detect apnea. As needed, use humidification and suction, and give supplemental oxygen. Give parenteral fluids to ensure adequate hydration. Chest physiotherapy may be required.

Geriatric pointers

Stiffness or deformity of the chest wall with aging may cause shallow respirations.

Patient counseling

Have the patient cough and deep-breathe every hour to clear secretions and counteract possible hypoventilation. Provide assistance with tracheal suctioning as needed.

REFERENCES

1. Taylor, M.M. "ARDS Diagnosis and Management: Implications for the Critical Care Nurse," *Dimensions of Critical Care Nursing* 24(5):197-207, September/October 2005.
2. Bershad, E.M., Feen, E.S., and Suarez, J.I. "Myasthenia Gravis Crisis," *Southern Medical Journal* 101(1):63-69, January 2008.
3. Pieracci, F.M., Barie, P.S., and Pomp, A. "Critical Care of the Bariatric Patient," *Critical Care Medicine* 34(6):1796-1804, June 2006.

RESPIRATIONS, STERTOROUS

Characterized by a harsh, rattling, or snoring sound, stertorous respirations usually result from the vibration of relaxed oropharyngeal structures during sleep or coma, causing partial airway obstruction. Less often, these respirations result from retained mucus in the upper airway.

This common sign occurs in about 10% of normal people, especially middle-aged, obese men. It may be aggravated by use of alcohol or a sedative before bed, which increases oropharyngeal flaccidity, and by sleeping in the supine position, which allows the relaxed tongue to slip back into the airway. The major pathologic causes of stertorous respirations are obstructive sleep apnea and life-threatening upper airway obstruction associated with an oropharyngeal tumor or with uvular or palatal edema. This obstruction also may occur during the postictal phase of a generalized seizure when mucous secretions or a relaxed tongue blocks the airway.

Occasionally, stertorous respirations are mistaken for stridor, which is another sign of upper airway obstruction. However, stridor indicates laryngeal or tracheal obstruction, whereas stertorous respirations signal higher airway obstruction.

If you detect stertorous respirations, check the patient's mouth and throat for edema, redness, masses, or foreign objects. If edema is marked, quickly take vital signs and check oxygen saturation. Observe the patient for evidence of respiratory distress, such as dyspnea, tachypnea, use of accessory muscles, intercostal muscle retractions, and cyanosis. Elevate the head of the bed 30 degrees to help ease breathing and reduce the edema. Then give supplemental oxygen by nasal cannula or face mask, and prepare to intubate the patient, perform a tracheostomy, or provide mechanical ventilation. Insert an I.V. line for fluid and drug access, and begin cardiac monitoring.

If you detect stertorous respirations while the patient is sleeping, observe his breathing pattern for 3 to 4 minutes. Do noisy respirations cease when he turns on his side and recur when he assumes a supine position?

Watch carefully for periods of apnea and note their length. When possible, question the patient's partner about his snoring habits. Is she frequently awakened by the patient's snoring? Does the snoring improve if the patient sleeps with the window open? Has she also observed the patient talk in his sleep or sleepwalk? Ask about signs of sleep deprivation, such as personality changes, headaches, daytime somnolence, or decreased mental acuity.

Medical causes

▶ *Airway obstruction.* Regardless of its cause, partial airway obstruction may lead to stertorous respirations with wheezing, dyspnea, tachypnea and, later, intercostal retractions and nasal flaring. If the obstruction becomes complete, the patient abruptly loses his ability to talk and displays diaphoresis, tachycardia, and inspiratory chest movement but absent breath sounds. Severe hypoxemia rapidly ensues, resulting in cyanosis, loss of consciousness, and cardiopulmonary collapse.

▶ *Obstructive sleep apnea (OSA).* Loud and disruptive snoring is a major characteristic of this syndrome, which commonly affects the obese. Typically, the snoring alternates with periods of sleep apnea, which usually end with loud gasping sounds. Alternating tachycardia and bradycardia may occur.

Episodes of snoring and apnea recur in a cyclic pattern throughout the night. Sleep disturbances, such as somnambulism and talking during sleep, also may occur. Some patients have hypertension and ankle edema. Most awaken in the morning with a generalized headache, feeling tired and unrefreshed. The most common complaint is excessive daytime sleepiness. Lack of sleep may cause depression, hostility, and decreased mental acuity.

Other causes

▶ *Endotracheal intubation, suction, or surgery.* These procedures may cause significant palatal or uvular edema, resulting in stertorous respirations.

Special considerations

Monitor the patient's respiratory status carefully. Give a corticosteroid or an antibiotic and cool, humidified oxygen to reduce palatal and uvular inflammation and edema. Laryngoscopy and bronchoscopy (to rule out airway obstruction) or formal sleep studies may be needed.

To decrease the occurrence of stertorous respirations in OSA, patients may be treated with continuous positive airway pressure or noninvasive positive pressure ventilation at night. These therapies help keep the airway open and ease ventilation, especially during perioperative and postoperative periods.[1]

Pediatric pointers

In children, stertorous respirations result most often from a foreign body or from nasal or pharyngeal obstruction caused by tonsillar or adenoid hypertrophy.

Geriatric pointers

Older adults with OSA have the chronic loud snoring and daytime drowsiness typical of the disorder, but they may attribute the snoring, sleepiness, and need for daytime naps to normal aging.[2] Urge the patient to seek treatment for sleep apnea if he has signs and symptoms.

Patient counseling

If the patient is overweight, discuss the importance and methods of weight loss. Explain the assembly and use of a continuous or bilevel positive airway pressure device for a patient with sleep apnea. Teach the patient to elevate his head while sleeping. If the patient smokes, provide information and recommend a smoking cessation program.

REFERENCES

1. Gross, J.B., et al. "Practice Guidelines for the Perioperative Management of Patients with Obstructive Sleep Apnea: A Report by the American Society of Anesthesiologists Task Force on Perioperative Management of Patients with Obstructive Sleep Apnea," *Anesthesiology* 104(5):1081-1093, May 2006.
2. Norman, D., and Loredo, J.S. "Obstructive Sleep Apnea in Older Adults," *Clinics in Geriatric Medicine* 24(1):151-165, February 2008.

RETRACTIONS, COSTAL AND STERNAL

A cardinal sign of respiratory distress in infants and children, retractions are visible indentations of the soft tissue covering the chest wall. They may be suprasternal (directly above the sternum and clavicles), intercostal (between the ribs), subcostal (below the lower costal margin of the rib cage), or substernal (just below the xiphoid process). Retractions may be mild or severe, producing barely visible to deep indentations.

Normally, infants and young children use abdominal muscles for breathing, unlike older children and adults, who use the diaphragm. Their chest walls are also more compliant due to their cartilaginous sternum and rib cage.[1] When breathing requires extra effort, accessory muscles assist respiration, especially inspiration. Retractions typically accompany accessory muscle use.

If you detect retractions in a child, check quickly for other signs of respiratory distress, such as cyanosis, tachypnea, tachycardia, and decreased oxygen saturation. Also, prepare the child for suctioning, insertion of an artificial airway, and oxygen administration.

Observe the depth and location of retractions. Also, note the rate, depth, and quality of respirations. Look for accessory muscle use, nasal flaring during inspiration, and grunting during expiration. If the child has a cough, record the color, consistency, and odor of any sputum. Note whether the child appears restless or lethargic. Finally, auscultate the child's lungs to detect abnormal breath sounds. (See *Observing retractions*, page 368.)

History and physical examination

If the child's condition permits, ask his parents about his medical history. Was he born prematurely? Was he born with a low birth weight? Was the delivery complicated? Ask about recent signs of an upper respiratory tract infection, such as a runny nose, cough, and low-grade fever. How often has the child had respiratory problems during the past year? Has he been in contact with anyone

Observing retractions

When you observe retractions in infants and children, be sure to note their exact location—an important clue to the cause and severity of respiratory distress. For example, subcostal and substernal retractions usually result from lower respiratory tract disorders. Suprasternal retractions usually result from upper respiratory tract disorders.

Mild intercostal retractions alone may be normal. Intercostal retractions with subcostal and substernal retractions may indicate moderate respiratory distress. Deep suprasternal retractions usually indicate severe distress.

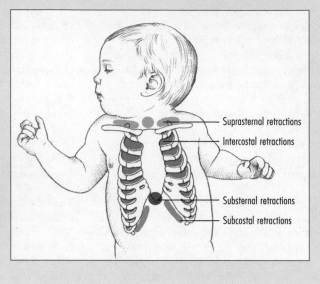

Suprasternal retractions
Intercostal retractions
Substernal retractions
Subcostal retractions

---

who has had a cold, the flu, or other respiratory ailments? Did he ever have respiratory syncytial virus? Did he aspirate any food, liquid, or foreign body? Inquire about any personal or family history of allergies or asthma.

Medical causes

▶ *Asthma attack.* Intercostal and suprasternal retractions may accompany an asthma attack. They're preceded by dyspnea, wheezing, a hacking cough, and pallor. Related features include cyanosis or flushing, crackles, rhonchi, diaphoresis, tachycardia, tachypnea, a frightened, anxious expression and, in patients with severe distress, nasal flaring.

▶ *Bronchiolitis.* Most common in children younger than age 2 and the leading cause of hospitalization in infants, this acute lower respiratory tract infection may cause intercostal and subcostal retractions, nasal flaring, tachypnea, dyspnea, cough, restlessness and a slight fever.[2] Periodic apnea may occur in infants younger than age 6 months.

▶ *Croup (spasmodic).* This disorder causes attacks of a barking cough, hoarseness, dyspnea, and restlessness. As distress worsens, the child may display suprasternal, substernal,

and intercostal retractions; nasal flaring; tachycardia; cyanosis; and an anxious, frantic expression. Croup attacks usually subside within a few hours but tend to recur.

▶ *Epiglottiditis.* This life-threatening bacterial infection may lead to severe respiratory distress with suprasternal, substernal, and intercostal retractions; stridor; nasal flaring; cyanosis; and tachycardia. Early features include sudden onset of a barking cough and high fever, sore throat, hoarseness, dysphagia, drooling, dyspnea, and restlessness. The child becomes panicky as edema makes breathing difficult. Total airway occlusion may occur in 2 to 5 hours.

▶ *Esophageal foreign body aspiration.* This disorder should be suspected in children younger than age 2 who have retractions, fever, wheezing, rhonchi, and stridor.[3]

▶ *Heart failure.* Usually linked to a congenital heart defect in children, this disorder may cause intercostal and substernal retractions with nasal flaring, progressive tachypnea, and—in severe respiratory distress—grunting respirations, edema, and cyanosis. Other findings include productive cough, crackles, jugular vein distention, tachycardia, right-upper-quadrant pain, anorexia, and fatigue.

▶ *Laryngotracheobronchitis (acute)*. With this viral infection, substernal and intercostal retractions typically follow a low to moderate fever, runny nose, poor appetite, a barking cough, hoarseness, and inspiratory stridor. Other signs and symptoms include tachycardia; shallow, rapid respirations; restlessness; irritability; and pale, cyanotic skin.

▶ *Pneumonia (bacterial)*. This disorder begins with signs and symptoms of acute infection, such as high fever and lethargy, which are followed by subcostal and intercostal retractions, nasal flaring, dyspnea, tachypnea, grunting respirations, cyanosis, and a productive cough. Auscultation may reveal diminished breath sounds, scattered crackles, and sibilant rhonchi over the affected lung. GI effects may include vomiting, diarrhea, and abdominal distention.

▶ *Respiratory distress syndrome*. Substernal and subcostal retractions are an early sign of this life-threatening syndrome, which affects premature infants shortly after birth. Other early signs include tachypnea, tachycardia, and expiratory grunting. As respiratory distress worsens, intercostal and suprasternal retractions typically occur, and apnea or irregular respirations replace grunting. Related effects include nasal flaring, cyanosis, lethargy, and eventual unresponsiveness as well as bradycardia and hypotension. Auscultation may detect crackles over the lung bases on deep inspiration and harsh, diminished breath sounds. Oliguria and peripheral edema may occur.

Special considerations

Continue to monitor the child's vital signs. Keep suction equipment and an airway of appropriate size at the bedside. If the infant weighs less than 15 lb (6.8 kg), place him in an oxygen hood. If he weighs more, place him in a cool mist tent instead. Perform chest physical therapy with postural drainage to help mobilize and drain excess lung secretions. (See *Positioning an infant for chest physical therapy*, pages 360 and 361.) A bronchodilator or, occasionally, a steroid also may be used.

Prepare the child for chest X-rays, cultures, pulmonary function tests, and arterial blood gas analysis. Explain the procedures to his parents, too, and have them calm and comfort the child.

Pediatric pointers

When examining a child for retractions, know that crying may accentuate the contractions.

Geriatric pointers

Although retractions may occur at any age, they're more difficult to assess in an older patient who's obese or who has chronic chest wall stiffness or deformity.

Patient counseling

Instruct the patient or a family member on proper drug administration at home. Teach them how to provide a humidified environment. Stress the need to maintain adequate hydration. Provide information on the use of respiratory equipment and techniques to administer respiratory therapies at home.

REFERENCES
1. McCaskey, M.S. "Pediatric Assessment: The Little Differences," *Home Healthcare Nurse* 25(1):20-24, January 2007.
2. Sterling, Y.M., and El-Dahr, J.M. "Wheezing and Asthma in Early Childhood: An Update," *Pediatric Nursing* 32(1):27-33, January/February 2006.
3. Louie, J.P., Alpern, E.R., and Windreich, R.M. "Witnessed and Unwitnessed Esophageal Foreign Bodies in Children," *Pediatric Emergency Care* 21(9):582-585, September 2005.

● RHONCHI

Rhonchi are continuous adventitious breath sounds detected by auscultation. They're usually louder and lower-pitched than crackles—more like a hoarse moan or a deep snore—though they may be described as rattling, sonorous, bubbling, rumbling, or musical. Sibilant rhonchi, or wheezes, are high pitched.[1]

Rhonchi are heard over large airways such as the trachea. They can occur in a patient with a pulmonary disorder when air flows

Differential diagnosis: Rhonchi

POSSIBLE CAUSES	SIGNS AND SYMPTOMS	DIAGNOSIS
Acute respiratory distress syndrome	• Crackles • Rapid, shallow respirations • Dyspnea • Intercostal and suprasternal retractions • Diaphoresis • Fluid accumulation	• Physical examination • Arterial blood gases (ABGs) • Chest X-ray
Bronchitis	• Wheezing • Exertional dyspnea • Barrel chest • Tachypnea • Clubbing • Decreased breath sounds *Additional in acute bronchitis* • Chills • Sore throat • Low-grade fever • Muscle and back pain • Substernal tightness *Additional in chronic bronchitis* • Coarse crackles • Prolonged expiration • Chronic productive cough • Increased accessory muscle use • Cyanosis • Fluid retention	• Physical examination • ABGs • Chest X-ray • Pulmonary function test (PFT)
Emphysema	• Wheezing • Exertional dyspnea • Barrel chest • Tachypnea • Clubbing • Decreased breath sounds • Weight loss • Mild, chronic productive cough • Accessory muscle use on inspiration • Grunting expirations	• Physical examination • ABGs • Serum alpha$_1$-antitrypsin level • Chest X-ray • PFT
Pneumonia	• Tachycardia • Tachypnea • Dyspnea • Cyanosis • Productive cough • Shaking chills • Fever • Myalgia • Headache • Pleuritic chest pain • Diaphoresis • Decreased breath sounds • Fine crackles	• Physical examination • Complete blood count • ABGs • Sputum Gram stain • Chest X-ray

TREATMENT AND FOLLOW-UP

- Oxygen therapy
- Treatment of underlying cause
Follow-up: Referral to pulmonologist

- Smoking cessation
- Antibiotics, if indicated
- Nebulizer treatment
- Oxygen therapy
- Chest physiotherapy
Follow-up: Referral to pulmonologist

- Smoking cessation
- Medication (diuretics, bronchodilators, corticosteroids)
Follow-up: Referral to pulmonologist

- Antibiotics
- Oxygen therapy
Follow-up: Reevaluation after 7 days

through passages that have been narrowed by secretions, a tumor or foreign body, bronchospasm, or mucosal thickening. The resulting vibration of airway walls produces the rhonchi.

History and physical examination

If you auscultate rhonchi, take the patient's vital signs, including oxygen saturation, and be alert for signs of respiratory distress. (See *Differential diagnosis: Rhonchi.*) Characterize the patient's respirations as rapid or slow, shallow or deep, and regular or irregular. Inspect the chest, noting the use of accessory muscles. Is the patient audibly wheezing or gurgling? Auscultate for other abnormal breath sounds, such as crackles and a pleural friction rub. If you detect these sounds, note their location. Are breath sounds diminished or absent? Next, percuss the chest. If the patient has a cough, note its frequency and characterize its sound. If it's productive, examine the sputum for color, odor, consistency, and blood.

Ask related questions: Does the patient smoke? If so, obtain a history in pack-years. Has he recently lost weight or felt tired or weak? Does he have asthma or other a pulmonary disorder? Is he taking any prescribed or over-the-counter drugs?

During the examination, keep in mind that thick or excessive secretions, bronchospasm, or inflammation of mucous membranes may lead to airway obstruction. If needed, suction the patient and keep equipment available for inserting an artificial airway. Keep a bronchodilator available to treat bronchospasm.

Medical causes

▶ *Acute respiratory distress syndrome.* Fluid accumulation with this life-threatening disorder produces rhonchi and crackles. Initial features include rapid, shallow respirations and dyspnea, sometimes after the patient's condition appears stable. Developing hypoxemia leads to intercostal and suprasternal retractions, diaphoresis, and fluid accumulation. As hypoxemia worsens, the patient displays increased difficulty breathing, restlessness, apprehension, decreased level of consciousness,

Differential diagnosis: Rhonchi *(continued)*

POSSIBLE CAUSES	SIGNS AND SYMPTOMS	DIAGNOSIS
Pulmonary edema	• Tachycardia • Tachypnea • Dyspnea • Cyanosis • Anxiety • Paroxysmal nocturnal dyspnea • Nonproductive cough • Dependent crackles • S_3	• Physical examination • ABGs • Chest X-ray • Computed tomography scan • Magnetic resonance imaging

cyanosis, motor dysfunction and, possibly, tachycardia.

▶ *Aspiration of a foreign body.* A retained foreign body in the bronchi can cause inspiratory and expiratory rhonchi and wheezing from increased secretions. You may auscultate reduced breath sounds over the obstructed area. Fever, pain, and cough also may occur.

▶ *Asthma.* An asthma attack can cause rhonchi, crackles and, commonly, wheezing. Other features include apprehension, a dry cough that later becomes productive, prolonged expirations, and intercostal and supraclavicular retractions on inspiration. The patient also may have increased accessory muscle use, nasal flaring, tachypnea, tachycardia, diaphoresis, and flushing or cyanosis.

▶ *Bronchiectasis.* This disorder causes lower-lobe rhonchi and crackles, which coughing may help relieve. The classic sign is a cough that produces mucopurulent, foul-smelling and, possibly, bloody sputum. Other findings include fever, weight loss, exertional dyspnea, fatigue, malaise, halitosis, weakness, and late-stage clubbing.

▶ *Bronchitis. Acute tracheobronchitis* produces sonorous rhonchi and wheezing from bronchospasm or increased mucus in the airways. Related findings include chills, sore throat, a low-grade fever (rising up to 102° F [38.9° C] in those with severe illness), muscle and back pain, and substernal tightness. A cough becomes productive as secretions increase.

With *chronic bronchitis,* auscultation may reveal scattered rhonchi, coarse crackles, wheezing, high-pitched piping sounds, and prolonged expirations. An early hacking cough later becomes productive. The patient also has exertional dyspnea, increased accessory muscle use, barrel chest, cyanosis, tachypnea, and clubbing (a late sign).

▶ *Emphysema.* This disorder may cause sonorous rhonchi, but faint, high-pitched wheezing is more typical, together with weight loss; a mild, chronic, productive cough with scant sputum; exertional dyspnea; accessory muscle use on inspiration; tachypnea; and grunting expirations. Other features include anorexia, malaise, barrel chest, peripheral cyanosis, and late-stage clubbing.

▶ *Esophageal foreign body aspiration.* Suspect this disorder in children younger than age 2 who have rhonchi, retractions, fever, wheezing, and stridor.[2]

▶ *Pneumonia.* Bacterial pneumonias can cause rhonchi and a dry cough that later becomes productive. Related signs and symptoms—shaking chills, high fever, myalgias, headache, pleuritic chest pain, tachypnea, tachycardia, dyspnea, cyanosis, diaphoresis, decreased breath sounds, and fine crackles—develop suddenly.

▶ *Pulmonary coccidioidomycosis.* This disorder causes rhonchi and wheezing. Other features include a cough with fever, occasional chills, pleuritic chest pain, sore throat, headache, backache, malaise, marked weak-

TREATMENT AND FOLLOW-UP

- Oxygen therapy
- Medication (diuretics, morphine)

Follow-up: Referral to cardiologist

ness, anorexia, hemoptysis, and an itchy macular rash.

Other causes

▶ *Diagnostic tests.* Pulmonary function tests or bronchoscopy can loosen secretions and mucus, causing rhonchi.

▶ *Respiratory therapy.* This may produce rhonchi from loosened secretions and mucus.

Special considerations

To ease the patient's breathing, place him in semi-Fowler's position and reposition him every 2 hours. Give an antibiotic, a bronchodilator, and an expectorant. Provide humidification to thin secretions, relieve inflammation, and prevent drying. Pulmonary physiotherapy with postural drainage and percussion can also help loosen secretions. Use tracheal suctioning, if needed, to help the patient clear secretions and to provide oxygenation and comfort. Promote coughing and deep breathing and incentive spirometry.

Prepare the patient for diagnostic tests, such as arterial blood gas analysis, pulmonary function studies, sputum analysis, and chest X-rays.

Pediatric pointers

Rhonchi in children can result from bacterial pneumonia, cystic fibrosis, and croup syndrome.

Because a respiratory tract disorder may begin abruptly and progress rapidly in an infant or a child, observe closely for signs of airway obstruction.

Patient counseling

If appropriate, encourage increased activity to promote drainage of secretions. Teach deep-breathing and coughing techniques and splinting, if needed. Urge the patient to drink plenty of fluids to help liquefy secretions and prevent dehydration. Advise him not to suppress a moist cough.

REFERENCES

1. McCormick, M. "Every Breath You Take: Making Sense of Breath Sounds," *Nursing Made Incredibly Easy!* 5(1):7-11, January/February 2007.
2. Louie, J.P., Alpern, E.R., and Windreich, R.M., "Witnessed and Unwitnessed Esophageal Foreign Bodies in Children," *Pediatric Emergency Care* 21(9):582-585, September 2005.

SEIZURES, GENERALIZED TONIC-CLONIC

Like other types of seizures, generalized tonic-clonic seizures are caused by the paroxysmal, uncontrolled discharge of central nervous system (CNS) neurons, leading to neurologic dysfunction. Unlike most other types of seizures, however, this cerebral hyperactivity isn't confined to the original focus or to a localized area but extends to the entire brain.

A generalized tonic-clonic seizure may start with or without an aura. As seizure activity spreads to the subcortical structures, the patient loses consciousness, falls to the ground, and may utter a loud cry caused by air rushing from the lungs through the vocal cords. His body stiffens (tonic phase), then undergoes rapid, synchronous muscle jerking and hyperventilation (clonic phase). Tongue biting, incontinence, diaphoresis, profuse salivation, and signs of respiratory distress also may occur. The seizure usually stops after 2 to 5 minutes. The patient regains consciousness fairly quickly or after a prolonged postictal period, but displays confusion. He may complain of headache, fatigue, muscle soreness, and arm and leg weakness.

Generalized tonic-clonic seizures usually occur singly. The patient may be asleep or awake and active. (See *What happens during a generalized tonic-clonic seizure*.) Possible complications include respiratory arrest due to airway obstruction from secretions, status epilepticus (occurring in 5% to 8% of pa-

tients), head or spinal injuries and bruises, Todd's paralysis and, rarely, cardiac arrest. Life-threatening status epilepticus is marked by prolonged seizure activity or by rapidly recurring seizures with no intervening periods of recovery. It's most commonly triggered by abrupt discontinuation of anticonvulsant therapy.

Generalized seizures may be caused by a brain tumor, vascular disorder, head trauma, infection, metabolic defect, drug or alcohol withdrawal syndrome, exposure to toxins, or a genetic defect. Generalized seizures also may result from a focal seizure. With recurring seizures, or epilepsy, the cause may be unknown. (See *What to do if your patient has a seizure*, page 376.)

History and physical examination

If you didn't see the seizure, obtain a description from a witness, if possible. Ask when the seizure started and how long it lasted. Did the patient report any unusual sensations before the seizure began? Did the seizure start in one area of the body and spread, or did it affect the entire body right away? Did the patient fall on a hard surface? Did his eyes or head turn? Did he turn blue? Did he lose bladder control? Did he have more than one seizure before recovering?

If the patient may have sustained a head injury, observe him closely for a decreasing level of consciousness (LOC), unequal or nonreactive pupils, and focal neurologic signs. Does he complain of headache and muscle sore-

What happens during a generalized tonic-clonic seizure

BEFORE THE SEIZURE

Prodromal signs and symptoms, such as my-oclonic jerks, throbbing headache, and mood changes, may occur over several hours or days. The patient may have premonitions of the seizure. For example, he may report an aura, such as seeing a flashing light or smelling a characteristic odor.

DURING THE SEIZURE

If a generalized seizure starts with an aura, it means that irritability in a specific area of the brain quickly became widespread. Common auras include palpitations, epigastric distress rapidly rising to the throat, head or eye turning, and sensory hallucinations.

Next, the patient loses consciousness as a sudden discharge of intense electrical activity overwhelms the brain's subcortical center. The patient falls and has brief, bilateral myoclonic contractures. Air forced through spasmodic vocal cords may produce a birdlike, piercing cry.

During the *tonic phase,* skeletal muscles contract for 10 to 20 seconds. The patient's eyelids are drawn up, his arms are flexed, and his legs are extended. His mouth opens wide, then snaps shut; he may bite his tongue. His respirations stop because of respiratory muscle spasm, and initial pallor of the skin and mucous membranes (the result of impaired venous return) changes to cyanosis secondary to apnea. The patient arches his back and slowly lowers his arms (as shown). Other effects include dilated, nonreactive pupils; greatly increased heart rate and blood pressure; increased salivation and tracheobronchial secretions; and profuse diaphoresis.

During the *clonic phase,* lasting about 60 seconds, mild trembling progresses to violent contractures or jerks. Other motor activity includes facial grimaces (with possible tongue biting) and violent expiration of bloody, foamy saliva from clonic contractures of thoracic cage muscles. Clonic jerks slowly decrease in intensity and frequency. The patient is still apneic.

AFTER THE SEIZURE

The patient's movements gradually cease, and he becomes unresponsive to external stimuli. Other postseizure features include stertorous respirations from increased tracheobronchial secretions, equal or unequal pupils (but becoming reactive), and urinary incontinence due to brief muscle relaxation. After about 5 minutes, the patient's level of consciousness increases, and he appears confused and disoriented. His muscle tone, heart rate, and blood pressure return to normal.

After several hours' sleep, the patient awakens exhausted and may have a headache, sore muscles, and amnesia about the seizure.

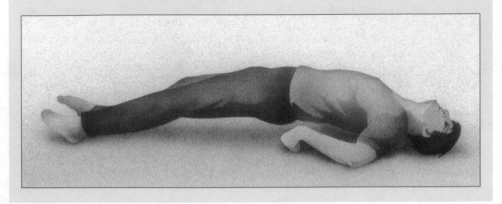

What to do if your patient has a seizure

If you see your patient start to have a seizure, first check his airway, breathing, and circulation, and make sure the cause isn't asystole or a blocked airway. Stay with the patient, and make sure his airway stays patent. Focus your care on observing the seizure and protecting the patient. Place a towel under his head to prevent injury, loosen his clothing, and move any sharp or hard objects out of his way. Don't try to restrain the patient or force a hard object into his mouth; you might chip his teeth or fracture his jaw.[1] Only at the start of the ictal phase can you safely insert a soft object into his mouth.

If possible, turn the patient to one side during the seizure to let secretions drain and prevent aspiration.[1] Otherwise, do this at the end of the clonic phase when respirations return. (If they don't return, check for airway obstruction and suction the patient if needed. Cardiopulmonary resuscitation, intubation, and mechanical ventilation may be needed.)

Protect the patient after the seizure by providing a safe area in which he can rest. As consciousness returns, reassure and reorient him. Check his vital signs and neurologic status. Be sure to carefully record these data and your observations during the seizure.

If the seizure lasts longer than 5 minutes or if a second seizure occurs before full recovery from the first, suspect status epilepticus. Establish an airway, start an I.V. line, give supplemental oxygen, and begin cardiac monitoring. Draw blood for appropriate studies, and check a blood glucose level. Turn the patient on his side with his head in a semi-dependent position, to drain secretions and prevent aspiration. Monitor oxygen saturation levels and give oxygen if needed. Give diazepam or lorazepam by slow I.V. push, repeated two or three times at 10- to 20-minute intervals, to stop the seizures. If the patient hasn't been diagnosed with epilepsy, an I.V. bolus of dextrose 50% may be ordered. Dextrose may stop the seizures if the patient has hypoglycemia. If his thiamine level is low, also give thiamine to guard against further damage.

If the patient is intubated, expect to insert a nasogastric tube to prevent vomiting and aspiration. Be aware that if the patient hasn't been intubated, the tube itself can trigger the gag reflex and cause vomiting. Be sure to record your observations and the intervals between seizures.

---

ness? Is he increasingly difficult to arouse when you check on him at 20-minute intervals? Examine his arms, legs, and face (including tongue) for injury, residual paralysis, or limb weakness.

Next, obtain a history. Has the patient ever had generalized or focal seizures before? If so, do they occur often? Do other family members also have them? Is the patient receiving drug therapy? Is he compliant? Ask about sleep deprivation and emotional or physical stress at the time the seizure occurred.

Medical causes

▶ *Alcohol withdrawal syndrome.* Sudden withdrawal from alcohol dependence may cause seizures 7 to 48 hours later as well as status epilepticus. The patient also may be restless and have hallucinations, profuse diaphoresis, and tachycardia.

▶ *Brain abscess.* Generalized seizures may occur in the acute stage of abscess formation or after the abscess disappears. Depending on the size and location of the abscess, LOC varies from drowsiness to deep stupor. Early signs and symptoms reflect increased intracranial pressure (ICP) and include constant headache, nausea, vomiting, and focal seizures. Typical later features include ocular disturbances, such as nystagmus, impaired vision, and unequal pupils. Other findings vary with the abscess site but may include aphasia, hemiparesis, abnormal behavior, and personality changes.

▶ *Brain tumor.* Generalized seizures may occur, depending on the tumor's location and type. Other findings include a slowly decreasing LOC, morning headache, dizziness, confusion, focal seizures, vision loss, motor and sensory disturbances, aphasia, and ataxia. Later findings include papilledema, vomiting, increased systolic blood pressure, widening pulse pressure, and (eventually) decorticate posture.

▶ *Cerebral aneurysm.* Occasionally, generalized seizures may occur with an aneurysmal rupture. Premonitory signs and symptoms may last several days, but onset is typically abrupt with severe headache, nausea, vomiting, and decreased LOC. Depending on the site and amount of bleeding, related signs and symptoms vary but may include nuchal rigidity, irritability, hemiparesis, hemisensory defects, dysphagia, photophobia, diplopia, ptosis, and unilateral pupil dilation.

▶ *Chronic renal failure.* End-stage renal failure produces rapid onset of twitching, trembling, myoclonic jerks, and generalized seizures. Related signs and symptoms include anuria or oliguria, fatigue, malaise, irritability, decreased mental acuity, muscle cramps, peripheral neuropathies, anorexia, and constipation or diarrhea. Skin effects include color changes (yellow, brown, or bronze), pruritus, and uremic frost. Other effects include ammonia breath odor, nausea and vomiting, ecchymoses, petechiae, GI bleeding, mouth and gum ulcers, hypertension, and Kussmaul's respirations.

▶ *Eclampsia.* Generalized seizures are a hallmark of this disorder, which occurs only during pregnancy and in the postpartal period. Related findings include severe frontal headache, nausea and vomiting, vision disturbances, increased blood pressure, temperature of up to 104° F (40° C), peripheral edema, and sudden weight gain. The patient also may exhibit oliguria, irritability, hyperactive deep tendon reflexes (DTRs), and decreased LOC.

▶ *Encephalitis.* Seizures are an early sign of this disorder, indicating a poor prognosis; they also may occur after recovery as a result of residual damage. Other findings include fever, headache, photophobia, nuchal rigidity, neck pain, vomiting, aphasia, ataxia, hemiparesis, nystagmus, irritability, cranial nerve palsies (causing facial weakness, ptosis, dysphagia), and myoclonic jerks.

▶ *Epilepsy (idiopathic).* In most cases, the cause of recurrent seizures is unknown. Ten percent to 39% of women with epilepsy are more prone to seizures at various points in their menstrual cycle.[2]

▶ *Head trauma.* In severe cases, generalized seizures may occur at the time of injury. (Months later, focal seizures may occur.) Severe head trauma also may cause a decreased LOC, leading to coma; soft-tissue injury of the face, head, or neck; clear or bloody drainage from the mouth, nose, or ears; facial edema; bony deformity of the face, head, or neck; Battle's sign; and lack of response to oculocephalic and oculovestibular stimulation. Motor and sensory deficits may occur along with altered respirations. Examination may reveal signs of increasing ICP, such as decreased response to painful stimuli, nonreactive pupils, bradycardia, increased systolic pressure, and widening pulse pressure. If the patient is conscious, he may exhibit vision deficits, behavioral changes, and headache.

▶ *Hepatic encephalopathy.* Generalized seizures may occur late in this disorder. Other late-stage findings in a comatose patient include fetor hepaticus, asterixis, hyperactive DTRs, and a positive Babinski's sign.

▶ *Hypertensive encephalopathy.* This life-threatening disorder may cause seizures along with severely increased blood pressure, decreased LOC, intense headache, vomiting, transient blindness, paralysis, and (eventually) Cheyne-Stokes respirations.

▶ *Hypoglycemia.* Generalized seizures usually occur with severe hypoglycemia, preceeded by blurred or double vision, motor weakness, hemiplegia, trembling, diaphoresis, tachycardia, myoclonic twitching, and decreased LOC.

▶ *Hyponatremia.* Seizures develop when serum sodium levels fall below 125 mEq/L, especially if the decrease is rapid. Hyponatremia also causes orthostatic hypotension, headache, muscle twitching and weakness, fatigue, oliguria or anuria, cold and clammy skin, decreased skin turgor, irritability, lethargy, confusion, and stupor or coma. Excessive thirst, tachycardia, nausea, vomiting, and abdominal cramps also may occur. Severe hyponatremia may cause cyanosis and vasomotor collapse, with a thready pulse.

▶ *Hypoparathyroidism.* Worsening tetany causes generalized seizures. Chronic hypoparathyroidism produces neuromuscular irritability and hyperactive DTRs.

▶ *Hypoxic encephalopathy.* Besides generalized seizures, this disorder may produce myoclonic jerks and coma. Later, if the patient has recovered, dementia, visual agnosia, choreoathetosis, and ataxia may occur.

▶ *Multiple sclerosis.* This disorder rarely produces generalized seizures. Characteristic findings include vision deficits, paresthesia, constipation, muscle weakness, paralysis, spasticity, hyperreflexia, intention tremor, ataxic gait, dysphagia, dysarthria, impotence, and emotional lability. Urinary frequency, urgency, and incontinence also may occur.

▶ *Neurofibromatosis.* Multiple brain lesions from this disorder cause focal and generalized seizures. Inspection reveals café-au-lait spots, multiple skin tumors, scoliosis, and kyphoscoliosis. Related findings include dizziness, ataxia, monocular blindness, and nystagmus.

▶ *Porphyria (intermittent acute).* Generalized seizures are a late sign of this disorder, indicating severe CNS involvement. Acute porphyria also causes severe abdominal pain, tachycardia, psychotic behavior, muscle weakness, and sensory loss in the trunk.

▶ *Sarcoidosis.* Lesions may affect the brain, causing generalized and focal seizures. Associated findings include a nonproductive cough with dyspnea, substernal pain, malaise, fatigue, arthralgia, myalgia, weight loss, tachypnea, dysphagia, skin lesions, and impaired vision.

▶ *Stroke.* Seizures (focal more often than generalized) may occur within 6 months of an ischemic stroke. Other signs and symptoms vary with the location and extent of brain damage. They include decreased LOC, contralateral hemiplegia, dysarthria, dysphagia, ataxia, unilateral sensory loss, apraxia, agnosia, and aphasia. The patient also may develop vision deficits, memory loss, poor judgment, personality changes, emotional lability, urine retention or urinary incontinence, constipation, headache, and vomiting.

Other causes

▶ *Arsenic poisoning.* Besides causing generalized seizures, arsenic poisoning may cause a garlicky breath odor, increased salivation, and generalized pruritus. GI effects include diarrhea, nausea, vomiting, and severe abdominal pain. Related effects include diffuse hyperpigmentation; sharply defined edema of the eyelids, face, and ankles; paresthesia of the extremities; alopecia; irritated mucous membranes; weakness; muscle aches; and peripheral neuropathy.

▶ *Barbiturate withdrawal.* In chronically intoxicated patients, barbiturate withdrawal may produce generalized seizures 2 to 4 days after the last dose. Status epilepticus is possible.

▶ *Diagnostic tests.* Contrast agents used in radiologic tests may cause generalized seizures.

DRUG WATCH *Toxic blood levels of some drugs, such as cimetidine, lidocaine, meperidine, penicillins, and theophylline may cause generalized seizures. Amphetamines, isoniazid, phenothiazines, tricyclic antidepressants, and vincristine may cause seizures in patients with epilepsy. Stimulants, such as cocaine and methamphetamine, may cause seizures when taken in large doses.*

Special considerations

Closely monitor the patient after the seizure for recurring seizure activity. Take seizure precautions for the patient's protection. Prepare him for a computed tomography scan or magnetic resonance imaging and EEG.

Pediatric pointers

Generalized seizures are common in children. In fact, 75% to 90% of epileptic patients have their first seizure before age 20. (See *Helping families cope with a child's epilepsy.*)

Many children between ages 3 months and 3 years have generalized seizures with fever, and few of them go on to develop a seizure disorder if they have no other risk factors (such as a positive family history or an underlying neurologic disorder).[3] Generalized seizures also may stem from inborn errors of metabolism, perinatal injury, brain infection, Reye's syndrome, Sturge-Weber syndrome, arteriovenous malformation, lead poisoning, hypoglycemia, and idiopathic causes. The per-

Helping families cope with a child's epilepsy

Question: *What concerns and needs are reported by children with epilepsy and their parents?*

Research: A diagnosis of epilepsy impacts a child's quality of life and increases parental stress. The authors used a qualitative focus group design to explore the concerns and needs of children with epilepsy and their parents. Two focus groups composed of children with epilepsy and two focus groups composed of parents of children with epilepsy were conducted. The focus group guide developed by the researchers aimed at generating discussion around concerns and fears related to diagnosis and prognosis, as well as quality of life issues. All sessions lasted about 90 minutes.

Conclusion: The study results suggest the need for assessing informational and emotional needs during diagnosis, as well as ongoing reassessment. The three categories of children's needs described are: talking at my level, feeling different from others, and parental perspective of children's needs (being informed, avoid-

ing misconceptions). Three major themes that emerged from the parent data include: difficulties dealing with their child's condition, need for information, and fears and concerns.

Application: Provide information to children using age-appropriate explanations and materials. Give written information to parents and explain all terms. Help parents navigate the healthcare system and provide appropriate referrals. Be available to answer questions and provide emotional support to parents and children as needed. Also, distribute educational materials to schools, pediatricians' offices, neurology offices, support groups, and camps.

Source: McNelis, A.M., Buelow, J., Myers, J., and Johnson, E. A. "Concerns and Needs of Children with Epilepsy and Their Parents," *Clinical Nurse Specialist: The Journal for Advanced Nursing Practice,* 21(4):195-202, 2007.

---

tussis component of the DPT vaccine may cause seizures; although this is rare.

Geriatric pointers

Simple partial or complex partial seizures are the most common seizure type in older patients.[2] Generalized tonic-clonic seizures aren't common in older patients, occuring in only 21% to 25% of seizure cases.[2] Auras also are less common in this population, and postictal states may be prolonged.[2]

Patient counseling

Teach the patient's family what to do if a seizure occurs.[1] Provide them with a written action plan if needed. Advise the patient's family to observe and record his seizure activity to facilitate management. If the patient is a child, encourage the parents to provide the child's caregivers with written information on

the drugs being used. Emphasize the importance of strict compliance with the drug regimen, and warn the patient about adverse reactions. Stress the need for regular follow-up appointments for blood studies. Counsel the patient against driving or other dangerous activities until he's under the care of a neurologist and his seizures are well controlled.

REFERENCES
1. Fagley, M.U. "Taking Charge of Seizure Activity," *Nursing* 37(9):42-47, September 2007.
2. Forcadas, M.I., Pena Mayor, P., and Puig, J.S. "Special Situations in Epilepsy: Women and the Elderly," *The Neurologist* 13(6):Supplement 1 S52-S61, November 2007.
3. Peterson, P. "Recognizing and Treating Seizure Disorders in Children," *LPN* 3(6):48-51, 53, 54, November/December 2007.

SKIN, CLAMMY

Clammy skin—moist, cool, and usually pale—is a sympathetic response to stress, which triggers release of the hormones epinephrine and norepinephrine. These hormones cause cutaneous vasoconstriction and secretion of cold sweat from eccrine glands, particularly on the palms, forehead, and soles.

Clammy skin typically accompanies shock as a sign of compensatory vasoconstriction.[1] It also may occur with acute hypoglycemia, anxiety reactions, arrhythmias, and heat exhaustion. It also occurs as a vasovagal reaction to severe pain associated with nausea, anorexia, epigastric distress, hyperpnea, tachypnea, weakness, confusion, tachycardia, and pupillary dilation or a combination of these findings. Marked bradycardia and syncope may follow.

History and physical examination

If you detect clammy skin, remember that rapid evaluation and intervention are paramount. (See *Clammy skin: A key finding.*) Ask the patient if he has a history of type 1 diabetes mellitus or a cardiac disorder. Is the patient taking any drugs, especially an antiarrhythmic? Is he experiencing pain, chest pressure, nausea, or epigastric distress? Does he feel weak? Does he have a dry mouth? Does he have diarrhea or increased urination?

Next, examine the pupils for dilation. Check for abdominal distention and increased muscle tension.

Medical causes

▶ *Acute myocardial infarction.* Cool clammy skin may stem from vasoconstriction.[2] Other findings may include chest pain, nausea, vomitting, palpitations, dyspnea, confusion, anxiety, and low-grade fever.

▶ *Anxiety.* An acute anxiety attack commonly produces cold, clammy skin on the forehead, palms, and soles. Other features include pallor, dry mouth, tachycardia or bradycardia, palpitations, and hypertension or hypotension. The patient also may develop tremors, breathlessness, headache, muscle tension, nausea, vomiting, abdominal distention, diarrhea, increased urination, and sharp chest pain.

▶ *Arrhythmias.* Cardiac arrhythmias may produce generalized cool, clammy skin along with mental status changes, dizziness, and hypotension.

▶ *Cardiogenic shock.* Generalized cool, moist, pale skin accompanies confusion, restlessness, hypotension, tachycardia, tachypnea, narrowing pulse pressure, cyanosis, and oliguria.[3]

▶ *Heat exhaustion.* In the acute stage of heat exhaustion, generalized cold, clammy skin accompanies an ashen appearance, headache, confusion, syncope, giddiness and, possibly, a subnormal temperature, with mild heat exhaustion. The patient may exhibit a rapid and thready pulse, nausea, vomiting, tachypnea, oliguria, thirst, muscle cramps, and hypotension.

▶ *Hypoglycemia (acute).* Generalized cool, clammy skin or diaphoresis may accompany irritability, tremors, palpitations, hunger, headache, tachycardia, and anxiety. Central nervous system disturbances include blurred vision, diplopia, confusion, motor weakness, hemiplegia, and coma. These signs and symptoms typically resolve after the patient is given glucose.

▶ *Hypovolemic shock.* With this common form of shock, generalized pale, cold, clammy skin accompanies subnormal body temperature, hypotension with narrowing pulse pressure, tachycardia, tachypnea, and rapid, thready pulse. Other findings are flat neck veins, increased capillary refill time, decreased urine output, confusion, and decreased level of consciousness.

▶ *Septic shock.* The cold shock stage causes generalized cold, clammy skin. Other findings include rapid and thready pulse, severe hypotension, persistent oliguria or anuria, and respiratory failure.

Special considerations

Take the patient's vital signs often, and monitor urine output. Offer fluids, if tolerated. If clammy skin occurs with an anxiety reaction or pain, offer the patient emotional support, give pain medication, and provide a quiet environment.

HEALTH & SAFETY

Clammy skin: A key finding

Be alert for clammy skin. Why? Because it commonly accompanies emergency conditions, such as shock, acute hypoglycemia, and arrhythmias. To know what to do, review these typical clinical situations.

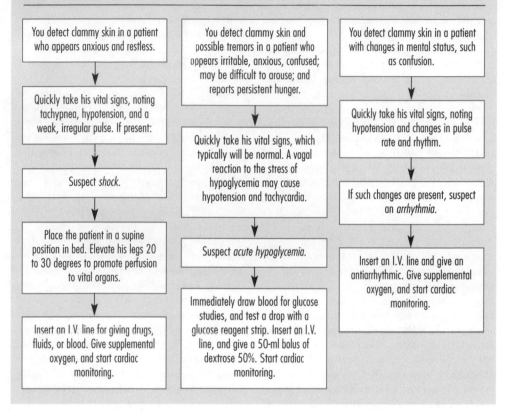

You detect clammy skin in a patient who appears anxious and restless.

↓

Quickly take his vital signs, noting tachypnea, hypotension, and a weak, irregular pulse. If present:

↓

Suspect *shock*.

↓

Place the patient in a supine position in bed. Elevate his legs 20 to 30 degrees to promote perfusion to vital organs.

↓

Insert an I.V. line for giving drugs, fluids, or blood. Give supplemental oxygen, and start cardiac monitoring.

You detect clammy skin and possible tremors in a patient who appears irritable, anxious, confused; may be difficult to arouse; and reports persistent hunger.

↓

Quickly take his vital signs, which typically will be normal. A vagal reaction to the stress of hypoglycemia may cause hypotension and tachycardia.

↓

Suspect *acute hypoglycemia*.

↓

Immediately draw blood for glucose studies, and test a drop with a glucose reagent strip. Insert an I.V. line, and give a 50-ml bolus of dextrose 50%. Start cardiac monitoring.

You detect clammy skin in a patient with changes in mental status, such as confusion.

↓

Quickly take his vital signs, noting hypotension and changes in pulse rate and rhythm.

↓

If such changes are present, suspect an *arrhythmia*.

↓

Insert an I.V. line and give an antiarrhythmic. Give supplemental oxygen, and start cardiac monitoring.

Pediatric pointers
Infants in shock don't have clammy skin because of their immature sweat glands.

Geriatric pointers
Elderly patients develop clammy skin easily because of decreased tissue perfusion. Always consider bowel ischemia in the differential diagnosis of older patients who have cool, clammy skin—especially if they also have abdominal pain or bloody stools.

Patient counseling
If an underlying illness is related to the patient's clammy skin, provide information on the condition. If the condition is related to an altered blood glucose level, provide information on management of hypoglycemia and early signs of a falling blood glucose level. Provide information on the importance of nutrition and hydration.

REFERENCES
1. Goodrich, C. "Endpoints of Resuscitation: What Should We Be Monitoring?" *AACN Advanced Critical Care* 17(3):306-316, July/September 2006.
2. Lackey, S.A. "Suppressing the Scourge of AMI," *Nursing* 36(5):36-41, May 2006.
3. Topalian, S., Ginsberg, F., and Parrillo, J.E. "Cardiogenic Shock," *Critical Care Medicine* 36(1):Suppl S66-S74, January 2008.

SKIN, MOTTLED

Mottled skin is patchy discoloration indicating primary or secondary changes of the deep, middle, or superficial dermal blood vessels. It can result from a hematologic, immune, or connective tissue disorder; chronic occlusive arterial disease; dysproteinemia; immobility; exposure to heat or cold; or shock. Mottled skin can be a normal reaction, such as the diffuse mottling that occurs when exposure to cold causes venous stasis in cutaneous blood vessels (cutis marmorata).

Mottling that occurs with other signs and symptoms usually affects the extremities, typically indicating restricted blood flow. For example, livedo reticularis, a characteristic network pattern of reddish blue discoloration, occurs when vasospasm of the middermal blood vessels slows local blood flow in dilated superficial capillaries and small veins. Shock causes mottling from systemic vasoconstriction.

History and physical examination

Mottled skin may indicate an emergency condition requiring rapid evaluation and intervention. (See *Mottled skin: Knowing what to do.*) However, if the patient isn't in distress, obtain a history. Ask if the mottling began suddenly or gradually. What precipitated it? How long has he had it? Does anything make it go away? Does the patient have other symptoms, such as pain, numbness, or tingling in an extremity? If so, do they disappear with temperature changes?

Observe the patient's skin color, and palpate his arms and legs for skin texture, swelling, and temperature differences between extremities. Check capillary refill. Palpate for the presence (or absence) of pulses and for their quality. Note breaks in the skin, muscle appearance, and hair distribution. Assess motor and sensory function.

Medical causes

▶ *Acrocyanosis.* With this rare disorder, anxiety or exposure to cold can cause vasospasm in small cutaneous arterioles. This yields persistent symmetrical blue and red mottling of the affected hands, feet, and nose.

▶ *Arterial occlusion (acute).* Initial signs include temperature and color changes. Pallor may change to blotchy cyanosis and livedo reticularis. Color and temperature demarcation develop at the level of obstruction. Other effects include sudden onset of pain in the limb and possibly paresthesia, paresis, and a sensation of cold in the affected area. Examination reveals diminished or absent pulses, cool limbs, increased capillary refill time, pallor, and reduced reflexes.

▶ *Arteriosclerosis obliterans.* Atherosclerotic buildup narrows intra-arterial lumina, resulting in reduced blood flow through the affected artery. Obstructed blood flow to the limbs (usually the legs) produces such peripheral signs and symptoms as leg pallor, cyanosis, blotchy erythema, and livedo reticularis. Related findings include intermittent claudication (most common symptom), reduced or absent pedal pulses, and leg coolness. Other symptoms include coldness and paresthesia.

▶ *Buerger's disease.* This form of vasculitis produces unilateral or asymmetrical color changes and mottling, particularly livedo networking in the legs. It also typically causes intermittent claudication and erythema along the blood vessels in the limbs. During exposure to cold, the feet are cold, cyanotic, and numb; later they're hot, red, and tingling. Other findings include impaired peripheral pulses and peripheral neuropathy. Buerger's disease typically is worsened by smoking.

▶ *Cryoglobulinemia.* This necrotizing disorder causes patchy livedo reticularis, petechiae, and ecchymoses. Other findings include fever, chills, urticaria, melena, skin ulcers, epistaxis, Raynaud's phenomenon, eye hemorrhages, hematuria, and gangrene.

▶ *Fibromyalgia.* Mottled skin may accompany the fatigue and widespread pain that are characteristic of this disorder.[1] Additional findings may include Raynaud's phenomenon, sleep disturbances, irritable bowel syndrome, and restless leg syndrome.

▶ *Hypovolemic shock.* Vasoconstriction from shock commonly produces skin mottling, initially in the knees and elbows. As shock worsens, mottling becomes generalized. Early signs

Mottled skin: Knowing what to do

If your patient's skin is pale, cool, clammy, and mottled at the elbows and knees or all over, he may be developing hypovolemic shock. Quickly take his vital signs, and be sure to note tachycardia or a weak, thready pulse. Observe the neck for flattened veins. Does the patient appear anxious? If you detect these signs and symptoms, place the patient in a supine position in bed with his legs elevated 20 to 30 degrees. Give oxygen by nasal cannula or face mask, and start cardiac monitoring. Insert a large-bore I.V. line for rapid delivery of fluids or blood products, and prepare to insert a central line or a pulmonary artery catheter. Prepare to catheterize the patient to monitor urine output.

Localized mottling in a pale, cool limb that the patient says feels painful, numb, and tingling may signal acute arterial occlusion. Immediately check the patient's distal pulses: If they're absent or diminished, you'll need to insert an I.V. line in an unaffected limb and prepare the patient for arteriography or immediate surgery.

include sudden onset of pallor, cool skin, restlessness, thirst, tachypnea, and slight tachycardia. As shock progresses, other findings include cool, clammy skin; rapid, thready pulse; hypotension; narrowed pulse pressure; decreased urine output; subnormal temperature; confusion; and decreased level of consciousness.

▶ *Livedo reticularis (idiopathic or primary).* Symmetrical, diffuse mottling can involve the hands, feet, arms, legs, buttocks, and trunk. Initially, networking is intermittent and most pronounced on exposure to cold or stress; eventually, mottling persists even with warming.

▶ *Periarteritis nodosa.* Skin findings include asymmetrical, patchy livedo reticularis, palpable nodules along the path of medium-sized arteries, erythema, purpura, muscle wasting, ulcers, gangrene, peripheral neuropathy, fever, weight loss, and malaise.

▶ *Polycythemia vera.* This hematologic disorder produces livedo reticularis, hemangiomas, purpura, rubor, ulcerative nodules, and scleroderma-like lesions. Other symptoms include headache, a vague feeling of fullness in the head, dizziness, vertigo, vision disturbances, dyspnea, and aquagenic pruritus.

▶ *Rheumatoid arthritis.* This disorder may cause skin mottling. Early nonspecific signs and symptoms progress to joint pain and stiffness with subcutaneous nodules, usually on the elbows.

▶ *Systemic lupus erythematosus.* This connective tissue disorder can cause livedo reticularis, most commonly on the outer arms. Other signs and symptoms include a butterfly rash, nondeforming joint pain and stiffness, photosensitivity, Raynaud's phenomenon, patchy alopecia, seizures, fever, anorexia, weight loss, lymphadenopathy, and emotional lability.

Other causes

▶ *Immobility.* Prolonged immobility may cause bluish mottling, most noticeably in dependent extremities.

▶ *Thermal exposure.* Prolonged thermal exposure, as from a heating pad or hot water bottle, may cause erythema ab igne—a localized, reticulated, brown-to-red mottling.

Special considerations

Assess for worsening of the underlying condition, and refer the patient for medical treatment. Maximize circulation to the affected areas by keeping them warm and in proper alignment.

Pediatric pointers

A common cause of mottled skin in children is systemic vasoconstriction from shock. Mottled skin also may occur as a complication of umbilical artery catheter placement in critically ill neonates as a result of vasospasm.[2] Other causes are the same as those for adults.

Geriatric pointers

In elderly patients, decreased tissue perfusion can easily cause mottled skin. Besides arterial occlusion and polycythemia vera, which are common in patients in this age-group, bowel ischemia is common in elderly patients who have livedo reticularis, especially if they also have abdominal pain or bloody stools.

Patient counseling

If the patient has a chronic condition, such as systemic lupus erythematosus, periarteritis nodosa, or cryoglobulinemia, advise him to watch for mottled skin because it may indicate a flare-up of his disorder. Teach patients to avoid tight clothing and overexposure to cold or to heating devices, such as hot water bottles and heating pads.

REFERENCES

1. Peterson, J. "Understanding Fibromyalgia and Its Treatment Options," *The Nurse Practitioner* 30(1):48-55, January 2005.
2. Furdon, S.A., Horgan, M.J., Bradshaw, W.T., and Clark, D.A. "Nurses' Guide to Early Detection of Umbilical Artery Catheter Complications in Infants," *Advances in Neonatal Care* 6(5):242-56, October 2006.

● STRIDOR

A loud, harsh, musical respiratory sound, stridor results from an obstruction in the trachea or larynx. Usually heard during inspiration, this sign also may occur during expiration in severe upper airway obstruction. It may begin as low-pitched "croaking" and progress to high-pitched "crowing" as respirations become more vigorous.

Life-threatening upper airway obstruction can stem from foreign-body aspiration, increased secretions, intraluminal tumor, localized edema or muscle spasms, and external compression by a tumor or aneurysm.

If you hear stridor, quickly check the patient's vital signs and oxygen saturation and examine him for other signs of partial airway obstruction—choking or gagging, tachypnea, dyspnea, shallow respirations, intercostal retractions, nasal flaring, tachycardia, cyanosis, and diaphoresis. (Be aware that abrupt cessation of stridor signals complete obstruction in which the patient has inspiratory chest movement but absent breath sounds. Unable to talk, he quickly becomes lethargic and loses consciousness.)

If you detect any signs of airway obstruction, try to clear the airway with back blows or abdominal thrusts (Heimlich maneuver). Next, give oxygen by nasal cannula or face mask, or prepare for emergency endotracheal intubation or tracheostomy and mechanical ventilation. (See *Emergency endotracheal intubation.*) Have equipment ready to suction any aspirated vomitus or blood through the endotracheal or tracheostomy tube. Connect the patient to a cardiac monitor, and position him upright to ease his breathing.

History and physical examination

When the patient's condition permits, obtain a history from him or a family member. First, find out when the stridor began. Has he had it before? Does he have an upper respiratory tract infection? If so, how long has he had it?

Ask about a history of allergies, tumors, and respiratory and vascular disorders. Note recent exposure to smoke or noxious fumes or gases. Next, explore related signs and symptoms. Does stridor occur with pain or a cough?

Then examine the patient's mouth for excessive secretions, foreign matter, inflammation, and swelling. Assess his neck for swelling, masses, subcutaneous crepitation, and scars. Observe the patient's chest for delayed, decreased, or asymmetrical chest expansion. Auscultate for wheezes, rhonchi, crackles, rubs, and other abnormal breath sounds. Percuss for dullness, tympany, or flatness. Finally, note any burns or signs of trauma, such as ecchymoses and lacerations.

Medical causes

▶ *Airway trauma.* Local trauma to the upper airway commonly causes acute obstruction, resulting in the sudden onset of stridor. Accompanying this sign are dysphonia, dysphagia, hemoptysis, cyanosis, accessory muscle use, intercostal retractions, nasal flaring, tachypnea, progressive dyspnea, and shallow

Emergency endotracheal intubation

For a patient with stridor, you may have to perform emergency endotracheal (ET) intubation to establish a patent airway and administer mechanical ventilation. Just follow these essential steps:
- Gather the necessary equipment.
- Explain the procedure to the patient.
- Place the patient flat on his back with a small blanket or pillow under his head. This position aligns the axis of the oropharynx, posterior pharynx, and trachea.
- Check the cuff on the ET tube for leaks.
- While holding the patient's mouth open with your right hand, grasp the laryngoscope handle in your left hand and gently slide the blade into the right side of the patient's mouth. Center the blade, and then push the patient's tongue to the left.
- Advance the blade to expose the epiglottis and lift the laryngoscope handle upward and away from your body at a 45-degree angle to reveal the vocal cords.
- Insert the ET tube into the right side of the patient's mouth.

- After intubation, inflate the cuff, using the minimal leak technique.
- Check tube placement by auscultating for bilateral breath sounds or using a capnometer; observe the patient for chest expansion and feel for warm exhalations at the ET tube's opening.
- Insert an oral airway or bite block.
- Secure the tube and airway with tape applied to skin treated with compound benzoin tincture.
- Suction secretions from the patient's mouth and the ET tube as needed.
- Administer oxygen or start mechanical ventilation (or both).

After the patient has been intubated, suction secretions as needed and check cuff pressure once every shift (correcting any air leaks with the minimal leak technique). Provide mouth care every 2 to 3 hours and as needed. Prepare the patient for chest X-rays to check tube placement, and restrain and reassure him as needed.

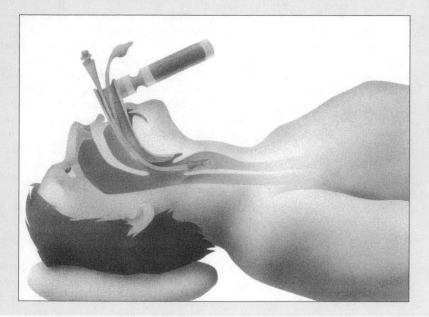

respirations. Palpation may reveal subcutaneous crepitation in the neck or upper chest.

▶ *Anaphylaxis*. With a severe allergic reaction, upper airway edema and laryngospasm cause stridor and other signs and symptoms of respiratory distress: nasal flaring, wheezing, accessory muscle use, intercostal retractions, and dyspnea.[1] The patient also may develop nasal congestion and profuse, watery rhinorrhea. Typically, these respiratory effects are preceded by a feeling of impending doom or fear, weakness, diaphoresis, sneezing, nasal pruritus, urticaria, erythema, and angioedema. Common related findings include chest or throat tightness, dysphagia and, possibly, signs of shock, such as hypotension, tachycardia, and cool, clammy skin.

▶ *Anthrax, inhalation*. Initial signs and symptoms are flulike and include fever, chills, weakness, cough, and chest pain. The disease typically occurs in two stages with a period of recovery after the initial symptoms. The second stage develops abruptly with rapid deterioration marked by stridor, fever, dyspnea, and hypotension generally leading to death within 24 hours. Radiologic findings include mediastinitis and symmetric mediastinal widening.

▶ *Aspiration of a foreign body*. Sudden stridor is characteristic in this life-threatening situation. Related findings include abrupt onset of dry, paroxysmal coughing, gagging or choking, hoarseness, tachycardia, wheezing, dyspnea, tachypnea, intercostal muscle retractions, diminished breath sounds, cyanosis, and shallow respirations. The patient typically appears anxious and distressed.

▶ *Epiglottiditis*. With this inflammatory condition, stridor is caused by an erythematous, edematous epiglottis that obstructs the upper airway. Stridor occurs along with fever, sore throat, and a croupy cough.

▶ *Hypocalcemia*. With this disorder, laryngospasm can cause stridor. Other findings include paresthesia, carpopedal spasm, and positive Chvostek's and Trousseau's signs.

▶ *Inhalation injury*. Within 48 hours after inhalation of smoke or noxious fumes, the patient may develop laryngeal edema and bronchospasms, resulting in stridor. Other signs and symptoms include singed nasal hairs, orofacial burns, coughing, hoarseness, sooty sputum, crackles, rhonchi, wheezes, and other signs and symptoms of respiratory distress, such as dyspnea, accessory muscle use, intercostal retractions, and nasal flaring.

▶ *Laryngeal tumor*. Stridor is a late sign and may be accompanied by dysphagia, dyspnea, enlarged cervical nodes, and pain that radiates to the ear.[2] Typically, stridor is preceded by hoarseness, minor throat pain, and a mild, dry cough.

▶ *Laryngitis (acute)*. This disorder may cause severe laryngeal edema, resulting in stridor and dyspnea. Its chief sign, however, is mild to severe hoarseness, perhaps with transient voice loss. Other findings include sore throat, dysphagia, dry cough, malaise, and fever.

▶ *Mediastinal tumor*. Commonly producing no symptoms at first, this type of tumor may eventually compress the trachea and bronchi, resulting in stridor. Its other effects include hoarseness, brassy cough, tracheal shift or tug, dilated neck veins, swelling of the face and neck, stertorous respirations, and suprasternal retractions on inspiration. The patient also may report dyspnea, dysphagia, and pain in the chest, shoulder, or arm.

▶ *Retrosternal thyroid*. This anatomic abnormality causes stridor, dysphagia, cough, hoarseness, and tracheal deviation. It can also cause signs of thyrotoxicosis.

▶ *Thoracic aortic aneurysm*. If this aneurysm compresses the trachea, it may cause stridor accompanied by dyspnea, wheezing, and a brassy cough. Other findings include hoarseness or complete voice loss, dysphagia, jugular vein distention, prominent chest veins, tracheal tug, paresthesia or neuralgia, and edema of the face, neck, and arms. The patient also may complain of substernal, lower back, abdominal, or shoulder pain.

Other causes

▶ *Diagnostic tests*. Bronchoscopy or laryngoscopy may precipitate laryngospasm and stridor.

▶ *Treatments*. After prolonged intubation, the patient may exhibit laryngeal edema and stridor when the tube is removed. Aerosol therapy with epinephrine may reduce stridor. Reintubation may be necessary in some cases.

Neck surgery, such as thyroidectomy, may cause laryngeal paralysis and stridor.

Special considerations
Continue to monitor the patient's vital signs closely. Prepare him for diagnostic tests, such as arterial blood gas analysis and chest X-rays.

Pediatric pointers
Stridor is the most prominent sign of airway obstruction in children.[3] When you hear this sign, you must intervene quickly to prevent total airway obstruction. This emergency can happen more rapidly in an infant or young child because his airway is narrower than an adult's.

Causes of stridor in infants and children include foreign-body aspiration, croup syndrome, laryngeal diphtheria, pertussis, retropharyngeal abscess, and congenital abnormalities of the larynx.

Therapy for partial airway obstruction typically involves hot or cold steam in a mist tent or hood, parenteral fluids and electrolytes, and plenty of rest.

Patient counseling
Instruct the patient and his family about safety measures in the home environment if the stridor is related to aspiration of a foreign object. If the stridor is related to croup, teach the parents techniques to manage the condition. Teach the patient and his family about signs and symptoms that require immediate attention.

REFERENCES
1. O'Brien, J.F. "The Keys to Quickly Identifying Anaphylaxis," *Journal of Respiratory Diseases* 26(7):308-309, 312-316, July 2005.
2. Schiech, L. "Looking at Laryngeal Cancer," *Nursing* 37(5):50-55, May 2007.
3. Zoumalan, R., Maddalozzo, J., and Holinger, L.D. "Etiology of Stridor in Infants," *Annals of Otology, Rhinology, & Laryngology* 116(5):329-334, May 2007.

● SYNCOPE

A common neurologic sign, syncope, or *fainting*, refers to transient loss of consciousness with impaired cerebral blood supply or cerebral hypoxia. It usually occurs abruptly and lasts for seconds to minutes. An episode of syncope usually starts as a feeling of light-headedness. A patient can usually prevent an episode of syncope by lying down or sitting with his head between his knees. Typically, the patient lies motionless with his skeletal muscles relaxed but sphincter muscles controlled. However, the depth of unconsciousness varies—some patients can hear voices or see blurred outlines; others are unaware of their surroundings.

During syncope, the patient is strikingly pale with a slow, weak pulse, hypotension, and almost imperceptible breathing. If severe hypotension lasts 20 seconds or longer, the patient also may develop convulsive, tonic-clonic movements.

Syncope may result from cardiac and cerebrovascular disorders, hypoxemia, and postural changes in the presence of autonomic dysfunction. It also may follow vigorous coughing (tussive syncope) and emotional stress, injury, shock, or pain (vasovagal syncope, or common fainting). Hysterical syncope also may follow emotional stress but isn't accompanied by other vasodepressor effects.

If you see a patient faint, ensure a patent airway and patient safety. Take vital signs. Then place the patient in a supine position, elevate his legs, and loosen any tight clothing. Be alert for tachycardia, bradycardia, or an irregular pulse. Meanwhile, place him on a cardiac monitor to detect arrhythmias. If an arrhythmia appears, give oxygen and insert an I.V. line for drugs or fluids. Be ready to start cardiopulmonary resuscitation. Cardioversion, defibrillation, or insertion of a temporary pacemaker may be needed.

History and physical examination
If the patient reports a fainting episode, gather information about the episode from him and his family. Did he feel weak, light-headed,

nauseous, or sweaty just before he fainted? Did he get up quickly from a chair or from lying down? During the fainting episode, did he have muscle spasms or incontinence? How long was he unconscious? When he regained consciousness, was he alert or confused? Did he have a headache? Has he fainted before? If so, how often does it occur?

Next, take the patient's vital signs and examine him for any injuries that may have occurred during his fall.

Medical causes

▶ *Aortic arch syndrome.* With this syndrome, the patient has syncope and may have weak or abruptly absent carotid pulses and unequal or absent radial pulses. Early signs and symptoms include night sweats, pallor, nausea, anorexia, weight loss, arthralgia, and Raynaud's phenomenon. He also may develop hypotension in the arms; neck, shoulder, and chest pain; paresthesia; intermittent claudication; bruits; vision disturbances; and dizziness.

▶ *Aortic stenosis.* A cardinal late sign, syncope is accompanied by exertional dyspnea and angina. Related findings include marked fatigue, orthopnea, paroxysmal nocturnal dyspnea, palpitations, and reduced carotid pulses. Typically, auscultation reveals atrial and ventricular gallops as well as a harsh, crescendo-decrescendo systolic ejection murmur that's loudest at the right sternal border of the second intercostal space.

▶ *Cardiac arrhythmias.* Any arrhythmia that decreases cardiac output and impairs cerebral circulation may cause syncope. Other effects—such as palpitations, pallor, confusion, diaphoresis, dyspnea, and hypotension—usually develop first. However, with Adams-Stokes syndrome, syncope may occur without warning. During syncope, the patient develops asystole, which may precipitate spasm and myoclonic jerks if prolonged. He also has an ashen pallor that progresses to cyanosis, incontinence, bilateral Babinski's reflex, and fixed pupils.

▶ *Carotid sinus hypersensitivity.* Syncope is triggered by compression of the carotid sinus, which may be caused by turning the head to one side or by wearing a tight collar. The fainting episode usually is brief.

▶ *Hypoxemia.* Regardless of its cause, severe hypoxemia may produce syncope. Common related effects include confusion, tachycardia, restlessness, and incoordination.

▶ *Orthostatic hypotension.* Syncope occurs when the patient rises quickly from a recumbent position. Look for a drop of 10 to 20 mm Hg or more in systolic or diastolic blood pressure as well as tachycardia, pallor, dizziness, blurred vision, nausea, and diaphoresis.

▶ *Transient ischemic attacks.* Marked by transient neurologic deficits, these attacks may produce syncope and decreased level of consciousness. Other findings vary with the affected artery but may include vision loss, nystagmus, aphasia, dysarthria, unilateral numbness, hemiparesis or hemiplegia, tinnitus, facial weakness, dysphagia, and staggering or uncoordinated gait.

▶ *Vagal glossopharyngeal neuralgia.* Vasovagal syncope is responsible for more than 80% of all syncopal events.[1] With vagal glossopharyngeal neuralgia, localized pressure may trigger pain in the base of the tongue, pharynx, larynx, tonsils, and ear, resulting in syncope that lasts for several minutes.

Other causes

DRUG WATCH *Quinidine may cause syncope—and possibly sudden death—from ventricular fibrillation. Prazosin may cause severe orthostatic hypotension and syncope, usually after the first dose. Occasionally, griseofulvin, indomethacin, and levodopa can produce syncope.*

Special considerations

Continue to monitor the patient's vital signs closely. Prepare him for an electrocardiogram, Holter monitor, carotid duplex, carotid Doppler, and electrophysiology studies.

Pediatric pointers

Syncope is much less common in children than adults. It may result from a cardiac or neurologic disorder, allergies, or emotional stress.

Children ages 6 to 17 may be at risk for syncope when receiving vaccinations. This population receives many vaccinations and may feel more nervous or fearful about receiving them.[2] Ask children about their feelings when receiving injections, and give vaccinations while they are sitting or laying down. Observe children at risk for syncope after vaccine administration for at least 15 minutes before they leave the office.[2]

Geriatric pointers

Postural hypotension is a common cause of syncope in older adults, and may stem from dehydration or multidrug therapy. Older adults are at particular risk for serious injury from syncope-induced falls.[1]

Patient counseling

Urge the patient to pace his activities, to rise slowly from a recumbent position, to avoid standing still for a prolonged time, and to sit or lie down as soon as he feels faint.

REFERENCES

1. Peterson, R., and Berns, S. "Prevention and Education to Decrease Patient Falls due to Syncope," *Journal of Nursing Quality Care* 21(4):331-334, October/December 2006.
2. Miller, E., and Woo, E.J. "Time to Prevent Injuries from Postimmunization Syncope," *Nursing* 36(12):20, December 2006.

TACHYCARDIA

Easily detected by counting the apical, carotid, or radial pulse rate, tachycardia is a heart rate greater than 100 beats/minute. The patient with tachycardia usually complains of palpitations or a "racing" heart. This common sign normally occurs in response to emotional or physical stress, such as excitement, exercise, pain, anxiety, and fever. It also may result from the use of stimulants, such as caffeine and tobacco. However, tachycardia may be an early sign of a life-threatening disorder, such as cardiogenic, hypovolemic, or septic shock. It also may result from a cardiovascular, respiratory, or metabolic disorder or from the effects of certain drugs, tests, or treatments. (See *What happens in tachycardia.*)

If you detect tachycardia, obtain an electrocardiogram (ECG) and check for evidence of reduced cardiac output, which may cause or be caused by tachycardia. Take the patient's other vital signs and determine his level of consciousness (LOC). If the patient has increased or decreased blood pressure and is drowsy or confused, give oxygen and start cardiac monitoring. Insert an I.V. line for delivery of fluids, blood products, and drugs, and gather emergency resuscitation equipment.

History and physical examination

If the patient's condition permits, take a focused history. Find out if he has had palpitations before. If so, how were they treated? Explore related symptoms. Is the patient dizzy or short of breath? Is he weak or fatigued? Is he experiencing episodes of syncope or chest pain? Next, ask about a history of trauma, diabetes, or cardiac, pulmonary, or thyroid disorders. Also, obtain an alcohol and drug history, including prescription, over-the-counter, and illicit drugs.

Inspect the patient's skin for pallor or cyanosis. Assess pulses, noting peripheral edema. Finally, auscultate the heart and lungs for abnormal sounds or rhythms.

Medical causes

▶ *Acute respiratory distress syndrome.* Besides tachycardia, this syndrome causes crackles, rhonchi, dyspnea, tachypnea, nasal flaring, and grunting respirations. Other findings include cyanosis, anxiety, decreased LOC, and abnormal chest X-ray findings.

▶ *Adrenocortical insufficiency.* In this disorder, tachycardia is commonly accompanied by a weak pulse as well as progressive weakness and fatigue, which may become so severe that the patient requires bed rest. Other signs and symptoms include abdominal pain, nausea and vomiting, altered bowel habits, weight loss, orthostatic hypotension, irritability, bronze skin, decreased libido, and syncope. Some patients report an enhanced sense of taste, smell, and hearing.

▶ *Alcohol withdrawal syndrome.* Tachycardia can occur with tachypnea, profuse diaphoresis, fever, insomnia, anorexia, and anxiety. The patient is characteristically anxious, irritable, and prone to visual and tactile hallucinations.

What happens in tachycardia

Tachycardia represents the heart's effort to deliver more oxygen to body tissues by increasing the rate at which blood passes through the vessels. This sign can reflect overstimulation in the sinoatrial node, atrium, atrioventricular node, or ventricles.

Because heart rate affects cardiac output (cardiac output = heart rate × stroke volume), tachycardia can lower cardiac output by reducing ventricular filling time and stroke volume (the output of each ventricle at every contraction). As cardiac output decreases, arterial pressure and peripheral perfusion do too. Tachycardia further aggravates myocardial ischemia by increasing the heart's demand for oxygen while reducing the duration of diastole—the period of greatest coronary blood flow.

▶ *Anaphylactic shock.* In life-threatening anaphylactic shock, tachycardia and hypotension develop within minutes after exposure to an allergen, such as penicillin or an insect sting. Typically, the patient is visibly anxious and has severe pruritus, perhaps with urticaria and a pounding headache. Other findings may include flushed and clammy skin, a cough, dyspnea, nausea, abdominal cramps, seizures, stridor, change or loss of voice associated with laryngeal edema, and urinary urgency and incontinence.

▶ *Anemia.* Tachycardia and bounding pulse are characteristic signs of anemia. Associated signs and symptoms include fatigue, pallor, dyspnea and, possibly, bleeding tendencies. Auscultation may reveal an atrial gallop, a systolic bruit over the carotid arteries, and crackles.

▶ *Anxiety.* A fight-or-flight response produces tachycardia, tachypnea, chest pain, nausea, and light-headedness. The symptoms dissipate as anxiety resolves.

▶ *Aortic insufficiency.* Accompanying tachycardia in this disorder are a "water-hammer" bounding pulse and a large, diffuse apical heave. Severe insufficiency also produces widened pulse pressure. Auscultation reveals a hallmark decrescendo, high-pitched, and blowing diastolic murmur that starts with the second heart sound and is heard best at the left sternal border of the second and third intercostal spaces. An atrial or ventricular gallop, an early systolic murmur, an Austin Flint murmur (apical diastolic rumble), or Duroziez's sign (a murmur over the femoral artery during systole and diastole) also may be heard. Other findings include angina, dyspnea, palpitations, strong and abrupt carotid pulsations, pallor, and signs of heart failure, such as crackles and jugular vein distention.

▶ *Aortic stenosis.* Typically, this valvular disorder causes tachycardia, an atrial gallop, and a weak, thready pulse. Its chief features, however, are exertional dyspnea, angina, dizziness, and syncope. Aortic stenosis also causes a harsh, crescendo-decrescendo systolic ejection murmur that's loudest at the right sternal border of the second intercostal space. Other findings include palpitations, crackles, and fatigue.

▶ *Cardiac arrhythmias.* Tachycardia may occur with many cardiac arrhythmias.[1,2,3] The patient may be hypotensive and report dizziness, palpitations, weakness, and fatigue. Depending on his heart rate, he also may have tachypnea, decreased LOC, and pale, cool, clammy skin.

▶ *Cardiac contusion.* The result of blunt chest trauma, a cardiac contusion may cause tachycardia, substernal pain, dyspnea, and palpitations. Assessment may detect sternal ecchymoses and a pericardial friction rub.

▶ *Cardiac tamponade.* In life-threatening cardiac tamponade, tachycardia is commonly accompanied by paradoxical pulse, dyspnea, and tachypnea. The patient is visibly anxious and restless and has cyanotic, clammy skin and distended jugular veins. He may develop muffled heart sounds, a pericardial friction rub, chest pain, hypotension, narrowed pulse pressure, and hepatomegaly.

▶ *Cardiogenic shock.* Although many features of cardiogenic shock appear in other types of shock, they're usually more profound in this type. Accompanying tachycardia are a weak, thready pulse; narrowed pulse pressure; hypotension; tachypnea; cold, pale, clammy, and cyanotic skin; oliguria; restlessness; and altered LOC.

▶ *Cholera.* This infectious disease is marked by abrupt watery diarrhea and vomiting. Severe fluid and electrolyte loss leads to tachycardia, thirst, weakness, muscle cramps, decreased skin turgor, oliguria, and hypotension. Without treatment, death can occur within hours.

▶ *Chronic obstructive pulmonary disease.* Although clinical findings vary widely in this disorder, tachycardia is a common sign. Other characteristic findings include cough, tachypnea, dyspnea, pursed-lip breathing, accessory muscle use, cyanosis, diminished breath sounds, rhonchi, crackles, and wheezing. Clubbing and barrel chest are usually late findings.

▶ *Diabetic ketoacidosis.* This life-threatening disorder commonly produces tachycardia and a thready pulse. Its cardinal sign, however, is Kussmaul's respirations—abnormally rapid, deep breathing. Other signs and symptoms of ketoacidosis include fruity breath odor, orthostatic hypotension, generalized weakness, anorexia, nausea, vomiting, and abdominal pain. The patient's LOC may vary from lethargy to coma.

▶ *Febrile illness.* Fever can cause tachycardia. Related findings reflect the specific disorder.

▶ *Heart failure.* Especially common in left-sided heart failure, tachycardia may be accompanied by a ventricular gallop, fatigue, dyspnea (exertional and paroxysmal nocturnal), orthopnea, and leg edema. Eventually, the patient develops widespread signs and symptoms, such as palpitations, narrowed pulse pressure, hypotension, tachypnea, crackles, dependent edema, weight gain, slowed mental response, diaphoresis, pallor and, possibly, oliguria. Late signs include hemoptysis, cyanosis, marked hepatomegaly, and pitting edema.

▶ *Hyperosmolar hyperglycemic nonketotic syndrome.* A rapidly deteriorating LOC is commonly accompanied by tachycardia, hypotension, tachypnea, seizures, oliguria, and severe dehydration marked by poor skin turgor and dry mucous membranes.

▶ *Hypertensive crisis.* A life-threatening hypertensive crisis is characterized by tachycardia, tachypnea, diastolic blood pressure that exceeds 120 mm Hg, and systolic blood pressure that may exceed 200 mm Hg. Typically, the patient develops pulmonary edema with jugular vein distention, dyspnea, and pink, frothy sputum. Related findings include chest pain, severe headache, drowsiness, confusion, anxiety, tinnitus, epistaxis, muscle twitching, seizures, nausea and vomiting and, possibly, focal neurologic signs such as paresthesia.

▶ *Hypoglycemia.* A common sign of hypoglycemia, tachycardia is accompanied by hypothermia, nervousness, trembling, fatigue, malaise, weakness, headache, hunger, nausea, diaphoresis, and moist, clammy skin. Central nervous system effects include blurred or double vision, motor weakness, hemiplegia, seizures, and decreased LOC.

▶ *Hyponatremia.* Tachycardia is a rare effect of this electrolyte imbalance. Other findings include orthostatic hypotension, headache, muscle twitching and weakness, fatigue, oliguria or anuria, poor skin turgor, thirst, irritability, seizures, nausea and vomiting, and decreased LOC that may progress to coma. Severe hyponatremia may cause cyanosis and signs of vasomotor collapse such as thready pulse.

▶ *Hypovolemia.* Tachycardia may occur with this disorder along with hypotension, decreased skin turgor, sunken eyeballs, thirst, syncope, and dry skin and tongue.

▶ *Hypovolemic shock.* Mild tachycardia, an early sign of life-threatening hypovolemic shock, may be accompanied by tachypnea, restlessness, thirst, and pale, cool skin. As shock progresses, the patient's skin becomes clammy and his pulse, increasingly rapid and thready. He also may develop hypotension, narrowed pulse pressure, oliguria, subnormal body temperature, and decreased LOC.

▶ *Hypoxemia.* Tachycardia may be accompanied by tachypnea, dyspnea, cyanosis, confusion, syncope, and incoordination.

▶ *Myocardial infarction (MI).* A life-threatening MI may cause tachycardia or bradycardia. Its classic symptom, however, is crushing substernal chest pain that may radiate to the left arm, jaw, neck, or shoulder. Auscultation may reveal an atrial gallop, a new murmur, and crackles. Other signs and symptoms include dyspnea, diaphoresis, nausea and vomiting, anxiety, restlessness, increased or decreased blood pressure, and pale, clammy skin.

▶ *Neurogenic shock.* Tachycardia or bradycardia may accompany tachypnea, apprehension, oliguria, variable body temperature, decreased LOC, and warm, dry skin.

▶ *Orthostatic hypotension.* Tachycardia accompanies the characteristic signs and symptoms of this condition, which include dizziness, syncope, pallor, blurred vision, diaphoresis, and nausea.

▶ *Pheochromocytoma.* Characterized by sustained or paroxysmal hypertension, this rare tumor also may cause tachycardia and palpitations. Other findings include headache, chest and abdominal pain, diaphoresis, paresthesia, tremors, nausea and vomiting, insomnia, extreme anxiety (possibly even panic), and pale or flushed, warm skin.

▶ *Pneumothorax.* Life-threatening pneumothorax causes tachycardia and other signs and symptoms of distress, such as severe dyspnea and chest pain, tachypnea, and cyanosis. Related findings include dry cough, subcutaneous crepitation, absent or decreased breath sounds, cessation of normal chest movement on the affected side, and decreased vocal fremitus.

▶ *Pulmonary embolism.* In this disorder, tachycardia is usually preceded by sudden dyspnea, angina, or pleuritic chest pain. Other common signs and symptoms include weak peripheral pulses, cyanosis, tachypnea, low-grade fever, restlessness, diaphoresis, and a dry cough or a cough producing blood-tinged sputum.

▶ *Septic shock.* Initially, septic shock produces chills, sudden fever, tachycardia, tachypnea and, possibly, nausea, vomiting, and diarrhea. The patient's skin is flushed, warm, and dry; his blood pressure is normal or slightly decreased. Eventually, he may display anxiety; restlessness; thirst; oliguria or anuria; cool, clammy, cyanotic skin; rapid, thready pulse; and severe hypotension. His LOC may decrease progressively, perhaps culminating in a coma.

▶ *Thyrotoxicosis.* Tachycardia is a classic feature of this thyroid disorder. Others include an enlarged thyroid gland, nervousness, heat intolerance, weight loss despite increased appetite, diaphoresis, diarrhea, tremors, palpitations, and sometimes exophthalmos. Because thyrotoxicosis affects virtually every body system, its associated features are diverse and numerous. Some examples include full and bounding pulse, widened pulse pressure, dyspnea, anorexia, nausea, vomiting, altered bowel habits, hepatomegaly, and muscle weakness, fatigue, and atrophy. The patient's skin is smooth, warm, and flushed; his hair is fine and soft and may gray prematurely or fall out. Women may have a reduced libido and oligomenorrhea or amenorrhea; men may have a reduced libido and gynecomastia.

Other causes

▶ *Diagnostic tests.* Cardiac catheterization and electrophysiologic studies may induce transient tachycardia.

DRUG WATCH *Various drugs affect the nervous system, circulatory system, or heart muscle, resulting in tachycardia. Examples of these include sympathomimetics; phenothiazines; anticholinergics such as atropine; thyroid drugs; vasodilators, such as hydralazine and nitroglycerin; alpha-adrenergic blockers such as phentolamine; and beta-adrenergic bronchodilators such as albuterol. Excessive caffeine intake and alcohol intoxication also may cause tachycardia.*

▶ *Surgery and pacemakers.* Cardiac surgery and pacemaker malfunction or wire irritation may cause tachycardia.

Special considerations

Continue to monitor the patient closely. Explain ordered diagnostic tests, such as a thyroid panel, electrolyte and hemoglobin levels, hematocrit, pulmonary function studies, and 12-lead ECG. If appropriate, prepare him for electrophysiology studies.

Pediatric pointers

When assessing a child for tachycardia, be aware that normal heart rates for children are higher than those for adults. (See *Normal pediatric vital signs,* pages 394 and 395.) Many of the adult causes described above also may cause tachycardia in children.

Normal pediatric vital signs

This chart lists the normal resting respiratory rate, blood pressure, and pulse rate for girls and boys up to age 16.

VITAL SIGNS	NEONATE	2 YEARS	4 YEARS	6 YEARS	8 YEARS	10 YEARS
Respiratory rate (breaths/minute)						
Girls	28	26	25	24	24	22
Boys	30	28	25	24	22	23
Blood pressure (mm Hg)						
Girls	—	98/60	98/60	98/64	104/68	110/72
Boys	—	96/60	98/60	98/62	102/68	110/72
Pulse rate (beats/minute)						
Girls	130	110	100	100	90	90
Boys	130	110	100	100	90	90

Patient counseling

Provide information about the possibility of the tachyarrhythmia recurring. Teach the patient to take his pulse and monitor his blood pressure at home. Explain the need to take drugs as prescribed, such as thyroid replacement or antiarrhythmics. Explain dietary limitations, such as caffeine and alcohol.

Explain that an antiarrhythmic and an internal defibrillator or ablation therapy may be indicated for symptomatic tachycardia.

REFERENCES

1. Foran, C.K. "Recognize Supraventricular Tachycardia," *Nursing Critical Care* 2(6):14-15, 17, November 2007.
2. Bosen, D.M. "Recognizing Atrioventricular Nodal Reentry Tachycardia," *Nursing* 35(1):32cc1-32cc5, January 2005.
3. Jacobson, C. "Narrow QRS Complex Tachycardias," *AACN Advanced Critical Care* 18(3):264-274, July/September 2007.

● TACHYPNEA

A common sign of cardiopulmonary disorders, tachypnea is an abnormally fast respiratory rate of 20 or more breaths per minute. Tachypnea may reflect the need to increase minute volume, which is the amount of air breathed each minute. If so, it may be accompanied by an increase in tidal volume—the volume of air inhaled or exhaled per breath—resulting in hyperventilation. However, tachypnea also may reflect stiff lungs or overloaded ventilatory muscles, in which case tidal volume may actually be reduced.

Tachypnea may result from reduced arterial oxygen tension or arterial oxygen content, decreased perfusion, or increased oxygen demand. Increased oxygen demand may result from fever, exertion, anxiety, or pain. It also may occur as a compensatory response to metabolic acidosis or may result from pulmonary irritation, stretch receptor stimula-

12 YEARS	14 YEARS	16 YEARS
20	18	16
20	16	16
114/74	118/76	120/78
112/74	120/76	124/78
90	85	80
85	80	75

tion, or a neurologic disorder that upsets medullary respiratory control. Typically, the respiratory rate increases by 4 breaths/minute for every 1° F (0.5° C) increase in body temperature.

If you detect tachypnea, quickly evaluate the patient's cardiopulmonary status; check vital signs and oxygen saturation; and assess for cyanosis, chest pain, dyspnea, tachycardia, and hypotension. If the patient has paradoxical chest movement, suspect flail chest and immediately splint his chest with your hands or with sandbags. Then give supplemental oxygen by nasal cannula or face mask and, if possible, place the patient in semi-Fowler's position to help ease his breathing. If respiratory failure occurs, intubation and mechanical ventilation may be needed. Also, insert an I.V. line for fluid and drug delivery, and start cardiac monitoring.

History and physical examination

If the patient's condition permits, obtain a medical history. Find out when the tachypnea began. Did it follow activity? Has he had it before? Does the patient have a history of asthma, chronic obstructive pulmonary disease (COPD), or any other pulmonary or cardiac conditions? Then have him describe associated signs and symptoms, such as diaphoresis, chest pain, and recent weight loss. Is he anxious about anything or does he have a history of anxiety attacks? Note whether he takes any drugs for pain relief. If so, how effective are they?

Begin the physical examination by taking the patient's vital signs, including oxygen saturation, if you haven't already done so, and observing his overall behavior. (See *Differential diagnosis: Tachypnea*, pages 396 to 399.) Does he seem restless, confused, or fatigued? Then auscultate the chest for abnormal heart and breath sounds. If the patient has a productive cough, record the color, amount, and consistency of sputum. Finally, check for jugular vein distention, and examine the skin for pallor, cyanosis, edema, and warmth or coolness.

Medical causes

▶ *Acute respiratory distress syndrome (ARDS).* Tachypnea and apprehension may be the earliest features of this life-threatening disorder. Tachypnea gradually worsens as fluid accumulates in the patient's lungs, causing them to stiffen. It's accompanied by accessory muscle use, grunting expirations, suprasternal and intercostal retractions, crackles, and rhonchi. Eventually, ARDS produces hypoxemia, resulting in tachycardia, dyspnea, cyanosis, respiratory failure, and shock.

▶ *Alcohol withdrawal syndrome.* A late sign in the acute phase of this syndrome, tachypnea typically accompanies anorexia, insomnia, tachycardia, fever, and diaphoresis. The patient also may experience anxiety, irritability, and bizarre visual or tactile hallucinations.

▶ *Anaphylactic shock.* In this life-threatening type of shock, tachypnea develops within minutes after exposure to an allergen, such as penicillin or insect venom. Other signs and symptoms include anxiety, pounding

Differential diagnosis: Tachypnea

Patients with tachypnea also commonly have tachycardia, dyspnea, and cyanosis. To help differentiate between underlying causes, consider any additional signs and symptoms, such as those listed here.

POSSIBLE CAUSES	SIGNS AND SYMPTOMS	DIAGNOSIS
Pulmonary embolism	• Acute dyspnea • Sudden pleuritic chest pain • Low-grade fever • Nonproductive cough or productive cough with blood-tinged sputum • Pleural friction rub • Crackles • Hemoptysis (possibly) • Wheezing • Dullness on percussion • Decreased breath sounds • Diaphoresis • Restlessness • Anxiety • Signs of shock (possibly)	• Imaging studies (chest X-rays, pulmonary V̇/Q̇ scan, spiral chest computed tomography scan, pulmonary angiography) • Electrocardiogram (ECG)
Pneumothorax	• Severe, sharp, usually unilateral chest pain that's aggravated by chest wall movement • Accessory muscle use • Dry cough • Anxiety • Restlessness	• Physical examination • Arterial blood gas (ABG) analysis • Chest X-rays
Pneumonia	• Hacking, dry cough that progresses to a productive cough • High-grade fever • Shaking chills • Headache • Pleuritic chest pain • Fatigue • Nasal flaring	• Chest X-rays • Sputum specimens • Bronchoscopy if needed
Asthma	• Acute dyspneic attacks • Audible or auscultated wheezing • Dry cough • Hyperpnea • Chest tightness • Accessory muscle use	• Laboratory tests (complete blood count [CBC], ABG analysis, allergy skin testing) • Chest X-rays • Pulmonary function tests

TREATMENT AND FOLLOW-UP

- Oxygen therapy
- Medication (anticoagulants, thrombolytic therapy)

Follow-up: Return visit within first week after hospitalization

- Chest tube insertion
- Analgesics
- Oxygen therapy

Follow-up: Referral to pulmonologist

- Medication (antibiotics, expectorants)
- Oxygen if needed
- Intubation if warranted

Follow-up: Referral to pulmonologist and hospitalization if needed

- Avoidance of allergens, tobacco, and beta blockers
- Medication (inhaled beta$_2$-agonists, inhaled corticosteroids [nedocromil or cromolyn if younger than age 12], leukotriene receptor agonists [possibly], systemic corticosteroids during infections and exacerbations)
- Peak expiratory flow monitoring

(continued)

headache, skin flushing, intense pruritus and, possibly, diffuse urticaria. The patient may have widespread edema of the eyelids, lips, tongue, hands, feet, and genitalia. Other findings include cool, clammy skin; rapid, thready pulse; cough; dyspnea; stridor; and change or loss of voice with laryngeal edema.

▶ *Anemia.* Tachypnea may occur in this disorder, depending on the duration and severity of anemia. Associated signs and symptoms include fatigue, pallor, dyspnea, tachycardia, orthostatic hypotension, bounding pulse, an atrial gallop, and a systolic bruit over the carotid arteries.

▶ *Anxiety.* Tachypnea may occur during high-anxiety states because of the "fight-or-flight" response. Other signs and symptoms include tachycardia, restlessness, chest pain, nausea, and light-headedness, all of which dissipate as the anxiety state resolves.

▶ *Aspiration of a foreign body.* A life-threatening upper airway obstruction may result from aspiration of a foreign body. In a partial obstruction, the patient abruptly develops a paroxysmal dry cough with rapid, shallow respirations. Other signs and symptoms include dyspnea, gagging or choking, intercostal retractions, nasal flaring, cyanosis, decreased or absent breath sounds, hoarseness, and stridor or coarse wheezing. Typically, the patient appears frightened and distressed. A complete obstruction may rapidly cause asphyxia and death.

▶ *Asthma.* Tachypnea is common in life-threatening asthma attacks, which commonly occur at night. These attacks usually begin with mild wheezing and a dry cough that progresses to mucus expectoration. Eventually, the patient becomes apprehensive and develops prolonged expirations, intercostal and supraclavicular retractions on inspiration, accessory muscle use, severe audible wheezing, rhonchi, flaring nostrils, tachycardia, diaphoresis, and flushing or cyanosis.

▶ *Bronchiectasis.* Although this disorder may produce tachypnea, its classic sign is a chronic productive cough that produces copious amounts of mucopurulent, foul-smelling sputum and, occasionally, hemoptysis. Related findings include coarse crackles on inspiration, exertional dyspnea, rhonchi, and halitosis. The patient also may have fever, malaise,

Differential diagnosis: Tachypnea *(continued)*

POSSIBLE CAUSES	SIGNS AND SYMPTOMS	DIAGNOSIS
Asthma (continued)	• Nasal flaring • Intercostal and supraclavicular retractions • Tachycardia • Diaphoresis • Prolonged expiration • Flushing or cyanosis • Apprehension	
Heart failure	• Gradually developing dyspnea • Chronic paroxysmal nocturnal dyspnea • Orthopnea • Tachycardia • Palpitations • S_3 • Fatigue • Dependent peripheral edema • Hepatomegaly • Dry cough • Anorexia • Weight gain • Loss of mental acuity • Hemoptysis *In acute onset heart failure* • Distended jugular veins • Bibasilar crackles • Oliguria • Hypotension	• Laboratory tests (CBC, cardiac enzymes, troponin) • Imaging studies (chest X-rays, echocardiogram) • ECG

weight loss, fatigue, and weakness. Clubbing is a common late sign.

▶ *Bronchitis (chronic).* Mild tachypnea may occur in this form of COPD, but it isn't typically a characteristic sign. Chronic bronchitis usually begins with a dry, hacking cough, which later produces copious amounts of sputum. Other characteristic findings include dyspnea, prolonged expirations, wheezing, scattered rhonchi, accessory muscle use, and cyanosis. Clubbing and barrel chest are late signs.

▶ *Cardiac arrhythmias.* Depending on the patient's heart rate, tachypnea may occur along with hypotension, dizziness, palpitations, weakness, and fatigue. The patient's level of consciousness (LOC) may be decreased.

▶ *Cardiac tamponade.* In life-threatening cardiac tamponade, tachypnea may accompany tachycardia, dyspnea, and paradoxical pulse. Related findings include muffled heart sounds, pericardial friction rub, chest pain, hypotension, narrowed pulse pressure, and hepatomegaly. The patient is noticeably anxious and restless. His skin is clammy and cyanotic, and his jugular veins are distended.

▶ *Cardiogenic shock.* Although many signs of cardiogenic shock appear in other types of shock, they're usually more severe in this type. Besides tachypnea, the patient commonly displays cold, pale, clammy, cyanotic skin; hypotension; tachycardia; narrowed pulse pressure; a ventricular gallop; oliguria; decreased LOC; and jugular vein distention.

TREATMENT AND FOLLOW-UP

Follow-up: For acute exacerbations, return visit within 24 hours, then every 3 to 5 days, and then every 1 to 3 months; referral to pulmonologist if treatment is ineffective

• Medication (angiotensin-converting enzyme inhibitors, diuretics, possibly carvedilol, possibly digoxin)
Follow-up: Return visit within 1 week after discharge, at 4 weeks, and then every 3 months; referral to cardiologist if condition is chronic

▶ *Emphysema.* This form of COPD commonly produces tachypnea with exertional dyspnea.[1] It also may cause anorexia, malaise, peripheral cyanosis, pursed-lip breathing, accessory muscle use, and a chronic productive cough. Percussion yields a hyperresonant tone; auscultation reveals wheezing, crackles, and diminished breath sounds. Clubbing and barrel chest are late signs.
▶ *Febrile illness.* Fever can cause tachypnea, tachycardia, and other signs.
▶ *Flail chest.* Tachypnea usually appears early in this life-threatening disorder. Other findings include paradoxical chest wall movement, rib bruises and palpable fractures, localized chest pain, hypotension, and diminished breath sounds. The patient also may de-

velop signs of respiratory distress, such as dyspnea and accessory muscle use.
▶ *Head trauma.* When trauma affects the brain stem, the patient may develop central neurogenic hyperventilation, a form of tachypnea marked by rapid, even, and deep respirations. The tachypnea may be accompanied by other signs of life-threatening neurogenic dysfunction, such as coma, unequal and nonreactive pupils, seizures, hemiplegia, flaccidity, and hypoactive or absent deep tendon reflexes.
▶ *Hyperosmolar hyperglycemic nonketotic syndrome.* Rapidly deteriorating LOC occurs along with tachypnea, tachycardia, hypotension, seizures, oliguria, and signs of dehydration.
▶ *Hypovolemic shock.* An early sign of life-threatening hypovolemic shock, tachypnea is accompanied by cool, pale skin; restlessness; thirst; and mild tachycardia. As shock progresses, the patient develops clammy skin and an increasingly rapid and thready pulse. Other findings include hypotension, narrowed pulse pressure, oliguria, subnormal body temperature, and decreased LOC.
▶ *Hypoxia.* Lack of oxygen from any cause increases the rate (and often the depth) of breathing. Associated symptoms are related to the cause of the hypoxia.
▶ *Interstitial fibrosis.* In this disorder, tachypnea develops gradually and may become severe. Related features include exertional dyspnea, pleuritic chest pain, a paroxysmal dry cough, crackles, late inspiratory wheezing, cyanosis, fatigue, and weight loss. Clubbing is a late sign.
▶ *Lung abscess.* In this type of abscess, tachypnea is usually paired with dyspnea and accentuated by fever. However, the chief sign is a productive cough with copious amounts of purulent, foul-smelling, usually bloody sputum. Other findings include chest pain, halitosis, diaphoresis, chills, fatigue, weakness, anorexia, weight loss, and clubbing.
▶ *Lung, pleural, or mediastinal tumor.* These types of tumors may cause tachypnea along with exertional dyspnea, cough, hemoptysis, and pleuritic chest pain. Other effects include anorexia, weight loss, and fatigue.
▶ *Mesothelioma (malignant).* Commonly related to asbestos exposure, this pleural mass

initially produces tachypnea and dyspnea on mild exertion. Other classic symptoms are persistent dull chest pain and aching shoulder pain that progresses to arm weakness and paresthesia. Later signs and symptoms include a cough, insomnia from pain, clubbing, and dullness over the malignant mesothelioma.

▶ *Neurogenic shock.* Tachypnea is characteristic in this life-threatening type of shock. It's commonly accompanied by apprehension, bradycardia or tachycardia, oliguria, fluctuating body temperature, and decreased LOC that may progress to coma. The patient's skin is warm, dry, and perhaps flushed. He may have nausea and vomiting.

▶ *Plague.* The onset of the pneumonic form of this virulent bacterial infection is usually sudden and marked by chills, fever, headache, and myalgia. Pulmonary signs and symptoms include tachypnea, a productive cough, chest pain, dyspnea, hemoptysis, increasing respiratory distress, and cardiopulmonary insufficiency. The pneumonic form may be contracted by inhaling respiratory droplets from an infected person. It also could be contracted from aerosolization and inhalation of the organism in biological warfare.

▶ *Pneumonia (bacterial).* A common sign in this infection, tachypnea usually is preceded by a painful, hacking, dry cough that rapidly becomes productive. Other signs and symptoms quickly follow, including high fever, shaking chills, headache, dyspnea, pleuritic chest pain, tachycardia, grunting respirations, nasal flaring, and cyanosis. Auscultation reveals diminished breath sounds and fine crackles; percussion yields a dull tone.

▶ *Pneumothorax.* Tachypnea, a common sign of life-threatening pneumothorax, typically is accompanied by severe, sharp, and commonly unilateral chest pain that's aggravated by chest movement. Other signs and symptoms include dyspnea, tachycardia, accessory muscle use, asymmetrical chest expansion, a dry cough, cyanosis, anxiety, and restlessness. Examination of the affected lung reveals hyperresonance or tympany, subcutaneous crepitation, decreased vocal fremitus, and diminished or absent breath sounds. A patient with tension pneumothorax also develops a deviated trachea.

▶ *Pulmonary edema.* An early sign of this life-threatening disorder, tachypnea is accompanied by exertional dyspnea, paroxysmal nocturnal dyspnea and, later, orthopnea. Tachypnea, tachycardia, hypoxia, and hypotension or hypertension are poor prognostic signs in pulmonary edema.[2] Other features include a dry cough, crackles, tachycardia, and a ventricular gallop. In severe pulmonary edema, respirations become increasingly rapid and labored, tachycardia worsens, crackles become more diffuse, and the cough produces frothy, bloody sputum. Signs of shock—such as hypotension, thready pulse, and cool, clammy skin—also may occur.

▶ *Pulmonary embolism (acute).* In pulmonary embolism, tachypnea occurs suddenly, usually with dyspnea.[3] The patient may complain of angina or pleuritic chest pain. Other characteristic findings include tachycardia, a dry or productive cough with blood-tinged sputum, low-grade fever, restlessness, and diaphoresis. Less common signs include massive hemoptysis, chest splinting, leg edema, and—with a large embolus—jugular vein distention and syncope. Other findings include pleural friction rub, crackles, diffuse wheezing, dullness on percussion, diminished breath sounds, and signs of shock, such as hypotension and a weak, rapid pulse.

▶ *Pulmonary hypertension (primary).* In this rare disorder, tachypnea is usually a late sign that's accompanied by exertional dyspnea, general fatigue, weakness, and episodes of syncope. The patient may complain of angina on exertion, which may radiate to the neck. Other effects include a cough, hemoptysis, and hoarseness.

▶ *Septic shock.* Early in septic shock, the patient usually develops tachypnea; sudden fever; chills; flushed, warm, dry skin; and possibly nausea, vomiting, and diarrhea. He also may develop tachycardia and normal or slightly decreased blood pressure. As this life-threatening type of shock progresses, the patient may have anxiety; restlessness; decreased LOC; hypotension; cool, clammy, cyanotic skin; rapid, thready pulse; thirst; and oliguria that may progress to anuria.

Other causes

▶ *Salicylates.* Tachypnea may result from an overdose of these drugs.

Special considerations

Continue to monitor the patient's vital signs closely. Be sure to keep suction and emergency equipment nearby. Prepare to intubate the patient and to provide mechanical ventilation if needed. If mechanical ventilation becomes necessary, monitor the patient's respiratory status closely and be prepared to wean as soon as possible to prevent complications such as pneumonia and trauma to the airways.[4] Prepare the patient for diagnostic studies, such as arterial blood gas analysis, blood cultures, chest X-rays, pulmonary function tests, and an electrocardiogram.

Pediatric pointers

When assessing a child for tachypnea, remember that the normal respiratory rate varies with a child's age. (See *Normal pediatric vital signs,* pages 394 and 395.) If you detect tachypnea, first rule out the causes listed above. Then consider these pediatric causes: congenital heart defects, meningitis, metabolic acidosis, and cystic fibrosis. Keep in mind, however, that hunger and anxiety also may cause tachypnea.

Geriatric pointers

Tachypnea may have a variety of causes in elderly patients, such as pneumonia, heart failure, COPD, anxiety, or failure to take cardiac and respiratory drugs correctly; mild increases in respiratory rate may be unnoticed.

Patient counseling

Reassure the patient that slight increases in respiratory rate may be normal.

REFERENCES
1. Gant, M.J. "COPD: The Lung-Crushing Culprit," *Nursing Critical Care* 2(3):50-56, May 2007.
2. Ezzone, S.A. "Pulmonary Edema," *Clinical Journal of Oncology Nursing* 11(3):457-459, June 2007.
3. Charlebois, D. "Early Recognition of Pulmonary Embolism: The Key to Lowering Mortality," *Journal of Cardiovascular Nursing* 20(4):254-259, July/August 2005.
4. Lindgren, V.A., and Ames, N.J. "Caring for Patients on Mechanical Ventilation: What Research Indicates is Best Practice," *AJN* 105(5):50-60, May 2005.

● THROAT PAIN

Throat pain, or sore throat, refers to discomfort in any part of the pharynx: nasopharynx, oropharynx, or hypopharynx. This common symptom ranges from a sensation of scratchiness to severe pain. It's commonly accompanied by ear pain because cranial nerves IX and X innervate the pharynx as well as the middle and external ear. (See *Anatomy of the throat,* page 402.)

Throat pain may result from infection, trauma, allergy, cancer, or a systemic disorder. It also may follow surgery and endotracheal intubation. Nonpathologic causes include dry mucous membranes associated with mouth breathing and laryngeal irritation associated with vocal strain, alcohol consumption, and inhalation of smoke or chemicals such as ammonia.

History and physical examination

Ask the patient when he first noticed the pain and have him describe it. Has he had throat pain before? Does he also have fever, ear pain, or dysphagia? Review the patient's medical history for throat problems, allergies, and systemic disorders.

Next, carefully examine the pharynx, noting redness, exudate, or swelling. Examine the oropharynx, using a warmed metal spatula or tongue blade, and the nasopharynx, using a warmed laryngeal mirror or a fiber-optic nasopharyngoscope. Laryngoscopic examination of the hypopharynx may be required. (If needed, spray the soft palate and pharyngeal wall with a local anesthetic to prevent gagging.) Observe the tonsils for redness, swelling, or exudate; if exudate is present, obtain a specimen for culture. Then examine the nose, using a nasal speculum. Also, check the patient's ears, especially if he reports ear pain. Finally, palpate the neck and oropharynx for nodules or lymph node enlargement.

Anatomy of the throat

The throat, or pharynx, is divided into three areas: the nasopharynx (the soft palate and the posterior nasal cavity), the oropharynx (the area between the soft palate and the upper edge of the epiglottis), and the hypopharynx (the area between the epiglottis and the level of the cricoid cartilage). A disorder affecting any of these areas may cause throat pain. Pinpointing the causative disorder begins with accurate assessment of the throat structures illustrated here.

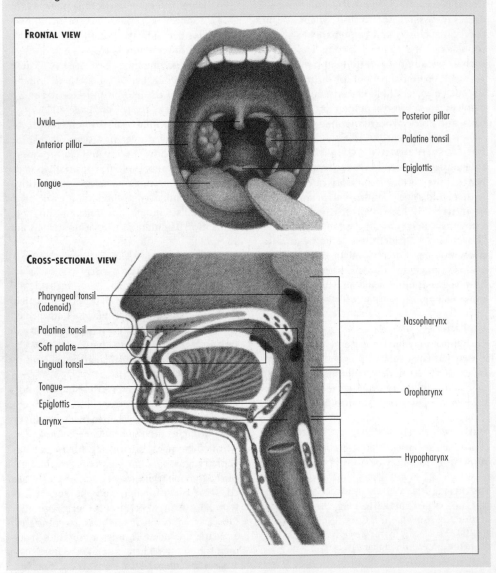

FRONTAL VIEW

Uvula

Anterior pillar

Tongue

Posterior pillar

Palatine tonsil

Epiglottis

CROSS-SECTIONAL VIEW

Pharyngeal tonsil (adenoid)

Palatine tonsil

Soft palate

Lingual tonsil

Tongue

Epiglottis

Larynx

Nasopharynx

Oropharynx

Hypopharynx

Medical causes

▶ *Agranulocytosis.* In this disorder, sore throat may accompany other signs and symptoms of infection, such as fever, chills, and headache. Typically, it follows progressive fatigue and weakness. Other findings include nausea and vomiting, anorexia, and bleeding tendencies. Rough-edged ulcers with gray or black membranes may appear on the gums, palate, or perianal area.

▶ *Allergic rhinitis.* Occurring seasonally or year-round, this disorder may produce sore throat as well as nasal congestion with a thin nasal discharge, postnasal drip, paroxysmal sneezing, decreased sense of smell, frontal or temporal headache, and itchy eyes, nose, and throat. Examination reveals pale and glistening nasal mucosa with edematous nasal turbinates, watery eyes, reddened conjunctivae and eyelids and, possibly, swollen eyelids.

▶ *Avian influenza.* Throat pain, muscle aches, cough, and fever are common early symptoms of avian influenza. The most virulent of these viruses, avian influenza A (H5N1), also may cause pneumonia, acute respiratory distress, and other life-threatening complications. A recent outbreak of the H5N1 virus among domesticated birds (chickens, turkeys, geese) in Asian countries has caused human sickness and death in those who contracted the virus from infected poultry and contaminated surfaces. Studies are underway to investigate the effectiveness of antiviral drugs and vaccines.

▶ *Bronchitis (acute).* This disorder may produce lower throat pain, fever, chills, cough, and muscle and back pain. Auscultation reveals rhonchi, wheezing, and sometimes crackles.

▶ *Chronic fatigue syndrome.* This nonspecific symptom complex is characterized by incapacitating fatigue. Other findings include sore throat, myalgia, and cognitive dysfunction.

▶ *Common cold.* Sore throat may accompany cough, sneezing, nasal congestion, rhinorrhea, fatigue, headache, myalgia, and arthralgia.

▶ *Contact ulcers.* Common in men with stressful jobs, contact ulcers appear symmetrically on the posterior vocal cords, resulting in sore throat. The pain is aggravated by talking and may be accompanied by referred ear pain and occasionally hemoptysis. Typically, the patient also has a history of chronic throat clearing or acid reflux.

▶ *Foreign body.* A foreign body lodged in the palatine or lingual tonsil and pyriform sinus may produce localized throat pain. The pain may persist after the foreign body is dislodged until mucosal irritation resolves.

▶ *Gastroesophageal reflux disease.* In this disorder, an incompetent gastroesophageal sphincter allows gastric juices to enter the hypopharynx and irritate the larynx, causing chronic sore throat and hoarseness. The arytenoid cartilage also may appear red and swollen, resulting in a sensation of a lump in the throat.

▶ *Glossopharyngeal neuralgia.* Triggered by a specific pharyngeal movement, such as yawning or swallowing, this condition causes unilateral, knifelike throat pain in the tonsillar fossa that may radiate to the ear.

▶ *Herpes simplex virus.* Sore throat may result from lesions on the oral mucosa, especially the tongue, gingivae, and cheeks. After causing brief prodromal discomfort, lesions erupt into erythematous vesicles that eventually rupture and leave a painful ulcer, followed by a yellowish crust. In generalized infection, the vesicles accompany submaxillary lymphadenopathy, halitosis, increased salivation, anorexia, and fever of up to 105° F (40.6° C).

▶ *Influenza.* Patients with the flu commonly complain of sore throat, fever with chills, headache, weakness, malaise, myalgia, cough and, occasionally, hoarseness and rhinorrhea.

▶ *Laryngeal cancer.* In extrinsic laryngeal cancer, the chief symptom is pain or burning in the throat when drinking citrus juice or hot liquids, or a lump in the throat; in intrinsic laryngeal cancer, it's hoarseness that persists for longer than 3 weeks. Later signs and symptoms of metastasis include dysphagia, dyspnea, a cough, enlarged cervical lymph nodes, and pain that radiates to the ear.

▶ *Laryngitis (acute).* This disorder produces sore throat, but its cardinal sign is mild to severe hoarseness, perhaps with temporary loss of voice. Other findings are malaise, low-grade fever, dysphagia, dry cough, and tender, enlarged cervical lymph nodes.

▶ *Monkeypox.* Early symptoms of this rare viral disease include sore throat, fever, lymphadenopathy, chills, myalgia, and rash. The virus exhibits some similarities to smallpox, but its symptoms tend to be milder. Monkeypox is spread primarily through contact with lesions or body fluids of infected animals. Although it occurs primarily in central and western Africa, the virus has also been reported in the United States since 2003. There's no specific treatment for monkeypox, which typically lasts 2 to 4 weeks.

▶ *Mononucleosis (infectious).* Sore throat is one of the three classic findings in this infection. The other two classic signs are cervical lymphadenopathy and fluctuating temperature with an evening peak of 101° to 102° F (38.3° to 38.9° C). Splenomegaly and hepatomegaly also may develop.

▶ *Necrotizing ulcerative gingivitis (acute).* Also known as trench mouth, this disorder usually begins abruptly with sore throat and tender gums that ulcerate and bleed. A gray exudate may cover the gums and pharyngeal tonsils. Related signs and symptoms include a foul taste in the mouth, halitosis, cervical lymphadenopathy, headache, malaise, and fever.

▶ *Peritonsillar abscess.* The most common deep infection of the head and throat, this abscess typically causes severe throat pain that radiates to the ear.[1] Accompanying the pain may be dysphagia, drooling, dysarthria, halitosis, fever with chills, malaise, and nausea. The patient usually tilts his head toward the side of the abscess. Examination also may reveal a deviated uvula, trismus, and tender, enlarged cervical lymph nodes.

▶ *Pharyngeal burns.* First- or second-degree burns of the posterior pharynx may cause throat pain and dysphagia.

▶ *Pharyngitis.* Whether bacterial, fungal, or viral, pharyngitis may cause sore throat and localized erythema and edema. *Bacterial pharyngitis* begins abruptly with a unilateral sore throat. Other signs and symptoms include dysphagia, fever, malaise, headache, abdominal pain, myalgia, and arthralgia. Inspection reveals an exudate on the tonsil or tonsillar fossa, uvular edema, soft palate erythema, and tender cervical lymph nodes.

Also called *thrush, fungal pharyngitis* causes diffuse sore throat—often described as a burning sensation—accompanied by pharyngeal erythema and edema. White plaques mark the pharynx, tonsil, tonsillar pillars, base of the tongue, and oral mucosa; scraping these plaques uncovers a hemorrhagic base.

Viral pharyngitis produces a diffuse sore throat, malaise, fever, and mild erythema and edema of the posterior oropharyngeal wall.

Tonsil enlargement and anterior cervical lymphadenopathy may be present.

▶ *Pharyngomaxillary space abscess.* A complication of untreated pharyngeal or tonsillar infection or tooth extraction, pharyngomaxillary space abscess causes mild throat pain. Inspection reveals a bulge in the medial wall of the pharynx accompanied by swelling of the neck and at the jaw angle on the affected side. Other signs and symptoms include fever, dysphagia, trismus and, possibly, signs of respiratory distress or toxemia.

▶ *Sinusitis (acute).* This disorder may cause sore throat with a purulent nasal discharge and postnasal drip, resulting in halitosis. Other effects include headache, malaise, cough, fever, and facial pain and swelling associated with nasal congestion.

▶ *Tongue cancer.* The patient with tongue cancer has localized throat pain that may occur around a raised white lesion or ulcer. The pain may radiate to the ear and be accompanied by dysphagia.

▶ *Tonsillar cancer.* Sore throat is the presenting symptom in tonsillar cancer. Unfortunately, the cancer is usually quite advanced before this symptom appears. The pain may radiate to the ear and is accompanied by a superficial ulcer on the tonsil or one that extends to the base of the tongue.

▶ *Tonsillitis.* Mild to severe sore throat is usually the first symptom of *acute tonsillitis.* The pain may radiate to the ears and be accompanied by dysphagia and headache. Related findings include malaise, fever with chills, halitosis, myalgia, arthralgia, and tender cervical lymph nodes. Examination reveals edematous, reddened tonsils with a purulent exudate.

Chronic tonsillitis causes a mild sore throat, malaise, and tender cervical lymph nodes. The tonsils appear smooth, pink and, possibly, enlarged, with purulent debris in the crypts. Halitosis and a foul taste in the mouth are other common findings.

Unilateral or bilateral throat pain occurs just above the hyoid bone in *lingual tonsillitis.* The lingual tonsils appear red and swollen and are covered with exudate. Other findings include a muffled voice, dysphagia, and tender cervical lymph nodes on the affected side.

▶ *Uvulitis*. This inflammation may cause throat pain or a sensation of something in the throat. The uvula is usually swollen and red but, in allergic uvulitis, it's pale.

Other causes

▶ *Treatments*. Endotracheal intubation and local surgery, such as tonsillectomy and adenoidectomy, commonly cause sore throat. Chemotherapy can cause mucositis that may affect any portion of the alimentary canal from the mouth to the anus.[2] If the throat is affected, the patient will have throat pain and ulcerations.

Special considerations

Provide analgesic sprays or lozenges to relieve throat pain. Also, prepare the patient for a throat culture, a complete blood count, and a mononucleosis spot test.

Pediatric pointers

Sore throat is a common complaint in children and may result from many of the same disorders that affect adults. Other pediatric causes of sore throat include acute epiglottidis, herpangina, scarlet fever, acute follicular tonsillitis, and retropharyngeal abscess.

Patient counseling

If the patient is taking antibiotics, stress the importance of completing the 10-day course of treatment, even if symptoms improve after only a few days. Tell the patient that he's presumed noninfectious after 24 hours of antibiotic coverage. Suggest gargling with salt water to soothe the throat.

REFERENCES

1. Kamienski, M. "When Sore Throat Gets Serious: Three Different Cases, Three Very Different Causes," *AJN* 107(10):35-38, October 2007.
2. Keefe, D.M., Rassias, G., O'Neil, L., and Gibson, R.J. "Severe Mucositis: How Can Nutrition Help?" *Current Opinion in Clinical Nutrition and Metabolic Care* 10(5):627-31, September 2007.

TINNITUS

About 17% of Americans develop tinnitus.[1] Although the term literally means ringing in the ears, it includes many other abnormal sounds as well. For example, tinnitus may sound like escaping air, running water, the inside of a seashell, or a sizzling, buzzing, or humming noise. Occasionally, it's described as a roaring or musical sound. *Acute tinnitus* may last days to weeks; *chronic tinnitus* lasts longer than 6 months.[1] This common symptom may be unilateral or bilateral and constant or intermittent. Although the brain may adjust to or suppress constant tinnitus, some patients are so disturbed by the sounds that they contemplate suicide as their only source of relief.

Tinnitus can be classified in several ways. *Subjective tinnitus* (the most common form) is heard only by the patient; *objective tinnitus* is also heard by an observer who places a stethoscope near the patient's affected ear.[1] *Tinnitus aurium* refers to noise that the patient hears in his ears; *tinnitus cerebri*, to noise that he hears in his head.

Tinnitus usually is associated with neural injury in the auditory pathway, resulting in spontaneous altered firing of sensory auditory neurons. It may stem from an ear disorder, a cardiovascular or systemic disorder, or the effects of certain drugs. Nonpathologic causes of tinnitus include acute anxiety and presbycusis. (See *Common causes of tinnitus,* page 406.)

History and physical examination

Ask the patient to describe the sound he hears, including its onset, pattern, pitch, location, and intensity. Ask whether it's accompanied by other symptoms, such as vertigo, headache, or hearing loss. Next, take a health history, including a complete drug history.

Using an otoscope, inspect the patient's ears and examine the tympanic membrane. To check for hearing loss, perform the Weber and Rinne tuning fork tests. (See *Differentiating conductive from sensorineural hearing loss,* page 218.)

Also, auscultate for bruits in the neck. Then compress the jugular vein or carotid ar-

Common causes of tinnitus

Tinnitus usually results from a disorder that affects the external, middle, or inner ear. Below are some of its more common causes and their locations.

EXTERNAL EAR
- Ear canal obstruction by cerumen or a foreign body
- Otitis externa
- Tympanic membrane perforation

MIDDLE EAR
- Ossicle dislocation
- Otitis media
- Otosclerosis

INNER EAR
- Acoustic neuroma
- Atherosclerosis of carotid artery
- Labyrinthitis
- Ménière's disease

tery to see if this affects the tinnitus. Finally, examine the nasopharynx for masses that might cause eustachian tube dysfunction and tinnitus.

Medical causes

▶ *Acoustic neuroma.* An early symptom of this eighth cranial nerve tumor, unilateral tinnitus precedes unilateral sensorineural hearing loss and vertigo. Facial paralysis, headache, nausea, vomiting, and papilledema also may occur.

▶ *Anemia.* Severe anemia may produce mild, reversible tinnitus. Other common effects include pallor, weakness, fatigue, exertional dyspnea, tachycardia, bounding pulse, atrial gallop, and a systolic bruit over the carotid arteries.

▶ *Atherosclerosis of the carotid artery.* In this disorder, the patient has constant tinnitus that can be stopped by applying pressure over the carotid artery. Auscultation over the upper part of the neck, on the auricle, or near the ear on the affected side may detect a bruit. Palpation may reveal a weak carotid pulse.

▶ *Cervical spondylosis.* In this degenerative disorder, osteophytic growths may compress the vertebral arteries, resulting in tinnitus. Typically, a stiff neck and pain aggravated by activity accompany tinnitus. Other features include brief vertigo, nystagmus, hearing loss, paresthesia, weakness, and pain that radiates down the arms.

▶ *Ear canal obstruction.* When cerumen or a foreign body blocks the ear canal, the patient may have tinnitus, conductive hearing loss, itching, and a feeling of fullness or pain in the ear.

▶ *Eustachian tube patency.* Normally, the eustachian tube remains closed, except during swallowing. However, persistent patency of this tube can cause tinnitus, audible breath sounds, loud and distorted voice sounds, and a sense of fullness in the ear. Examination with a pneumatic otoscope reveals movement of the tympanic membrane with respirations. At times, breath sounds can be heard with a stethoscope placed over the auricle.

▶ *Glomus jugulare or glomus tympanicum tumor.* A pulsating sound usually is the first symptom of these tumors. Other early features include a reddish blue mass behind the tympanic membrane and progressive conductive hearing loss. Later, total unilateral deafness is accompanied by ear pain and dizziness. Otorrhagia also may occur if the tumor breaks through the tympanic membrane.

▶ *Hypertension.* Severe hypertension (diastolic blood pressure exceeding 120 mm Hg) may cause bilateral high-pitched tinnitus, a severe throbbing headache, restlessness, nausea, vomiting, blurred vision, seizures, and decreased level of consciousness.

▶ *Intracranial arteriovenous malformation.* A large malformation may cause pulsating tinnitus accompanied by a bruit over the mastoid process.

▶ *Labyrinthitis (suppurative).* In this disorder, tinnitus may accompany sudden, severe attacks of vertigo, unilateral or bilateral sensorineural hearing loss, nystagmus, dizziness, nausea, and vomiting.

▶ *Ménière's disease.* Most common in adults—especially men ages 30 to 60—this labyrinthine disease is characterized by attacks of tinnitus, vertigo, a feeling of fullness or blockage in the ear, and fluctuating sensorineural hearing loss. Attacks last 10 minutes to several hours; they occur over a few days or weeks and are followed by a remission. Severe nausea, vomiting, diaphoresis, and nystagmus also may occur during attacks.

▶ *Ossicle dislocation.* Acoustic trauma, such as a slap on the ear, may dislocate the ossicle, resulting in tinnitus and sensorineural hearing loss. Bleeding from the middle ear also may occur.

▶ *Otitis externa (acute).* Although not a major complaint in this disorder, tinnitus may result if debris in the external ear canal impinges on the tympanic membrane. More typical findings include pruritus, a foul-smelling purulent discharge, and severe ear pain that's aggravated by manipulation of the tragus or auricle, teeth clenching, mouth opening, and chewing. The external ear canal typically appears red and edematous and may be occluded by debris, causing partial hearing loss.

▶ *Otitis media.* This infection may cause tinnitus and conductive hearing loss. However, its more typical features include ear pain, a red and bulging tympanic membrane, high fever, chills, and dizziness.

▶ *Otosclerosis.* In this disorder, the patient may describe ringing, roaring, or whistling tinnitus or a combination of these sounds. He also may report progressive hearing loss, which may lead to bilateral deafness, and vertigo.

▶ *Palatal myoclonus.* In this disorder, muscles of the palate contract rhythmically, either intermittently or continuously, causing a clicking sound in the ear and vibratory tinnitus. The contractions are visible with a nasopharyngeal mirror.

▶ *Presbycusis.* This otologic effect of aging produces tinnitus and progressive, symmetrical, bilateral sensorineural hearing loss, usually of high-frequency tones.

▶ *Tympanic membrane perforation.* Tinnitus and hearing loss go hand-in-hand in this disorder. Tinnitus is usually the chief complaint in a small perforation; hearing loss, in a larger perforation. These symptoms typically develop suddenly and may be accompanied by pain, vertigo, and a feeling of fullness in the ear.

Other causes

DRUG WATCH *Indomethacin, quinine, and excessive use of salicylates may cause reversible tinnitus. Common drugs that may cause irreversible tinnitus include the aminoglycoside antibiotics (especially kanamycin, streptomycin, and gentamicin) and vancomycin.*

▶ *Alcohol use.* Consumption of alcohol may cause reversible tinnitus.

▶ *Noise.* Chronic exposure to noise, especially high-pitched sounds, can damage the ear's hair cells, causing tinnitus and bilateral hearing loss. These symptoms may be temporary or permanent.

Special considerations

Tinnitus is typically difficult to treat successfully. If reversible causes have been ruled out, educate the patient about strategies for adapting to the tinnitus, including biofeedback and masking devices. In addition, a hearing aid may be prescribed to amplify environmental sounds, thereby obscuring tinnitus. For some patients, a device that combines the features of a masker and a hearing aid may be used to block out tinnitus.

Pediatric pointers

An expectant mother's use of ototoxic drugs during the third trimester of pregnancy can cause labyrinthine damage in the fetus, resulting in tinnitus. Many of the disorders described above can also cause tinnitus in children.

Geriatric pointers

About 25% to 30% of adults over age 65 develop chronic tinnitus.[1]

Patient counseling

Advise the patient to avoid exposure to excessive noise, ototoxic agents, and other factors that may cause cochlear damage. Instruct the patient to avoid caffeine, nicotine, and alchol, which can worsen fluid imbalance of the inner ear.[1,2] Inform him that even people with normal hearing may have intermittent periods of mild, high-pitched tinnitus that can last for several minutes.

REFERENCES
1. Daugherty, J.A. "The Latest Buzz on Tinnitus," *The Nurse Practitioner* 32(10):42-47, October 2007.
2. Pullen, R.L. "Spin Control: Caring for A Patient with Inner Ear Disease," *Nursing* 36(5):48-51, May 2006.

TRACHEAL DEVIATION

Normally, the trachea is located at the midline of the neck—except at the bifurcation, where it shifts slightly toward the right. Visible deviation from its normal position signals a condition that can compromise pulmonary function and, possibly, cause respiratory distress. A hallmark of life-threatening tension pneumothorax, tracheal deviation occurs in disorders that produce a mediastinal shift from asymmetrical thoracic volume or pressure. (See *Detecting slight tracheal deviation.*)

If you detect tracheal deviation, be alert for signs and symptoms of respiratory distress (tachypnea, dyspnea, decreased or absent breath sounds, stridor, nasal flaring, accessory muscle use, asymmetrical chest expansion, restlessness, and anxiety). If possible, place the patient in semi-Fowler's position to aid respiratory excursion and improve oxygenation. Give supplemental oxygen, and intubate the patient if needed. Insert an I.V. line for fluid and drug administration. In addition, palpate the neck and chest for subcutaneous crepitation, a sign of tension pneumothorax. Chest tube insertion may be needed to release trapped air or fluid and restore normal intrapleural and intrathoracic pressure gradients.[1]

History

If the patient doesn't have signs of distress, ask about a history of pulmonary or cardiac disorders, surgery, trauma, or infection. If he smokes, determine how much. Ask about related signs and symptoms, especially breathing difficulty, pain, and cough.

Medical causes

▶ *Atelectasis.* Extensive lung collapse can produce tracheal deviation toward the affect-

Detecting slight tracheal deviation

Although gross tracheal deviation is visible, slight deviation can be detected only by palpation or sometimes an X-ray. Try palpation first.

With the tip of your index finger, locate the patient's trachea by palpating between the sternocleidomastoid muscles. Then compare the trachea's position to an imaginary line drawn vertically through the suprasternal notch. Any deviation from midline usually is considered abnormal.

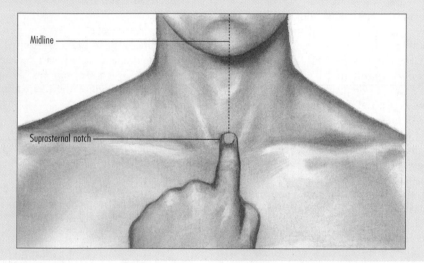

Midline

Suprasternal notch

ed side. Respiratory findings include dyspnea, tachypnea, pleuritic chest pain, a dry cough, dullness on percussion, decreased vocal fremitus and breath sounds, inspiratory lag, and substernal or intercostal retraction.

▶ *Hiatal hernia.* Intrusion of abdominal viscera into the pleural space causes tracheal deviation toward the unaffected side. The degree of attendant respiratory distress depends on the extent of herniation. Other effects include pyrosis, regurgitation or vomiting, and chest or abdominal pain.

▶ *Kyphoscoliosis.* This disorder can cause rib cage distortion and mediastinal shift, producing tracheal deviation toward the compressed lung. Respiratory effects include a dry cough, dyspnea, asymmetrical chest expansion and, possibly, asymmetrical breath sounds. Backache and fatigue are also common.

▶ *Mediastinal tumor.* This type of tumor commonly produces no symptoms in its early stages; however, a large mediastinal tumor can press against the trachea and nearby structures, causing tracheal deviation and dys-

phagia. Other late findings include stridor, dyspnea, a brassy cough, hoarseness, and stertorous respirations with suprasternal retraction. The patient may have shoulder, arm, or chest pain as well as edema of the neck, face, or arm. His neck and chest wall veins may be dilated.

▶ *Pleural effusion.* A large pleural effusion can shift the mediastinum to the contralateral side, producing tracheal deviation. Related effects include a dry cough, dyspnea, pleuritic chest pain, pleural friction rub, tachypnea, decreased chest motion, decreased or absent breath sounds, egophony, flatness on percussion, decreased tactile fremitus, fever, and weight loss.

▶ *Pulmonary fibrosis.* Asymmetrical fibrosis can cause tracheal deviation as the mediastinum shifts toward the affected side. Related findings reflect the underlying condition and pattern of fibrosis. Dyspnea, cough, clubbing, malaise, and fever commonly occur.

▶ *Pulmonary tuberculosis.* In a large cavitation, tracheal deviation toward the affected side accompanies asymmetrical chest excursion, dullness on percussion, increased tactile fremitus, amphoric breath sounds, and inspiratory crackles. Insidious early effects include fatigue, anorexia, weight loss, fever, chills, and night sweats. A productive cough, hemoptysis, pleuritic chest pain, and dyspnea develop as the disease progresses.

▶ *Retrosternal thyroid.* This anatomic abnormality can displace the trachea. The gland is felt as a movable neck mass above the suprasternal notch. Dysphagia, cough, hoarseness, and stridor are common. Signs of thyrotoxicosis may be present.

▶ *Tension pneumothorax.* This acute, life-threatening condition produces tracheal deviation toward the unaffected side.[2] It's marked by a sudden onset of respiratory distress with sharp chest pain, a dry cough, severe dyspnea, tachycardia, wheezing, cyanosis, accessory muscle use, nasal flaring, air hunger, and asymmetrical chest movement. Restless and anxious, the patient also may develop subcutaneous crepitation in the neck and upper chest, decreased vocal fremitus, decreased or absent breath sounds on the affected side, jugular vein distention, and hypotension.

▶ *Thoracic aortic aneurysm.* This disorder usually causes the trachea to deviate to the right. Highly variable related findings may include stridor, dyspnea, wheezing, a brassy cough, hoarseness, and dysphagia. Edema of the face, neck, or arm may occur with distended chest wall and jugular veins. The patient also may have substernal, neck, shoulder, or low back pain as well as paresthesia or neuralgia.

Special considerations

Because tracheal deviation usually signals a severe underlying disorder that can cause respiratory distress at any time, monitor the patient's respiratory and cardiac status constantly, and make sure that emergency equipment is readily available. Prepare the patient for diagnostic tests, such as chest X-rays, bronchoscopy, an electrocardiogram, and arterial blood gas analysis.

Pediatric pointers

Keep in mind that respiratory distress typically develops more rapidly in children than in adults.

Geriatric pointers

In elderly patients, tracheal deviation to the right commonly stems from an elongated, atherosclerotic aortic arch, but this deviation isn't considered abnormal.

Patient counseling

Teach the patient the techniques required to perform coughing and deep-breathing exercises. Explain the signs and symptoms of respiratory difficulty that require immediate attention.

REFERENCES

1. Coughlin, A.M. "Go With The Flow of Chest Tube Therapy," *Nursing* 36(3):36-42, March 2006.
2. Ryan, B. "Pneumothorax: Assessment and Diagnostic Testing," *Journal of Cardiovascular Nursing* 20(4):251-253, July/August 2005.

● TREMORS

The most common type of involuntary muscle movement, tremors are regular rhythmic oscillations that result from alternating contraction of opposing muscle groups. They're typical signs of extrapyramidal or cerebellar disorders and can also result from the use of certain drugs.

Tremors can be characterized by their location, amplitude, and frequency. They're classified as resting, intention, or postural. *Resting tremors* occur when a limb is at rest and subside with movement. They include the classic pill-rolling tremor of Parkinson's disease. Conversely, *intention tremors* occur only with movement and subside with rest. *Postural (or action) tremors* appear when a limb or the trunk is actively held in a particular posture or position.

Tremorlike movements also may occur—for example, asterixis, the characteristic flapping tremor seen in hepatic failure.

Stress, emotional upset, fatigue, or stimulant use tend to aggravate tremors. Alcohol commonly diminishes postural tremors.

History and physical examination

Begin the patient history by asking about the tremor's onset (sudden or gradual) and about its duration, progression, and any aggravating or alleviating factors. Does the tremor interfere with the patient's normal activities? Does he have other symptoms? Has he noticed any behavioral changes or memory loss? (The patient's family or friends may provide more accurate information on this.)

Explore the patient's personal and family medical history for a neurologic (especially seizures), endocrine, or metabolic disorder. Obtain a complete drug history, noting especially the use of phenothiazines. Also, ask about alcohol use.

Assess the patient's overall appearance and demeanor, noting mental status. Test range of motion and strength in all major muscle groups while observing for chorea, athetosis, dystonia, and other involuntary movements. Check deep tendon reflexes and, if possible, observe the patient's gait.

Medical causes

▶ *Alcohol withdrawal syndrome.* Acute alcohol withdrawal after long-term dependence may cause resting and intention tremors that appear within 8 hours after the last drink and progressively worsen.[1] Other early signs and symptoms include diaphoresis, tachycardia, elevated blood pressure, anxiety, restlessness, irritability, insomnia, headache, nausea, and vomiting. Severe withdrawal may produce profound tremors, agitation, confusion, hallucinations, and seizures.

▶ *Alkalosis.* Severe alkalosis may produce a severe intention tremor along with twitching, carpopedal spasms, agitation, diaphoresis, and hyperventilation. The patient may complain of dizziness, tinnitus, palpitations, and peripheral and circumoral paresthesia.

▶ *Benign familial essential tremor.* This disorder of early adulthood produces a bilateral essential tremor that typically begins in the fingers and hands and may spread to the head,

jaw, lips, and tongue. The tremors gradually increase in amplitude over time.[2] Laryngeal involvement may result in a quavering voice.

▶ *Cerebellar tumor.* An intention tremor is a cardinal sign of this disorder; related findings may include ataxia, nystagmus, incoordination, muscle weakness and atrophy, and hypoactive or absent deep tendon reflexes.

▶ *General paresis.* This effect of neurosyphilis may cause an intention tremor accompanied by clonus, a positive Babinski's sign, ataxia, Argyll Robertson pupils, and a diffuse, dull headache.

▶ *Graves' disease.* Fine tremors of the hand, nervousness, weight loss, fatigue, palpitations, dyspnea, and increased heat intolerance are typical signs and symptoms of this most common form of hyperthyroidism.[3] An enlarged thyroid gland (goiter) and exophthalmos are also characteristic.

▶ *Hypercapnia.* Elevated partial pressure of carbon dioxide may result in a rapid, fine intention tremor. Other common findings include headache, fatigue, blurred vision, weakness, lethargy, and decreasing level of consciousness (LOC).

▶ *Hypoglycemia.* Acute hypoglycemia may produce a rapid, fine intention tremor accompanied by confusion, weakness, tachycardia, diaphoresis, and cold, clammy skin. Early patient complaints typically include a mild generalized headache, profound hunger, nervousness, and blurred or double vision. The tremor may disappear as hypoglycemia worsens and hypotonia and decreased LOC become evident.

▶ *Kwashiorkor.* Coarse intention and resting tremors may occur in the advanced stages of this disease. Examination reveals myoclonus, rigidity of all limbs, hyperreflexia, hepatomegaly, and pitting edema in the hands, feet, and sacral area. Other signs include a flat affect, pronounced hair loss, and dry, peeling skin.

▶ *Multiple sclerosis (MS).* An intention tremor that waxes and wanes may be an early sign of MS, but visual and sensory impairments are usually the earliest findings. Other effects vary greatly and may include nystagmus, muscle weakness, paralysis, spasticity, hyperreflexia, ataxic gait, dysphagia, and dysarthria. Constipation, urinary frequency and urgency, incontinence, impotence, and emotional lability also may occur.

▶ *Parkinson's disease.* Tremors, the first symptom in 70% of patients with this degenerative disease, usually begin in the fingers and may eventually affect the foot, eyelids, jaw, lips, and tongue.[4] The slow, regular, rhythmic resting tremor takes the form of flexion-extension or abduction-adduction of the fingers or hand, or pronation-supination of the hand. Flexion-extension of the fingers combined with abduction-adduction of the thumb is known as the characteristic pill-rolling tremor.

Leg involvement produces flexion-extension foot movement. Lightly closing the eyelids causes them to flutter. The jaw may move up and down, and the lips may purse. The tongue, when protruded, may move in and out of the mouth in tempo with tremors elsewhere in the body. The rate of the tremor remains constant over time, but its amplitude varies.

Other characteristic findings include cogwheel or lead-pipe rigidity, bradykinesia, propulsive gait with forward-leaning posture, monotone voice, masklike facies, drooling, dysphagia, dysarthria, and occasionally oculogyric crisis (eyes fix upward, with involuntary tonic movements) or blepharospasm (eyelids close completely).

▶ *Porphyria.* Involvement of the basal ganglia in porphyria can produce a resting tremor with rigidity accompanied by chorea and athetosis. As the disease progresses, generalized seizures may appear along with aphasia and hemiplegia.

▶ *Thalamic syndrome.* Central midbrain syndromes are heralded by contralateral ataxic tremors and other abnormal movements along with Weber's syndrome (oculomotor palsy with contralateral hemiplegia), paralysis of vertical gaze, and stupor or coma.

Anteromedial-inferior thalamic syndrome produces varying combinations of tremor, deep sensory loss, and hemiataxia. However, the main effect of this syndrome may be an extrapyramidal dysfunction, such as hemiballismus or hemichoreoathetosis.

▶ *Thyrotoxicosis.* Neuromuscular effects of this disorder include a rapid, fine intention tremor of the hands and tongue, along with clonus, hyperreflexia, and Babinski's reflex. Other common signs and symptoms include tachycardia, cardiac arrhythmias, palpitations, anxiety, dyspnea, diaphoresis, heat intolerance, weight loss despite increased appetite, diarrhea, an enlarged thyroid and, possibly, exophthalmos.

▶ *Wernicke's encephalopathy.* An intention tremor is an early sign of this thiamine deficiency. Other features include ocular abnormalities (such as gaze paralysis and nystagmus), ataxia, apathy, and confusion. Orthostatic hypotension and tachycardia also may develop.

▶ *West Nile encephalitis.* This brain infection is caused by West Nile virus, a mosquito-borne flavivirus endemic in Africa, the Middle East, western Asia, and the United States. Mild infections are common and include fever, headache, and body aches, commonly accompanied by rash and swollen lymph glands. More severe infections are marked by headache, high fever, neck stiffness, stupor, disorientation, coma, tremors, occasional seizures, and paralysis.

▶ *Wilson's disease.* This disorder of abnormal copper metabolism produces slow "wing-flapping" tremors in the arms and pill-rolling tremors in the hands; these tremors appear early in the disease and progressively worsen. The most characteristic sign, however, is Kayser-Fleischer rings—rusty brown rings around the corneas. Other signs and symptoms include incoordination, dysarthrial chorea, ataxia, muscle spasms and rigidity, abdominal distress, fatigue, personality changes, hypotension, syncope, and seizures. Liver and spleen enlargement, ascites, jaundice, and hyperpigmentation also may occur.

Other causes

◉ **DRUG WATCH** *Phenothiazines (particularly piperazine derivatives such as fluphenazine) and other antipsychotics may cause resting and pill-rolling tremors. Metoclopramide and metyrosine also cause these tremors occasionally. Amphetamines, lithium toxicity, phenytoin, and sympatho-*

mimetics *(such as terbutaline and pseudoephedrine) can all cause tremors that disappear when the dosage is decreased.*

▶ *Herbs.* Herbal products, such as ephedra (banned by the FDA), have been known to cause serious adverse reactions, which may include tremors.

▶ *Manganese toxicity.* Early signs of manganese poisoning include resting tremor, chorea, propulsive gait, cogwheel rigidity, personality changes, amnesia, and masklike facies.

▶ *Mercury poisoning.* The chronic form of mercury poisoning is characterized by irritability, copious amounts of saliva, loose teeth, gum disease, slurred speech, and tremors.

Special considerations

Severe intention tremors may interfere with the patient's ability to perform activities of daily living. Help the patient with these activities as needed, and take precautions against possible injury during such activities as walking and eating.

Pediatric pointers

A normal neonate may display coarse tremors with stiffening—an exaggerated hypocalcemic startle reflex—in response to noises and chills. Pediatric-specific causes of pathologic tremors include cerebral palsy, fetal alcohol syndrome, and maternal drug addiction.

Patient counseling

Advise a patient with Parkinson's disease and excessive tremors that he may achieve partial control of his body by sitting on a chair and using its arms to steady himself. Encourage the patient to be as independent as possible. Help the patient learn adaptive techniques to perform activities of daily living.

REFERENCES

1. Phillips, S., Haycock, C., and Boyle, D. "Development of an Alchol Withdrawal Protocol: CNS Collaborative Exemplar," *Clinical Nurse Specialist* 20(4):190-198, July/August 2006.
2. Louis, E.D. "Treatment of Tremor," *CONTINUUM: Lifelong Learning in Neurology. Movement Disorders* 13(1):58-71, February 2007.
3. Weeks, B.H. "Graves' Disease: The Importance of Early Diagnosis," *The Nurse Practitioner* 30(11):34-45, November 2005.
4. McCarron, K. "The Shakedown on Parkinson's Disease," *Nursing Made Incredibly Easy!* 4(6):40-49, November/December 2006.

URINARY FREQUENCY

Urinary frequency refers to an increased urge to void without an increase in the total volume of urine produced. Usually resulting from decreased bladder capacity, urinary frequency is a cardinal sign of urinary tract infection (UTI). However, it also can stem from another urologic disorder, neurologic dysfunction, or pressure on the bladder from a nearby tumor or from organ enlargement (as occurs in pregnancy).

History and physical examination

Ask the patient how many times a day he voids and how this compares to his previous pattern of voiding. Also ask about the onset and duration of the increased frequency and about any associated urinary signs or symptoms, such as dysuria, urgency, incontinence, hematuria, discharge, or lower abdominal pain during urination.

Also ask about neurologic symptoms, such as muscle weakness, numbness, and tingling. Explore the patient's medical history for UTIs or other urologic problems, recent urologic procedures, and neurologic disorders. Ask a male patient about a history of prostatic enlargement. Ask a female patient of childbearing age whether she is or could be pregnant.

Obtain a clean-catch midstream urine specimen for urinalysis and culture and sensitivity tests. Then palpate the patient's suprapubic area, abdomen, and flanks, noting any tenderness. Examine the urethral meatus for redness, discharge, or swelling. The physician may palpate the prostate gland of a male patient.

If the patient's history or symptoms suggest a neurologic disorder, perform a neurologic examination.

Medical causes

▶ *Anxiety neurosis.* Morbid anxiety produces urinary frequency and other types of genitourinary dysfunction, such as dysuria, impotence, and female sexual dysfunction. Other findings may include headache, diaphoresis, hyperventilation, palpitations, muscle spasm, generalized motor weakness, dizziness, polyphagia, and constipation or other GI complaints.

▶ *Benign prostatic hyperplasia.* Prostatic enlargement causes urinary frequency along with nocturia and possibly incontinence and hematuria. Initial effects are those of prostatism: reduced caliber and force of the urine stream, urinary hesitancy and tenesmus, inability to stop the urine stream, a feeling of incomplete voiding, and occasionally urine retention. Assessment reveals bladder distention.

▶ *Bladder calculus.* Bladder irritation from a calculus may lead to urinary frequency and urgency, dysuria, terminal hematuria, and suprapubic pain from bladder spasms. If the calculus lodges in the bladder neck, the patient may have overflow incontinence and referred pain to the lower back or heel.

▶ *Bladder cancer.* Urinary frequency, urgency, dribbling, and nocturia may develop from bladder irritation. The first sign of bladder cancer commonly is intermittent gross, painless hematuria (often with clots). Patients with invasive lesions commonly have suprapubic or pelvic pain from bladder spasms.

▶ *Multiple sclerosis (MS)*. Urinary frequency, urgency, and incontinence are common urologic findings in patients with MS, but these effects widely vary and tend to wax and wane. Vision problems (such as diplopia and blurred vision) and sensory impairment (such as paresthesia) are usually the earliest symptoms. Other findings may include constipation, muscle weakness, paralysis, spasticity, hyperreflexia, intention tremor, ataxic gait, dysarthria, impotence, and emotional lability.

▶ *Prostate cancer*. In advanced prostate cancer, urinary frequency may occur along with hesitancy, dribbling, nocturia, dysuria, bladder distention, perineal pain, constipation, and a hard, irregularly shaped prostate.[1]

▶ *Prostatitis*. Acute prostatitis commonly produces urinary frequency and urgency, dysuria, nocturia, and a purulent urethral discharge. Other findings include fever, chills, lower back pain, myalgia, arthralgia, and perineal fullness. The prostate may be tense, boggy, tender, and warm. Prostate massage to obtain prostatic fluid is contraindicated. Signs and symptoms of chronic prostatitis are usually the same as those of the acute form, but to a lesser degree. The patient also may have pain on ejaculation.

▶ *Rectal tumor*. The pressure that this tumor exerts on the bladder may cause urinary frequency. Early findings include altered bowel elimination habits, commonly starting with an urgent need to defecate on arising or obstipation alternating with diarrhea; blood or mucus in the stool; and a sense of incomplete evacuation.

▶ *Reiter's syndrome*. In this self-limiting syndrome, urinary frequency and other symptoms of acute urethritis occur 1 to 2 weeks after sexual contact. Other symptoms of Reiter's syndrome include asymmetrical arthritis of the knees, ankles, and metatarsophalangeal joints; unilateral or bilateral conjunctivitis; and small painless ulcers on the mouth, tongue, glans penis, palms, and soles.

▶ *Reproductive tract tumor*. A tumor in the female reproductive tract may compress the bladder, causing urinary frequency. Other findings vary but may include abdominal distention, menstrual disturbances, vaginal bleeding, weight loss, pelvic pain, and fatigue.

▶ *Spinal cord lesion*. Incomplete cord transection results in urinary frequency, continuous overflow, dribbling, urgency when voluntary control of sphincter function weakens, urinary hesitancy, and bladder distention. Other effects occur below the level of the lesion and include weakness, paralysis, sensory disturbances, hyperreflexia, and impotence.

▶ *Urethral stricture*. Bladder decompensation produces urinary frequency, urgency, and nocturia. Early signs include hesitancy, tenesmus, and reduced caliber and force of the urine stream. Eventually, overflow incontinence, urinoma, and urosepsis may develop.

▶ *UTI*. Affecting the urethra, the bladder, or the kidneys, this common cause of urinary frequency also may produce urgency, dysuria, hematuria, cloudy urine and, in males, a urethral discharge. The patient may report a fever and bladder spasms or a feeling of warmth during urination. Women may have suprapubic or pelvic pain. In young men, a UTI usually is related to sexual contact.

Other causes

▶ *Diuretics*. These substances, which include caffeine, reduce the body's total volume of water and salt by increasing urine excretion. Excessive intake of coffee, tea, and other caffeinated beverages leads to urinary frequency.

▶ *Treatments*. Radiation therapy may cause bladder inflammation, leading to urinary frequency.

Special considerations

Prepare the patient for diagnostic tests, such as urinalysis, culture and sensitivity tests, imaging tests, ultrasonography, cystoscopy, cystometry, postvoid residual tests, and a complete neurologic workup. If the patient's mobility is impaired, keep a bedpan or commode near his bed. Carefully and accurately document the patient's daily intake and output.

Pediatric pointers

UTIs are a common cause of urinary frequency in children, especially girls. Congenital anomalies that can cause UTIs include a duplicated ureter, congenital bladder diverticulum, and an ectopic ureteral orifice.

Geriatric pointers

Men older than age 50 have an increased risk of urinary frequency and incontinence.[2] Decreased estrogen levels in postmenopausal women cause urinary frequency, urgency, and nocturia.[3]

Patient counseling

Instruct sexually active men in safer sex practices. Advise girls and women to clean the genital area from front to back to reduce contamination by *Escherichia coli*. Also urge them to drink plenty of fluids, especially water, and to void often during the day.

REFERENCES
1. Hsiao, C.P., Loescher, L.J., and Moore, I.M. "Symptoms and Symptom Distress in Localized Prostate Cancer," *Cancer Nursing* 30(6):E19-E32, November/December 2007.
2. Crestodina, L.R. "Assessment and Management of Urinary Incontinence in the Elderly Male," *The Nurse Practitioner* 32(9):26-34, September 2007.
3. Palmer, M.H., and Newman, D.K. "Urinary Incontinence and Estrogen," *AJN* 107(3):35-37, March 2007.

● URINARY INCONTINENCE

Incontinence, the uncontrollable passage of urine, can result from a bladder abnormality, a neurologic disorder, or an alteration in pelvic muscle strength. A common urologic sign, incontinence may be transient or permanent and may involve large volumes of urine or scant dribbling. It can be classified as stress, overflow, urge, or total incontinence. *Stress incontinence* refers to intermittent leakage resulting from a sudden physical strain, such as a cough, sneeze, laugh, or quick movement. *Overflow incontinence* is a dribble resulting from urine retention, which fills the bladder and prevents it from contracting with sufficient force to expel a urine stream. *Urge incontinence* refers to the inability to suppress a sudden urge to urinate. *Total incontinence* is continuous leakage resulting from the bladder's inability to retain urine.

History and physical examination

Ask the patient when he first noticed the incontinence and whether it began suddenly or gradually. Have him describe his typical urinary pattern: Does incontinence usually occur during the day or at night? Does he have any urinary control, or is he totally incontinent? If can control urination occasionally, ask him the usual times and amounts voided. Determine his normal fluid intake. Ask about other urinary problems, such as hesitancy, frequency, urgency, nocturia, and decreased force or interruption of the urine stream. Also ask if he's ever sought treatment for incontinence or found a way to deal with it himself.

Obtain a medical history, especially noting urinary tract infection (UTI), prostate conditions, spinal injury or tumor, stroke, or surgery involving the bladder, prostate, or pelvic floor. Ask a woman how many pregnancies and childbirths she has had.

After completing the history, have the patient empty his bladder. Inspect the urethral meatus for obvious signs of inflammation or an anatomic defect. Have female patients bear down, and note any urine leakage. Gently palpate the abdomen for bladder distention, which signals urine retention. Perform a complete neurologic assessment, noting motor and sensory function and obvious muscle atrophy.

Medical causes

▶ *Benign prostatic hyperplasia (BPH)*. Overflow incontinence is common in this disorder as a result of urethral obstruction and urine retention. BPH begins with a group of signs and symptoms known as *prostatism*: reduced caliber and force of the urine stream, urinary hesitancy, and a feeling of incomplete voiding. As the obstruction increases, the patient may develop urinary frequency, nocturia and, possibly, hematuria. Examination reveals bladder distention and an enlarged prostate.
▶ *Bladder calculus*. Overflow incontinence may occur if the calculus lodges in the bladder

Correcting incontinence with bladder retraining

An incontinent patient typically feels frustrated, embarrassed, and sometimes hopeless. Fortunately, however, his problem may be corrected by bladder retraining—a program that aims to establish a regular voiding pattern. Here are some guidelines for establishing such a program:

• Before you start the program, assess the patient's intake pattern, voiding pattern, and behavior (for example, restlessness or talkativeness) before each voiding episode.

• Encourage the patient to use the toilet 30 minutes before he's usually incontinent. If this isn't successful, adjust the schedule. Once he can stay dry for 2 hours, increase the time between voidings by 30 minutes each day until he achieves a 3- to 4-hour voiding schedule.

• When your patient voids, make sure the sequence of conditioning stimuli is always the same.

• Make sure the patient has privacy while voiding, and avoid any inhibiting stimuli.

• Keep a record of continence and incontinence for 5 days; this may reinforce your patient's efforts to remain continent.

TIPS FOR SUCCESS

Remember that both you and your patient need a positive attitude to ensure his successful bladder retraining. Here are some additional tips that may help your patient succeed:

• Make sure the patient is close to a bathroom or portable toilet. Leave a light on at night, and make sure that the pathway to the bathroom is clear.

• If your patient needs help getting out of his bed or chair, answer his call promptly.

• Urge the patient to wear his usual clothing as an indication that you're confident he can remain continent. Acceptable alternatives to diapers include condoms for men and incontinence pads or panties for women.

• Encourage the patient to drink 2 to 2½ qt (2 to 2.5 L) of fluid each day. Less fluid doesn't prevent incontinence but does promote bladder infection. Limiting his intake after 5 p.m., however, will help him remain continent during the night.

• Reassure your patient that episodes of incontinence don't signal a failure of the program. Encourage him to maintain a positive attitude.

neck. Associated findings vary but may include those of an irritable bladder: urinary frequency and urgency, dysuria, hematuria, and suprapubic pain from bladder spasms. Pelvic pain may be referred to the tip of the penis, vulva, lower back, or heel and may be worsened by movement.

▶ *Bladder cancer.* Urge incontinence and hematuria are common findings in bladder cancer; obstruction by a tumor may produce overflow incontinence. The early stages can be asymptomatic. Other urinary signs and symptoms include frequency, dysuria, nocturia, dribbling, and suprapubic pain from bladder spasms after voiding. A mass may be palpable on bimanual examination.

▶ *Diabetic neuropathy.* Autonomic neuropathy may cause painless bladder distention with overflow incontinence. Related findings include episodic constipation or diarrhea (which is commonly nocturnal), impotence and retrograde ejaculation, orthostatic hypotension, syncope, and dysphagia.

▶ *Guillain-Barré syndrome.* Urinary incontinence may occur early in this disorder as a result of peripheral and autonomic nerve dysfunction. The cardinal sign is progressive, profound muscle weakness, which typically starts in the legs and extends to the arms and facial nerves within 24 to 72 hours. Other findings include paresthesia, dysarthria, nasal speech, dysphagia, orthostatic hypotension, tachycardia, fecal incontinence, diaphoresis, drooling, and pain in the shoulders, thighs, or lumbar region.

▶ *Multiple sclerosis (MS).* Urinary incontinence, urgency, and frequency are common urologic findings in MS. Vision problems and sensory impairment are usually the first symptoms. Other findings include constipation, muscle weakness, paralysis, spasticity, hyperreflexia, intention tremor, ataxic gait, dysarthria, impotence, and emotional lability.

Effectiveness of PFMT in treating urinary incontinence in women

Question: *How much of an effect does pelvic floor muscle training (PFMT) have on incontinent episodes, amount of urine leakage, and perceived severity of urine loss?*

Research: Urinary incontinence (UI) is a major health concern with high financial costs and significant impact on women's health. PFMT is commonly used as a conservative form of treatment for UI. Twelve randomized controlled trials were included in this meta-analysis. All 12 studies met inclusion criteria established by the authors, who then performed the review.

The authors created a codebook for data collection. Five dimensions were coded for each study: report identification, subject parameters (sample size, mean and range of age, types of UI, and baseline perceived severity of UI), methodology, treatment parameters (length of PFMT training period, the number of daily PFMT contractions, velocity of contractions, holding time, combined treatments with PFMT, and time-to-outcome measure), and information for effect size (mean and standard deviation).

Conclusion: PFMT is effective for all women; however, the treatment effect on incontinent episodes may be greater in younger women who have only stress incontinence. Findings regarding the effect on amount of urine leakage and perceived severity were inconclusive.

Application: As part of patient teaching, instruct women with UI on the proper technique for performing PFMT and encourage them to perform PFMT exercises with at least 24 contractions daily. Also, tell patients that improvement in symptoms may not be noticed until after 6 weeks.

Source: Choi, H., Palmer, M. H., and Park, J. "Meta-Analysis of Pelvic Floor Muscle Training: Randomized Controlled Trials in Incontinent Women," *Nursing Research,* 56(4):226-234, 2007.

▶ *Prostate cancer.* Urinary incontinence usually occurs only in the advanced stages of prostate cancer. Urinary frequency and hesitancy, nocturia, dysuria, bladder distention, perineal pain, constipation, and a hard, irregularly shaped, nodular prostate are other common late findings.

▶ *Prostatitis (chronic).* Urinary incontinence may occur as a result of urethral obstruction from an enlarged prostate. Other findings include urinary frequency and urgency, dysuria, hematuria, bladder distention, a persistent urethral discharge, dull perineal pain that may radiate to other areas, ejaculatory pain, and decreased libido.

▶ *Spinal cord injury.* Complete cord transection above the sacral level causes flaccid paralysis of the bladder. Overflow incontinence follows rapid bladder distention. Other findings include paraplegia, sexual dysfunc-

tion, sensory loss, muscle atrophy, anhidrosis, and loss of reflexes distal to the injury.

▶ *Stroke.* Urinary incontinence may be transient or permanent in a stroke patient. Associated findings reflect the site and extent of the lesion and may include impaired mentation, emotional lability, behavioral changes, altered level of consciousness, and seizures. Sensorimotor effects may include contralateral hemiplegia, dysarthria, dysphagia, ataxia, apraxia, agnosia, aphasia, and unilateral sensory loss. Headache, vomiting, visual deficits, and decreased visual acuity also may occur.

▶ *Urethral stricture.* Partial obstruction of the lower urinary tract from trauma or infection produces urinary hesitancy, tenesmus, and decreased force and caliber of the urine stream. Urinary frequency and urgency, nocturia, and eventually overflow incontinence also may occur. As the obstruction increases, urine extravasation may lead to formation of urinomas and urosepsis.

▶ *UTI.* Besides incontinence, a UTI may produce urinary urgency, dysuria, hematuria, cloudy urine and, in males, a urethral discharge. Bladder spasms or a feeling of warmth during urination may occur.

Other causes

▶ *Surgery.* Urinary incontinence may occur after prostatectomy as a result of urethral sphincter damage.

Special considerations

Prepare the patient for diagnostic tests, such as cystoscopy, cystometry, and a complete neurologic workup. Obtain a urine specimen.

If the patient's incontinence has a neurologic cause, monitor him for urine retention, which may require periodic catheterizations. A patient with permanent urinary incontinence may need surgical creation of a urinary diversion.

Pediatric pointers

Incontinence in children may be caused by infrequent or incomplete voiding, which also may lead to a UTI. Ectopic ureteral orifice is an uncommon congenital anomaly that causes incontinence. A complete diagnostic evaluation usually is needed to rule out organic disease.

Geriatric pointers

Risk factors for urinary incontinence increase with age. Urinary incontinence occurs in 13% to 17% of men older than age 60.[1] In a recent study of women, about 50% of those ages 50 to 90 experienced urinary incontinence every month.[2]

Patient counseling

Begin management of incontinence by implementing a bladder retraining program. (See *Correcting incontinence with bladder retraining,* page 417.) To prevent stress incontinence, teach the patient Kegel exercises to help strengthen the pelvic floor muscles. (See *Effectiveness of PFMT in treating urinary incontinence in women.*) If appropriate, teach the patient self-catheterization techniques.

REFERENCES

1. Crestodina, L.R. "Assessment and Management of Urinary Incontinence in the Elderly Male," *The Nurse Practitioner* 32(9):26-34, September 2007.
2. Melville, J.L., Katon, W., Delaney, K., and Newton, K. "Urinary Incontinence in U.S. Women: A Population-Based Study," *Archives of Internal Medicine* 165(5):537-42, March 2005.

● URTICARIA

Urticaria, or *hives,* presents as transient pruritic wheals that appear as smooth, slightly elevated patches with well-defined erythematous margins and pale centers of various shapes and sizes.[1] They result from a vascular skin reaction caused by local release of histamine or other vasoactive substances as part of a hypersensitivity reaction.

Acute urticaria evolves rapidly and usually has a detectable cause, such as hypersensitivity to certain drugs, foods, insect bites, inhalants, or contactants; emotional stress; or environmental factors. Although individual lesions usually subside within 12 to 24 hours, new crops of lesions may erupt continuously, thus prolonging the attack.

Urticaria lasting longer than 6 weeks is known as *chronic urticaria.* The lesions may recur for months or years, and the underlying cause usually is unknown. Occasionally, a diagnosis of psychogenic urticaria is made.

Angioedema, or *giant urticaria,* is characterized by the acute eruption of wheals involving the mucous membranes and occasionally the arms, legs, or genitals.

In a patient with acute urticaria, quickly evaluate his respiratory status and take his vital signs. Ensure patent I.V. access if you note respiratory difficulty or signs of impending anaphylactic shock. Also, as appropriate, give local epinephrine or apply ice to the affected site to decrease absorption of the irritating agent through vasoconstriction. Clear and maintain the airway, give oxygen as needed, and institute cardiac monitoring. Have resuscitation equipment at hand, and be prepared to start cardiopulmonary resuscitation. Intubation or a tracheostomy may be needed.

History

If the patient isn't in distress, obtain a complete history. Does he have any known allergies? Does the urticaria follow a seasonal pattern? Do certain foods or drugs seem to aggravate it? Is it related to physical exertion? Is the patient routinely exposed to chemicals on the job or at home? Has he recently used new skin products? Obtain a detailed drug history, including prescription and over-the-counter drugs. Note any history of chronic or parasitic infection, skin disease, or a GI disorder.

Medical causes

▶ *Anaphylaxis.* This life-threatening reaction is marked by rapid eruption of diffuse urticaria and angioedema, with wheals ranging from pinpoint to palm-size or larger. Lesions usually are pruritic and stinging and preceded by paresthesia. Other acute findings include profound anxiety, weakness, diaphoresis, sneezing, shortness of breath, profuse rhinorrhea, nasal congestion, dysphagia, and warm, moist skin.

▶ *Lyme disease.* Urticaria may result from the characteristic skin lesion (erythema chronicum migrans) produced by this tick-borne disease. Later effects include constant malaise and fatigue, intermittent headache, fever, chills, lymphadenopathy, neurologic and cardiac abnormalities, and arthritis.

Other causes

▶ *Drugs.* Many drugs can produce urticaria, the second most common cutaneous adverse drug reaction after a morbilliform rash.[2] Among the most common are aspirin, atropine, codeine, dextrans, immune serums, insulin, morphine, penicillin, quinine, sulfonamides, and vaccines. In addition, radiographic contrast media commonly produce urticaria, especially when given I.V.[3]

Special considerations

To help relieve the patient's discomfort, apply a bland skin emollient or one containing menthol and phenol. Expect to give an antihistamine, a systemic corticosteroid or, if stress is a suspected contributing factor, a tranquilizer. Tepid baths and cool compresses also may enhance vasoconstriction and decrease pruritus..

Pediatric pointers

Pediatric forms of urticaria include acute papular urticaria (usually after insect bites) and urticaria pigmentosa (rare).

Patient counseling

Urge the patient to avoid the causative stimulus if it's identified. Emphasize the need to wear or carry medical identification that identifies his allergies. Explain the risks of delayed symptoms and which signs and symptoms to report. Discuss methods and techniques to prevent anaphylaxis. Instruct the patient on the proper use of an anaphylaxis kit and epinephrine administration.

REFERENCES

1. Pullen, R.L. "Assessing Skin Lesions: Learn to Identify the Different Types and Document Their Characteristics," *Nursing* 37(8):44-45, August 2007.
2. Hayden, M.L. "Did That Medication Cause This Rash?" *Nursing* 35(9):62-64, September 2005.
3. Kohtz, C., and Thompson, M. "Preventing Contrast Medium-Induced Nephropathy," *AJN* 107(9):40-49, September 2007.

VERTIGO

Vertigo is an illusion of movement in which the patient feels that he's revolving in space (*subjective vertigo*) or that his surroundings are revolving around him (*objective vertigo*). He may complain of feeling pulled sideways, as though drawn by a magnet.

A common symptom, vertigo usually begins abruptly and may be temporary or permanent and mild or severe. It may worsen when the patient moves and subside when he lies down. It's commonly confused with dizziness—a nonspecific sensation of imbalance and light-headedness. However, unlike dizziness, vertigo commonly is accompanied by nausea, vomiting, nystagmus, and tinnitus or hearing loss. Although the patient's limb coordination is unaffected, he may have a vertiginous gait.

Vertigo may result from a neurologic or otologic disorder that affects the equilibratory apparatus (the vestibule, semicircular canals, eighth cranial nerve, vestibular nuclei in the brain stem and their temporal lobe connections, and eyes). However, this symptom also may result from alcohol intoxication, hyperventilation, postural changes (benign postural vertigo), and the effects of certain drugs, tests, or procedures.

History and physical examination

Ask your patient to describe the onset and duration of his vertigo, being careful to distinguish this symptom from dizziness. Does he feel that he's moving or that his surroundings are moving around him? How often do the attacks occur? Do they follow position changes, or are they unpredictable? Find out if the patient can walk during an attack, if he leans to one side, and if he's ever fallen. Ask if he gets motion sickness and if he prefers one position during an attack. Obtain a recent drug history, and note any evidence of alcohol abuse.

Perform a neurologic assessment, focusing particularly on eighth cranial nerve function. Observe the patient's gait and posture for abnormalities.

Medical causes

▶ *Acoustic neuroma.* This tumor of the eighth cranial nerve causes mild, intermittent vertigo and unilateral sensorineural hearing loss. Other findings include tinnitus, postauricular or suboccipital pain, and—with cranial nerve compression—facial paralysis.

▶ *Benign paroxysmal positional vertigo.* In this disorder, the most common cause of recurrent vertigo, debris in a semicircular canal produces vertigo lasting a few minutes when the patient changes head position.[1] This type of vertigo usually is temporary and can be effectively treated with positional maneuvers.

▶ *Brain stem ischemia.* This condition produces sudden, severe vertigo that may become episodic and later persistent. Other findings include ataxia, nausea, vomiting, increased blood pressure, tachycardia, nystagmus, and lateral deviation of the eyes toward the side of the lesion. Hemiparesis and paresthesia also may occur.

▶ *Head trauma.* Persistent vertigo, occurring soon after a head injury, accompanies spontaneous or positional nystagmus and, if the temporal bone is fractured, hearing loss. Other findings include headache, nausea, vomiting, and decreased level of consciousness. Behavioral changes, diplopia or blurred vision, seizures, motor or sensory deficits, and signs of increased intracranial pressure also may occur.

▶ *Herpes zoster.* Infection of the eighth cranial nerve produces sudden onset of vertigo accompanied by facial paralysis, hearing loss in the affected ear, and herpetic vesicular lesions in the auditory canal.

▶ *Labyrinthitis.* Severe vertigo begins abruptly in this inner ear infection. Vertigo may occur in a single episode or may recur over months or years. Other findings include nausea, vomiting, progressive sensorineural hearing loss, and nystagmus.

▶ *Ménière's disease.* In this disease, labyrinthine dysfunction causes abrupt onset of vertigo, lasting minutes, hours, or days. Unpredictable episodes of severe vertigo and unsteady gait may cause the patient to fall. During an attack, any sudden motion of the head or eyes can precipitate nausea and vomiting.

▶ *Motion sickness.* This condition is characterized by vertigo, nausea, vomiting, and headache in response to rhythmic or erratic motions.

▶ *Multiple sclerosis (MS).* Episodic vertigo may occur early and become persistent in MS. Other early findings include diplopia, blurred vision, and paresthesia. MS also may produce nystagmus, constipation, muscle weakness, paralysis, spasticity, hyperreflexia, intention tremor, and ataxia.

▶ *Posterior fossa tumor.* This type of tumor may produce positional vertigo that lasts for a few seconds as well as papilledema, headache, memory loss, nausea, vomiting, nystagmus, apneustic or ataxic respirations, and increased blood pressure. The patient also may fall sideways.

▶ *Seizures.* Temporal lobe seizures may produce vertigo, usually associated with other symptoms of partial complex seizures.

▶ *Vestibular neuritis.* In this disorder, severe vertigo usually begins abruptly, lasts several days, and isn't accompanied by tinnitus or hearing loss. Other findings include nausea, vomiting, and nystagmus.

Other causes

▶ *Diagnostic tests.* Caloric testing (irrigating the ears with warm or cold water) can induce vertigo.

▶ *Drugs and alcohol.* High or toxic doses of certain drugs or alcohol may produce vertigo. These drugs include salicylates, aminoglycosides, antibiotics, quinine, and hormonal contraceptives.

▶ *Surgery and other procedures.* Ear surgery may cause vertigo that lasts for several days. Administration of overly warm or cold eardrops or irrigating solutions can also cause vertigo.

Special considerations

Place the patient in a comfortable position, and monitor his vital signs and level of consciousness. Keep the side rails up if he's in bed, or help him to a chair if he's standing when vertigo occurs. Darken the room and keep him calm. Give diazepam, promethazine, dexamethasone, or meclizine to treat acute vertigo, and drugs to control nausea and vomiting.

Prepare the patient for diagnostic tests, such as electronystagmography, EEG, and X-rays of the middle and inner ears.

Pediatric pointers

Ear infection is a common cause of vertigo in children. Vestibular neuritis also may cause this symptom.

Patient counseling

A patient with vertigo is at risk for falling. Educate the patient and his family on how to maintain a safe environment to prevent injury.[2] Teach the patient strategies to manage an acute attack of vertigo, such as getting to a safe place right away, taking his antivertigo medication, lying on a firm bed or sofa with a pillow on either side of his head to prevent head movement, and staying as still as possible while staring straight ahead to reduce the sensation of movement.[3] Advise the patient who must move during an acute vertigo attack, such as to use the bathroom, to crawl with his head held low near the floor.[3]

REFERENCES

1. Neuhauser, H.K. "Epidemiology of Vertigo," *Current Opinion in Neurology* 20(1):40-46, February 2007.
2. Hendrich, A. "Predicting Patient Falls," *AJN* 107(11):50-58, November 2007.
3. Pullen, R.L. "Spin Control: Caring for a Patient with Inner Ear Disease," *Nursing* 36(5):48-51, May 2006.

VISION LOSS

Vision loss—the inability to perceive visual stimuli—can be sudden or gradual and temporary or permanent. The deficit can range from a slight impairment of vision to total blindness. It can result from an ocular, a neurologic, or a systemic disorder or from trauma or the use of certain drugs. The ultimate visual outcome may depend on early, accurate diagnosis and treatment.

History and physical examination

Sudden vision loss can signal an ocular emergency. Don't touch the eye if the patient has a perforating or penetrating ocular trauma. (See *Managing sudden vision loss,* page 424.)

If the patient's vision loss occurred gradually, ask him if it affects one eye or both and all or only part of the visual field. Is the vision loss transient or persistent? Did it occur abruptly or develop over hours, days, or weeks? What is the patient's age? Ask the patient if he has experienced photosensitivity, and ask about the location, intensity, and duration of any eye pain. Also, obtain an ocular history and a family history of eye problems or systemic diseases that may lead to eye problems, such as hypertension; diabetes mellitus; thyroid, rheumatic, or vascular disease; infections; and cancer.

The first step in performing the eye examination is to assess visual acuity with the best available correction in each eye.

Carefully inspect both eyes, noting edema, foreign bodies, drainage, or conjunctival or scleral redness. Observe whether lid closure is complete or incomplete, and check for ptosis. Using a flashlight, examine the cornea and iris for scars, irregularities, and foreign bodies. Observe the size, shape, and color of the pupils, and test the direct and consensual light reflex and the effect of accommodation. Evaluate extraocular muscle function by testing the six cardinal fields of gaze.

Medical causes

▶ *Amaurosis fugax.* In this disorder, recurrent attacks of unilateral vision loss may last from a few seconds to a few minutes. Vision is normal at other times. Other findings may include transient unilateral weakness, hypertension, and elevated intraocular pressure (IOP) in the affected eye.

▶ *Cataract.* Typically, painless and gradual blurred vision precedes vision loss. As the cataract progresses, the pupil turns milky white.

▶ *Concussion.* Immediately or shortly after blunt head trauma, the patient may develop blurred, double, or lost vision. Vision loss is usually temporary. Other findings include headache, anterograde and retrograde amnesia, transient loss of consciousness, nausea, vomiting, dizziness, irritability, confusion, lethargy, and aphasia.

▶ *Corneal dystrophies, hereditary.* Some corneal dystrophies cause vision loss with associated pain, photophobia, tearing, and corneal opacities.

▶ *Diabetic retinopathy.* Retinal edema and hemorrhage lead to blurred vision, which may progress to blindness.

▶ *Endophthalmitis.* Typically, this intraocular inflammation follows penetrating trauma, I.V. drug use, or intraocular surgery, causing unilateral vision loss that may be permanent; a sympathetic inflammation may affect the other eye.

▶ *Glaucoma.* This disorder produces gradual blurred vision that may progress to total blindness. It's the second leading cause of blindness in the United States.[1] *Acute angle-closure glaucoma* is an ocular emergency that may produce blindness within 3 to 5 days. It's characterized by rapid onset of unilateral inflammation and pain, pressure over the eye, moderate pupil dilation, nonreactive pupillary response, a cloudy cornea, reduced visual acu-

Managing sudden vision loss

Sudden vision loss can signal central retinal artery occlusion or acute angle-closure glaucoma—ocular emergencies that require immediate intervention. If your patient reports sudden vision loss, immediately notify an ophthalmologist for an emergency examination, and perform the following interventions.

For a patient with suspected central retinal artery occlusion, perform light massage over his closed eyelid. Increase his carbon dioxide level by giving a set flow of oxygen and carbon dioxide through a Venturi mask, or have the patient rebreathe in a paper bag to retain exhaled carbon dioxide. These steps will dilate the artery and may restore blood flow to the retina.

For a patient with suspected acute angle-closure glaucoma, measure intraocular pressure (IOP) with a tonometer. (You also can estimate IOP without a tonometer by placing your fingers over the patient's closed eyelid. A rock-hard eyeball usually indicates increased IOP.) Expect to instill timolol drops and to give I.V. acetazolamide to help decrease IOP.

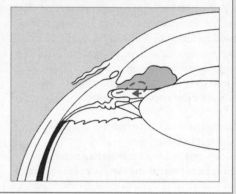

SUSPECTED CENTRAL RETINAL ARTERY OCCLUSION

SUSPECTED ACUTE ANGLE-CLOSURE GLAUCOMA

ity, photophobia, and perception of blue or red halos around lights. Nausea and vomiting also may occur.

Chronic angle-closure glaucoma has a gradual onset and usually produces no symptoms, although blurred or halo vision may occur. If untreated, it progresses to blindness and extreme pain.

Chronic open-angle glaucoma usually has an insidious onset, progresses slowly, and affects both eyes. It causes peripheral vision loss, aching eyes, halo vision, and reduced visual acuity (especially at night).

▶ *Herpes zoster.* When this disorder affects the nasociliary nerve, bilateral vision loss is accompanied by eyelid lesions, conjunctivitis, skin lesions (usually on the nose), and ocular muscle palsies.

▶ *Hyphema.* Blood in the anterior chamber can reduce vision to light perception only. Most hyphemas are the direct result of blunt trauma to the normal eye.

▶ *Keratitis.* This inflammation of the cornea may lead to complete unilateral vision loss. Other findings include an opaque cornea, increased tearing, irritation, and photophobia.

▶ *Macular degeneration, age-related.* Age-related macular degeneration (ARMD), occuring most commonly in adults older than age 60, is the most common cause of central vision loss in the United States.[2] It occurs in two forms, dry ARMD (most common) and wet ARMD. In both conditions, drusen (whitish yellow deposits) develop under the retina and progressively increase in number and size.[3] In early stages, slightly blurred vision occurs. Advancing stages produce central blurred or distorted spots that get larger and darker. These enlarging blind spots can cause a total loss of vision.

▶ *Ocular trauma.* Sudden unilateral or bilateral vision loss may occur after an eye injury. Vision loss may be total or partial and permanent or temporary. The eyelids may be reddened, edematous, and lacerated; intraocular contents may be extruded.

▶ *Optic atrophy.* Degeneration of the optic nerve, optic atrophy can develop spontaneously or follow inflammation or edema of the nerve head, causing irreversible loss of the visual field with changes in color vision. Pupillary reactions are sluggish, and optic disk pallor is evident.

▶ *Optic neuritis.* An umbrella term for inflammation, degeneration, or demyelinization of the optic nerve, optic neuritis usually produces temporary but severe unilateral vision loss, pain around the eye (especially with movement of the globe), a sluggish pupillary response to light and, possibly, visual field defects. Ophthalmoscopic examination commonly reveals hyperemia of the optic disk, blurred disk margins, and filling of the physiologic cup.

▶ *Paget's disease.* In this disorder, bony impingements on the cranial nerves may cause bilateral vision loss, which may be accompanied by hearing loss, tinnitus, vertigo, and severe, persistent bone pain. Cranial enlargement may be noticeable frontally and occipitally, and headaches may occur. Sites of bone involvement are warm and tender, and impaired mobility and pathologic fractures are common.

▶ *Papilledema.* Papilledema is characterized by swelling of both optic disks from increased intracranial pressure. Acute papilledema may lead to momentary blurring or transiently obscured vision, whereas chronic papilledema may lead to vision loss.

▶ *Pituitary tumor.* As a pituitary adenoma grows, blurred vision progresses to hemianopsia and, possibly, unilateral blindness. Double vision, nystagmus, ptosis, limited eye movement, and headaches also may occur.

▶ *Retinal artery occlusion (central).* This painless ocular emergency causes sudden unilateral vision loss, which may be partial or complete. Pupil examination reveals a slug-

gish direct pupillary response and a normal consensual response. Permanent blindness may occur within hours.

▶ *Retinal detachment.* Depending on the degree and location of detachment, painless vision loss may be gradual or sudden and total or partial. Macular involvement causes total blindness. Other effects include visual floaters, light flashes, and a sensation of a shadow or curtain over the visual field.

▶ *Retinal vein occlusion (central).* Most common in geriatric patients, this painless disorder causes a unilateral decrease in visual acuity with variable vision loss. IOP may be elevated in both eyes.

▶ *Rift Valley fever.* Inflammation of the retina is a complication of this viral disease that may result in some degree of permanent vision loss. Typical signs and symptoms include fever, myalgia, weakness, dizziness, and back pain. A small percentage of patients may develop encephalitis or hemorrhagic fever that can lead to shock and hemorrhage.

▶ *Stevens-Johnson syndrome.* Corneal scarring from conjunctival lesions produces marked vision loss and possibly purulent conjunctivitis, eye pain, and trouble opening the eyes. Other findings include widespread bullae, fever, malaise, cough, drooling, inability to eat, sore throat, chest pain, vomiting, diarrhea, myalgia, arthralgia, hematuria, and signs of renal failure.

▶ *Temporal arteritis.* Vision loss and blurred vision with a throbbing, unilateral headache characterize this disorder. Other findings include malaise, anorexia, weight loss, weakness, low-grade fever, generalized muscle aches, and confusion.

▶ *Trachoma.* This rare disorder may initially produce varying degrees of vision loss and a mild infection resembling bacterial conjunctivitis. Conjunctival follicles, red and edematous eyelids, pain, photophobia, tearing, and exudation also occur. After about 1 month, conjunctival follicles enlarge into inflamed yellow or gray papillae.

▶ *Uveitis.* Inflammation of the uveal tract may result in unilateral vision loss. Anterior uveitis produces moderate to severe eye pain, severe conjunctival injection, photophobia, and a small, nonreactive pupil. Posterior uveitis may produce insidious onset of blurred vision, conjunctival injection, visual floaters, pain, and photophobia. Associated posterior scar formation distorts the shape of the pupil.

▶ *Vitreous hemorrhage.* This condition, which may result from intraocular trauma, ocular tumors, or systemic disease (especially diabetes, hypertension, sickle cell anemia, or leukemia), can cause sudden unilateral vision loss, visual floaters, and a reddish haze. The vision loss may be permanent.

Other causes

DRUG WATCH *Chloroquine may cause patchy retinal pigmentation that typically leads to blindness. Digoxin derivatives, ethambutol, indomethacin, methanol toxicity, and quinine sulfate, also may cause vision loss.*

Phosphodiesterase type 5 (PDE-5) inhibitors, such as sildenafil, vardenafil, and tadalafil, may cause vision loss from nonarteritic anterior ischemic optic neuropathy.[4] Any patient prescribed a PDE-5 inhibitor should be instructed to stop the drug immediately and inform his healthcare provider if he has any new vision problems or vision loss.

Special considerations

Any degree of vision loss can be extremely frightening. To ease your patient's fears, orient him to his environment, make sure it's safe, and announce your presence each time you approach him. If the patient reports photophobia, darken the room and suggest that he wear sunglasses during the day. Obtain cultures of any drainage, and instruct him not to touch the unaffected eye with anything that has come in contact with the affected eye. Instruct him to wash his hands often and to avoid rubbing his eyes. If necessary, prepare him for surgery.

Pediatric pointers

Children who complain of slowly progressive vision loss may have an optic nerve glioma (a slow-growing, usually benign tumor) or retinoblastoma (a malignant tumor of the retina). Congenital rubella and syphilis may cause vision loss in infants. Retrolental fibroplasia may cause vision loss in premature infants. Other congenital causes of vision loss include Marfan syndrome, retinitis pigmentosa, and amblyopia.

Geriatric pointers

In elderly patients, reduced visual acuity may be caused by morphologic changes in the choroid, pigment epithelium, or retina or by decreased function of the rods, cones, or other neural elements. Major causes of vision loss in older adults include age-related macular degeneration, cataracts, glaucoma, and diabetic retinopathy.[5]

Patient counseling

Discuss safety measures to prevent injury. If the patient has an infectious process, emphasize the importance of frequent hand washing and to avoid rubbing the eyes. If the loss is progressive or permanent, refer the patient to the appropriate social service agencies, community support services, and related associations for assistance with adaptation and equipment.

REFERENCES

1. Kowing, D., and Kester, E. "Keep An Eye Out for Glaucoma," *The Nurse Practitioner* 32(7):18-23, July 2007.
2. Schexnaydre, M., and Carruth, A.K. "My Father's Experience with Macular Degeneration: Implications for the Home Healthcare Nurse," *Home Healthcare Nurse* 26(1):8-14, January 2008.
3. Covell, C.A., Graziano, J.A., Rich, D., and Tobin, K.A. "New Outlook for Age-Related Macular Degeneration," *Nursing* 37(3):22-24, March 2007.
4. O'Malley, P. "Viagra and Vision Loss: What Is Known and Unknown," *Clinical Nurse Specialist* 20(5):227-28, September/October 2006.
5. Whiteside, M.M., Wallhagen, M.I., and Pettengill, E. "Sensory Impairment in Older Adults: Part 2: Vision Loss," *AJN* 106(11):52-61, November 2006.

● VISION, BLURRED

Blurred vision is a common symptom that refers to the loss of visual acuity with indistinct visual details. It may result from an eye injury, a neurologic or eye disorder, or a disorder with vascular complications, such as diabetes mellitus. Blurred vision also may result from mucus passing over the cornea, a refractive error, improperly fitted contact lenses, or the use of certain drugs.

History and physical examination

If your patient has blurred vision with sudden, severe eye pain, a history of trauma, or sudden vision loss, order an ophthalmologic examination. If he has a penetrating or perforating eye injury, don't touch the eye. (See *Managing sudden vision loss,* page 424.)

If the patient isn't in distress, ask him how long he has had blurred vision. Does it occur only at certain times? Ask about associated signs and symptoms, such as pain or discharge. If blurred vision followed injury, obtain details of the accident, and ask if vision was impaired immediately after the injury. Obtain a medical and drug history.

Inspect the patient's eye, noting lid edema, drainage, or conjunctival or scleral redness. Also note an irregularly shaped iris, which may indicate previous trauma, and excessive blinking, which may indicate corneal damage. Assess the patient for pupillary changes, and test visual acuity in both eyes.

Medical causes

▶ *Brain tumor.* A brain tumor may cause blurred vision, decreased level of consciousness (LOC), headache, apathy, behavioral changes, memory loss, decreased attention span, dizziness, confusion, aphasia, seizures, ataxia, and signs of hormonal imbalance. Its later effects may include papilledema, vomiting, increased systolic blood pressure, widened pulse pressure, and decorticate posture.
▶ *Cataract.* This painless disorder causes gradual blurred vision. Other effects include halo vision (an early sign), visual glare in bright light, progressive vision loss, and a gray pupil that later turns milky white.
▶ *Concussion.* Immediately or shortly after blunt head trauma, the patient may develop blurred, double, or temporarily lost vision. Other findings include changes in LOC and behavior.
▶ *Conjunctivitis.* Blurred vision may be accompanied by photophobia, pain, burning,

tearing, itching, and a feeling of fullness around the eyes. Other findings include redness near the fornices (brilliant red suggests a bacterial cause; milky red, an allergic cause) and drainage (copious, mucopurulent, and flaky in bacterial conjunctivitis; stringy in allergic conjunctivitis). Copious tearing, minimal exudate, and an enlarged preauricular lymph node occur in viral conjunctivitis.
▶ *Corneal abrasions.* Blurred vision may occur with severe eye pain, photophobia, redness, and excessive tearing.
▶ *Corneal dystrophies, hereditary.* Blurring may remain stable or may worsen progressively throughout life in this disorder. Some corneal dystrophies cause pain, vision loss, photophobia, tearing, and corneal opacities.
▶ *Corneal foreign bodies.* Blurred vision may accompany a foreign-body sensation, excessive tearing, photophobia, intense eye pain, miosis, conjunctival injection, and a dark corneal speck.
▶ *Diabetic retinopathy.* Retinal edema and hemorrhage produce gradual blurring, which may progress to blindness.
▶ *Dislocated lens.* Dislocation of the lens, especially beyond the line of vision, causes blurred vision and (with trauma) redness.
▶ *Eye tumor.* If the tumor involves the macula, blurred vision may be the presenting symptom. Related findings include varying visual field losses.
▶ *Glaucoma.* In *acute angle-closure glaucoma,* an ocular emergency, unilateral blurred vision and severe pain begin suddenly. Other findings include halo vision; a moderately dilated, nonreactive pupil; conjunctival injection; a cloudy cornea; and decreased visual acuity. Severely elevated intraocular pressure may cause nausea and vomiting.

In *chronic angle-closure glaucoma,* transient blurred vision and halo vision may precede pain and blindness.
▶ *Hypertension.* This disorder may cause blurred vision and a throbbing morning headache that decreases in severity during the day. However, if diastolic blood pressure exceeds 120 mm Hg, the headache may persist. Other findings include restlessness, confusion, nausea, vomiting, seizures, and decreased LOC.

▶ *Hyphema.* Blunt eye trauma with hemorrhage into the anterior chamber causes blurred vision. Other effects include moderate pain, diffuse conjunctival injection, visible blood in the anterior chamber, ecchymosis, eyelid edema, and a hard eye.

▶ *Iritis.* Acute iritis causes sudden blurred vision, moderate to severe eye pain, photophobia, conjunctival injection, and a constricted pupil.

▶ *Macular degeneration, age-related.* Age-related macular degeneration (ARMD) occurs most commonly in adults over age 60.[1] It occurs in two forms, dry ARMD (most common) and wet ARMD. In both conditions, drusen (whitish yellow deposits) develop under the retina and progressively increase in number and size.[2] In early stages, vision is slightly blurred. Advancing stages produce central blurring or distorted spots that get larger and darker. These enlarging blind spots can cause a total loss of vision.

▶ *Migraine headache.* This disorder may cause blurred vision and paroxysmal attacks of severe, throbbing, unilateral or bilateral headache. Other effects include nausea, vomiting, sensitivity to light and noise, and sensory or visual auras.

▶ *Multiple sclerosis (MS).* Blurred vision, diplopia, and paresthesia may occur in the early stages of MS. Later effects vary and may include nystagmus, muscle weakness, paralysis, spasticity, hyperreflexia, intention tremor, and ataxic gait. Urinary frequency, urgency, and incontinence also may occur.

▶ *Optic neuritis.* Inflammation, degeneration, or demyelinization of the optic nerve usually causes an acute attack of blurred vision and vision loss. Related findings include scotomas and eye pain. Ophthalmoscopic examination reveals hyperemia of the optic disk, large vein distention, blurred disk margins, and filling of the physiologic cup.

▶ *Retinal detachment.* Sudden blurred vision may be the initial symptom of a detached retina. Other effects include visual floaters and recurring flashes of light. As the detachment progresses, the patient has gradual vision loss, likened to a curtain covering the visual field.

▶ *Retinal vein occlusion (central).* This disorder causes gradual unilateral blurred vision and varying degrees of vision loss.

▶ *Serous retinopathy (central).* Blurring may accompany darkened vision in the affected eye.

▶ *Stroke.* Brief attacks of bilateral blurred vision may precede or accompany a stroke. Other findings include a decreased LOC, contralateral hemiplegia, dysarthria, dysphagia, ataxia, unilateral sensory loss, and apraxia. Stroke also may cause agnosia, aphasia, homonymous hemianopsia, diplopia, disorientation, memory loss, and poor judgment. Other features include urine retention or urinary incontinence, constipation, personality changes, emotional lability, headache, vomiting, and seizures.

▶ *Temporal arteritis.* Most common in women older than age 60, this disorder causes sudden blurred vision accompanied by vision loss and a throbbing unilateral headache in the temporal or frontotemporal region. Prodromal signs and symptoms include malaise, anorexia, weight loss, weakness, low-grade fever, and generalized muscle aches. Other findings include confusion; disorientation; swollen, nodular, tender temporal arteries; and erythema of overlying skin.

▶ *Uveitis (posterior).* This disorder may produce insidious onset of blurred vision, conjunctival injection, visual floaters, pain, and photophobia.

▶ *Vitreous hemorrhage.* This condition may cause sudden unilateral blurred vision, varying degrees of vision loss, visual floaters, or dark streaks.

Other causes

DRUG WATCH *Blurred vision may stem from the effects of cycloplegics, reserpine, clomiphene, thiazide diuretics, antihistamines, anticholinergics, and phenothiazines. Antidepressants such as tricyclic antidepressants and mirtazapine also may produce blurred vision.[3]*

Special considerations

Prepare the patient for diagnostic tests, such as tonometry, slit-lamp examination, X-rays of the skull and orbit and, if a neurologic lesion is suspected, a computed tomography scan. As necessary, teach him how to instill ophthalmic drugs. If blurred vision leads to permanent vision loss, provide emotional support, orient him to his surroundings, and provide for his safety. If necessary, prepare him for surgery.

Pediatric pointers

Blurred vision in children may stem from congenital syphilis, congenital cataracts, refractive errors, eye injuries or infections, or increased intracranial pressure. Refer the child to an ophthalmologist if appropriate.

Test vision in school-age children as you would in adults; test children ages 3 to 6 with the Snellen symbol chart. Test toddlers with Allen cards, each illustrated with a familiar object such as an animal. Ask the child to cover one eye and identify the objects as you flash them. Then ask him to identify them as you gradually back away. Record the maximum distance at which he can identify at least three pictures.

Patient counseling

Discuss safety measures to prevent injury. Refer the patient to an ophthalmologist that specializes in low vision services, and teach the patient about adaptive devices that are available to facilitate reading, view the television, and use the computer.[1]

REFERENCES

1. Schexnaydre, M., and Carruth, A.K. "My Father's Experience with Macular Degeneration: Implications for the Home Healthcare Nurse," *Home Healthcare Nurse* 26(1):8-14, January 2008.
2. Covell, C.A., Graziano, J.A., Rich, D., and Tobin, K.A. "New Outlook for Age-Related Macular Degeneration," *Nursing* 37(3):22-24, March 2007.
3. Blake, T. "Tracking the Ups and Downs of Antidepressants," *Nursing* 37(4):49-51, April 2007.

● VOMITING

Vomiting is the forceful expulsion of gastric contents through the mouth. Characteristically preceded by nausea, vomiting results from a coordinated sequence of abdominal muscle contractions and reverse esophageal peristalsis.

A common sign of GI disorders, vomiting also occurs with fluid and electrolyte imbalances; infections; and metabolic, endocrine, labyrinthine, central nervous system (CNS), and cardiac disorders. It can also result from drug therapy, surgery, or radiation.

Vomiting occurs normally during the first trimester of pregnancy, but its subsequent development may signal complications. It can also result from stress, anxiety, pain, alcohol intoxication, overeating, or ingestion of distasteful foods or liquids.

History and physical examination

Ask your patient to describe the onset, duration, and intensity of his vomiting. What started it? What makes it subside? If possible, collect, measure, and inspect the character of the vomitus. (See *Vomitus: Characteristics and causes,* page 430.) Explore any related complaints, particularly nausea, abdominal pain, anorexia and weight loss, changes in bowel elimination patterns or the appearance of stools, excessive belching or flatus, and bloating or fullness.

Obtain a medical history, noting GI, endocrine, and metabolic disorders; recent infections; and cancer, including chemotherapy or radiation therapy. Ask about current drug use and alcohol consumption. If the patient is a female of childbearing age, ask if she is or could be pregnant and which contraceptive method she uses.

Inspect the abdomen for distention, and auscultate for bowel sounds and bruits. Palpate for rigidity and tenderness, and test for rebound tenderness. Next, palpate and percuss the liver for enlargement. Assess other body systems as appropriate.

During the examination, keep in mind that projectile vomiting *unaccompanied by nausea* may indicate increased intracranial pressure, a life-threatening emergency. If this occurs in a patient with a CNS injury, quickly check his vital signs. Be alert for widened pulse pressure or bradycardia.

Medical causes

▶ *Adrenal insufficiency.* Common GI findings in the disorder include nausea and vomiting, anorexia, and diarrhea. Other findings in-

Vomitus: Characteristics and causes

When you collect a specimen of a patient's vomitus, observe it carefully for clues to the underlying disorder.

Bile-stained (greenish) vomitus	Obstruction below the pylorus, as from a duodenal lesion
Bloody vomitus	Upper GI bleeding (if bright red, may result from gastritis or a peptic ulcer; if dark red, from esophageal or gastric varices)
Brown vomitus with a fecal odor	Intestinal obstruction or infarction
Burning, bitter-tasting vomitus	Excessive hydrochloric acid in gastric contents
Coffee-ground vomitus	Digested blood from a slowly bleeding gastric or duodenal lesion
Undigested food	Gastric outlet obstruction, as from a gastric tumor or ulcer

clude weakness, fatigue, weight loss, bronze skin, orthostatic hypotension, and a weak, irregular pulse.

▶ *Anthrax, GI.* Initial signs and symptoms after ingestion of contaminated meat from an infected animal include nausea and vomiting, anorexia, and fever. Later, abdominal pain, severe bloody diarrhea, and hematemesis may occur.

▶ *Appendicitis.* Nausea and vomiting may follow or accompany abdominal pain. Pain typically begins as vague epigastric or periumbilical discomfort and rapidly progresses to severe, stabbing pain in the right lower quadrant. The patient typically has a positive McBurney's sign—severe pain and tenderness at a point two-thirds the distance from the umbilicus to the right anterior superior spine of the ilium. Other findings usually include abdominal rigidity and tenderness, anorexia, constipation or diarrhea, cutaneous hyperalgesia, fever, tachycardia, and malaise.

▶ *Bulimia.* Most common in women ages 18 to 29, bulimia is characterized by polyphagia that alternates with self-induced vomiting, fasting, or diarrhea. It's commonly accompanied by anorexia. The patient may weigh less than normal but has a morbid fear of obesity. Self-induced vomiting may be evidenced by calloused knuckles and changes in teeth (enamel loss).

▶ *Cholecystitis (acute).* With this disorder, nausea and mild vomiting commonly follow severe right-upper-quadrant pain that may radiate to the back or shoulders. Other findings include abdominal tenderness and, possibly, rigidity and distention, fever, and diaphoresis.

▶ *Cholelithiasis.* Nausea and vomiting accompany severe unlocalized right-upper-quadrant or epigastric pain after ingestion of fatty foods. Other findings include abdominal tenderness and guarding, flatulence, belching, epigastric burning, pyrosis, tachycardia, and restlessness.

▶ *Cholera.* Signs and symptoms of cholera include vomiting and abrupt watery diarrhea. Severe water and electrolyte loss leads to thirst, weakness, muscle cramps, decreased skin turgor, oliguria, tachycardia, and hypotension. Without treatment, death can occur within hours.

▶ *Cirrhosis.* Insidious early signs and symptoms of cirrhosis typically include nausea and vomiting, anorexia, aching abdominal pain, and constipation or diarrhea. Later findings include jaundice, hepatomegaly, and abdominal distention.

▶ *Escherichia coli O157:H7.* The signs and symptoms of this infection include nausea and vomiting, watery or bloody diarrhea, fever, and abdominal cramps. Children younger than age 5 and elderly people may develop hemolytic uremic syndrome, which causes red blood cell destruction and may eventually lead to acute renal failure.

▶ *Ectopic pregnancy.* Nausea, vomiting, vaginal bleeding, and lower abdominal pain occur in this potentially life-threatening disorder.

▶ *Electrolyte imbalances.* Such disturbances as hyponatremia, hypernatremia, hypokalemia, and hypercalcemia commonly cause nausea and vomiting. Other effects include arrhythmias, tremors, seizures, anorexia, malaise, and weakness.

▶ *Food poisoning.* Vomiting, diarrhea, and fever are common findings in food poisoning, which is caused by ingestion of preformed toxins produced by bacteria typically found in foods, such as *Bacillus cereus*, *Clostridium*, and *Staphylococcus*.

▶ *Gastric cancer.* This rare type of cancer may produce mild nausea, vomiting (possibly of mucus or blood), anorexia, upper abdominal discomfort, and chronic dyspepsia. Fatigue, weight loss, melena, and altered bowel elimination habits are also common.

▶ *Gastritis.* Nausea and vomiting of mucus or blood are common in gastritis, especially after ingestion of alcohol, aspirin, spicy foods, or caffeine. Epigastric pain, belching, and fever also may occur.

▶ *Gastroenteritis.* This disorder causes nausea, vomiting (often of undigested food), diarrhea, and abdominal cramping. Fever, malaise, hyperactive bowel sounds, and abdominal pain and tenderness also may occur.

▶ *Heart failure.* Nausea and vomiting may occur, especially in right-sided heart failure. Associated findings include tachycardia, ventricular gallop, fatigue, dyspnea, crackles, peripheral edema, and jugular vein distention.

▶ *Hepatitis.* Vomiting commonly follows nausea as an early sign of viral hepatitis. Other early findings include fatigue, myalgia, arthralgia, headache, photophobia, anorexia, pharyngitis, cough, and fever.

▶ *Hyperemesis gravidarum.* Unremitting nausea and vomiting that last beyond the first trimester characterize this disorder of pregnancy. Vomitus contains undigested food, mucus, and small amounts of bile early in the disorder; later, it has a coffee-ground appearance. Other findings include weight loss, headache, delirium and, possibly, thyroid dysfunction.

▶ *Increased intracranial pressure.* Projectile vomiting that isn't preceded by nausea is a sign of increased intracranial pressure. The patient may have a decreased level of consciousness (LOC) and Cushing's triad (bradycardia, hypertension, and respiratory pattern changes). He also may have a headache, widened pulse pressure, impaired movement, visual disturbances, pupillary changes, and papilledema.

▶ *Infection.* Acute localized or systemic infection may cause vomiting and nausea. Other common findings include fever, headache, malaise, and fatigue.

▶ *Intestinal obstruction.* Nausea and vomiting (bilious or fecal) are common in this type of obstruction, especially of the upper small intestine. Abdominal pain is usually episodic and colicky but can become severe and steady. Constipation occurs early in large intestinal obstruction and late in small intestinal obstruction. Obstipation, however, may signal complete obstruction. In partial obstruction, bowel sounds are typically high pitched and hyperactive; in complete obstruction, hypoactive or absent. Abdominal distention and tenderness also occur, possibly with visible peristaltic waves and a palpable abdominal mass.

▶ *Labyrinthitis.* Nausea and vomiting commonly occur in this acute inner ear inflammation. Other findings include severe vertigo, progressive hearing loss, nystagmus and, possibly, otorrhea.

▶ *Listeriosis.* After ingesting food contaminated with the bacterium *Listeria monocytogenes*, the patient develops nausea, vomiting, abdominal pain, diarrhea, fever, and myalgia. If the infection spreads to the nervous system, he may develop meningitis. Signs and symptoms may include fever, headache, nuchal rigidity, and altered LOC. This food-borne illness primarily affects pregnant women, newborns, and those with weakened immune systems.

▶ *Ménière's disease.* This disorder results in sudden, brief, recurrent attacks of nausea and vomiting, dizziness, vertigo, hearing loss, tinnitus, diaphoresis, and nystagmus.

▶ *Mesenteric artery ischemia.* This life-threatening disorder may cause nausea and vomiting and severe, cramping abdominal pain, especially after meals. Other findings include diarrhea or constipation, abdominal tenderness and bloating, anorexia, weight loss, and abdominal bruits.

▶ *Mesenteric venous thrombosis.* Insidious or acute onset of nausea, vomiting, and abdominal pain occurs along with diarrhea or constipation, abdominal distention, hematemesis, and melena.

▶ *Metabolic acidosis.* This imbalance may produce nausea, vomiting, anorexia, diarrhea, Kussmaul's respirations, and decreased LOC.

▶ *Migraine headache.* Prodromal signs and symptoms of migraine include nausea and vomiting, fatigue, photophobia, light flashes, increased noise sensitivity and, possibly, partial vision loss and paresthesia.

▶ *Motion sickness.* Nausea and vomiting may be accompanied by headache, vertigo, dizziness, fatigue, diaphoresis, and dyspnea.

▶ *Myocardial infarction.* Nausea and vomiting may occur, but the cardinal symptom is severe substernal chest pain, which may radiate to the left arm, jaw, or neck. Dyspnea, pallor, clammy skin, diaphoresis, and restlessness also occur.

▶ *Norovirus infection.* Violent vomiting may occur frequently and without warning in this infection. Children infected with noroviruses tend to experience acute-onset vomiting more often than adults. Additional symptoms include nausea, diarrhea, and abdominal pain or cramping. There are no drugs or vaccines for noroviruses, but symptomatic therapy may be necessary to replace fluids and correct electrolyte disturbances resulting from frequent vomiting and diarrhea. Young children, elderly people, and those who are otherwise ill are at increased risk for dehydration.

▶ *Pancreatitis (acute).* Vomiting, usually preceded by nausea, is an early sign of pancreatitis. Associated findings include steady, severe epigastric or left-upper-quadrant pain that may radiate to the back; abdominal tenderness and rigidity; hypoactive bowel sounds; anorexia; vomiting; and fever. Severe pancreatitis may result in tachycardia, restlessness, hypotension, skin mottling, and cold, sweaty extremities.

▶ *Peptic ulcer.* Nausea and vomiting may follow sharp, burning or gnawing epigastric pain, especially when the stomach is empty or after ingestion of alcohol, caffeine, or aspirin. Attacks are relieved by eating or taking antacids. Hematemesis or melena also may occur.

▶ *Peritonitis.* Nausea and vomiting usually accompany acute abdominal pain in the area of inflammation. Other findings include high fever with chills; tachycardia; hypoactive or absent bowel sounds; abdominal distention, rigidity, and tenderness; weakness; pale, cold skin; diaphoresis; hypotension; signs of dehydration; and shallow respirations.

▶ *Preeclampsia.* Nausea and vomiting are common in this disorder of pregnancy. Rapid weight gain, epigastric pain, generalized edema, elevated blood pressure, oliguria, a severe frontal headache, and blurred or double vision also occur.

▶ *Q fever.* Signs and symptoms of this rickettsial infection include nausea and vomiting, fever, chills, severe headache, malaise, chest pain, and diarrhea. Fever may last up to 2 weeks. In severe cases, the patient may develop hepatitis or pneumonia.

▶ *Renal and urologic disorders.* Cystitis, pyelonephritis, calculi, and other renal and urologic disorders can cause vomiting. Accompanying findings reflect the specific disorder. Persistent nausea and vomiting are typical findings in patients with acute or worsening chronic renal failure.

▶ *Rhabdomyolysis.* Signs and symptoms of this disorder include nausea and vomiting, muscle weakness or pain, fever, malaise, and dark urine. Acute renal failure, the most commonly reported complication of rhabdomyolysis, results from renal structure obstruction and injury during the kidneys' attempt to filter the myoglobin from the bloodstream.

▶ *Thyrotoxicosis.* Nausea and vomiting may accompany the classic findings of severe anxiety, heat intolerance, weight loss despite increased appetite, diaphoresis, diarrhea, tremors, tachycardia, and palpitations. Other findings include exophthalmos, ventricular or atrial gallop, and an enlarged thyroid gland.

▶ *Typhus.* Typhus is a rickettsial disease transmitted to humans by fleas, mites, or body louse. Initial symptoms include headache, myalgia, arthralgia, and malaise, followed by an abrupt onset of nausea, vomiting, chills, and fever. A maculopapular rash may be present in some cases.

▶ *Ulcerative colitis.* Nausea, vomiting, and anorexia may occur, but the most common sign is recurrent diarrhea with blood, pus, and mucus. Fever, chills, and weight loss are other common signs and symptoms.

Other causes

DRUG WATCH *Drugs that commonly cause vomiting include anesthetics, antibiotics, chloride replacements, estrogens, ferrous sulfate, levodopa, opioids, oral potassium, quinidine, sulfasalazine, and overdoses of cardiac glycosides and theophylline. Chemotherapy-induced nausea and vomiting occurs in 30% to 90% of patients.[1] Syrup of ipecac, a mixture of ipecac fluid extract, glycerin, and syrup, is used to treat drug overdoses by inducing vomiting.*

▶ *Radiation and surgery.* Radiation therapy may cause nausea and vomiting if it disrupts the gastric mucosa. Postoperative nausea and vomiting are the most common adverse effects of anesthesia.[2]

Special considerations

Initiate nothing-by-mouth status as ordered.[3] Draw blood to determine fluid, electrolyte, and acid-base balance because prolonged vomiting can cause dehydration, electrolyte imbalances, and metabolic alkalosis.[1] Have the patient breathe deeply to ease his nausea and help prevent further vomiting. Keep his room fresh and clean smelling by removing bedpans and emesis basins promptly after use. Elevate his head or position him on his side to prevent aspiration of vomitus. Continuously monitor vital signs and intake and output (including vomitus and liquid stools). If needed, give I.V. fluids or have the patient sip clear liquids to maintain hydration.

Because pain can cause or worsen nausea and vomiting, give analgesics promptly. If possible, give them by injection or suppository to avoid worsening nausea. If an opioid is used to treat pain, monitor bowel sounds, flatus, and bowel movements carefully because they may slow GI motility and exacerbate vomiting. If you give an antiemetic, be alert for abdominal distention and hypoactive bowel sounds, which may indicate gastric retention. If this occurs, insert a nasogastric tube.

Pediatric pointers

In a neonate, pyloric obstruction may cause projectile vomiting, and Hirschsprung's disease may cause fecal vomiting. Intussusception may lead to vomiting of bile and fecal matter in an infant or toddler. Because an infant may aspirate vomitus as a result of his immature cough and gag reflexes, position him on his side or abdomen and clear any vomitus immediately.

Geriatric pointers

Although elderly patients can develop several of the disorders mentioned earlier, always rule out intestinal ischemia first—it's especially common in this age-group and has a high mortality.

Patient counseling

Advise patients to replace fluid losses to avoid dehydration. If vomiting is persistent, give an antiemetic; consider hospitalizing the patient for I.V. fluid replacement or parenteral nutrition therapy. Advise patients with from migraine headaches that vomiting may be a prodromal symptom and that they should take their antimigraine drug. To reduce the risk of nausea and vomiting, advise the patient to eat small, frequent, low-fat meals and to avoid carbonated beverages.[3]

REFERENCES

1. Viale, P.H. "Update on the Mangement of Chemotherapy-Induced Nausea and Vomiting," *Journal of Infusion Nursing* 29(5):283-291, September/October 2006.
2. Gan, T.J. "Risk Factors for Postoperative Nausea and Vomiting," *Anesthesia & Analgesia* 102(6)1884-1898, June 2006.
3. Steele, A., and Carlson, K.K. "Nausea and Vomiting: Applying Research to Bedside Practice," *AACN Advanced Critical Care* 18(1):61-73, January/March 2007.

VULVAR LESIONS

Vulvar lesions are cutaneous lumps, nodules, papules, vesicles, or ulcers that result from benign or malignant tumors, dystrophies, dermatoses, or infection. They can appear anywhere on the vulva and may go undetected until a gynecologic examination. Usually, however, the patient notices the lesions because of related symptoms, such as pruritus, dysuria, or dyspareunia.

History and physical examination

Ask the patient when she first noticed a vulvar lesion, and find out about related features, such as swelling, pain, tenderness, itching, or discharge. Does she have lesions elsewhere on her body? Ask about signs and symptoms of systemic illness, such as malaise, fever, or a rash on other body areas. Is the patient sexually active? Could she have been exposed to a sexually transmitted infection (STI)?

Also, examine the lesion, do a pelvic examination, and obtain cultures. (See *Recognizing common vulvar lesions.*) Examine other areas of the skin and mucous membranes (such as the eyes and mouth), which also may be affected in some cases.[1]

Medical causes

▶ *Basal cell carcinoma.* Most common in postmenopausal women, this nodular tumor has a central ulcer and a raised, poorly rolled border. Although it typically produces no symptoms, basal cell carcinoma occasionally causes pruritus, bleeding, discharge, and a burning sensation.

▶ *Benign cysts. Epidermal inclusion cysts,* the most common vulvar cysts, appear primarily on the labia majora. They're usually round and cause no symptoms; occasionally, they become erythematous and tender.

Bartholin's duct cysts are usually unilateral, tense, nontender, and palpable; they appear on the posterior labia minora and may cause minor discomfort during intercourse or, when large, difficulty with intercourse or even walking. Bartholin's abscess, an infected Bartholin's duct cyst, causes gradual pain and tenderness and possibly vulvar swelling, redness, and deformity.

▶ *Benign vulvar tumors.* Cystic or solid benign vulvar tumors usually produce no symptoms.

▶ *Chancroid.* This rare STI causes painful vulvar lesions. Other findings may include headache, malaise, fever up to 102.2° F (39° C), and enlarged, tender inguinal lymph nodes.

▶ *Dermatoses (systemic).* Psoriasis, seborrheic dermatitis, and other skin conditions may produce vulvar lesions that resemble the causative lesions found in other body areas.

▶ *Genital warts.* This STI is characterized by painless warts on the vulva, vagina, and cervix. The warts start as tiny red or pink swellings that grow and become pedunculated. Multiple swellings with a cauliflower-like appearance are common. Other findings include pruritus, erythema, burning or paresthesia in the vaginal introitus, and a profuse mucopurulent vaginal discharge. (See *Understanding HPV vaccine,* page 436.)

▶ *Gonorrhea.* Although most women with gonorrhea are asymptomatic, some develop vulvar lesions, which are usually confined to Bartholin's glands and may be accompanied by pruritus, a burning sensation, pain, and a green-yellow vaginal discharge. Other findings include dysuria and urinary incontinence; vaginal redness, swelling, bleeding, and engorgement; and severe pelvic and lower abdominal pain.

▶ *Granuloma inguinale.* This rare, chronic venereal infection begins with a single painless macule or papule on the vulva that ulcerates into a raised, beefy-red lesion with a granulated, friable border. Later, other painless and possibly foul-smelling lesions may erupt on the labia, vagina, or cervix. Eventually, they become infected and painful and may be accompanied by enlarged and tender regional lymph nodes, fever, weight loss, and malaise.

▶ *Herpes simplex (genital).* In this disorder, fluid-filled vesicles appear on the cervix and, possibly, on the vulva, labia, perianal skin, vagina, or mouth. The vesicles, initially painless, may rupture and develop into extensive shallow, painful ulcers, with redness, marked edema, and tender inguinal lymph nodes. Other findings include fever, malaise, and dysuria.

Recognizing common vulvar lesions

Various disorders can cause vulvar lesions. Sexually transmitted infections account for most vulvar lesions in premenopausal women, whereas vulvar tumors and cysts account for most lesions in women ages 50 to 70. The illustrations below will help you recognize some of the most common lesions.

Primary genital herpes produces multiple ulcerated lesions surrounded by red halos.

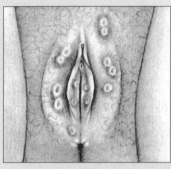

Basal cell carcinoma can produce an ulcerated lesion with raised, poorly rolled edges.

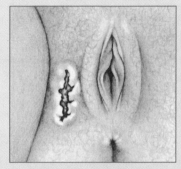

Primary syphilis produces chancres that appear as ulcerated lesions with raised borders.

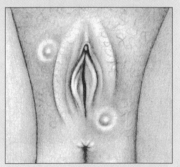

Epidermal inclusion cysts produce a round lump that usually appears on the labia majora.

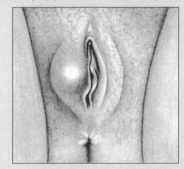

Squamous cell carcinoma can produce a large, granulomatous-appearing ulcer.

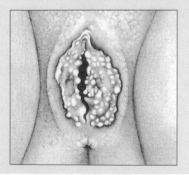

Bartholin's duct cysts produce a tense, non-tender, palpable lump that usually appears on the labia majora.

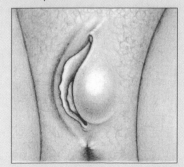

Understanding HPV vaccine

Gardasil, a recombinant vaccine that protects against cervical cancer, precancerous cervical dysplasia, genital lesions, and genital warts caused by four human papillomavirus (HPV) strains, was approved by the Food and Drug Administration in June 2006 for girls and women ages 9 to 26. According to the Centers for Disease Control and Prevention (CDC), HPV is the most common sexually transmitted infection (STI), affecting more than 6 million Americans each year.[2] HPV types 6, 11, 16, and 18 (the strains covered by the HPV vaccine) cause 70% of all cervical cancers and 90% of all genital warts.[3]

The CDC Advisory Committee on Immunization Practices and the American Academy of Pediatrics recommend routine vaccination of girls ages 11 and 12, as well as those ages 13 through 26 who haven't yet received or completed the full vaccine series. However, the vaccine isn't mandated or required for school entry in any state at this time. It's administered I.M. over 6 months, with doses two and three given 2 months and 6 months after the first dose.

The HPV vaccine is currently the most expensive pediatric vaccine, costing $360 for the full series of three injections.[2] Insurance reimbursement and coverage vary widely, although this may change if the vaccine becomes a required series.

Thus far, the HPV vaccine has caused no serious adverse reactions. The main adverse effect reported has been pain at the injection site. It's contraindicated in patients with immediate hypersensitivity to yeast or any components of the vaccine. Further research is needed to determine the vaccine's overall effectiveness, its duration of protection, and any possible long-term adverse reactions.[4]

If your patient receives the HPV vaccine, remind her to keep having her regular cervical cancer screenings because the vaccine doesn't protect against all types of HPV. Also advise her to keep practicing safer sex because the vaccine doesn't prevent all cases of genital warts or other STIs.

▶ *Herpes zoster.* This viral infection may produce vulvar lesions, although other areas are more commonly affected. Small, red nodular lesions erupt on painful erythematous areas. The lesions quickly evolve into vesicles or pustules, which dry and form scabs about 10 days later. Other findings include fever, malaise, paresthesia or hyperesthesia, and pain.

▶ *Lymphogranuloma venereum.* Most patients with this bacterial infection initially exhibit a single painless papule or ulcer on the posterior vulva that heals in a few days. Painful, swollen lymph nodes, usually unilateral, develop 2 to 6 weeks later. Other findings include fever, chills, headache, anorexia, myalgia, arthralgia, weight loss, and perineal edema.

▶ *Malignant melanoma.* This type of skin cancer may cause irregular, pigmented vulvar or clitoral lesions that enlarge rapidly and may ulcerate and bleed.

▶ *Molluscum contagiosum.* This viral infection produces raised, umbilicated, pearly or flesh-colored vulvar papules that are 1 to 2 mm in diameter and have a white core. Pruritic lesions also may appear on the face, eyelids, breasts, and inner thighs.

▶ *Pediculosis pubis.* This parasitic infection produces erythematous vulvar papules with pruritus and skin irritation. Adult pubic lice and nits are visible on pubic hair with magnification.

▶ *Squamous cell carcinoma.* Squamous cell carcinoma accounts for 90% of all cases of cancer of the vulva.[5] Invasive carcinoma occurs mainly in postmenopausal women and may produce a painful, pruritic vulvar tumor. As the tumor enlarges, it may encroach on the vagina, anus, and urethra, causing bleeding, discharge, or dysuria. Carcinoma in situ is most common in premenopausal women and produces a vulvar lesion that may be white or red, raised, well defined, moist, crusted, and isolated.

▶ *Squamous cell hyperplasia.* Formerly known as *hyperplastic dystrophy,* this disorder produces vulvar lesions that may be well delineated or poorly defined; localized or extensive; and red, brown, white, or red and white. However, its cardinal symptom is intense pruritus, possibly with vulvar pain, intense burning, and dyspareunia. In lichen sclerosis, a type of vulvar dystrophy, vulvar skin has a parchmentlike appearance. Fissures may develop between the clitoris and urethra or other vulvar areas.

▶ *Syphilis.* In this STI, chancres may appear on the vulva, vagina, or cervix 10 to 90 days after initial contact. They usually start as painless papules and then erode to form indurated ulcers with raised edges and clear bases. Condylomata lata develop after these ulcers clear up. These highly contagious secondary vulvar lesions are raised, gray, flat topped, and commonly ulcerated. Other findings include a maculopapular, pustular, or nodular rash; headache; malaise; anorexia; weight loss; fever; nausea and vomiting; generalized lymphadenopathy; and sore throat.

▶ *Viral diseases (systemic).* Varicella, measles, and other systemic viral diseases may produce vulvar lesions.

Special considerations

Expect to give a systemic antibiotic, an antiviral, a topical corticosteroid, topical testosterone, or an antipruritic.

Pediatric pointers

Vulvar lesions in children may result from congenital syphilis or gonorrhea. Evaluate for sexual abuse.

Geriatric pointers

Vulvar dystrophies and neoplasia become more common with advancing age. All persistent vulvar lesions should be biopsied for cancer detection.[6] Many women remain sexually active well into their older years, so be sure to question them about sexual activities and teach them safer sex practices.

Patient counseling

Show the patient how to give herself a sitz bath to promote healing and comfort. If she has an STI, encourage her to inform her sexual partners and urge them to be treated. Advise her to avoid sexual contact until the lesions are no longer contagious. Provide information about safer sex practices.

REFERENCES

1. Lewis, F.M., and Velangi, S.S. "An Overview of Vulvar Ulceration," *Clinical Obstetrics and Gynecology* 48(4):824-837, December 2005.
2. Centers for Disease Control and Prevention. "HPV and HPV vaccine: Information for Healthcare Providers." Revised August 2006. Retrieved January 22, 2007 from *http://www.cdc.gov/std/hpv/STDFact-HPV-vaccine-hcp.htm.*
3. Snow, M. "HPV Vaccine: New Treatment for an Old Disease," *Nursing* 37(3):67, March 2007.
4. Nelson, R. "Politics and Power Plays Behind the HPV Vaccine," *AJN* 107(8):23-24, August 2007.
5. Stehman, F.B., and Look, K.Y. "Carcinoma of the Vulva." *Obstetrics & Gynecology* 107(3):719-733, March 2006.
6. Summers, P.R., and Hunn, J. "Unique Dermatologic Aspects of the Postmenopausal Vulva," *Clinical Obstetrics and Gynecology* 50(3):745-751, September 2007.

WEIGHT GAIN, EXCESSIVE

Weight gain occurs when ingested calories exceed body requirements for energy, causing adipose tissue storage to increase. Weight also may increase when fluid retention causes edema. When weight gain results from overeating, emotional factors—usually anxiety, guilt, and depression—and social factors may be the main causes.

Among elderly people, weight gain commonly reflects a sustained food intake with a normal, progressive decline in basal metabolic rate. Among women, progressive weight gain occurs in pregnancy, whereas periodic weight gain usually occurs with menstruation.

A primary sign of many endocrine disorders, weight gain also occurs in conditions that limit activity, especially cardiovascular and pulmonary disorders. It also can result from drug therapy that increases appetite or causes fluid retention or from cardiovascular, hepatic, and renal disorders that cause edema.

History and physical examination

Determine your patient's previous patterns of weight gain and loss. Does he have a family history of obesity, thyroid disease, or diabetes mellitus? Assess his eating and activity patterns. Has his appetite increased? Does he exercise regularly or at all? Next, ask about associated symptoms. Has he had vision disturbances, hoarseness, paresthesia, or increased urination and thirst? Has he become impotent? If the patient is female, has she had menstrual irregularities or had weight gain during menstruation?

Form an impression of the patient's mental status. Is he anxious or depressed? Does he respond slowly? Is his memory poor? What drugs does he use?

During your physical examination, measure skin-fold thickness to estimate fat reserves. (See *Evaluating nutritional status,* pages 440 and 441.) Note fat distribution, the presence of localized or generalized edema, and overall nutritional status. Examine the patient for other abnormalities, such as abnormal body hair distribution or hair loss and dry skin. Take and record the patient's vital signs.

Medical causes

▶ *Acromegaly.* This disorder causes moderate weight gain. Other findings include coarsened facial features, prognathism, enlarged hands and feet, increased sweating, oily skin, deep voice, back and joint pain, lethargy, sleepiness, heat intolerance and, occasionally, hirsutism.

▶ *Cushing's syndrome (hypercortisolism).* Excessive weight gain, usually over the trunk and the back of the neck (buffalo hump), characteristically occurs in this disorder. Other cushingoid features include slender extremities, moon face, weakness, purple striae, emotional lability, and increased susceptibility to infection. Gynecomastia may occur in men; hirsutism, acne, and menstrual irregularities may occur in women.

▶ *Diabetes mellitus.* The increased appetite caused by this disorder may lead to weight

Treating metabolic syndrome with a reduced-carbohydrate diet

Question: *What's the impact of a reduced-carbohydrate diet on outcomes associated with metabolic syndrome?*

Research: Metabolic syndrome is diagnosed based on the presence of three or more of the following abnormalities: abdominal obesity, elevated blood pressure, elevated serum triglycerides, decreased high-density lipoprotein (HDL) cholesterol, and elevated fasting glucose. This syndrome increases the risk of cardiovascular disease mortality and type 2 diabetes mellitus.

Twenty-one adults who met the criteria for metabolic syndrome were recruited for this study. The participants received two sessions of nutritional counseling. The first session was for 60 minutes during which phase I of the diet was taught; the second session was 30 minutes long during which phase II of the diet was taught. In phase I, the diet was structured to be very low in carbohydrates (10% of energy). The diet in phase II consisted of 27% of energy from carbohydrates. Low glycemic index carbohydrates were encouraged and participants were also encouraged to pay attention to feelings of satiety.

Data collection included obtaining the following information at each of 4 visits: body weight, waist circumference, fasting glucose, insulin, lipoproteins, blood pressure, medications, physical activity, and dietary intake. Energy expenditure was assessed using the Seven-Day Physical Activity Recall interview and dietary intake was assessed using 24-hour dietary recall phone interviews, which were unannounced to study subjects.

Conclusion: At the end of the study, the mean weight loss was 5 kg, which was significantly different from baseline. Other significant changes included reduction in waist circumference, body mass index, and systolic and diastolic blood pressure. Only 50% of the subjects met the criteria for metabolic syndrome at the end of the study. It's important to note, however, that the subjects didn't meet the dietary goals of phase I or phase II of the prescribed diet.

Application: When educating patients, stress that lifestyle modifications are important to anyone at risk for chronic disease. While a reduced-carbohydrate diet can be effective in promoting weight loss, the long term benefits in preventing metabolic syndrome weren't documented in this study. Tell patients with metabolic syndrome to consult their health care provider before beginning any special diet. Also, refer patients for more extensive nutritional counseling as needed.

Source: Miller, C.K., Ulbrecht, J. S., Lyons, J., Parker-Klees, L., Gutschall, M. D., Smiciklas-Wright, H., Mitchell, D. C., Covasa, M., and Hayes, M. A. "Reduced-Carbohydrate Diet Improves Outcomes in Patients with Metabolic Syndrome: A Translational Study," *Topics in Clinical Nutrition,* 22(1):82-91, 2007.

gain, although weight loss sometimes occurs instead. Other findings include fatigue, polydipsia, polyuria, nocturia, weakness, polyphagia, and somnolence.

▶ *Heart failure.* Despite anorexia, weight gain may result from edema. Other typical findings include paroxysmal nocturnal dyspnea, orthopnea, and fatigue.

▶ *Hyperinsulinism.* This disorder increases appetite, leading to weight gain. Emotional lability, indigestion, weakness, diaphoresis, tachycardia, vision disturbances, and syncope also occur.

▶ *Hypogonadism.* Weight gain is common in this disorder. Prepubertal hypogonadism causes eunuchoid body proportions with relatively sparse facial and body hair and a high-pitched voice. Postpubertal hypogonadism causes loss of libido, impotence, and infertility.

Evaluating nutritional status

If your patient gains or loses excessive weight, you can help assess his nutritional status by measuring his skin-fold thickness and midarm circumference and by calculating his midarm muscle circumference. Skin-fold measurement reflects adipose tissue mass (subcutaneous fat accounts for about 50% of the body's adipose tissue). Midarm measurement reflects both skeletal muscle and adipose tissue mass.

Use these steps to gather the measurements. Then express them as a percentage of standard measurements by using this formula:

$$\frac{\text{actual measurement}}{\text{standard measurement}} \times 100 = \underline{\hspace{2cm}}\%$$

Standard anthropometric measurements vary according to the patient's age and gender and can be found in a table of normal anthropometric values. The abridged table below lists standard arm measurements for adult men and women.

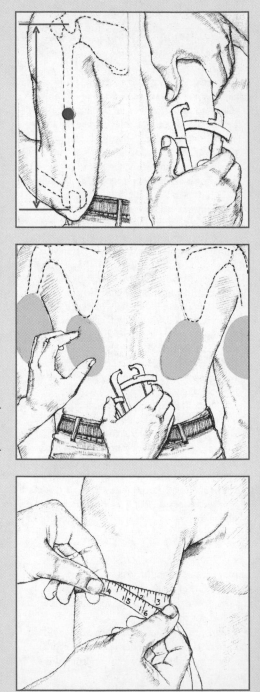

TEST	STANDARD	STANDARD
Triceps skin fold	Men	12.5 mm
	Women	16.5 mm
Midarm circumference	Men	29.3 mm
	Women	28.5 mm
Midarm muscle circumference	Men	25.3 mm
	Women	23.2 mm

A triceps or subscapular skin-fold measurement less than 60% of the standard value indicates severe depletion of fat reserves; measurement between 60% and 90% indicates moderate to mild depletion; and greater than 90% indicates significant fat reserves. A midarm circumference less than 90% of the standard value indicates caloric deprivation; greater than 90% indicates adequate or ample muscle and fat. A midarm muscle circumference less than 90% indicates protein depletion; greater than 90% indicates adequate or ample protein reserves.

To measure the triceps skin fold, locate the midpoint of the patient's upper arm using a nonstretch tape measure, and mark it with a felt-tip pen. Then grasp the skin with your thumb and forefinger about 1 cm above the midpoint. Place the calipers at the midpoint and squeeze them for about 3 seconds. Record the measurement registered on the handle gauge to the nearest 0.5 mm. Take two more readings and average all three to compensate for any measurement error.

To measure the subscapular skin fold, use your thumb and forefinger to grasp the skin just below the angle of the scapula, in line with the natural cleavage of the skin. Apply the calipers and proceed as when measuring the triceps skin fold. Both subscapular and triceps skin-fold measurements are reliable measurements of fat loss or gain during hospitalization.

To measure midarm circumference, return to the midpoint you marked on the patient's upper arm, and use a tape measure to determine the arm circumference at this point. This measurement reflects both skeletal muscle and adipose tissue mass and helps evaluate protein and calorie reserves. To calculate midarm muscle circumference, multiply the triceps skin-fold thickness (in centimeters) by 3.143, and subtract this figure from the midarm circumference. Midarm muscle circumference reflects muscle mass alone, providing a more sensitive index of protein reserves.

▶ *Hypothalamic dysfunction.* Conditions such as Laurence-Moon-Biedl syndrome cause a voracious appetite and subsequent weight gain along with altered body temperature and sleep rhythms.

▶ *Hypothyroidism.* In this disorder, weight gain occurs despite anorexia. Related signs and symptoms include fatigue; cold intolerance; constipation; menorrhagia; slowed intellectual and motor activity; dry, pale, cool skin; dry, sparse hair; and thick, brittle nails. Myalgia, hoarseness, hypoactive deep tendon reflexes, bradycardia, and abdominal distention may occur. Eventually, the face assumes a dull expression with periorbital edema.

▶ *Metabolic syndrome.* This syndrome, previously called *syndrome X,* consists of a group of disorders that affect metabolism, including excessive weight gain (usually in the central abdomen), hypertension (blood pressure greater than 135/85 mm Hg), abnormal cholesterol levels (high low-density lipoprotein and triglyceride levels, low high-density lipoprotein level), and high insulin levels. Inefficient use of insulin in the body may be a major contributor to metabolic syndrome, along with physical inactivity, poor diet, and genetic factors. Those with metabolic syndrome are at significantly increased risk of heart disease, stroke, and diabetes. Treatment typically involves exercising, following a heart-healthy diet, and refraining from smoking; medical therapy may be prescribed for individual disorders. (See *Treating metabolic syndrome with a reduced-carbohydrate diet,* page 439.)

▶ *Nephrotic syndrome.* In this syndrome, weight gain results from edema. Severe edema (anasarca) can increase body weight by up to 50%. Related effects include abdominal distention, orthostatic hypotension, and lethargy.

▶ *Pancreatic islet cell tumor.* This type of tumor causes excessive hunger, which leads to weight gain. Other findings include emotional lability, weakness, malaise, fatigue, restlessness, diaphoresis, palpitations, tachycardia, visual disturbances, and syncope.

▶ *Preeclampsia.* In this disorder, rapid weight gain (exceeding the normal weight gain of pregnancy) may accompany nausea and vomiting, epigastric pain, elevated blood pressure, and blurred or double vision.

▶ *Sheehan's syndrome.* Most common in women who experience severe obstetric hemorrhage, this syndrome may cause weight gain caused by impaired pituitary gland function.

Other causes
DRUG WATCH *Corticosteroids, phenothiazines, and tricyclic antidepressants cause weight gain from fluid retention and increased appetite. Other drugs that can lead to weight gain include cyproheptadine, which increases appetite; hormonal contraceptives, which cause fluid retention; and lithium, which can induce hypothyroidism.*

Special considerations
Psychological counseling may be needed for patients with excessive weight gain, particularly when it's caused by emotional problems or alters body image. If the patient is obese or has a cardiopulmonary disorder, any exercise should be monitored closely. Further study to rule out possible secondary causes should include thyroid-stimulating hormone determination and dexamethasone suppression testing. Laboratory test results of all patients ideally include cardiac risk factors: cholesterol, triglyceride, and glucose levels.

Pediatric pointers
Weight gain in children can result from an endocrine disorder such as Cushing's syndrome or from disorders that cause inactivity, such as Prader-Willi syndrome, Down syndrome, Werdnig-Hoffmann disease, late stages of muscular dystrophy, and severe cerebral palsy.

Obesity is increasing among children. Non-pathologic causes include poor eating habits, sedentary lifestyles, and emotional problems, especially among adolescents. Regardless of the cause, encourage good nutrition and healthy food choices, discourage fad diets, and provide a balanced weight loss program.

Geriatric pointers
Desired weights (those with the lowest mortality rates) increase with age.

Patient counseling
Educating the patient about weight control is extremely important. Stress the benefits of behavior modification and dietary compliance. Help the patient plan an appropriate exercise routine.

Advise a patient with heart failure to weigh himself and record his weight every morning, and to report any changes.[1]

REFERENCES
1. Lesperance, M.E., Bell, S.E., and Ervin, N.E. "Heart Failure and Weight Gain Monitoring," *Lippincott's Case Management* 10(6):287-293, November/December 2005.

WEIGHT LOSS, EXCESSIVE

Weight loss can reflect decreased food intake, decreased food absorption, increased metabolic requirements, or a combination of the three. It may be caused by endocrine, neoplastic, GI, and psychiatric disorders; nutritional deficiencies; infections; or neurologic lesions that cause paralysis and dysphagia. Weight loss also may result from conditions that prevent sufficient food intake, such as painful oral lesions, ill-fitting dentures, and loss of teeth, or from the metabolic effects of poverty, fad diets, excessive exercise, or certain drugs.

Weight loss may be a late sign in such chronic diseases as heart failure and renal disease, usually as the result of anorexia (see "Anorexia," page 20).

History and physical examination
Begin with a thorough diet history because weight loss almost always resutls from inadequate caloric intake. If the patient hasn't been eating properly, try to determine why. Ask about his previous weight and whether the recent loss was intentional. Be alert for lifestyle or occupational changes that may be causing anxiety or depression. For example, has he separated or divorced? Has he recently changed jobs?

Inquire about recent changes in bowel habits, such as diarrhea or bulky, floating stools. Has the patient had nausea, vomiting, or abdominal pain, which may indicate a GI disorder? Has he had excessive thirst, excessive urination, or heat intolerance, which may signal an endocrine disorder? Take a careful drug history, noting especially the use of diet pills or laxatives.

Carefully check the patient's height and weight, and ask about exact weight changes with approximate dates. Take his vital signs and note his general appearance: Is he well nourished? Do his clothes fit? Is muscle wasting evident?

Next, examine the patient's skin for turgor and abnormal pigmentation, especially around the joints. Does he have pallor or jaundice? Examine his mouth, including the condition of his teeth or dentures. Look for signs of infection or irritation on the roof of the mouth, and note any hyperpigmentation of the buccal mucosa. Also, check the patient's eyes for exophthalmos and his neck for swelling; auscultate his lungs for adventitious sounds. Inspect his abdomen for signs of wasting, and palpate for masses, tenderness, and an enlarged liver.

Conventional laboratory and radiologic tests, such as complete blood count, serum albumin levels, urinalysis, chest X-rays, and upper GI series, usually reveal the cause. Almost all physical causes can be found during the initial evaluation. Cancer, GI disorders, and depression are the most common pathologic causes.

Medical causes

▶ *Adrenal insufficiency.* Weight loss occurs in this disorder along with anorexia, weakness, fatigue, irritability, syncope, nausea, vomiting, abdominal pain, and diarrhea or constipation. Hyperpigmentation may occur at the joints, belt line, palmar creases, lips, gums, tongue, and buccal mucosa.

▶ *Anorexia nervosa.* This psychogenic disorder, most common in young women, is characterized by a severe, self-imposed weight loss ranging from 10% to 50% of premorbid weight, which typically was normal or no more than 5 lb (2.3 kg) over ideal weight. Related findings include skeletal muscle atrophy, loss of fatty tissue, hypotension, constipation, dental caries, susceptibility to infection, blotchy or sallow skin, cold intolerance, hairiness on the face and body, dryness or loss of scalp hair, and amenorrhea. The patient usually shows restless activity and vigor and may have a morbid fear of becoming fat. Self-induced vomiting or use of laxatives or diuretics may lead to dehydration or to metabolic alkalosis or acidosis.

▶ *Cancer.* Weight loss can be a sign of many types of cancer. Other findings reflect the type, location, and stage of the tumor and can include fatigue, pain, nausea, vomiting, anorexia, abnormal bleeding, and a palpable mass.

▶ *Crohn's disease.* Weight loss occurs with chronic cramping, abdominal pain, and anorexia. Other signs and symptoms include diarrhea, nausea, fever, tachycardia, hyperactive bowel sounds, and abdominal distention, tenderness, and guarding. Perianal lesions and a palpable mass in the right or left lower quadrant also may occur.

▶ *Cryptosporidiosis.* This opportunistic protozoan infection may cause weight loss, profuse watery diarrhea, abdominal cramping, flatulence, anorexia, nausea, vomiting, malaise, fever, and myalgia.

▶ *Depression.* Severe depression may cause weight loss or weight gain along with insomnia or hypersomnia, anorexia, apathy, fatigue, and feelings of worthlessness. Indecisiveness, incoherence, and suicidal thoughts or behavior also may occur.

▶ *Diabetes mellitus.* In this disorder, weight loss may occur despite increased appetite. Other findings include polydipsia, weakness, fatigue, and polyuria with nocturia.

▶ *Esophagitis.* Painful inflammation of the esophagus leads to temporary avoidance of eating and subsequent weight loss. Intense pain in the mouth and anterior chest is accompanied by hypersalivation, dysphagia, tachypnea, and hematemesis. If a stricture develops, dysphagia and weight loss will recur.

▶ *Gastroenteritis.* Malabsorption and dehydration cause weight loss in this disorder. The weight loss may be sudden in acute viral infections or reactions or gradual in parasitic infection. Other findings include poor skin turgor, dry mucous membranes, tachycardia, hypotension, diarrhea, abdominal pain and tenderness, hyperactive bowel sounds, nausea, vomiting, fever, and malaise.

▶ *Herpes simplex type 1.* Painful fluid-filled blisters in and around the mouth make eating painful, causing decreased food intake and weight loss.

▶ *Leukemia. Acute leukemia* causes progressive weight loss accompanied by severe prostration; high fever; swollen, bleeding gums; and other bleeding tendencies. Dyspnea, tachycardia, palpitations, and abdominal or bone pain may occur. As the disease progresses, neurologic symptoms may eventually develop.

Chronic leukemia, which occurs insidiously in adults, causes progressive weight loss with malaise, fatigue, pallor, enlarged spleen, bleeding tendencies, anemia, skin eruptions, anorexia, and fever.

▶ *Lymphomas.* Hodgkin's disease and malignant lymphoma cause gradual weight loss. Associated findings include fever, fatigue, night sweats, malaise, hepatosplenomegaly, and lymphadenopathy. Scaly rashes and pruritus may develop.

▶ *Pulmonary tuberculosis.* This disorder causes gradual weight loss with fatigue, weakness, anorexia, night sweats, and low-grade fever. Other effects include a cough with bloody or mucopurulent sputum, dyspnea, and pleuritic chest pain. Examination may reveal dullness on percussion, crackles after coughing, increased tactile fremitus, and amphoric breath sounds.

▶ *Stomatitis.* Inflammation of the oral mucosa (which are usually red, swollen, and ulcerated) in this disorder causes weight loss due to decreased eating. Other findings include fever, increased salivation, malaise, mouth pain, anorexia, and swollen, bleeding gums.

▶ *Thyrotoxicosis.* In this disorder, increased metabolism causes weight loss. Other characteristic signs and symptoms include nervousness, heat intolerance, diarrhea, increased appetite, palpitations, tachycardia, diaphoresis, a fine tremor, and possibly an enlarged thyroid gland and exophthalmos. A ventricular or atrial gallop may be heard.

▶ *Ulcerative colitis.* Weight loss is a late sign of this disorder, which is initially characterized by bloody diarrhea with pus or mucus. Other findings include weakness, crampy lower abdominal pain, hyperactive bowel sounds, tenesmus, anorexia, low-grade fever and, oc-

casionally, nausea and vomiting. Constipation may occur late. Fulminant colitis causes severe and steady abdominal pain and diarrhea, high fever, and tachycardia.

▶ *Whipple's disease.* This rare disease causes progressive weight loss along with abdominal pain, diarrhea, steatorrhea, arthralgia, fever, hyperpigmentation, lymphadenopathy, and splenomegaly.

Other causes

DRUG WATCH *Amphetamines and inappropriate dosage of thyroid replacement commonly lead to weight loss. Laxative abuse may cause a malabsorptive state that leads to weight loss. Chemotherapy drugs may cause weight loss from severe stomatitis.*

Special considerations

Refer your patient for psychological counseling if weight loss negatively affects his body image. If the patient has a chronic disease, administer total parenteral nutrition or tube feedings to maintain adequate nutrition and to prevent edema, poor healing, and muscle wasting. Count his caloric intake daily and weigh him weekly. Consult a nutritionist to determine an appropriate diet with adequate calories.

Pediatric pointers

In infants, weight loss may be caused by failure-to-thrive syndrome. In children, severe weight loss may be the first indication of diabetes mellitus. Chronic, gradual weight loss occurs in children with marasmus—nonedematous protein-calorie malnutrition.

Weight loss also may result from child abuse or neglect; an infection causing high fevers; hand-foot-and-mouth disease, which causes painful oral sores; a GI disorder causing vomiting or diarrhea; or celiac disease.

Geriatric pointers

Some elderly patients experience mild, gradual weight loss due to changes in body composition (such as loss of height and lean body mass) and lower basal metabolic rate, leading to decreased energy requirements. Rapid, unintentional weight loss, however, is highly predictive of morbidity and mortality in the elderly.[1] Other nonpathologic causes of weight loss in this age-group include tooth loss, difficulty chewing, social isolation, and alcoholism.

REFERENCES

1. Chau, D., Cho, L.M., Jani, P., and St. Jeor, S.T. "Individualizing Recommendations for Weight Management in the Elderly," *Current Opinion in Clinical Nutrition and Metabolic Care* 11(1):27-31, January 2008.

WHEEZING

Wheezes (also called *sibilant rhonchi*) are adventitious breath sounds with a high-pitched, musical, squealing, creaking, or groaning quality. They're caused by air flowing at a high velocity through a narrowed airway. When they originate in the large airways, they can be heard by placing an unaided ear over the chest wall or at the mouth. When they originate in smaller airways, they can be heard by placing a stethoscope over the anterior or posterior chest. Unlike crackles and rhonchi, wheezes can't be cleared by coughing.

Usually, prolonged wheezing occurs during expiration when bronchi are shortened and narrowed. Causes of airway narrowing include bronchospasm; mucosal thickening or edema; partial obstruction from a tumor, a foreign body, or secretions; and extrinsic pressure, as in tension pneumothorax or goiter. In airway obstruction, wheezing occurs during inspiration.

Assess whether the patient is in respiratory distress. Is he responsive? Is he restless, confused, anxious, or afraid? Are his respirations abnormally fast, slow, shallow, or deep? Are they irregular? Can you hear wheezing through his mouth? Does he exhibit increased use of accessory muscles; increased chest wall motion; intercostal, suprasternal, or supraclavicular retractions; stridor; or nasal flaring? Take his other vital signs, noting hypotension or hypertension, decreased oxygen saturation, and an irregular, weak, rapid, or slow pulse.

Help the patient relax. Administer humidified oxygen by face mask, and encourage slow, deep breathing. Have endotracheal intubation and emergency resuscitation equipment readily available. Call the respiratory therapy department to supply intermittent positive-pressure breathing and nebulization treatments with bronchodilators. Insert an I.V. line for administration of drugs, such as diuretics, steroids, bronchodilators, and sedatives. Perform the abdominal thrust maneuver, as indicated, for airway obstruction.

History and physical examination

If the patient isn't in respiratory distress, obtain a history. What provokes his wheezing? Does he have asthma or allergies? Does he smoke or have a history of a pulmonary, cardiac, or circulatory disorder? Does he have cancer? Ask about recent surgery, illness, or trauma and recent changes in appetite, weight, exercise tolerance, or sleep patterns. Obtain a drug history. Ask about exposure to toxic fumes or any respiratory irritants. If he has a cough, ask how it sounds, when it starts, and how often it occurs. Does he have paroxysms of coughing? Is his cough dry, sputum producing, or bloody?

Ask the patient about chest pain. If he reports pain, determine its quality, onset, duration, intensity, and radiation. Does it increase with breathing, coughing, or certain positions?

Examine the patient's nose and mouth for congestion, drainage, or signs of infection such as halitosis. If he produces sputum, obtain a specimen for examination. Check for cyanosis, pallor, clamminess, masses, tenderness, swelling, distended jugular veins, and enlarged lymph nodes. Inspect his chest for abnormal configuration and asymmetrical motion, and determine if the trachea is midline. (See *Detecting slight tracheal deviation,* page 409.) Percuss for dullness or hyperresonance, and auscultate for crackles, rhonchi, or pleural friction rub. Note absent or hypoactive breath sounds, abnormal heart sounds, gallops, or murmurs. Also note arrhythmias, bradycardia, or tachycardia. (See *Evaluating breath sounds,* pages 446 and 447 and *Differ-*

Evaluating breath sounds

Reduced or absent breath sounds indicate some interference with airflow. If pus, fluid, or air fills the pleural space, breath sounds will be quieter than normal. If a foreign body or secretions obstruct a bronchus, breath sounds will be reduced or absent over distal lung tissue. Increased thickness of the chest wall, as occurs in a patient who is obese or extremely muscular, may cause breath sounds to be decreased, distant, or inaudible. Absent breath sounds typically indicate loss of ventilation power.

When air passes through narrowed airways or through moisture, or when the membranes lining the chest cavity become inflamed, you'll hear adventitious breath sounds. These include crackles, rhonchi, wheezes, and pleural friction rubs. Usually, these sounds indicate pulmonary disease.

Follow the auscultation sequences shown to assess the patient's breath sounds. Have the patient take full, deep breaths, and compare sound variations from one side to the other. Note the location, timing, and character of any abnormal breath sounds.

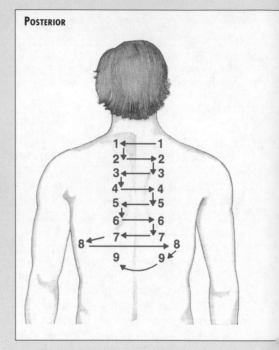

POSTERIOR

ential diagnosis: Wheezing, pages 448 and 449.)

Medical causes

▶ *Anaphylaxis.* This allergic reaction can cause tracheal edema or bronchospasm, resulting in severe wheezing and stridor.[1] Initial signs and symptoms include apprehension, weakness, sneezing, dyspnea, nasal pruritus, urticaria, erythema, and angioedema. Respiratory distress occurs with nasal flaring, accessory muscle use, and intercostal retractions. Other findings include nasal edema and congestion, profuse watery rhinorrhea, chest or throat tightness, and dysphagia. Cardiac effects include arrhythmias and hypotension.

▶ *Aspiration of a foreign body.* Partial obstruction by a foreign body produces sudden onset of wheezing and possibly stridor; a dry, paroxysmal cough; gagging; and hoarseness. Other findings include tachycardia, dyspnea, decreased breath sounds, and possibly cyanosis. A retained foreign body may cause inflammation leading to fever, pain, and swelling.

▶ *Aspiration pneumonitis.* In this disorder, wheezing may accompany tachypnea, marked dyspnea, cyanosis, tachycardia, fever, a productive (eventually purulent) cough, and frothy pink sputum.

▶ *Asthma.* Wheezing, coughing, and shortness of breath are the cardinal signs and symptoms of asthma.[2] Wheezing is heard at the mouth during expiration. An initially dry cough later becomes productive with thick mucus. Other findings include apprehension, prolonged expiration, intercostal and supraclavicular retractions, rhonchi, accessory muscle use, nasal flaring, and tachypnea. Asthma also produces tachycardia, diaphoresis, and flushing or cyanosis.

▶ *Blast lung injury.* Wheezing is a common symptom of this condition, which is characterized by hypoxia and respiratory difficulty. The forceful blast wave that follows an explosive detonation can cause serious lung injury,

ANTERIOR **LEFT LATERAL** **RIGHT LATERAL**

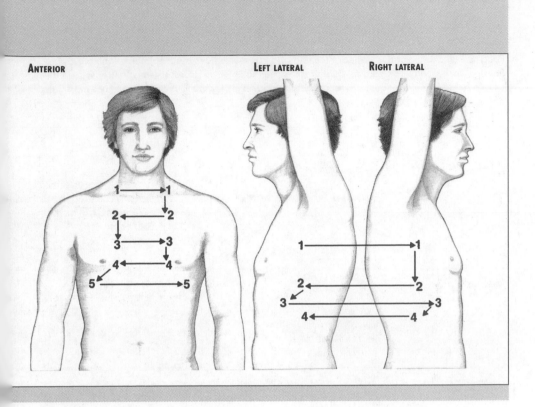

including hemorrhage, contusion, edema, and tearing. In addition to wheezing, patients may have chest pain, dyspnea, cyanosis, and hemoptysis. The diagnosis is confirmed by chest X-rays that show a classic "butterfly" pattern.

▶ *Bronchial adenoma.* This insidious disorder produces unilateral, possibly severe wheezing. Common features are a chronic cough and recurring hemoptysis. Symptoms of airway obstruction may occur later.

▶ *Bronchiectasis.* In this disorder, excessive mucus commonly causes intermittent and localized or diffuse wheezing. Characteristic findings include a chronic cough that produces copious amounts of foul-smelling, mucopurulent sputum; hemoptysis; rhonchi; and coarse crackles. Weight loss, fatigue, weakness, exertional dyspnea, fever, malaise, halitosis, and late-stage clubbing also may occur.

▶ *Bronchitis (chronic).* This disorder causes wheezing that varies in severity, location, and intensity. Related findings include prolonged expiration, coarse crackles, scattered rhonchi,

and a hacking cough that later becomes productive. Other effects include dyspnea, accessory muscle use, barrel chest, tachypnea, clubbing, edema, weight gain, and cyanosis.

▶ *Bronchogenic carcinoma.* Obstruction may cause localized wheezing. Typical findings include a productive cough, dyspnea, hemoptysis (initially blood-tinged sputum, possibly leading to massive hemorrhage), anorexia, and weight loss. Arm edema and chest pain also may occur.

▶ *Chemical pneumonitis (acute).* Mucosal injury causes increased secretions and edema, leading to wheezing, dyspnea, orthopnea, crackles, malaise, fever, and a productive cough with purulent sputum. The patient also may have signs of conjunctivitis, pharyngitis, laryngitis, and rhinitis.

▶ *Emphysema.* Mild to moderate wheezing may occur in this form of chronic obstructive pulmonary disease. Related findings include dyspnea, tachypnea, reduced breath sounds, peripheral cyanosis, pursed-lip breathing,

Differential diagnosis: Wheezing

Patients with audible or auscultated wheezing also commonly have dyspnea, chest tightness, apprehension, tachypnea, tachycardia, diaphoresis, nasal flaring, and accessory muscle use. To help differentiate between underlying causes, consider any additional signs and symptoms, such as those listed here.

POSSIBLE CAUSES	SIGNS AND SYMPTOMS	DIAGNOSIS
Asthma	• Dry or productive cough • Prolonged expiration • Intercostal and supraclavicular retractions • Rhonchi	• Allergy skin testing • Pulmonary function tests (PFTs) • Laboratory tests (complete blood cou[?] arterial blood gas [ABG] analysis) • Chest X-rays
Anaphylaxis	• Stridor • Weakness • Angioedema • Intercostal retractions • Nasal edema and congestion • Watery rhinorrhea	• Physical examination • History of allergen exposure
Chronic bronchitis	• Wheezing that varies in severity, location, and intensity • Prolonged expiration • Coarse crackles • Scattered rhonchi • Hacking, productive cough • Dyspnea • Clubbing • Accessory muscle use • Cyanosis • Edema	• PFTs • Laboratory tests (CBC, ABG analysis) • Chest X-rays
Gastroesophageal reflux disease	• Hematemesis • Abdominal pain • Pyrosis • Flatulence • Dyspepsia • Postural regurgitation	• Laboratory tests (electrolyte levels, C[?] guaiac) • Imaging studies (barium swallow, upp[?] ries, endoscopy) • Biopsy

anorexia, and malaise. Accessory muscle use, barrel chest, a chronic productive cough, and clubbing also may occur.

▶ *Inhalation injury.* Early findings include hoarseness and coughing, singed nasal hairs, orofacial burns, and soot-stained sputum.

Later effects may include wheezing, crackles, rhonchi, and respiratory distress.

▶ *Pneumothorax (tension).* This life-threatening disorder causes respiratory distress with possible wheezing, dyspnea, tachycardia, tachypnea, and sudden, severe, sharp chest

TREATMENT AND FOLLOW-UP

- Avoidance of allergens, tobacco, and beta blockers
- Medication (inhaled beta$_2$ agonists, inhaled corticosteroids, leukotriene receptor agonists, systemic steroids [during infections and exacerbations])
- Peak expiratory flow monitoring

Follow-up: Reevaluation in 24 hours; then every 3 to 5 days; then every 1 to 3 months

- Symptomatic treatment
- Airway and oxygenation maintenance
- Allergy testing (after treatment)
- Medication (I.V. or subQ epinephrine, antihistamines, nebulized albuterol)

Follow-up: Reevaluation within 24 hours

- Smoking cessation
- Medication (pneumococcal and influenza vaccines, beta$_2$ agonist, bronchodilator, corticosteroids)
- Avoidance of environmental irritants
- Avoidance of beta-adrenergic blockers and antihistamines
- Early treatment of infections
- Oxygen therapy

Follow-up: Return visit within 48 hours after acute exacerbation; then every 3 months

- Diet and lifestyle modification
- Medication (histamine$_2$ blockers, antacids, proton pump inhibitors)
- Blood transfusion (if indicated)

Follow-up: Reevaluation every 6 months unless the condition worsens; then referral to a gastroenterologist

pain (often unilateral). Other findings include a dry cough, cyanosis, accessory muscle use, asymmetrical chest wall movement, anxiety, and restlessness. Examination reveals hyperresonance or tympany and diminished or absent breath sounds on the affected side, subcutaneous crepitation, decreased vocal fremitus, and tracheal deviation.

▶ *Pulmonary coccidioidomycosis.* This disorder may cause wheezing and rhonchi along with cough, fever, chills, pleuritic chest pain, headache, weakness, malaise, anorexia, and macular rash.

▶ *Pulmonary edema.* This life-threatening disorder may cause wheezing, coughing, exertional and paroxysmal nocturnal dyspnea and, later, orthopnea. Examination reveals tachycardia, tachypnea, dependent crackles, and a diastolic gallop. Severe pulmonary edema produces rapid, labored respirations; diffuse crackles; a productive cough with frothy, bloody sputum; arrhythmias; cold, clammy, cyanotic skin; hypotension; and a thready pulse.

▶ *Pulmonary embolus.* Diffuse, mild wheezing rarely occurs in this disorder, which is characterized by dyspnea, chest pain, and cyanosis.

▶ *Pulmonary tuberculosis.* In late stages, fibrosis causes wheezing. Common findings include a mild to severe productive cough with pleuritic chest pain and fine crackles, night sweats, anorexia, weight loss, fever, malaise, dyspnea, and fatigue. Examination reveals dullness on percussion, increased tactile fremitus, and amphoric breath sounds.

▶ *Respiratory syncytial virus (RSV).* Infected individuals commonly develop wheezing and other symptoms within 4 to 6 days of exposure to this virus. Healthy adults and children older than age 3 usually have mild cases of RSV and experience wheezing along with other common cold-like symptoms of runny nose, cough, and low-grade fever. In children age 3 and younger, high-pitched expiratory wheezing can accompany a severe cough, rapid breathing, and high-grade fever. RSV is the primary cause of lower respiratory tract infection in infants, who may develop pneumonia or bronchiolitis. Infection-control practices help prevent the spread of this virus, which can be inactivated by disinfectants or soap and water. A vaccine is being researched for this common condition that affects most children by age 2.

▶ *Thyroid goiter.* This disorder may produce no symptoms, or it may cause wheezing, dysphagia, and respiratory difficulty related to a compressed airway.

▶ *Tracheobronchitis*. Auscultation may detect wheezing, rhonchi, and crackles. The patient also has a cough, a slight fever, sudden chills, muscle and back pain, and substernal tightness.

▶ *Wegener's granulomatosis*. This disorder may cause mild to moderate wheezing if it compresses major airways. Other findings include a cough (possibly bloody), dyspnea, pleuritic chest pain, hemorrhagic skin lesions, and progressive renal failure. Epistaxis and severe sinusitis are common.

Special considerations

Prepare the patient for diagnostic tests, such as chest X-rays, arterial blood gas analysis, pulmonary function tests, and sputum culture. Ease the patient's breathing by placing him in semi-Fowler's position and repositioning him frequently. Perform pulmonary physiotherapy as necessary.

Give an antibiotic to treat infection, a bronchodilator to relieve bronchospasm and maintain patent airways, a steroid to reduce inflammation, and a mucolytic or an expectorant to increase the flow of secretions. Provide humidification to thin secretions.

Pediatric pointers

Children are especially susceptible to wheezing because their small airways allow rapid obstruction. Primary causes of wheezing include bronchospasm, mucosal edema, and accumulation of secretions.[3] These may occur with such disorders as bronchiolitis, cystic fibrosis, aspiration of a foreign body, and pulmonary hemosiderosis.

Patient counseling

If appropriate, encourage increased activity to promote drainage and prevent pooling of secretions. Encourage regular deep breathing and coughing. Also urge the patient to drink fluids to liquefy secretions and prevent dehydration.

REFERENCES

1. Bryant, H. "Anaphylaxis: Recognition, Treatment, and Education," *Emergency Nurse* 15(2):24-28, May 2007.
2. Conboy-Ellis, K. "Asthma Pathogenesis and Management," *The Nurse Practitioner* 31(11):24-44, November 2006.
3. McCaskey, M.S. "Pediatric Assessment: The Little Differences," *Home Healthcare Nurse* 25(1):20-24, January 2007.

Appendices and index

EVIDENCE-BASED NURSING PRACTICE

Evidence-based practice is nursing practice built on information obtained from research. The basic steps involved in evidence-based nursing practice include:
▶ formulating the clinical question
▶ searching for peer-reviewed evidence-articles on the clinical question
▶ analyzing and comparing data by critically evaluating and comparing articles
▶ applying the information from the studies.

Step 1: Formulating the clinical question

Follow these steps to help you formulate the clinical question:
▶ Start with a specific and concrete question.
▶ Formulate the question in terms of a relationship between:
   – a patient or patient population
   – an intervention (typically a treatment, a diagnostic test, or a nursing procedure)
   – the result of the intervention
   – what else could be done instead.

Step 2: Searching for evidence

Your goal in doing a database search is to find published reports of the results of research projects. First and foremost is to use only articles that are published in peer-reviewed journals. These journals require outside experts to review articles submitted for publication. If the title of the article leaves you unsure of whether the article is a report of a research project, read the abstract carefully. Look for evidence from the following resources:
▶ library
▶ Internet websites
▶ electronic databases–web based tools such as CINAHL, MEDLINE, and PubMed (see International Evidence-Based Resources, page 454).

A standard format for research reports includes these sections:
▶ abstract
▶ introduction or review of the literature (a brief summary of past related research)
▶ methods
▶ results
▶ discussion.

Step 3: Analyzing and comparing data

Evaluating the quality of a research report can be difficult if you haven't had training in research methodology. In fact, even seasoned researchers debate the quality of studies and how to interpret and apply the results. However, if you follow a few basic rules, you can be sure that the study you read has met a baseline standard of quality.

▶ *Validity* refers to whether the research project actually measures what it claims to measure.

▶ *Reliability* refers to whether the results of the study will be repeatable. Ideally, you shouldn't accept the results of any study as true without finding at least one attempt to repeat it with the same results.

▶ *Randomizing* is a hallmark of high-quality research. Ideally, researchers assign people randomly to either a study or control group.

▶ *Group size* is important. Research on large numbers of subjects produces more reliable results than smaller studies.

However, not all types of research can use randomization, double-blinding, control groups, and large populations. Understanding the acceptable alternatives requires training and experience.

Comparing the studies you have gathered is the next step, and this can be challenging. You must weigh variables, such as patient population characteristics and quality of the study design. Final decisions usually require discussion and compromise.

Levels of evidence

Weighing and leveling the degree of evidence that a study has can be a daunting task. A systematic approach to leveling the evidence can be found below.

▶ Leveling the evidence is based on these questions:
▶ Was the study randomized?
▶ What was the study population?
▶ What criteria needed to be met by participants?
▶ Was the intervention described properly?
▶ Was the study blinded?
▶ How was the data collected?
▶ How was the data analyzed?
▶ What were the end results?
▶ What conclusions were achieved?
▶ Did the study have any limitations?

Leveling the evidence

LEVEL AND QUALITY OF EVIDENCE	TYPE OF EVIDENCE
Level 1	Evidence from a systematic review or meta-analysis of all relevant randomized controlled trials (RCTs), or evidence-based clinical practice guidelines based on systematic reviews of RCT, or three or more high-quality RCTs with similar results
Level 2	Evidence from at least one well-designed RCT
Level 3	Evidence from well-designed controlled trials with no randomization
Level 4	Evidence from well-designed case-control and cohort studies
Level 5	Evidence from systematic reviews of descriptive and qualitative studies
Level 6	Evidence from a single descriptive or qualitative study
Level 7	Evidence from the opinion of authorities and/or reports of expert committees

Adapted from Melnyk, B.M., and Fineout-Overholt, E. *Evidence-Based Practice in Nursing & Healthcare: A Guide to Best Practice.* Philadelphia: Lippincott Williams & Wilkins, 2005.

Step 4: Applying the data

After the evidence has been evaluated, the next step is to determine whether the evidence supports rejecting or implementing the intervention. If the evidence supports a change, procedures or policies can be changed or created to implement the new evidence.

INTERNATIONAL EVIDENCE-BASED RESOURCES

Academic Center for Evidence-Based Nursing: *www.acestar.uthscsa.edu/About.htm*

American Academy of Pediatrics: *http://aappolicy.aappublications.org/*

American Association of Clinical Endocrinologists: *www.aace.com*

American Association of Critical Care Nurses: *www.aacn.org/AACN/practice Alert.nsf/vwdoc/pa2?opendocument*

American Association of Respiratory Care: *www.rcjournal.com*

American Cancer Society: *www.cancer.org/docroot/ped/content/ped_2_3x_acs_cancer_detection_guidelines_36.asp?sitearea=ped*

American College of Cardiology: *www.acc.org*

American College of Physicians: *www.acponline.org*

American Medical Directors Association: *www.amda.com*

American Psychiatric Association: *www.psych.org*

Association of Women's Health, Obstetric and Neonatal Nurses: *http://awhonn.org*

Clinical Trials: *www.clinicaltrials.gov*

CMA InfoBase: *http://mdm.ca/cpgsnew/cpgs/index.asp*

Cochrane Library: *www.cochrane.org/*

Education Resources Information Center database: *www.eric.ed.gov/*

Guidelines Advisory Committee: *www.gacguidelines.ca*

Health Services/Technology Assessment Text (HSTAT): *http://hstat.nlm.nih.gov*

Healthlinks at University of Washington: *http://healthlinks.washington.edu*

Infusion Nursing Society: *www.ins1.org*

Institute for Clinical Systems Improvement: *www.icsi.org/guidelines_and_more/*

Institute for Scientific Information: *http://scientific.thomson.com/isi/*

Joanna Briggs Institute: *www.joanna briggs.edu.au/about/home.php*

Ministry of Health Services, British Columbia, Canada: *www.healthservices. gov.bc.ca/msp/protoguides*

National Association of Neonatal Nurses: *www.nann.org*

National Cancer Institute: *www.cancer. gov/search/cancer_literature/*

National Guideline Clearinghouse (NGC): *www.guideline.gov*

National Institute for Clinical Excellence (NICE): *www.nice.org.uk/catcg2.asp? c=20034*

National Kidney Foundation: *www.kidney.org/professionals/doqi/ guidelineindex/cfm*

New York Academy of Medicine: *www.ebmny.org/cpg.html*

NLM Gateway: *http://gateway.nlm.nih. gov/gw/Cmd*

Oncology Nursing Society: *www.ons.org*

Ovid CINAHL: *www.ovid.com/site/ products/ovidguide/nursing.htm*

Primary Care Practice Guidelines: *www.medscape.com/pages/ editorial/public/pguidelines/index- primarycare*

PubMed: *www.pubmed.gov*

Registered Nurses Association of Ontario: *www.rnao.org/bestpractices*

Resources for Evidence-Based Nursing at McMaster University: *http://hsl.lib. mcmaster.ca/education/nursing/ebn/ index.htm*

Scottish Intercollegiate Guideline Network (SIGN): *www.sign.ac.uk/ guidelines/index.html*

Teaching/Learning Resources for Evidence-Based Practice: *www.mdx. ac.uk/www/rctsh/ebp/main.htm*

University of Iowa College of Nursing Evidence-Based Practice Guidelines: *www.nursing.uiowa.edu/products_ services/evidence_based.htm*

Veterans Administration: *www.oqp. med.va.gov/cpg/cpg.htm*

Virginia Henderson International Nursing Library: *www.nursinglibrary. org/portal/main.aspx*

Wound, Ostomy, and Continence Nurses Society: *www.wocn.org/WOCN_ Library/Position_Statements*

INDEX

i refers to an illustration; t refers to a table.

i refers to an illustration; t refers to a table.

i refers to an illustration; t refers to a table.

i refers to an illustration; t refers to a table.

i refers to an illustration; t refers to a table.

i refers to an illustration; t refers to a table.

i refers to an illustration; t refers to a table.

i refers to an illustration; t refers to a table.

i refers to an illustration; t refers to a table.